Essentials of Surgical Specialties

Associate Editors
Mitchell H. Goldman, M.D.
Professor and Chief
Division of Vascular/Transplant Surgery
Department of Surgery
University of Tennessee Research Center and Hospital
Knoxville, Tennessee

James M. Hassett, Jr., M.D.
Associate Professor of Surgery
Coordinator, Undergraduate Surgical Education
State University of New York at Buffalo
Buffalo, New York

James C. Hebert, M.D.
Associate Professor of Surgery
College of Medicine
The University of Vermont
Burlington, Vermont

Illustrated by Lydia Kibiuk

About the Cover (detail from the Agnew Clinic)

"The Agnew Clinic," 1889, painted by Thomas Eakins, was created as a tribute to Dr. David Hayes Agnew, the first John Rhea Barton Professor of Surgery at the University of Pennsylvania. Dr. Agnew was a beloved and respected surgeon in 19th century Philadelphia. The painting was commissioned by Dr. Agnew's students to honor him on the occasion of his designation as professor emeritus in May 1889.

Approximately 6 feet high and 11 feet wide, "The Agnew Clinic" depicts the surgical amphitheater of the University of Pennsylvania. Included in the portrait is a likeness of all 25 students who commissioned the painting and paid the $750 fee; their attention to Dr. Agnew is varied. Agnew has stepped back from the table after performing a mastectomy ("mammectomy") and may be explaining to the students the procedure or the dismal prognosis for the young woman patient. A likeness of the artist, painted by Susan Macdowell (Mrs. Eakins), is shown at the right edge of the painting.

A comparison of "The Agnew Clinic" and "The Gross Clinic," which Eakins had painted 14 years earlier, reveals some major advances in surgery: the physician is gowned and the patient is draped (although no gloves or masks are worn); there is artificial lighting; and a nurse is assisting with the surgery. Like "The Gross Clinic," owned by the Jefferson Medical College, "The Agnew Clinic" remains with its original owner, The University of Pennsylvania School of Medicine.

(Courtesy of The University of Pennsylvania School of Medicine, Philadelphia, Pennsylvania.)

Essentials of Surgical Specialties

Senior Editor
Peter F. Lawrence, M.D.
Professor of Surgery
Department of Surgery
The University of Utah School of Medicine
Salt Lake, City, Utah

Editors
Richard M. Bell, M.D.
Professor of Surgery
Department of Surgery
University of South Carolina School of Medicine
Columbia, South Carolina

Merril T. Dayton, M.D.
Associate Professor of Surgery
Department of Surgery
The University of Utah School of Medicine
Salt Lake City, Utah

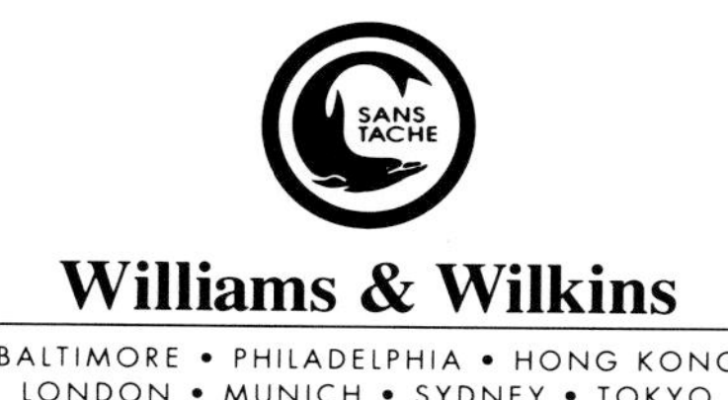

Williams & Wilkins
BALTIMORE • PHILADELPHIA • HONG KONG
LONDON • MUNICH • SYDNEY • TOKYO
A WAVERLY COMPANY

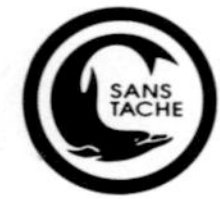

Editor: Timothy S. Satterfield
Managing Editor: Linda S. Napora
Copy Editor: S. Gillian Casey
Designer: JoAnne Janowiak
Illustration Planner: Ray Lowman
Production Coordinator: Charles E. Zeller
Cover Designer: Michael Kotarba

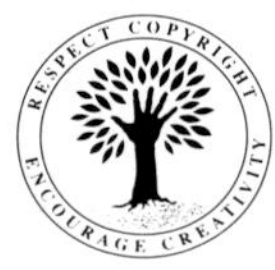

Accurate indications, adverse reactions, and dosage schedules for drugs are provided in this book, but it is possible that they may change. The reader is urged to review the package information data of the manufacturers of the medications mentioned.

Printed in the United States of America

Library of Congress Cataloging-in-Publication Data

Essentials of surgical specialties / senior editor, Peter F. Lawrence;
editors, Richard M. Bell, Merril T. Dayton.
p. cm.
Includes index.
ISBN 0-683-04871-6
1. Surgery. I. Lawrence, Peter F.
[DNLM: 1. Surgery, Operative. WO 500 E783]
RD31.E737 1993
617—dc20
DNLM/DLC
for Library of Congress 92-21071
CIP

93 94 95 96 97
1 2 3 4 5 6 7 8 9 10

To our parents—

Howard and Peg
W.R. and Macky
Reed and Lois

Who have taught us the lasting value of education, and who have sacrificed their own personal comfort to help us achieve our educational goals. Hopefully, this textbook partially fulfills our obligation to pass this philosophy on to the next generation.

Preface

Essentials of Surgical Specialties (along with *Essentials of General Surgery*) completes the teaching program in surgery that has been designed to provide medical students with the knowledge and skills to become competent physicians.

Because the potential knowledge in each surgical specialty is vast, we have used the same approach for this text that was used in *Essentials in General Surgery:* the material is limited to essential information that all students need to master. Each surgical specialty (through its national organization) was asked to select a physician or group of physicians who have an interest in surgical education to help determine the knowledge and skills required in that specialty. These specialty surgeons then used their own societies, as well as the Association for Surgical Education, to determine the content and rank the importance of fundamental information in their specialty. Based on this information, objectives were written (e.g., "A student should be able to describe the causes of hearing loss."). These objectives became the basis for this textbook, *Essentials in Surgical Specialties,* which was then written by nationally recognized experts in each surgical specialty. Each author was asked to emphasize the most important diseases and principles; uncommon diseases are not discussed. We have limited the length of each chapter so that it can be reasonably read during a specialty rotation.

Once the textbook was written, each chapter was reviewed by other specialists to assure that the authors had successfully and accurately conveyed the information. Each chapter was also reviewed by several medical students for clarity and content. By determining content through a scientific process, soliciting surgical educators to write the text, and having others independently review it, we have attempted to produce a readable textbook that presents the material all students should master. The book has been designed (by length and style) to be read in six weeks, which is the time that is usually assigned to students in the 3rd and 4th years of medical school for surgical specialties.

To complement the text, we have also developed clinical cases that use computer software to teach the evaluation and management of common problems in each surgical specialty. Once a student has read the text, he or she has the knowledge to begin solving clinical problems. Although a patient rarely presents with a disease such as a malignant bone tumor (patients present with bone pain or a pathologic bone fracture), most texts are organized with a disease and organ system approach. Using our clinical cases, or Patient Management Problems, students go through the initial presentation, diagnosis, treatment, and follow-up of each of the common clinical problems in a surgical specialty as they would present in a real surgical practice. These clinical problems are not intended to be a test, but rather an opportunity to learn the process of problem solving. The Patient Management Problems (PMPs) are written in a format similar to that used in the American College of Surgeons SESAP, a highly successful program for surgeons in practice.

The evaluation of students' knowledge in surgery can be divided into two areas: mastery of information from the text and ability to apply that information in a clinical setting (as has been taught by the PMPs). We have developed multiple choice examination questions, based on the text, to test factual knowledge. These questions (>1000) have been placed in a question bank, and can be generated with computer software into an exam in any or all surgical specialties. The exam is unique in that it is based on the text, so that students prepare for it by reading the text. The exam can identify deficiencies and the missed questions can be used to focus students back to the segment of the textbook that is not fully understood.

In addition, we have developed a standardized set of oral examination questions for each specialty, so students can be assured that the level and complexity of each question is similar for all students, and that the questions originate from the textbook and computerized Patient Management Problems. Oral exams are a test of problem solving, which is taught by the PMPs, although a range of factual information is also necessary to excel in an oral exam. Consequently, students can prepare for the oral exam by reading the textbook and reviewing PMPs, rather than preparing by undirected readings, which is the usual way to prepare for oral exams.

We believe that our approach, with a textbook and the PMPs, provides a flexible, yet structured approach to surgical education. Students have a textbook that addresses the types of problems and depth of knowledge that they need in each specialty. The Patient Management Problems allow students to test their problem solving ability on common surgical problems. The Oral and Written Examinations are keyed to the textbook and PMPs, so that students know how to prepare for the final exam and how to correct any deficiencies they identify.

Faculty and students benefit from an organized approach to medical education. We hope that *Essentials of Surgical Specialties*—an integrated educational package—will facilitate the development of outstanding teaching programs at all medical schools.

Acknowledgments

This project was nurtured by many members of the Association for Surgical Education (ASE), whose advice and expertise I would like to acknowledge. At its annual meetings the ASE provided an excellent forum for discussion and testing of ideas about the content of the surgical curriculum. In addition, the Curriculum Committee and Testing and Evaluation Committee were responsible for helping to write the objectives for each organ system and developing both oral and written examination questions.

My thanks go as well to Cathy Council and Beckie Bos, our editors at The University of Utah, who have spent 2 years editing, revising, and coordinating all components of this project. We would also like to acknowledge Linda Napora, Vicki Vaughn, and Tim Satterfield, our indefatigable editors at Williams & Wilkins, who have guided this project for the last 10 years.

Finally, I owe thanks to the many medical students, particularly Wayne Young, at The University of Utah School of Medicine, and Alyson Buckner, at Washington University, who took time to review the text, oral examination questions, and patient management problems, offering valuable suggestions for improvement and making many of the changes that have enhanced all components of the package.

Contributors

Richard L. Anderson, M.D.
Professor of Ophthalmology
The University of Utah School of Medicine
Salt Lake City, Utah

Robert A. Badalament, M.D.
Assistant Professor and Chief
Division of Urology
Ohio State University College of Medicine
Columbus, Ohio

Eugene E. Berg, M.D.
Associate Professor of Orthopaedic Surgery
The University of South Carolina School of Medicine
Columbia, South Carolina

Larry B. Conochie, M.D.
Assistant Professor of Orthopaedic Surgery
McGill University
Montreal, Quebec, Canada

Alan S. Crandall, Jr., M.D.
Professor of Ophthalmology
The University of Utah School of Medicine
Salt Lake City, Utah

Gregory S. Doren, M.D.
Head, Cornea Service
Department of Ophthalmology
Catherine McAuley Health Center
St. Joseph Mercy Hospital
Ann Arbor, Michigan

Russell W. Faria, D.O.
Clinical Assistant Professor
Department of Anesthesia and Critical Care
University of Chicago
Chicago, Illinois

Richard H. Feins, M.D.
Assistant Professor, Cardiothoracic Surgery
University of Rochester School of Medicine
Rochester, New York

Toni M. Ganzel, M.D.
Associate Professor of Surgery
Division of Otolaryngology
Department of Surgery
University of Louisville
Louisville, Kentucky

John R.F. Guy, M.D.
Private Practice
Mississauga, Ontario, Canada

Mary Alice Helikson, M.D.
Clinical Assistant Professor of Surgery
Assistant Professor of Child Health
University of Missouri Health Sciences Center
Columbia, Missouri

Constance H. Hill, M.D.
Clinical Associate Professor of Anesthesia
State University of New York Health Sciences Center at Brooklyn
New York, New York

Ralph A.W. Lehman, M.D.
Professor of Surgery
Division of Neurosurgery
Medical College of The Pennsylvania State University
Hershey, Pennsylvania

Robert P. Liss, M.D.
Private Practice
West Chester, Pennsylvania

John J. Marota, Ph.D., M.D.
Assistant Professor of Anesthesia
Harvard Medical School
Cambridge, Massachusetts

Serge A. Martinez, M.D.
Professor of Surgery
Division of Otolaryngology
Department of Surgery
University of Louisville
Louisville, Kentucky

William M. McLeish, M.D.
Private Practice
Jacksonville, Florida

Gordon T. McMurry, M.D.
Clinical Associate Professor of Surgery
Division of Otolaryngology
Department of Surgery
University of Louisville
Louisville, Kentucky

John A. Nesbitt, M.D.
Private Practice
Columbia, South Carolina

Michael B. Nolph, M.D.
Associate Professor of Surgery
Division of Otolaryngology
Department of Surgery
University of Louisville
Louisville, Kentucky

Robert B. Page, M.D.
Professor of Surgery and Anatomy
Division of Neurosurgery
Medical College of The Pennsylvania State University
Hershey, Pennsylvania

Susan L. Polk, M.D., M.S.Ed.
Assistant Professor, Director of Education
Department of Anesthesia and Critical Care
University of Chicago
Chicago, Illinois

Irving Raber, M.D.
Clinical Assistant Professor of Ophthalmology
Wills Eye Hospital
Jefferson Medical College
Philadelphia, Pennsylvania

David B. Reath, M.D.
Associate Professor of Surgery
Division of Plastic Surgery
The University of Tennessee Graduate School of Medicine
Knoxville, Tennessee

Arthur J.L. Schneider, M.D.
Professor of Anesthesiology
Medical College of The Pennsylvania State University
Hershey, Pennsylvania

Joseph A. Smith, Jr., M.D.
Professor and Chairman
Department of Urology
Vanderbilt University
Nashville, Tennessee

Norman J. Snow, M.D.
Associate Professor, Cardiothoracic Surgery
Case Western Reserve University School of Medicine
Cleveland, Ohio

William J. Somers, M.D.
Assistant Professor of Surgery
Division of Urology
Ohio State University College of Medicine
Columbus, Ohio

Michael L. Spector, M.D.
Assistant Professor, Cardiothoracic Surgery
Case Western Reserve University School of Medicine
Cleveland, Ohio

Brent V. Stromberg, M.D.
Senior Active Staff
St. Joseph Hospital
Omaha, Nebraska

Michael P. Teske, M.D.
Clinical Associate Professor of Ophthalmology
The University of Utah School of Medicine
Salt Lake City, Utah

George L. White, Jr., Ph.D.
Associate Professor of Public Health
The University of Southern Mississippi
Hattiesburg, Mississippi

Welby Winstead, M.D.
Assistant Professor of Surgery
Division of Otolaryngology
Department of Surgery
University of Louisville
Louisville, Kentucky

Philip J. Wolfson, M.D.
Associate Professor of Surgery
Director of Undergraduate Education
Jefferson Medical College
Philadelphia, Pennsylvania

Bruce E. Woodworth, M.D.
Private Practice
Columbus, Ohio

Jeffrey P. York, M.D.
Assistant Professor of Surgery
Division of Urology
Ohio State University College of Medicine
Columbus, Ohio

Contents

1 Anesthesiology

Susan L. Polk, M.D., M.S.Ed., Russell W. Faria, D.O., Constance H. Hill, M.D., John J. Marota, Ph.D., M.D., and Arthur J.L. Schneider, M.D.

ASSUMPTIONS

The student has completed courses in physiology and pathology and understands basic disorders of the cardiovascular, respiratory, renal, nervous, and endocrine systems.

The student is familiar with common surgical procedures and understands their physiologic impact on the patient.

The student understands the pharmacology of the common drugs used to treat cardiovascular, central nervous system, respiratory, and endocrine disorders.

The student appreciates the need to provide understanding and psychological support to patients who are frightened, ill, and/or in pain.

OBJECTIVES

1. Describe the information the anesthesiologist should obtain from the patient during the preanesthetic visit.
2. Differentiate among types of anesthesia and give the indications for selection of type, based on the various surgical procedures.
3. Distinguish between general and regional anesthetics on the basis of time course, general pharmacology, and toxicology.
4. Describe the pharmacologic and physiologic properties of commonly used anesthetic agents and their effects on patients who are undergoing surgery.
5. Discuss the basic principles of airway management.
6. Describe the methods and devices used in anesthesiology to monitor the patient's oxygenation, circulation, respiration, and temperature.
7. Describe the immediate complications of anesthesia that occur in the postanesthesia care unit (PACU) and their management.
8. Discuss the management of postoperative pain.
9. Discuss the ways in which chronic medical conditions affect the patient in the perioperative period; describe any special preoperative testing and preparation required.

Introduction

In 1842, Crawford W. Long used diethyl ether to produce surgical anesthesia. From that time to the present, anesthesiology has advanced tremendously and has developed into a recognized medical discipline. Anesthesiologists render patients insensitive to surgery, manage their medical problems, and maintain their physiology near normal during and immediately after the operative period. They are also involved in caring for patients in intensive care units, managing the pain of labor and delivery, treating acute pain in the postoperative or postinjury period, and managing chronic pain syndromes. Much of the basic knowledge in anesthesiology is derived from the fields of pharmacology and physiology and is helpful to physicians who deal with patients requiring surgery. This chapter will discuss the role of the anesthesiologist in perioperative care, specific intraoperative drugs and anesthesia techniques, monitoring in the operative period, the management of acute postoperative pain, and (in the appendix) the implications of concurrent medical conditions in the perioperative period. The intent of the chapter is to familiarize students with the risks and hazards of anesthesia so that they can learn to safely prepare a patient physically and psychologically for anesthesia and surgery. Students will also become acquainted with problems peculiar to anesthesia so that they will be able to consult with the anesthesiologist regarding medical problems that may affect the patient's response to anesthesia and surgery.

Preoperative Evaluation

Except in an emergency, no patient should undergo surgery until in optimum medical condition. Before surgery, the anesthesiologist must evaluate the patient's risk for the anesthetic and facilitate plans for anesthetic technique, monitoring, and postoperative care. During the preoperative evaluation, the anesthesiologist must also provide the patient and family with appropriate psychological preparation for upcoming procedures and establish doctor-patient rapport. The anesthesiologist should discuss the planned anesthetic technique with the patient and document that the risks and benefits of that technique have been reviewed. The patient is informed of the time after which no food or liquids should be consumed, the projected time and length of surgery, the premedication planned, and the monitors that will be used in the operating room. The patient should be prepared for the recovery room and be made aware of the possible need for ventilatory assistance, prolonged endotracheal intubation, or invasive monitoring. The patient should be told to expect some discomfort, be aware of postanesthesia procedures, and understand how to contribute to restoring normal function (by coughing and deep breathing, for example). Finally, the patient is asked to give informed consent for the anesthetic and monitoring interventions.

Traditionally, the preoperative evaluation for anesthesia was performed in the hospital on the day before surgery. Early preoperative evaluation is desirable, because it allows the anesthesiologist and surgeon time for appropriate laboratory tests and consultations. Today, many patients arrive at the hospital on the day of surgery and must be evaluated either as outpatients or immediately before surgery. Test results or consultations may be difficult to obtain on short notice. In emergency procedures, the preoperative visit is made just prior to surgery, with little time to test or adjust the patient's condition.

On completion of the preoperative visit, a summary of pertinent findings is written in the patient's record. Included in the summary are details of past medical history, medication history, physical examination, and laboratory data. Healthy, asymptomatic female patients under 40 years of age with a normal physical examination need few lab tests (e.g., complete blood count (CBC) or hematocrit (Hct)), while male patients with a similar profile frequently require no tests. The laboratory data traditionally requested for healthy patients over 40 years of age include CBC, urinalysis, serum electrolytes, renal function tests, electrocardiogram, and chest x-ray. Recent recommendations for patients aged 40–49 do not include a chest x-ray (unless there is a history of cardiac or pulmonary disease) or CBC, unless major blood loss is anticipated. Further tests should be requested on any patient when indicated by history, symptoms, or surgical procedure. Finally, a physical status classification is assigned based on criteria established by the American Society of Anesthesiologists (ASA). The ASA classification is not a prediction of anesthetic risk (of death) per se, but rather a description of the overall condition of the patient for purposes of comparison with other patients (see Table 1.1). In cases of elective surgery, if the patient is not in optimal medical condition the anesthesiologist should discuss postponing surgery with the patient's primary physician or surgeon.

Table 1.1.
American Society of Anesthesiologists (ASA) Physical Status Classification

ASA I	Healthy patient
ASA II	Patient with mild systemic disease
ASA III	Patient with severe systemic disease limiting activity but not incapacitating
ASA IV	Patient with incapacitating systemic disease that is a constant threat to life
ASA V	Moribund patient not expected to survive 24 hours with or without surgery
ASA VI	Organ donor for harvest already declared brain dead
E	Notation added to the classification if the procedure is performed as an emergency

History

The preanesthetic history should include a review of the following systems: cardiovascular, pulmonary, renal, hepatic, endocrine, metabolic, hematologic, and central nervous. For a thorough discussion of the interaction between disease and anesthesia see the appendix, "Patient Factors Influencing Anesthesia." A brief dental history should also be obtained and the presence of dentures, loose teeth, and chipped, missing, or capped teeth noted. The time, composition, and amount of the last oral intake should be determined. In females, an obstetric and gynecologic history that includes the date of the last menstrual period should be obtained. A social history should include drug, alcohol, and tobacco use. A history of previous surgical and anesthetic procedures is important, including type of anesthesia and complications. A family history of anesthetic problems should also be obtained to rule out inherited conditions such as cholinesterase abnormalities, malignant hyperthermia, and porphyria. The medication history should include the names of drugs, dosage and schedule, and allergies or unusual reactions. Time of last dose should also be noted. Most medications should be continued up until the time of surgery.

Physical Examination

The physical examination is usually confined to the upper airway, the lungs, and the cardiovascular system. To assess possible difficulties in airway management, the head and neck evaluation should include the size of the mouth, tongue, dentition, and range of motion of the temporomandibular joint and cervical spine. Obesity, short neck, and tracheal deviation signal potential difficulties. The lungs are auscultated for the presence of abnormal breath sounds, rales, and wheezing. The cardiovascular examination consists of measurements of blood pressure, skin turgor, heart rate and rhythm, auscultation for cardiac murmurs and carotid bruits, and, in appropriate situations, assessment of intravascular volume status. If nasotracheal intubation is anticipated, the patency of both nasal passages should be assessed. Sites for intravenous access, invasive monitoring, and regional anesthesia should be examined for infection and anatomical abnormalities.

Psychological Preparation and Preoperative Medication

The goals of premedication are sedation, anxiolysis, and pain relief. In the immediate preoperative period, the patient should be calm and pain free but easy to arouse and cooperative. There is no "recipe" for this mental state, and drugs and doses must be tailored to the individual patient. Some anesthesiologists feel that the psychological preparation provided by the preoperative visit should address the patient's fear and preclude the need for pharmacological premedication. Elderly and debilitated patients usually require reduced or no premedication. Patients with increased intracranial pressure, chronic or acute lung disease, blood volume depletion, or altered levels of consciousness should not be premedicated. Premedicants are classified as sedatives, narcotics, and anticholinergics.

Sedatives. Barbiturates, benzodiazepines, butyrophenones, and antihistamines are all used as preanesthetic sedatives.

Barbiturates. Barbiturates provide excellent sedation for the surgical patient in the preoperative period; these drugs may be used alone or in combination with narcotics. Unless given in large doses, barbiturates cause minimal ventilatory and circulatory depression and rarely cause nausea and vomiting. Patients with acute intermittent porphyria should not receive these drugs since they may trigger an acute exacerbation of this disease. The most commonly used barbiturates are pentobarbital (Nembutal) and secobarbital (Seconal).

Benzodiazepines. These drugs are tranquilizers that produce minimal cardiorespiratory depression when used in appropriate doses. They usually produce anterograde amnesia and may cause prolonged sedation. Diazepam (Valium), 5–10 mg orally (p.o.) with a sip of water for an adult, or 5 mg intravenously (i.v.) in the immediate preinduction period when the patient is under the anesthesiologist's observation, and midazolam (Versed), 1–2 mg i.v. for an adult immediately prior to surgery, are the most frequently used benzodiazepines. Diazepam should not be given intramuscularly (i.m.) because of excessive pain on injection as well as poor and unpredictable absorption. Injectable midazolam may be given orally or intranasally in infants and children.

Butyrophenones. Droperidol (Inapsine) produces long-acting sedation in most patients but may cause dysphoria in some. It is an excellent antiemetic, and in low doses it prevents postoperative narcotic-induced nausea and vomiting. It produces mild systemic vasodilation secondary to its α-adrenergic blocking effect and may cause extrapyramidal symptoms, such as rigidity and tremor, because of its dopaminergic receptor blockade effect. It is administered intravenously immediately preoperatively, 1.25 mg in a normal adult, or during the anesthetic itself.

Antihistamines. These drugs provide both sedation and antiemetic properties. Antihistamines potentiate the sedative and analgesic properties of narcotics. The phenothiazine, promethazine (Phenergan), 25 mg i.m., and the piperazine, hydroxyzine (Vistaril), 25–50 mg i.m., are antihistamines frequently used for premedication.

Narcotics. Narcotics produce analgesia in patients with preoperative pain. They may also be used to reduce discomfort in patients who are undergoing insertion of invasive monitoring lines or regional anesthesia. Since narcotics produce respiratory depression, they are best avoided in patients with decreased pulmonary reserve and those in whom respiratory depression may be harmful, such as patients with increased intracranial pressure. Undesired side effects include nausea, vomiting, orthostatic hypotension, and smooth muscle constriction. Morphine, 5–10 mg i.m., and meperidine (Demerol), 25–50 mg i.m., are the narcotics most frequently used for premedication.

Anticholinergics. These drugs are administered for their antisialagogue (salivation reducing) effect, for prevention of reflex bradycardia (especially in children), and for their sedative and amnesic effects. They include atropine (0.02 mg/kg up to 0.6 mg), scopolamine (0.02 mg/kg up to 0.4 mg), and glycopyrrolate (Robinul, 0.01 mg/kg up to 0.2 mg). Their i.m. administration 1 hour before surgery has fallen into disfavor with many anesthesiologists because all are as effective, and much more comfortable for the patient, when given i.v. immediately before induction of anesthesia. An antisialagogue effect is useful for intraoral surgery or when intraoral or nasal topical anesthesia is employed. Glycopyrrolate and scopolamine are more effective antisialagogues than atropine. Atropine and glycopyrrolate have a greater vagolytic action than scopolamine, and they can be given to prevent the bradycardia that may result from administration of succinylcholine or from laryngoscopy and endotracheal intubation. Scopolamine and, to a lesser degree, atropine cross the blood-brain barrier and produce sedation and amnesic effects. Glycopyrrolate does not affect the central nervous system.

Undesirable side effects of anticholinergic drugs include central nervous system toxicity (manifested as delirium or prolonged somnolence after anesthesia), tachycardia, elevation of body temperature, relaxation of the lower esophageal sphincter resulting in passive gastric reflux, mydriasis, and cycloplegia. Patients usually complain of a dry mouth when the drugs are in effect while they are conscious.

Table 1.2.
When to Assume a Full Stomach

Solid food intake within 6–8 hours in normal adult
Pregnancy, regardless of last oral intake
Trauma victim, regardless of last oral intake
Bowel obstruction
Peritonitis
Ascites
Septic shock
Morbid obesity
Elderly with autonomic dysfunction
Diabetic with autonomic dysfunction
Parkinson's disease
Hiatus hernia
Esophageal abnormalities (achalasia, diverticula)
Hypothyroidism
Addison's disease
Chronic neuromuscular disorders

Prophylaxis for Pulmonary Aspiration

Sedation or anesthesia causes a decrease of both gastroesophageal sphincter integrity and airway protective reflexes, and this increases the risk of aspiration. Patients at high risk for aspiration pneumonitis are listed in Table 1.2. Gastric contents flow into the pharynx either actively or passively, and then are inhaled into the trachea during spontaneous or controlled respiration. An endotracheal tube with the cuff inflated is not a reliable seal of the trachea. The adverse effect of aspiration pneumonitis is markedly reduced by decreasing the acidity and volume of gastric contents.

Acid Reduction. The H_2 antagonists, cimetidine (Tagamet), 300 mg p.o. the night before surgery and i.v. or i.m. the morning of surgery, or ranitidine (Zantac), 50 mg i.m. the morning of surgery, increase gastric fluid pH by inhibiting the ability of histamine to induce secretion of gastric acid. Cimetidine has been shown to prolong the elimination of many drugs, including diazepam, lidocaine, theophylline, and propranolol. To be effective, H_2 antagonists must be given at least an hour before the induction of anesthesia. *Particulate* antacids (e.g., Maalox) can produce serious pneumonitis when aspirated and are not used in this setting. Sodium citrate (Bicitra), 10–30 mL p.o. on call to the OR, is an effective and safe means of increasing the pH of gastric contents when a full stomach is anticipated. In contrast to the H_2 blockers, antacids do increase the volume of gastric contents and so are used only in emergency situations when there is not enough time for H_2 antagonists to become effective.

Volume Reduction. Metoclopramide (Reglan), 10 mg i.v., i.m., or p.o., a cholinergic stimulant, speeds gastric emptying by increasing motility of the upper GI tract and decreasing pyloric sphincter tone. While it results in decreased intragastric volume, it has no effect on gastric fluid pH. It should be included in the preoperative preparation of patients suspected of having a significant volume of gastric contents.

Operative Anesthetic Techniques

Anesthetic techniques fall into one of three categories: general, regional, or local. These may be used either alone or in combination. General anesthesia is maintained by the use of gas, volatile anesthetics, intravenous drugs (narcotics, sedatives), and muscle relaxants. Regional anesthesia is achieved by central or regional techniques. Central techniques include spinal, epidural, and caudal anesthesia, while peripheral techniques include nerve, plexus, and intravenous (Bier) blocks. Local anesthesia (infiltration of the tissues at the surgical site) is usually performed by the surgeon, although the anesthesiologist may stand by to monitor and sedate the patient, thus managing his ongoing medical condition during surgery. The choice of anesthetic technique is the combined responsibility of the anesthesiologist, surgeon, and patient; frequently there are several comparable options. After the alternatives, risks, and benefits of each are explained, the patient should be allowed to choose a technique. When deciding on anesthetic technique, several factors are taken into consideration. Most important is whether a local or regional technique will provide adequate analgesia given the site of surgery. The duration of the procedure and the position of the patient during the procedure must also be considered. Patient factors influencing choice of anesthetic include the presence and type of coexisting diseases, bleeding tendencies, infection, the patient's age, and the possibility of a full stomach. Finally, the surgeon's and anesthesiologist's personality and skill are important to consider when suggesting that a patient be conscious during surgery.

General Anesthesia

General anesthesia should provide analgesia, unconsciousness, muscle relaxation, and autonomic control. It is used whenever complete insensitivity is required, when the surgery is going to involve a part of the body not amenable to regional or local anesthesia, when mechanical ventilation is necessary, or when the position required for the procedure does not allow the patient to be comfortable when awake. General anesthesia is achieved using a combination of inhalational anesthetics and other drugs such as narcotics, sedatives, and muscle relaxants.

Induction. Before induction, the patient is preoxygenated to minimize hypoxemia on induction. Induction begins with the intravenous injection of an ultrashort-acting drug, usually a barbiturate. Other drugs causing rapid loss of consciousness that may be used are listed in Table 1.3. When intubation of the trachea is planned, a depolarizing (succinylcholine) or nondepolarizing (pancuronium, atracurium, vecuronium, mivacurium) muscle relaxant is given to facilitate the process. An alternative to intravenous induction is an inhalation induction, which is more gradual and may not be as pleasant for the patient. For inhalation induction the patient breathes nitrous oxide with oxygen and a gradually increasing concentration of volatile agent,

Table 1.3.
Characteristics of Induction Anesthetics

Drug	Route	Dose (mg/kg)	Onset of Sleep	Duration of Sleep (min)	Elimination Half-Life (hr)
Thiopental (Pentothal)	i.v.	3–5	1 circulation time	5–10	5–12
Methohexital (Brevital)	i.v.	1–1.5	1 circulation time	5–10	1.5–4
	Rectal	15–25	10–15 min	30–40	
Thiamylal	i.v.	3–5	1 circulation time	5–10	5–12
Etomidate	i.v.	0.3	1 circulation time	3–5	1.2–4.5
Ketamine	i.v.	1–2	1 circulation time	10–15	2–3
	i.m.	4–6	5–15 min	20–30	2–3
Propofol (Diprivan)	i.v.	2–2.5	1 circulation time	3–5	0.9
Diazepam (Valium)	i.v.	0.3–0.6	2–3 min	6–15	20–40
Midazolam (Versed)	i.v.	0.15–0.4	3 min	6–15	2–4

usually halothane. Enflurane and isoflurane may also be used for inhalation inductions but are often even less pleasant for the patient.

Intravenous Induction Agents. Intravenous induction agents cause rapid loss of consciousness as their early peak plasma levels are delivered directly to the brain. Consciousness returns when the drug is redistributed to other tissues. Differences in their elimination half-lives result in lingering mild sedation after one dose with some agents, and, in most cases, prolonged effects when continuous infusions or repeated doses are administered. Specific agents and their characteristics are listed in Table 1.3.

The barbiturates thiopental, thiamylal, and methohexital are most frequently used because they are inexpensive, do not irritate veins, act rapidly, and because their mechanism of action, half-life, metabolism, and elimination are well known. The nonbarbiturate etomidate causes less cardiovascular depression than barbiturates and so is used to induce anesthesia in patients who have severely compromised cardiovascular systems or who are in shock. Propofol, a new agent, has utility because of its rapid, complete elimination and is especially useful as a continuous infusion throughout the anesthetic because its effects are totally dissipated moments after it is discontinued. The benzodiazepines diazepam and midazolam also cause less cardiac depression than the barbiturates, but are longer acting and prolong recovery from anesthesia. Ketamine has sympathetic stimulating effects and so does not cause hypotension on induction. It has detrimental effects on myocardial oxygen supply-demand and on intracranial pressure. It is sometimes used as an induction agent in children, because it can be given intramuscularly while the parents are still holding the child. It is also useful for inducing anesthesia in patients with hypovolemia from trauma or bleeding, but will impart no benefit if the patient has been in shock long enough to have depleted catecholamine stores. Pharmacologic differences among the induction agents are summarized in Table 1.4.

The choice of an induction agent depends on the patient's preexisting medical condition, the length of the surgery, the anticipated length of hospital stay, and the particular needs of the anesthetic. Slow intravenous injection of the barbiturates etomidate or propofol will induce sleep without causing apnea. The effects of an inhalation agent introduced gradually can be maintained without endotracheal intubation and controlled ventilation. Rapid induction with larger doses of intravenous agents requires immediate injection of muscle relaxant and intubation while the patient is unconscious. Intravenous induction agents have no toxic effects, and when used as part of anesthesia for delivery their effect on the fetus is limited to varying degrees of sedation.

Rectal or i.m. induction is used in children who will not allow an intravenous catheter; it also avoids a mask induction with inhalation agents. Either route allows a young patient to fall asleep outside the operating room while held by the parents. The child can then be transported into the operating room, monitors and an intravenous catheter established, and anesthesia begun without frightening the child. Induction by these alternative routes has the disadvantage of prolonging the recovery period.

Ketamine is different from the other induction agents, whether used i.m. or i.v., because of its unique central nervous system (CNS) actions. The drug is a hallucinogen in adults and causes signs of excitement in children. Anesthetic depth is difficult to assess because there are often neuromuscular excitatory signs such as nystagmus, purposeful and nonpurposeful movements, and myoclonus. During the recovery period, auditory stimulation causes excitement in children, which may be secondary to nightmares. Although ketamine induces signs of CNS stimulation, paradoxically it has been shown to suppress seizure activity. When administered in very small doses, ketamine is an excellent sedative for use with local or regional anesthesia. Its profound analgesic effect has not been seen in any other nonnarcotic intravenous anesthetic, so it is often used for short, painful procedures such as dressing changes, suture removal or insertion, and fracture reductions in children.

In sum, barbiturates remain the most popular induction agents (porphyrias and allergy are the only contraindications). While etomidate, the benzodiazepines, and ketamine have a blood pressure supporting effect on normal patients, this effect does not extend to patients with hypovolemia or little cardiac reserve. The search for new induction agents results from a desire to

Table 1.4.
Advantages and Disadvantages of Intravenous Induction Agents

Agent	Advantages	Disadvantages
Thiopental and Thiamylal	Inexpensive Rapid acting May be given rectally in children Decreases ICP profoundly Brain protection Onset in 1 circulation time Excellent anticonvulsant No muscle relaxation	Long elimination half-life; postoperative sedation Myocardial depression Hypotension No analgesic effect Difficult to use as sedative Causes apnea and hypotension at sedative and anticonvulsant doses Contraindicated in porphyria
Methohexital	Rapid acting Shorter duration of sedation Used to unmask or potentiate seizures, i.e., for ECTs or brain mapping May be given rectally in children Onset in 1 circulation time No muscle relaxation	Myocardial depression Hypotension No analgesic effect Difficult to use as sedative Contraindicated in porphyria
Diazepam	Less myocardial and respiratory depression than barbiturates Amnesia Muscle relaxant Excellent sedative in low doses Excellent anticonvulsant	Pain on injection Phlebitis Prolonged sedation Longer time to onset of sleep, difficult to use alone as induction agent Questionably safe in porphyria
Midazolam	Less myocardial and respiratory depression than barbiturates No pain on injection or phlebitis Retrograde and antegrade amnesia Excellent sedative in low doses Excellent anticonvulsant	More myocardial depression than diazepam Prolonged sedation Prolongs opioid action, apnea Slow onset time Questionably safe in porphyria
Etomidate	Little effect on cardiovascular system Safe in porphyria Onset in 1 circulation time Less respiratory depression than barbiturates Less postoperative sedation than barbiturates or benzodiazepines Decreases ICP Decreases cerebral O_2 consumption	Postoperative nausea and vomiting No analgesia Pain on injection Depresses adrenal steroid production May cause myoclonus on induction No evidence of analgesic effect Probably safe in porphyria
Propofol	Shortest duration of sedation of any i.v. agent Onset in 1 circulation time Safe in porphyria Very rare nausea and vomiting	Pain on injection Involuntary muscle action Most cardiovascular depression of any i.v. induction agent No analgesia Difficult to use as sedative
Ketamine	Excellent analgesic Increases BP and pulse rate in intact patient Little if any respiratory depression Maintains protective airway reflexes No muscle relaxation Probably safe in porphyria Very rare nausea and vomiting	Causes hallucinations in adults May cause myocardial ischemia in susceptible patients Causes increased secretions Difficult to assess level of anesthesia Increases intracranial pressure Causes myocardial depression when sympathetic NS is depressed

Table 1.5.
Physical Characteristics of Inhaled Anesthetics

Agent	Minimum alveolar concentration (%)	Vapor Pressure	Blood/Gas Solubility	Lipid/Gas Solubility
Nitrous Oxide	104.00	—	0.47	1.40
Halothane	0.74	243	2.30	224.00
Enflurane	1.68	175	1.80	96.50
Isoflurane	1.15	239	1.40	90.80

Table 1.6.
Physiological Effects of Inhaled Anesthetics

Agent	Cardiac Effects		Vascular Effects		Nervous System Effects	
	Contractility	Rate	Arteriolar	Venous	Sympathetic	Neuromuscular
N_2O	Decrease or no change	No change or increase	No change or constrict	No change	Stimulate	No effect or increased tone
Halothane	Decrease	Decrease or no change	Dilate	Dilate	Abolish reflexes	Relax
Enflurane	Decrease	Increase	Dilate	Dilate	Decrease reflexes	Relax
Isoflurane	Decrease	No change or increase	Dilate	Dilate	Slight decrease of reflexes	Relax

identify one that has a very short elimination period, a good analgesic effect, and no undesirable emergence effects. Propofol is enjoying increasing popularity, especially in the ambulatory setting, because it approaches the ideal in its characteristics.

Maintenance. Anesthesia can be maintained by *inhalation agents, intravenous agents* (discussed above), or a combination of both. These agents may be supplemented with a *muscle relaxant*, depending on the need for operative exposure and controlled ventilation. All drugs used for anesthesia are selected according to their pharmacologic effects on the patient's physiologic function, keeping in mind the patient's medical condition and the surgical requirements. The anesthesiologist's goal is to maintain the patient's cardiovascular system as close to the preoperative state as possible.

Inhalation Agents. The inhalation agents have the most profound effects on the physiology of the patient, adding to or even potentiating the effects of other drugs used. The four agents used most often are nitrous oxide, halothane, enflurane, and isoflurane. The physical characteristics of these agents are compared in four areas: the minimum alveolar concentration (MAC), vapor pressure, blood/gas solubility, and lipid/gas solubility. The MAC is the alveolar concentration of gas at 1 atmosphere that prevents movement in response to a surgical stimulus such as skin incision in 50% of patients. It is the standard by which anesthetics are compared with respect to their potencies, and is roughly proportional to the lipid solubility. The vapor pressure determines the concentration of agent in the carrying gas. The blood/gas solubility is a measure of how much of the agent remains dissolved in the blood as it is carried to the brain and other tissues of the body. The lipid/gas solubility determines how easily the agent enters brain and neural tissue to exert its anesthetic effect and is roughly proportional to its potency. Table 1.5 summarizes the important physical characteristics of inhaled agents currently in use and gives the MAC of each. Table 1.6 summarizes the physiological effects of the commonly used inhalation agents. All of the agents depress respiration (N_2O less than the volatile agents), and all depress the cardiovascular system, although these effects are moderated by varying degrees of autonomic reflex depression.

Nitrous oxide is different from the other inhaled agents (see Tables 1.5 and 1.6). First, it is a gas while the others are volatile agents—they are supplied as liquids and are vaporized in a carrier gas. In most hospitals N_2O is piped in through a central system. Otherwise, it is supplied in blue cylinders that attach to the anesthesia machine. Its MAC of 104%, determined under hyperbaric conditions (under greater than atmospheric pressure), indicates its relative impotency. Since anesthetic gas mixtures should deliver at least 30% oxygen to ensure adequate tissue oxygenation, it is possible to administer safely a maximum of only 70% N_2O at sea level, and less at high altitudes. It is evident, then, that nitrous oxide cannot be used as the sole anesthetic in most patients. It must be supplemented with narcotics or a volatile agent in order to cause unconsciousness and analgesia. When administered in high concentrations under hyperbaric conditions it has unique physiological effects in that it acts as a central and sympathetic nervous system stimulant. Because it has few effects on the cardiovascular system and is an excellent analgesic, it is often used to potentiate the effects of other anesthetic agents. Its principal drawback is that it diffuses into closed air spaces much faster than it diffuses out, and so causes a rapid increase in volume of entrapped air. It is thus not indicated for use in obstructed bowel surgery or any other abdominal surgery where an increased volume of bowel gas would interfere with the surgical procedure, increase trauma, or make closure difficult. Nitrous oxide is contraindicated in patients with pneumothorax, large alveolar bullae, and pneumocephalus. It must be used with caution in patients who need a high inspired oxygen concentration for any reason. It is also the only inhaled anesthetic that has been shown to have toxic effects with prolonged exposure. Bone marrow depression, chronic neuropathies, and possible teratogenicity have been reported. It has been shown to inactivate methionine synthetase, which in turn inhibits vitamin B_{12} for up to 4 days after exposure. This inhibition is postulated to be the reason for its toxicity. It must be emphasized, however, that N_2O is still used in up to 90% of all general anesthetics, and frequently as an analgesic of choice for dental and other procedures. When patient outcomes are compared, it is found to be the safest of all anesthetics. The advantages of N_2O are that it is not metabolized, is rapidly taken up and exhaled, is easy to administer, and causes minimal cardiovascular and respiratory depression at concentrations used clinically.

In vitro, all three commonly used *volatile anesthetics*—halothane, enflurane, and isoflurane—depress myocardial contractility to the same degree. In contrast to enflurane and isoflurane, halothane decreases myocardial contractility with very little decrease in peripheral resistance. Isoflurane causes the greatest decrease in peripheral resistance. When halothane is used, the heart rate is unchanged or decreases secondary to an almost complete depression of baroreceptor reflexes. At and above 1 MAC, isoflurane and enflurane may cause increases in the resting heart rate. Arrhythmias are common during halothane anesthesia because they increase the sensitivity of the myocardial conduction system to the effects of endogenous and exogenous catecholamines. A moderate rise in partial arterial carbon dioxide pressure (Pa_{CO_2}) or the injection of a relatively small amount of epinephrine-containing local anesthetic results in frequent premature ventricular contractions (PVCs) or ventricular tachycardia in patients receiving halothane. Right atrial pressure remains higher with halothane than with enflurane and isoflurane because of less arteriolar dilation and hence less peripheral sequestration of blood volume. The blood pressure fall seen with halothane is due to myocardial depression rather than vasodilation. Halothane is thought to be the most protective anesthetic for myocardial oxygenation since it reduces demand but not supply. Baroreceptor and other sympathetic reflexes remain more active with enflurane and isoflurane, and cardiac output is better preserved under surgical conditions.

All three volatile anesthetics depress the respiratory response to CO_2 in a dose-dependent fashion, enflurane more so than the other two. Surgical stimulation partially reverses this depression, if the patient is allowed to ventilate spontaneously during anesthesia and if other factors such as position do not interfere. Respiration tends to be shallow but rapid. The pattern of respiration coupled with the position of the body contribute to intraoperative atelectasis. Furthermore, all inhaled agents interfere with mucociliary flow over the respiratory epithelium. The resulting lung consolidation can be prevented with frequent expansion, humidifying the inspired gas mixtures, and frequent sterile suctioning. Enflurane alone preserves the sigh mechanism, and one often observes an occasional deep sigh made by patients spontaneously breathing this agent.

All three agents cause bronchodilation and are particularly useful in reversing acute reactive bronchoconstriction because of their relaxing effect on bronchial smooth muscle and their inhibitory effect on airway reflexes. Because of an ether linkage in their structure, enflurane and isoflurane are more irritating to the airway than halothane. This is evidenced clinically by coughing, breath holding, and laryngospasm during attempted inhalational induction of anesthesia with either enflurane or isoflurane. Halothane is much less irritating and therefore the agent of choice for inhalational induction in children.

Hypoxic pulmonary vasoconstriction is an important mechanism by which the lung compensates for ventilation-perfusion inequalities, shutting off blood flow to alveoli that are not ventilated. Unfortunately, this mechanism is abolished by all three agents and probably also by N_2O, accounting for the almost universal findings of increased alveolar-arterial difference in partial pressure of oxygen ($P_{AO_2} - Pa_{O_2}$) and lower than expected arterial partial pressure of oxygen (Pa_{O_2}) seen in patients during and following general anesthesia.

The volatile agents all produce dose-dependent relaxation of skeletal and smooth muscle and potentiate the action of muscle relaxants given simultaneously. Surgical relaxation required for abdominal procedures cannot be achieved with volatile agents alone except at concentrations that produce unacceptable cardiovascular depression, and thus the addition of muscle relaxing agents is required.

All inhaled agents, including N_2O, increase cerebral blood flow and abolish autoregulation, again in a dose-dependent fashion. In the face of intracranial hypertension, these effects may cause significant increases in intracranial pressure and irreversible damage from herniation. Hyperventilation of the patient exerts some protection, but does not completely negate the effect. In high concentrations, enflurane may cause further brain damage by inducing seizure activity and increasing the metabolic demand for oxygen and hence regional blood flow. Seizure activity has been seen at inspired concentrations of 3%, and at lower concentrations in the presence of hypocapnia or previously existing seizure foci. N_2O has also been seen to cause seizures, but only at high inspired partial pressures under hyperbaric conditions. Conversely, at 2 MAC isoflurane completely silences the electroencephalogram (EEG) and may actually protect the brain from the effects of hypoxia or reduced perfusion because of the resultant reduced metabolic demand for oxygen.

All the volatile agents are metabolized to varying degrees by the hepatic microsomal enzymatic system, and most of the metabolites are excreted by the kidneys. The unmetabolized drug is excreted by the lungs. Up to 25% of halothane is metabolized. It is the only agent whose metabolites reach significant blood concentrations. In contrast, only 3% of enflurane and less than 1% of isoflurane are metabolized. In conditions of hepatic hypoxia, halothane may be metabolized by a reductive pathway. It is postulated that it is the metabolites from this reductive metabolism that cause hepatocyte toxicity and thus halothane has the undeserved reputation of liver toxin. In the national halothane study of the 1960s, "halothane hepatitis" or massive hepatic necrosis was found to occur in 1 in 35,000 administrations. Besides the direct toxicity, in some patients there appears to be an immune component to halothane-related liver dysfunction. Current recommendations are that halothane not be administered to any patient who has a history of unexplained liver dysfunction following a previous halothane anesthetic, or to one who for any reason has altered liver perfusion. Cases of hepatic dysfunction following administration of the other inhaled anesthetics are felt to be related to global or surgical effects on liver perfusion rather than to the agent itself.

The metabolites of all three volatile agents include small amounts of inorganic fluoride ion, but in concentrations that are too low to cause renal toxicity. Halothane metabolism may also result in a measurable blood level of bromine, which may have some sedative effects of its own. Halothane itself is measurable in exhaled air many hours after the anesthesia has been discontinued. Its metabolites are measurable in urine up to several days postoperatively.

In summary, with the exception of halothane the inhaled anesthetics are remarkably inert metabolically. It is extremely rare for them to cause toxicity. Despite their causing profound cardiovascular, respiratory, and neurological system depression, they are safe when used under controlled conditions. Combining volatile agents with N_2O, and all inhaled agents with the adjunctive drugs discussed below, results in profound general anesthesia with little interference to tissue perfusion and oxygenation.

Muscle Relaxants. Muscle relaxants allow a much lighter plane of anesthesia in order to provide conditions required for surgery. They facilitate such procedures as endotracheal intubation and abdominal surgery, which require a degree of muscle relaxation that often cannot be safely achieved by inhalation agents alone. Controlled ventilation is also facilitated by muscle relaxants, extending their use beyond the operating room and into intensive care units.

The normal reflex response to a noxious stimulus is withdrawal. If a patient moves during anesthesia, it indicates that the depth of anesthesia is not sufficient to prevent this motor response. Because muscle relaxants might mask a sign of inadequate anesthesia, the anesthesiologist relies on autonomic (cardiovascular, metabolic) rather than motor reflexes as a sign of depth of anesthesia. The use of muscle relaxants is thus a safe method of reducing inhalational anesthetic requirements to a level that does not cause dangerous cardiovascular depression and other ill effects.

Two classes of muscle relaxants are in use today. The *depolarizing relaxants* cause activation of the postsynaptic cholinergic receptor of the neuromuscular junction, then dissociate only slowly from that receptor, binding it so that it will not fire again until it is free. The *nondepolarizing relaxants* prevent muscle contraction by competitively blocking the postsynaptic receptor from binding with acetylcholine, but do not activate the receptor. Monitoring the response to single and repeated supramaximal twitch stimuli and tetanic stimulation differentiates the two types (Table 1.7) and determines the percentage of receptors blocked at any one time.

Of the *depolarizing agents,* succinylcholine is the only one currently in use. It consists of two acetylcholine molecules joined together; it produces relaxation of short duration after initial generalized contraction, which is clinically visible as fasciculations. Succinylcholine is not metabolized at the neuromuscular junction by acetylcholinesterase, but diffuses into the blood where it is rapidly hydrolyzed by plasma cholinesterase (pseudocholinesterase). Its onset of action is almost immediate, and a single dose of 1 mg/kg has a duration of around 10 minutes. Despite its side effects (see Table 1.8), the drug has continued to be the choice of many anesthesiologists for endotracheal intubation because of its rapid onset. Many of these side effects can be ameliorated by preceding the injection with a small, defasciculating dose of a nondepolarizing relaxant, but this action also increases the time to onset, the duration, and the dose of succinylcholine required to suppress neuromuscular transmission. Nondepolarizing relaxants do not have these undesirable side effects.

Hyperkalemia following succinylcholine injection occurs as a consequence of depolarization, and can be clinically significant in patients with recent massive soft tissue injury, acute and chronic denervation injuries, renal failure, or preexisting hyperkalemia. In these situations, cardiac arrest is not uncommon and is not effectively prevented by pretreatment with nondepolarizing agents. Intracranial and intraocular pressure rises with succinylcholine have been shown to occur even in the absence of both fasciculations and increased venous pressure. The reason for the intracranial pressure increase has not been determined, but the rise in intraocular pressure is initiated by contracture of extraocular muscles and perhaps enhanced by transient dilation of choroidal blood vessels. The result may lead to extrusion of vitreous in patients with an open globe injury. The rise in intra-abdominal pressure is the consequence of contractions of the abdominal muscles, and may be significant enough to cause regurgitation of stomach contents and their aspiration into the lungs if protective measures are not taken. Nonetheless, succinylcholine is still the favorite relaxant of many anesthesiologists for rapid endotracheal intubation, especially in patients with a full stomach, because of its rapid, reliable onset of action.

The action of succinylcholine is prolonged in patients with abnormal or deficient plasma cholinesterase and in those with chronic neuromuscular disease. Severe liver failure results in low levels of plasma cholinesterase. Succinylcholine may be safely used as a continuous infusion relaxant for short procedures with constant as-

Table 1.7.
Monitoring Neuromuscular Blockade

Type of Relaxant	Single Twitch	Train of Four[a]	Tetanic (50 Hz) Stimulation	Posttetanic Twitch
Depolarizing	Decreased height in proportion to dose	No fade, all four equally decreased	No fade, tetany depressed in proportion to dose	No facilitation, twitch same as pretetany
EMG	Drug injection			
Nondepolarizing	Decreased height in proportion to dose	Fade, in proportion to dose	Rapid fade	Posttetanic facilitation: first twitches greater in height than pretetanic twitch
EMG	Drug injection			

[a]Train of four is four twitches delivered at a rate of one every 0.5 second.

Table 1.8.
Side Effects of Succinylcholine

Vagal stimulation (common in children)
  Bradycardia (especially with repeat injections)
Sympathetic stimulation
  Tachycardia and hypertension in adults
Increased intracranial pressure
Increased intraocular pressure
Fasciculations
  Hyperkalemia
  Increased intraabdominal pressure
  Further increase in intracranial pressure
  Further increase in intraocular pressure
  Postoperative myalgia

sessment of its effect with a twitch monitor. Large doses of the drug result in the development of a Phase II (or desensitization) block, a postjunctional effect that cannot reliably be reversed pharmacologically and must be allowed to wear off gradually. Monitoring the twitch shows the onset of signs of a nondepolarizing blockade when this Phase II block develops.

Nondepolarizing agents are used for prolonged relaxation during the surgical procedure. While they can be used for endotracheal intubation, they take longer than succinylcholine to complete relaxation of the jaw (around 2 minutes) when twice the ED_{95} (dose required to block 95% of receptors) is administered. When intubating doses of curare, gallamine, metocurine, atracurium, pancuronium, and mivacurium are used, the autonomic and histamine-related side effects may be significant. Vecuronium, doxacurium, and pipecuronium have not been associated with significant cardiovascular effects. The duration of effect is also prolonged with higher doses and may limit their use for this purpose in short procedures. The nondepolarizing agents currently in use and their dose, duration, and side effects are listed in Table 1.9.

The cardiovascular effects of nondepolarizing relaxants are the result of ganglionic blockade, vagal stimulation, and histamine release. Ganglionic blockade and histamine release result in hypotension, while vagal stimulation results in tachycardia.

Gallamine is 90% dependent on the kidney for elimination, and is not appreciably metabolized. Pancuronium, doxacurium, pipecuronium, and metocurine are metabolized somewhat in the liver, but 60–90% of injected doses are recovered unchanged in the urine. Between 40–60% of curare is recovered unmetabolized in the urine, while less than 25% of vecuronium and atracurium is recovered. Atracurium is unique among the nondepolarizing relaxants in that it undergoes Hofmann elimination (spontaneous degradation in plasma) and does not rely on either the kidney or the liver for termination of its effect. Mivacurium is metabolized in the blood by plasma cholinesterase, but may undergo some metabolism in the liver as well.

Most anesthesiologists monitor the twitch response when using neuromuscular blocking agents, since their effect is potentiated by the concurrent administration of inhalational agents, and their metabolism and excretion may be affected by many physiological factors. As shown in Table 1.7, 75–80% of receptors must be blocked before there is a depression of twitch response, while 90–95% of receptors must be blocked before there is no response to a single twitch. Fade (a progressive decrease in height of successive twitches) may be seen in the train-of-four stimulation sequence when 70–75% of receptors are blocked. A train-of-four sequence consists of four supramaximal stimuli delivered at a rate of 2 cycles per second (2 Hz). Tetanic stimulation at 30 Hz results in appreciable fade when 75–80% of receptors are blocked, and at 100 Hz fade is seen when 50% of receptors are blocked. Even though relaxation may be antagonized by the administration of neostigmine, pyridostigmine, or edrophonium, this effect is not reliable when doses of nondepolarizing relaxants sufficient to block all twitch responses at the time of antagonist administration have been used.

Airway Maintenance. The patient's airway must be maintained when a general anesthetic is being adminis-

Table 1.9.
Characteristics of Nondepolarizing Relaxants

Relaxant	ED_{95} (mg/kg)	Intubating Dose (mg/kg)	Time to 5% Recovery (min)[a]	Side Effects
d-Tubocurarine	0.51	0.6	30–45	+ + + Histamine release Blocks ganglionic transmission No effect on vagus
Metocurine	0.28	0.4	30–45	+ + Histamine release Blocks ganglionic transmission less than curare No effect on vagus
Pancuronium	0.07	0.1 0.2	45 129	+ + Vagal blockade (tachycardia) No histamine release No ganglionic effect
Vecuronium	0.05	0.1	20–30	No effect on vagus No ganglionic effect No histamine release
Atracurium	2.8	3.5	20–30	No effect on vagus No ganglionic effect + Histamine release
Gallamine	2.8	3.5	30–45	+ + + Vagal blockade (tachycardia) No ganglionic effect No histamine release
Mivacurium	0.08	0.2–0.4	16–19	+ Histamine release No effect on vagus No ganglionic effect
Pipecuronium	0.05–0.06	0.1	80–120	No histamine release No vagal effect No ganglionic effect
Doxacurium	0.025	0.06	80–120	No histamine release No vagal effect No ganglionic effect

[a]After intubating dose.

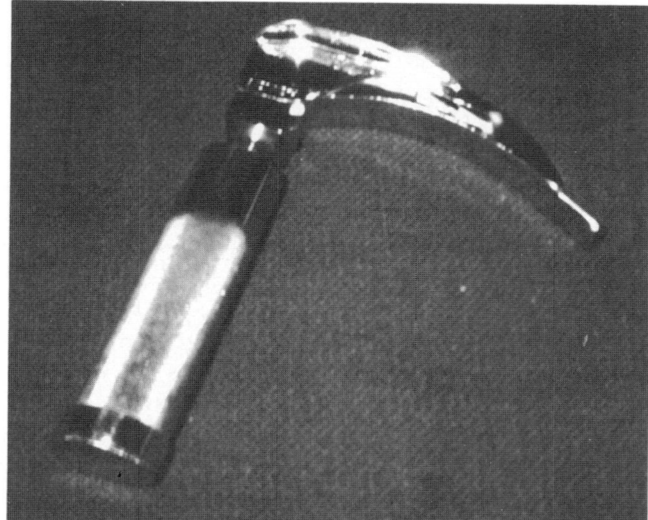

Figure 1.1. A battery-operated laryngoscope with a Macintosh-3 blade.

tered. As soon as the patient loses consciousness, the upper airway structures relax and the tongue falls backward, obstructing the glottis. This obstruction can be corrected by pulling the lower jaw upward and forward and hyperextending the neck, and also by inserting an oropharyngeal airway. However, if an oropharyngeal airway is inserted before the pharyngeal and laryngeal reflexes are obtunded, laryngospasm may occur. Obese patients or those with a short, muscular neck tend to obstruct easier and earlier during the induction. If the patient is not anesthetized deeply enough for the mouth to be opened, a nasopharyngeal airway may be inserted.

If the patient's airway cannot be maintained with a mask, or if a long period of airway control is anticipated, endotracheal intubation becomes necessary. Muscle relaxants facilitate intubation, but, because they inhibit spontaneous ventilation, should not be given until the anesthesiologist can manually ventilate the patient through a mask. If mask ventilation is impossible, the depth of anesthesia must be lessened, and the endotracheal tube must be inserted with the patient awake and breathing spontaneously. Intubation is facilitated by the use of a laryngoscope. Figure 1.1 illustrates a laryngoscope with a curved, Macintosh-3 blade. There is a small light bulb on the side of the blade that is powered by batteries in the handle. The operator holds the handle in the left hand and opens the patient's mouth with the right hand. The blade is inserted from the right side of the mouth and slides back along the right margin of the tongue to the vallecula (the area between the base of the tongue and the epiglottis). With the blade in the proper position and the patient's

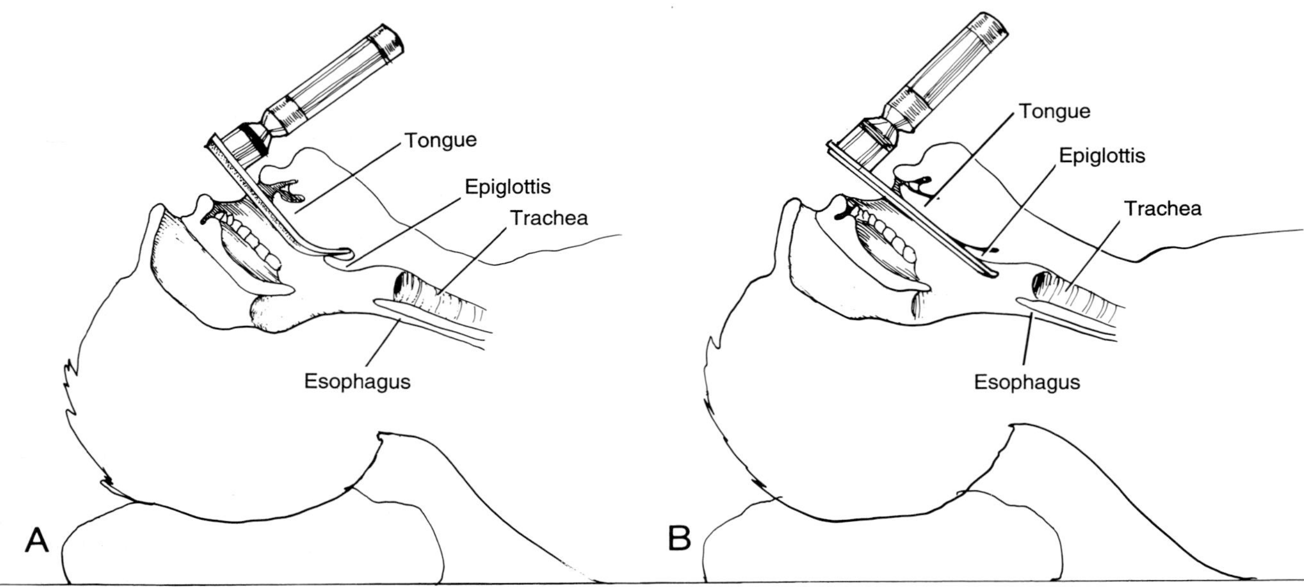

Figure 1.2. Position of the curved blade (**A**) and straight blade (**B**) in exposing the larynx.

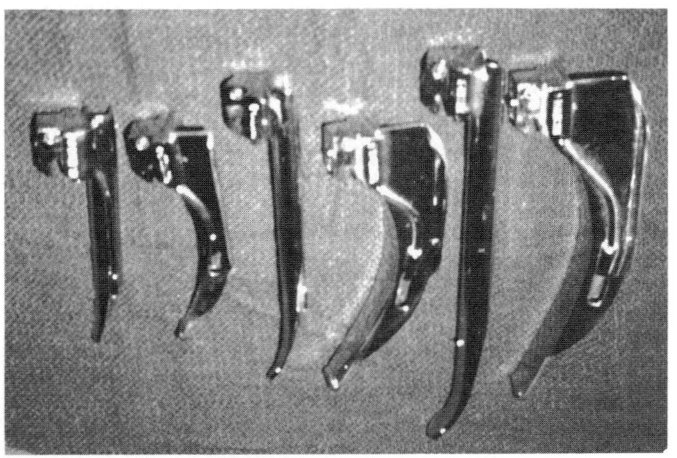

Figure 1.3. Curved and straight laryngoscope blades of various sizes. From left to right: 1½-Wis-Hipple and 1-Macintosh (MAC) for small children; 3-Miller and 3-MAC for most intubations; 4-Miller and 4-MAC for very large adults.

neck slightly extended in the sniffing position, lifting the handle raises the epiglottis and brings the vocal cords into direct vision (Fig. 1.2). Figure 1.3 shows the difference between the curved and the straight blades in various sizes. In all except the newborn, the straight blade should be placed over the epiglottis to lift it along with the base of the tongue in order to expose the larynx.

In general, intubation is required whenever the anesthesiologist does not have immediate access to the airway, when mechanical ventilation is required because of muscle relaxation or physical characteristics of the patient, or when there is risk of aspiration. Intubation of the trachea in a poorly anesthetized patient results in massive autonomic stimulation seen as hypertension, tachycardia or bradycardia, arrhythmias, and bronchoconstriction. It is important to remember that endotracheal intubation never guarantees an adequate airway. The tube may become obstructed by secretions or kinking, it may become displaced either out of the trachea or down into a bronchus, and patients may aspirate pharyngeal contents despite the presence of an inflated cuff. In order to minimize the risk of aspiration of gastric contents, patients who are suspected of having a full stomach can be intubated either awake under topical anesthesia or after being anesthetized with a rapid sequence or "crash" induction. In the rapid sequence induction, the patient is preoxygenated for 3–5 minutes and then anesthesia is rapidly induced with the induction agent and muscle relaxant, while an assistant provides downward pressure on the cricoid cartilage of the neck. This pressure is applied to compress the lumen of the esophagus between the posterior ring of that cartilage and the vertebral body; it prevents passive regurgitation of gastric contents through the esophagus. The anesthesiologist intubates the trachea without ventilating the patient with the mask, to avoid pushing air into the stomach and increasing gastric pressure. When the position of the tube in the trachea is verified and the cuff is inflated, the assistant releases the cricoid pressure. Indications and complications of endotracheal intubation for general anesthesia are listed in Table 1.10.

If the uvula and tonsillar pillars are easily visible when the patient opens his mouth and sticks out his tongue, the anesthesiologist can safely assume intubation will be possible with direct laryngoscopy. A difficult intubation may be anticipated in patients who present with a short, muscular "bull" neck, a receding chin, protruding upper incisors, or a high arched palate in a narrow mouth. Inability to open the mouth wide or to extend the neck also predicts difficult laryngoscopy. Finally, any space-occupying lesion of the mouth, pharynx, larynx, or neck makes direct laryngoscopy difficult. In those cases, conventional induction and intuba-

Table 1.10.
Endotracheal Intubation During Anesthesia

Indications	Complications
Inability to maintain airway	Trauma to teeth and oropharyngeal soft tissue
Requirement by surgeon for muscle relaxation	Aspiration
Inaccessibility of the airway, or shared airway with surgeon	Hypoxemia:
Patient with a full stomach, or at risk for aspiration	Obstruction by secretions
Need for tracheal toilet	Endobronchial intubation
Patients requiring positive pressure ventilation	Accidental extubation
Massive upper airway secretions or bleeding	Autonomic response:
	Hypertension, tachycardia, bradycardia, arrhythmias
	Bronchospasm
	Endotracheal tube obstruction

Table 1.11.
Criteria for Postanesthesia Extubation

Adequate spontaneous respiration:
- Normal respiratory rate
- Adequate tidal volume
- Vital capacity >15 mL/kg
- Expired CO_2 <45–50 mm Hg

Return of protective reflexes (gag and cough)
Responsive to verbal commands
Cardiovascular stability
Metabolic stability (temperature >35°C)
No residual neuromuscular blockade
- By nerve stimulator
- Able to sustain head lift for 5 seconds
- Good muscle tone
- Negative inspiratory force (NIF) > −20 cm H_2O

tion may not be appropriate. Alternative methods include awake intubation under direct vision with topical anesthesia, awake blind nasal intubation, intubation over a fiberoptic bronchoscope inserted into the trachea with the patient either awake or asleep, or tracheotomy under local anesthesia.

Emergence. A noncritically ill patient should be returning to a normal state when leaving the operating room. In this condition, respiratory obstruction, pulmonary aspiration, and cardiovascular instability are unlikely. Recovery from anesthesia begins when anesthetic drugs are discontinued. Oxygen at 100% should be administered while the anesthetic gases are being excreted through the lungs. The patient's alveolar ventilation, the lipid solubility of the agent, and the duration of the anesthetic determine how quickly gases are eliminated. An agent that is highly lipid soluble tends to remain sequestered in body fat, dissolving only very slowly and providing a long period of low blood concentration as it does so. The recovery rate from intravenous anesthetics depends on the amount administered, time of last injection, lipid solubility, hepatic metabolism, and renal excretion. If muscle relaxants have been used, the degree of remaining blockade should be monitored using a nerve stimulator, and the effects neutralized by neuromuscular antagonists if necessary. All monitoring continues until the patient leaves the operating room; it commences again in the recovery room. In unstable patients monitoring continues during transportation. Because hypoxemia has been documented consistently in the immediate postanesthesia period, oxygen is administered as the patient is transported to the recovery room.

Extubation of the Trachea. Patients are safely extubated when the criteria in Table 1.11 are met. Before extubation, the patient breathes 100% oxygen for at least 5 minutes and the oropharynx is suctioned. The endotracheal tube may be suctioned if necessary. The cuff is deflated to allow easy removal of the endotracheal tube. Complications that may follow extubation postanesthesia include laryngospasm, aspiration, pharyngitis or laryngitis, and vocal cord dysfunction. The most frequent and the most serious is laryngospasm, which occurs when the vocal cords are irritated. Laryngospasm is treated by administering positive pressure oxygen by mask and by maintaining an unobstructed airway. Occasionally, a small amount of muscle relaxant is necessary to relax the vocal cords sufficiently to allow air entry; the patient's respirations then need to be controlled until the relaxant wears off.

Regional Anesthesia

Regional anesthesia provides loss of pain perception in the area of surgical intervention. The patient usually remains awake and is able to breathe adequately. The patient is monitored and observed in the operating room and recovery room in a manner identical to that of the patient who undergoes general anesthesia. The most commonly used regional anesthetics are those of the lower spinal nerve roots (spinal, epidural, and caudal blocks) and of the brachial plexus.

Figure 1.4 diagrams the lower spinal canal and illustrates the different needle placements for subarachnoid (spinal), epidural, and caudal blocks. Each of these approaches provides adequate anesthesia and operating conditions for surgical procedures below the waist. If the procedure is to be performed in the upper abdomen, or if extensive manipulation of the viscera is required, adequate analgesia may be achieved only with the addition of a celiac plexus block (to denervate the viscera) to the regional technique.

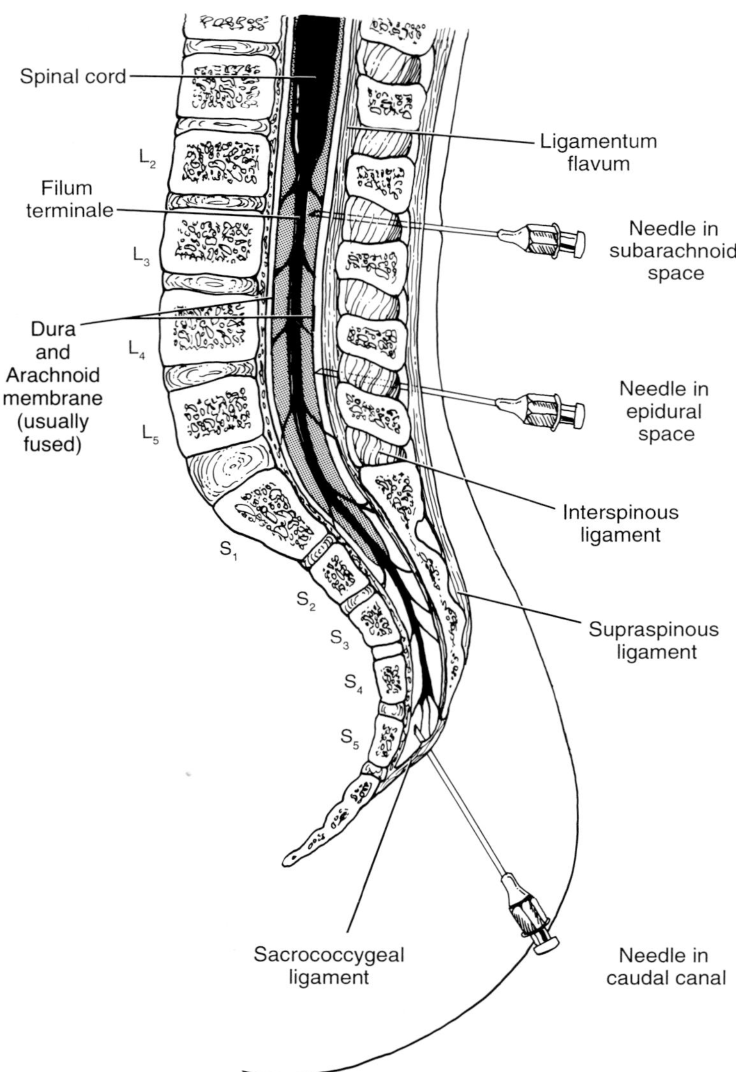

Figure 1.4. Diagram of the lumbosacral spinal canal illustrating needle placement for subarachnoid, epidural, and caudal block. Note the spinal cord terminates at about L2 and the dural sac at about S2. Below S2 the sacral canal contains only the dura-enclosed sacral nerve roots.

Spinal Anesthesia. Spinal anesthesia is an ideal technique for surgery on the lower part of the body. When a small amount of local anesthetic is injected into the subarachnoid space at a level below L2, it diffuses through the cerebrospinal fluid (CSF) to a height determined by the specific gravity and concentration of the anesthetic solution and the position of the patient. After the drug is injected, there is an almost immediate sympathetic blockade that results in vasodilation, blood pooling in dependent areas, and decreased cardiac output. This sympathetic effect is best treated by administering fluids and raising the patient's legs to increase venous return. Trendelenburg position is contraindicated soon after a spinal injection, because it will elevate the level of block to higher than desired in the case of a hyperbaric (specific gravity greater than that of CSF) anesthetic solution and to stay lower than expected in the case of a hypobaric (specific gravity less than that of CSF) solution. If the level of sympathetic blockade is higher than T1 to T4, the cardioaccelerator sympathetic nerves are blocked and bradycardia will ensue.

During a spinal anesthetic, the sympathetic blockade is several levels higher than the sensory blockade, and the motor blockade is several levels lower than the sensory level. If the level of motor blockade is higher than C3, the diaphragm as well as the intercostal muscles will be paralyzed, and the patient will not be able to breathe adequately. Apnea may also occur secondary to ischemia of the medullary centers caused by profound hypotension induced by the anesthesia. If respiration is compromised, the patient should be intubated and ventilated until the level recedes enough for spontaneous respiration to resume. The anesthesiologist must ensure that the patient receiving a spinal anesthetic is fully monitored during and after the block, that a reliable i.v. is running, that oxygen is available, and that all anesthetic drugs and equipment are within arm's reach as the block is being performed. Patient preparation should be as complete for a regional technique as for a general anesthetic, i.e., the patient should be in optimal medical condition, have an empty stomach, and be psychologically prepared.

Headache, the most common complication of a spinal anesthetic, occurs in 20–30% of cases, mostly among younger patients. It usually begins the day after the spinal and is posture related, occurring when the patient is upright and disappearing when the patient lies down. The headache probably is caused by leakage of CSF through the dural puncture. Using a 25- or 27-gauge needle for the puncture reduces the probability of spinal headache. Hydration and bed rest are usually adequate treatment, but if the headache is prolonged (1–2 days), it should be treated by injecting 5–10 mL of the patient's own blood in the epidural space at the level of the previous spinal injection (epidural blood patch).

Epidural Anesthesia. When anesthesia is needed in the lower half of the body, epidural anesthesia is another option. The epidural space is that area within the spinal canal outside the dura and arachnoid. In the area below L2 it contains fat, an extensive venous plexus, and the dura-enclosed cauda equina. A large volume of local anesthetic is injected into the space, with the level of the block depending on the actual volume injected. Continuous analgesia can be obtained by giving additional doses of the anesthetic through a catheter inserted through the needle at the time the epidural space is identified. The concentration of anesthetic determines whether the block is sympathetic, sensory, or complete (i.e., including motor fibers).

The onset of epidural anesthesia is slower than of spinal anesthesia, but the level and characteristics of the block are much more controllable because anesthetic can be added in small increments through the indwelling catheter placed in the epidural space. Because of anatomical abnormalities that may be present in the space, a "patchy" block is much more likely to result from an epidural than from a spinal block. Hypotension and respiratory insufficiency may develop, but less frequently than with a spinal anesthetic because of the more gradual onset of blockade. Because the needle used in an epidural block is larger than the one used in a spinal block, if the dura is accidentally punctured during its insertion, a spinal headache is more apt to ensue. Backache also is more likely following an epidural block: tissues are more likely to be injured when inserting the larger, blunter needle through the ligaments supporting the spinal column. Anesthetic unknowingly injected into the subarachnoid space because of unrecognized dural puncture results in a "total spinal," with total blockade of all the spinal nerves. If the anesthetic reaches the brainstem level, unconsciousness and apnea occur. If the anesthetic is injected into one of the numerous epidural veins, systemic toxicity occurs. These complications are rare, and epidural anesthesia is the gold standard for many lower extremity, pelvic, and lower abdominal surgeries as well as for analgesia during labor and delivery.

Caudal Anesthesia. The caudal block is a variation of the epidural block, in which the needle is inserted through the sacral hiatus at the bottom of the sacrum and anesthetic injected into the epidural space. Larger volumes of anesthetic are required to achieve the same level of analgesia using this route, but there is virtually no possibility of an unrecognized subarachnoid injection. Because of anatomical variations present in a large percentage of the population, however, reliable anesthesia is often difficult to achieve with this technique. It consequently is used less frequently than the epidural block.

Brachial Plexus Blocks. The brachial plexus may be blocked in the interscalene area, the supraclavicular area, or the axilla. Any of these approaches results in reliable anesthesia of the forearm and hand. Anesthesia of the upper arm using a brachial plexus block is less reliable. The plexus is identified with a needle by eliciting paresthesia or by motor response to stimulation by a nerve stimulator attached to the needle. A relatively large volume (35–50 mL) of local anesthetic, usually 1.5–2% lidocaine, 0.5% bupivacaine, or 2% chloroprocaine, is injected when the plexus is located. Anesthesia of all the nerves in the plexus depends on the volume and concentration injected. Complications of brachial plexus blocks are related to the volume of anesthetic or the proximity of the injection site to the carotid or axillary artery, the dome of the pleura, and the spinal canal.

Intravenous Regional Block (Bier Block). When the surgical procedure can be performed with a tourniquet on the extremity, a Bier block provides reliable anesthesia of an extremity. The block is achieved by exsanguinating the extremity with an elastic compression bandage, inflating a proximal tourniquet above arterial pressure, and replacing the blood volume of the extremity with a dilute solution of local anesthetic (usually 0.5% lidocaine). Complete blockade occurs almost immediately and continues until the tourniquet is released. If a second tourniquet is placed just distal to the first and inflated after the block is effective, the distal tourniquet may be deflated and tourniquet pain (ischemic pain under the tourniquet) is avoided. If the tourniquet is not inflated to a sufficiently high pressure, or if it is released or leaks during the procedure, the block fades as anesthetic escapes into the circulation. If this occurs within half an hour of the injection, systemic toxicity may occur because of the large load of anesthetic that may be released. At the end of the procedure, the tourniquet is released and the block diminishes rapidly. If the procedure has lasted less than half an hour, the tourniquet is released slowly and intermittently in order to minimize systemic blood levels of local anesthetic.

Nerve Blocks and Local Infiltration Anesthesia

Nerve Blocks. Peripheral nerves that are easily blocked with injections of local anesthetic to provide ad-

Table 1.12.
Characteristics of Local Anesthetic Agents

Agent	Linkage	Uses	Concentration Used—Dose	Onset[a] (min)	Duration[a] (min)
Benzocaine	Ester	Topical	20% Ointment	Immediate	30
			20% Aerosol	Immediate	30
Chloroprocaine	Ester	Infiltration	1–2 %, up to 1 g	5	30
		Epidural/Caudal	2%, 5–10 mL increments up to 25 mL	15	30–90
Cocaine	Ester	Topical	4%, up to 4 mL	Immediate	60
Dibucaine	Ester	Spinal	0.07 to 0.5%, 1–2 mL	Immediate	30
Procaine	Ester	Infiltration	1 & 2%, up to 1 g	Immediate	20
		Spinal	10%, 1–2 mL	5	30
Tetracaine	Ester	Spinal	1%, 1–2 mL	5–10	60–140
Bupivacaine	Amide	Infiltration	0.25–0.5%, up to 200 mg	15	200±33
		Spinal	0.5–0.75%, up to 1 mL	10	120–240
		Epidural/Caudal	0.25–0.55%, 5–10 mL increments up to 25 mL	17	195±30
Etidocaine	Amide	Infiltration	0.25–1%, up to 300 mg	4–5	300
		Epidural/Caudal	0.5–1%, 5–10 mL increments up to 25 mL	11	170±57
Lidocaine	Amide	Topical	1–5%, up to 500 mg	3	30
		Infiltration	0.5–2%, up to 500 mg	Immediate	75–127
		Spinal	5%, up to 1 mL	3–6	30–45
		Epidural/Caudal	0.5–2%, 5–10 mL increments up to 25 mL	15	100±20
Mepivacaine	Amide	Infiltration	1–2%, up to 500 mg	30–60	60–180
		Epidural/Caudal	2%, 5–10 mL increments up to 25 mL	15	115±15
Prilocaine	Amide	Infiltration	1–3%, up to 900 mg	10	100–150

[a]Onset and duration of surgical analgesia when anesthetic used without vasoconstrictors.

equate analgesia for limited surgery include the following: digital for finger or toe surgery, intercostal for thoracic or abdominal wall procedures, sciatic and femoral for lower leg procedures, mandibular for lower jaw procedures, retrobulbar for eye procedures, penile for circumcisions, and ankle blocks for foot procedures. Nerve blocks are effective for distal procedures that include skin, subcutaneous tissue, muscle, fascia, bone, joints, and periosteum. Peritoneum, pleura, and pericardium cannot be rendered insensitive by peripheral nerve block because they have autonomic innervation as well as somatic. Nerve blocks on digits should not contain an epinephrine local anesthetic solution, since epinephrine could cause local vasoconstriction, resulting in peripheral ischemia. The only contraindications to nerve blocks for appropriate procedures are unacceptability to the patient, local infection at the injection site, coagulopathy, and allergy to both kinds of local anesthetic.

Local Anesthesia. Local anesthesia is achieved by infiltrating a local anesthetic into the skin and underlying tissue around the operative site. Local infiltration of anesthetic is sufficient for limited superficial procedures that involve skin, subcutaneous tissue, muscle, and fascia. It is difficult to desensitize bone and periosteum with local infiltration. The same contraindications apply as to nerve blocks.

For a drier surgical field and prolongation of the block, epinephrine should be added to the local anesthetic.

Local Anesthetics. Local anesthetics may be administered by several routes: topically (directly on skin, cornea, or mucous membrane), by infiltration around a peripheral nerve or a plexus, in the subarachnoid space, in the epidural space, or even intravenously. Because virtually every practitioner uses local anesthetics to some extent, a working knowledge of their pharmacology and toxicity is important. All local anesthetics except cocaine consist of a tertiary amine and an unsaturated aromatic ring separated by either an ester or an amide link. The benzene ring imparts lipid solubility necessary to permeate nerve sheaths and coverings, while the amine imparts water solubility necessary to diffuse and bind to the axonal site of action. The amide or ester link determines the route and speed of drug metabolism: those with an ester linkage are metabolized rapidly by serum cholinesterase and acetylcholinesterase, while those with an amide linkage are metabolized more slowly by the hepatic microsomal system. Table 1.12 lists local anesthetics currently in use, the ways in which they are used, and their important characteristics.

Local anesthetics are classified according to their duration of action—the drugs in each category are similar with respect to their toxicities and potencies. Adding epinephrine or another vasoconstrictor to the injected solution usually prolongs the duration of action by one-third to one-half, and reduces the toxicity of the drug secondary to retarding its rapid vascular uptake. Because epinephrine causes vasoconstriction, it should not be used in areas prone to ischemia, such as nose, ear, digits, or penis.

True allergic reactions to local anesthetic agents, especially those with an amide linkage, are rare but life threatening. A patient with a history of allergy to local anesthesia should be skin tested with several agents in order to determine if they are truly contraindicated. While not 100% reliable, skin testing (applying an intradermal patch and looking for wheal and flare) is accepted as adequate screening for local anesthetic allergy. True allergy to lidocaine and other amides has been reported only a few times in millions of administrations. Distinguishing an allergic reaction from systemic toxicity is difficult because most reactions to local anesthetics are the result of accidental intravascular injections or overdoses rather than of true allergies. The maximum recommended dose of commonly used local anesthetic agents is included in Table 1.12. Systemic toxicity of local anesthetics is the greatest potential risk associated with their use. Symptoms are ringing in the ears, perioral numbness, and a metallic taste in the mouth, signaling the onset of central nervous system excitation that may then progress to jitteriness, shivering, convulsions, and coma. Treatment of local anesthetic toxicity consists of oxygenation and injection of anticonvulsants, preferably short-acting intravenous agents such as Pentothal, diazepam, or midazolam. Prevention is easily accomplished by calculating the dose to be administered, making sure that the injection is not into a vessel by aspirating frequently during injection, and premedicating with a benzodiazepine to reduce CNS toxicity whenever it is anticipated that large doses of local anesthetics will be used.

All local anesthetics with the exception of cocaine cause myocardial depression, peripheral vasodilation, and depression of autonomic responses in a dose-related fashion. Lidocaine is associated with a short-lived blockade of the myocardial conduction system. Bupivacaine causes a more prolonged blockade associated with malignant reentrant dysrhythmia, which is difficult to reverse and occurs at blood levels only slightly above those that cause CNS excitement. Emergency lifesaving support may be necessary, including prolonged CPR, bretylium rather than lidocaine for ventricular ectopy, and often large doses of epinephrine. If convulsions also occur after bupivacaine injection, they are controlled with a short-acting muscle relaxant such as succinylcholine. Anticonvulsants are contraindicated as they may cause further cardiac depression.

Cocaine is different from the other local anesthetics because it blocks the presynaptic uptake of norepinephrine into sympathetic nerve terminals. Because of this, it has local vasoconstrictive effects that make it useful as topical anesthesia for surgery of the nose and throat. Cocaine also has profound CNS effects, similar to those of antidepressants or amphetamines, accompanied by cardiovascular stimulation. The drug has fallen out of favor among many anesthesiologists because of the difficulty in keeping it "off the street," and because the same effects can be achieved with the combination of other topical anesthetics with vasoconstrictors, such as phenylephrine.

Anesthetic Supplements

Opioids are used to supplement local or regional anesthesia, to supplement inhalational anesthetics so that lower concentrations may be used, and with other drugs as a part of total intravenous anesthesia. Fentanyl, sufentanil, and alfentanil are often given as a continuous i.v. infusion or in small frequent doses after an initial bolus dose. The longer acting opioids are given as incremental small doses near the beginning of the anesthetic to establish a baseline narcosis that will continue through the immediate postoperative period. Opioids are all metabolized by the liver and the metabolites are excreted through the kidneys. Table 1.13 characterizes the opioid receptors and identifies their commonly used agonists and antagonists. The opioids used intravenously in the operating room, their relative potencies, onset times, and their elimination half-times are summarized in Table 1.14.

The CNS effects of opioids include analgesia, euphoria, drowsiness, miosis, depression of the cough reflex, nausea, and vomiting. The analgesia is caused by a reduction in transmission of noxious stimuli at both spinal and central levels, and perhaps in peripheral nerves as well. The nausea and vomiting originate from stimulation of both the vestibular system and the central chemoreceptor trigger zone in the medulla. High doses of opioids cause drowsiness and sedation, but since they do not reliably cause unconsciousness, anesthesia must include other agents.

Cardiovascular effects include bradycardia that is caused by stimulation of vagal nuclei in the medulla and easily treated with atropine. Meperidine may cause tachycardia in large i.v. doses, presumably because its chemical structure is similar to that of atropine. Only meperidine causes myocardial depression in clinically useful doses, which can be as low as 2–2.5 mg/kg. Morphine and meperidine stimulate the release of histamine in clinical doses, resulting in arteriolar and venous dilation and hypotension. Because fentanyl, sufentanil, and alfentanil do not show this effect, they are the narcotics most frequently used in high doses during anesthesia.

All opioid agonists produce a dose-dependent respiratory depression, causing an equivalent right shift of the CO_2 response curve without altering its slope. Lower doses decrease the respiratory rate without changing the tidal volume, but at higher doses the tidal volume is also smaller. Pontine and medullary centers are depressed at still higher doses, and breathing becomes irregular with eventual apnea ensuing in the unstimulated patient.

Contrary to previous belief, opioids alone do not affect renal function or antidiuretic hormone (ADH) secretion. Their effects on the liver are limited to contraction of the sphincter of Oddi and rise in pressure in the biliary tree. Opioids decrease the motility of the gastrointestinal tract, causing ileus, delayed gastric emptying, and constipation.

All agonists can cause skeletal muscle rigidity when given in high i.v. doses, but only fentanyl, sufentanil, and alfentanil are given in sufficiently large boluses for this to be clinically significant. There is large individual variation in this effect; it has been reported with doses as small as 1 μg/kg fentanyl. Rigidity is not caused by an action at the neuromuscular junction but rather by a central effect. Nonetheless, sometimes a patient who has developed truncal rigidity after i.v. narcotics cannot

Table 1.13.
Opioid Receptors, Agonists, and Antagonists

Receptor	Actions	Agonists	Partial Agonist/Antagonist		Antagonists
μ	Supraspinal analgesia Respiratory depression Euphoria Physical dependence	All morphine-like drugs	3/1 2–3/2 1/3	Buprenorphine (Buprenex) Butorphanol (Stadol) Pentazocine (Talwin) Nalbuphine (Nubain) Levallorphan (Lorphan) Nalorphine (Nalline)	Nalorphine Naloxone
κ	Spinal analgesia Respiratory depression	All morphine-like drugs Nalorphine (partial) Butorphanol Nalbuphine Pentazocine			Naloxone
Σ	Dysphoria Hallucinations Vasomotor stimulation	Nalorphine Butorphanol Nalbuphine			Naloxone

Table 1.14.
Opioids Used Intravenously During Anesthesia

Drug	Relative Potency	Time to Peak Effect[a] (min)	Duration of Action	Elimination Half-Life (hr)
Morphine	1	10	Long	2.9
Meperidine	0.1	10	Intermediate	4.2
Methadone	1	30	Long	35
Fentanyl	100	5	Intermediate	3.7
Sufentanyl	500–1000	2–5	Intermediate	2.7
Alfentanyl	25	1–2	Short	1.5

[a]When given intravenously.

be ventilated until a muscle relaxant has been administered. Muscle rigidity is rarely seen when opioids are given after an inhalation anesthetic has been started.

In general, the narcotics used in the perioperative period are safe. The most common problems are respiratory depression and resultant hypoxemia. Hypotension is encountered mainly with morphine because of its histamine-releasing effects, or in severely hypovolemic patients. There is no evidence of teratogenicity, organ toxicity, or other delayed effects. Overdose is easily reversed with antagonists, although these drugs have serious side effects of their own (see below). Allergic reactions are rare, and usually result in urticaria rather than in anaphylactoid reactions. Because of their ability to stimulate histamine release, morphine and meperidine may cause local wheal and flare formation at and near the site of injection.

Narcotic Antagonists. Naloxone and naltrexone are competitive antagonists at the μ, κ, and Σ receptors, for all opioid effects including analgesia. Naltrexone, a long-acting antagonist used only in an oral preparation, has no use in the perioperative period. Naloxone is used to reverse narcotic-induced ventilatory depression and sedation in the immediate postoperative period, and for unwanted side effects of epidural, subarachnoid, or continuous-infusion narcotics. Unfortunately, doses that rapidly reverse ventilatory depression may result in such rapid onset of pain that the accompanying sympathetic stimulation causes tachycardia, hypertension, and CNS excitement. Doses of 0.1–0.4 mg naloxone have been associated with atrial and ventricular dysrhythmia, pulmonary edema, cardiac arrest, and convulsions. In order to balance the desired effect of analgesia with the undesirable effect of respiratory depression, ventilation should be supported while reversal is titrated with small incremental doses of naloxone, so that a balance can be achieved between analgesia and acceptable respiration. The best course is to tailor the administration of narcotic so that patients do not develop respiratory depression in the first place.

Monitoring the Anesthetized Patient

Continuous assessment of the surgical patient's physiological function is essential to maintain homeostasis and to return the patient to the preanesthetic state. The anesthesiologist monitors the patient's oxygenation, level of consciousness, ventilation, circulation, and body temperature. Other monitors may also be necessary, depending on the patient and the surgical procedure. Table 1.15 summarizes monitors used in the operating room.

Table 1.15.
Intraoperative Monitors of the Body Systems

Cardiovascular System	Blood pressure
	Pulse palpation
	Auscultation
	Oscillometry
	Doppler
	Automated sphygmomanometers
	Intra-arterial measurement
	Cardiac rhythm and rate
	Auscultation
	Lead II ECG
	Pulse palpation
	Pulse oximetry
	Myocardial perfusion
	Lead V ECG
	Pressure wave form
	ST segment trending
	Transesophageal echocardiography
	Peripheral perfusion
	Pulse palpation
	Pulse oximetry
	Arterial blood gases
Respiratory System	Observation and auscultation
	Inspired pressure gauge
	Spirometry
	Pneumotachograph
	Oxygenation
	Observation
	Pulse oximetry
	Transcutaneous oxygen analysis
	Mass spectrometry
	Arterial blood gases
	Carbon dioxide excretion
	Capnography
	Mass spectrometry
	Transcutaneous CO_2 analyzers
	Arterial blood gases
Central Nervous System	Observation
	Eye signs
	Respiration and heart rate
	Intracranial pressure monitoring
	EEG, evoked potentials
Renal Function	Urine output
	Electrolytes
Metabolic System	Body temperature
	Blood glucose
	Electrolytes
	Arterial blood gases
Circulating Volume	Blood pressure
	Pulse characteristics
	Right and left ventricular filling pressures
	Urine output
	Arterial blood gases
	Electrolytes and hematocrit
Coagulation	Observation
	Laboratory tests
Integumentary and Neuromuscular System	Direct observation of position and padding
	Nerve stimulator

Basic Intraoperative Monitoring. Basic intraoperative monitoring for patients under the care of the anesthesiologist is described in standards published by the American Society of Anesthesiologists (Table 1.16). Certain states and insurance carriers also require basic monitoring.

Oxygenation. In order to prevent administration of a hypoxic gas mixture, the concentration of oxygen in the inspired gas is measured by an oxygen analyzer. Several devices are available; most measure oxygen content by an electrochemical process in which a current is produced that is proportional to the partial pressure of oxygen. These sensors, requiring frequent calibration, are attached to the anesthesia machine directly in line with the patient's inspired or expired gases in the breathing circuit, which connects the anesthesia machine to the patient. Among the sensors is an audible alarm, which is set to the desired minimum concentration, usually 30%, before anesthetic delivery is begun.

Adequate oxygen content in the patient's blood is a major concern during administration of an anesthetic. Several methods are available to evaluate oxygenation. The color of the patient's skin and of blood in the surgical field are the simplest and most direct monitors. Although the least quantitative, they should be evaluated continuously. Cyanosis usually is apparent when the concentration of deoxygenated hemoglobin reaches 5 g/dL. This assessment of color requires that the operating room be adequately illuminated and that a portion of the patient be exposed and available for observation. Skin color observation may be unreliable in dark-skinned or anemic patients, but blood can usually be evaluated in the surgical field.

The development of the pulse oximeter has greatly improved the adequacy and accuracy of patient monitoring. Pulse oximeters measure changes in the ratio of bright red, oxygenated hemoglobin to darker, deoxygenated hemoglobin, and display this ratio as percentage of oxygen saturation. To accomplish this, two different wave forms of light are projected through a translucent portion of tissue, such as fingertip or earlobe, to a detection cell on the other side. One frequency of light is absorbed by oxygenated hemoglobin, and the other by both oxygenated and deoxygenated hemoglobin. As hemoglobin enters the tissue with arterial pulsation, more light is absorbed. Microelectronics interpret the change in light absorption as a pulse, and, using the ratio of absorption of the two light waves, calculate the percentage of oxygen saturation in hemoglobin entering the tissue. The anesthesiologist is provided with a pulse-to-pulse update of the adequacy of oxygenation as well as with a monitor of tissue perfusion.

Less common is the transcutaneous oxygen analyzer, which measures oxygen partial pressure through the skin with an electrode that arterializes the underlying capillary blood with heat. Unlike the pulse oximeter, this device requires frequent change in position to avoid burning the underlying skin, as well as frequent recalibration. It becomes unreliable when skin perfusion decreases. If it were easier to use and more reliable, it would be advantageous because it measures partial pressure of oxygen rather than hemoglobin saturation, and so gives a more quantitative evaluation of

Table 1.16.
Standards for Basic Intraoperative Monitoring

1. Qualified anesthesia personnel present at all times	
2. Continual evaluation of the patient's oxygenation, ventilation, circulation and temperature	
Oxygenation	Inspired oxygen concentration
	Pulse oximetry
	Skin color
Ventilation	Observation, auscultation
	Capnography (CO_2 content of expired air) to verify endotracheal tube placement and strongly urged throughout anesthetic
	Spirometry
	Disconnect alarm when ventilator used
Circulation	ECG
	Blood Pressure
	Heart Rate
	Peripheral Perfusion: palpation of pulse, heart auscultation, pulse oximetry, plethysmography, or intra-arterial pressure tracing
Temperature	A means of evaluation should be readily available

oxygenation. It also provides a more sensitive evaluation of tissue microperfusion.

Arterial blood may also be sampled for blood gas analysis. This invasive technique is made easier by inserting an indwelling arterial cannula. Blood gas analysis is frequently used to check the accuracy of other monitors, as well as to assess acid-base and electrolyte status and hematocrit.

Ventilation. Adequacy of ventilation must be monitored continually throughout an anesthetic administration. Several direct methods are available, the most direct being observation of chest excursion and change in volume in the reservoir bag of the breathing circuit during respiration. There is no substitute for auscultation of breath sounds, however, in evaluating respiratory status. A precordial stethoscope is a heavily weighted bell placed over the precordium or sternal notch during anesthesia. When the trachea is intubated, an esophageal stethoscope can be substituted. This instrument is a plastic tube with a soft balloon at the end, and it is placed directly into the esophagus. The anesthesiologist usually listens through a monaural ear piece, allowing him to simultaneously hear ventilation and communicate with operating room personnel.

More quantitative monitors of ventilation are also employed. The best monitor of ventilatory adequacy is arterial blood gas analysis, and this technique is also frequently used to assess the accuracy of the other monitors. Many operating room electrocardiogram (ECG) monitors are able to provide a pneumotachogram, which is a respiratory trace of both chest motion and respiratory rate. A spirometer attached to the expiratory limb of the breathing circuit gives a breath-to-breath record of expired volume. The best constant monitor of adequate ventilation is the expired CO_2 pressure ($P_{E}CO_2$), which is determined by a capnograph or a mass spectrometer. Unless there is a large ventilation-perfusion abnormality, the end expired CO_2, which reflects the alveolar CO_2 concentration, is very close to the arterial CO_2 concentration. Expired gas is monitored at the patient's endotracheal tube with a small infrared device or at the monitoring unit after a small quantity of expired gas has been aspirated through a small catheter in the breathing circuit. Usually the monitor provides a plot of CO_2 partial pressure against time, displayed as a capnogram, and allows the anesthesiologist to assess the pattern of respiration. A slow rise in exhaled CO_2 pressure indicates obstructive airway dysfunction that may be caused by chronic disease, acute bronchospasm, or tube kinking. If the curve does not return to zero during inspiration, there is CO_2 in the inspired gas. A sudden drop in expired CO_2 may be caused by acute pulmonary embolism with air, blood clot or other substance, or an acute drop in cardiac output resulting in failure of pulmonary perfusion and CO_2 excretion. Also available are transcutaneous CO_2 analyzers, which measure the partial pressure of CO_2 in arterialized capillary blood. Like transcutaneous oxygen analyzers, they are not currently reliable or simple enough to have achieved much popularity.

Correct placement of the endotracheal tube must be verified after every intubation: undetected esophageal placement results in hypoxemia in apneic patients and is rapidly fatal. Evaluation of chest excursion and breath sounds occasionally are misleading. A normal capnogram is the strongest evidence that the tube is in the trachea. Endobronchial placement can be reliably detected by noting a large, otherwise unexplained difference in the partial pressure of oxygen between alveolar (inspired) and arterial measurements ($P_{A}O_2 - P_{a}O_2$), or by noting diminished breath sounds in one hemithorax compared to the other while auscultating the lateral chest walls. The only absolutely foolproof method of confirming proper endotracheal tube placement is by direct observation of the carina through a fiberoptic bronchoscope inserted through the endotracheal tube past the tip.

During general anesthesia, the patient's ventilation is often controlled by a mechanical ventilator. Disconnection of the ventilator from the breathing circuit will be fatal if the patient is paralyzed, hypocapnic, or is apneic because of anesthetic respiratory depressant effects. The anesthesia machine must be equipped with a low pressure alarm in the breathing circuit that will activate if positive pressure is not sensed within a certain period of time. Many machines also have a high pressure sensing system that sounds or automatically relieves pressure if a preset pressure is exceeded during the ventilatory cycle, as might happen when the endotracheal tube becomes obstructed by kinking or a mucus plug, or if the patient's lung compliance suddenly decreased markedly because of tension pneumothorax.

Circulation. Without instrumentation, circulation can be measured continuously by listening to the heart and palpating a peripheral pulse. The speed of pulse upstroke provides a qualitative assessment of the force of myocardial contraction and of the cardiac output. The volume of heart sounds provides the same information. Changes in rhythm also are evident using these methods.

The ECG, a required operating room monitor, is used to evaluate heart rate and rhythm as well as to indicate myocardial oxygenation. Modern ECG monitors provide a four- or five-lead system with one or two standard leads continuously monitored on a cathode ray tube. Most have extensive filtering systems to reduce interference by other electrical equipment in the operating room. Many are able to store tracings so that comparisons can be made when change occurs or a hard copy is needed for later analysis. An audible heart sound is provided and QRS complexes counted to provide an averaged heart rate (displayed on the screen). Lead II is most often used for rhythm analysis because the P wave is most evident in that lead. If ischemic episodes are of concern, Lead V5 is preferred because it monitors the anterolateral wall of the left ventricle where most ischemic episodes occur. If the area of the ventricle at risk is known preoperatively, a five-lead system allows the anesthesiologist to choose which area to monitor for ST segment changes. Continuous simultaneous monitoring of Leads II and V5 detects approximately 75% of intraoperative myocardial ischemic events. Computer software is available in many ECG monitors to provide an analysis of ST segment depression or elevation, and is more accurate than the anesthesiologist's observational skills in detecting incipient events.

Various instruments are available to monitor peripheral circulation continuously. The most commonly used is the pulse oximeter discussed previously. Doppler pulse monitors placed directly over a peripheral pulse are also used. They detect changes in sound wave transmission of arterial pulsation and are monitored by an audible sound. Pulse plethysmography measures changes in light absorption in the tissue as blood volume changes with arterial pulsation. It is similar to the pulse oximeter but lacks the added second light wave needed to calculate oxygen saturation.

Systemic blood pressure must be assessed at least every 5 minutes and, along with the heart rate, recorded on the anesthesia record in graphic form. The 5-minute standard is generally accepted as the minimum interval to permit detection of trends early enough to allow successful intervention. The standard method of determining blood pressure uses a cuff over the brachial artery (although other peripheral arteries are occasionally used), an aneroid manometer, and a stethoscope affixed over the artery. Oscillometry can produce reliable measurement, but error in diastolic pressure is more likely. A finger on the pulse, a Doppler probe, or a plethysmograph can be placed distal to the cuff to detect systolic blood pressure, but, again, determining diastolic pressure is difficult without a stethoscope. Whatever the detection technique, in order for a sphygmomanometer to function accurately and reliably, the full cuff pressure must be transmitted to the artery beneath it. Ideally the cuff should be 20% wider than the diameter of the limb on which it is positioned: if too narrow, an artificially high pressure will be obtained, and if too wide, the pressure will be underestimated. The inflatable rubber bladder within the cuff should just encircle the limb without overlapping and be no shorter than half the limb circumference.

Several automated noninvasive blood pressure monitors are available and have almost replaced the manual devices in the operating and recovery rooms. These devices use either a Doppler or oscillometric technique and display the systolic, diastolic, and mean pressures. They can also display the heart rate at an interval set by the user, which can be as frequent as 1 minute. Most are equipped with audible alarms for high or low values, and for changes from the previously determined values. These automated monitors are more accurate than manual techniques and function reliably even when the patient is profoundly hypotensive. They are valuable also because they free the anesthesiologist to perform other functions while they perform blood pressure determinations during busy or critical times.

Temperature. During surgery and anesthesia, a patient can lose a significant amount of body heat and become hypothermic. Severe hypothermia results in hemodynamic compromise, cardiac irritability, metabolic change, decreased coagulation, and postoperative shivering with a corresponding increase in oxygen consumption. Almost all patients lose some body heat, but infants and geriatric patients are particularly at risk. An intraoperative rise in temperature is much less frequent, but must be detected early and treated because of the metabolic consequences, such as marked increase in oxygen consumption and carbon dioxide production. Malignant hyperthermia is a rare hypermetabolic response to anesthesia and surgery that results in profound morbidity and frequent death. It is best detected by continuous temperature monitoring, although temperature rise is sometimes only a late manifestation of the syndrome, following earlier signs of tachycardia, hypertension, and increased CO_2 production.

Because these conditions must be treated early, continuous temperature monitoring is desirable in the operating room. The most common method in the intubated patient is with an esophageal temperature probe, which may be incorporated into the esophageal stethoscope. Temperature probes can also be inserted in the rectum, the nasopharynx, the axilla, or in the external auditory canal near the tympanic membrane. Skin patches, usually placed on the forehead, are available with a continuous digital display using liquid crystal thermography. While they are useful for determining trends, they are not as accurate as probes placed nearer the core.

The Anesthesiologist. In spite of sophisticated technology, the anesthesiologist remains the principal monitor and should be present and alert at all times. The anesthesiologist should also keep an accurate, timely, and inclusive record of all of the events in the operating room; that record should become a part of the patient's permanent medical record. The anesthesia record should include information regarding positioning and padding, anesthetic technique, monitors employed and information gathered from them, drugs and doses, fluids administered including blood products, airway maintenance techniques, and all events related to the surgery. Vital signs and other physiologic data should be recorded graphically at 5-minute intervals. This record is useful in determining trends during the course of the anesthetic, and provides invaluable information for postoperative care of the patient.

Figure 1.5 shows a typical anesthesia record generated during an uncomplicated surgical procedure. All drugs administered are noted, with the anesthetic agents (other than induction agents) listed on top of the graph and doses or concentrations noted at the appropriate times. Vital signs recorded at 5-minute intervals are noted as symbols that are explained in the left margin. Running totals of blood loss, fluid administration, and urine output are noted on the bottom, as are ventilation parameters. The commentary at the bottom explains induction and emergence, with symbols noted as explained in the left margin. In the Position and Remarks area there is documentation of the patient's condition on arrival in the postanesthesia care unit.

Additional and Optional Monitors

Neuromuscular Blockade. Neuromuscular-blocking drugs are often administered during general anesthesia to provide relaxation essential for the surgery, to facilitate controlled ventilation, or to provide optimal conditions without the cardiovascular depression associated with deep anesthesia. Monitoring the extent of the blockade helps determine subsequent doses, adequacy of reversal, and criteria for extubation at the end of the procedure. The extent of blockade can be estimated without the use of instrumentation. Observation of the surgical field gives an indication of how well the muscles are relaxed. During abdominal surgery the contents of the peritoneal cavity are extruded through the incision when abdominal wall tone is high, and the surgeon has difficulty approximating the wound edges at closure. Increased tone of abdominal and respiratory muscles is evident as decreased compliance (increased inspiratory pressure) during controlled ventilation. The recovery from blockade can be estimated by respiratory tidal volume, vital capacity, and negative inspiratory force. In the conscious patient, the strength of the hand grip and the ability to hold the head off the table for at least 5 seconds indicate adequate return of muscle function.

The extent of neuromuscular function can be measured using a nerve stimulator to deliver a small electrical stimulus to skin electrodes placed over a motor nerve (usually ulnar) and observing the response (flexion of the fourth and fifth digits). If the arm is not accessible, the forehead or foot can be used. The train-of-four stimulus pattern is usually chosen, because it is most sensitive to varying levels of blockade with a nondepolarizing relaxant (see Table 1.7). Other parameters monitored include the single twitch response at a rate of one per 1, 5, or 10 seconds and the response to tetanic stimulation at a rate of 50–200 Hz.

Respiratory Gases. In addition to capnography and an oxygen analyzer in the circuit, other methods may be used to monitor respiratory gases. The mass spectrometer is used to sample and analyze both inspired and expired gases, and to measure the content of oxygen, carbon dioxide, nitrogen, and each of the inhaled anesthetics. A small sample of the respiratory gas is withdrawn into a vacuum chamber through a catheter placed at the junction of the patient's endotracheal tube and the breathing circuit. The sample is then analyzed by ion or infrared detection. Most instruments provide a numerical display of inspired partial pressures or percent concentrations, as well as a continuous capnogram or graphical display of other gas concentrations. Because nitrogen and the inhaled anesthetics are also analyzed, mass spectrometry provides more information about the anesthetic state and general status of the patient than do individual oxygen and carbon dioxide analyzers.

Urine Output. To avoid overdistension of the bladder during long surgeries and to provide a monitor of renal function, Foley catheters are often positioned in the bladder prior to surgery. Frequently measured urine output is a good indicator of blood volume and renal and perfusion function. Intraoperative oliguria may be the result of decreased renal perfusion because of blood volume depletion, circulatory failure, the antidiuretic effects of anesthetics or other drugs, or the hormonal response to stress. It can also be caused by mechanical obstruction of the ureters or of the catheter itself.

The quality of the urine is also a good monitor of the physiological status of the patient. The specific gravity can often be easily estimated from changes in color of the urine, giving a good indication of renal perfusion. If the urine becomes reddish, a microscopic exam and quick dipstick test will tell if there is blood, hemoglobin, or myoglobin in the urine. Blood indicates trauma to the kidneys, ureters, or bladder. Hemoglobin or myoglobin indicates a serious systemic problem that may easily result in renal or other end-organ damage. The cause should be found and treatment instituted immediately. Electrolyte and glucose content of the urine provides valuable information about the volume status and renal concentrating ability. The benefits of continuous urine output monitoring must be weighed against

FORM 71.16-402-2B

THE UNIVERSITY OF CHICAGO HOSPITALS

ANESTHESIA RECORD

OPERATING ROOM # 1D — MACHINE # 47

Name ——— Sex M Age 24 Date 2/15 1990
Unit No. ——— Location ——— Surgeons ———

Diagnosis preop. R INGUINAL HERNIA, HYDROCOELE
postop. Same
Operation proposed REPAIR HERNIA, HYDROCOELE
performed Same
Wt. 75 kg. BP 120-130/60-80 P 62-70 R 14 T 37 °C. Hgb. 15 Hct. 45 Allergies: ō
Resp. Circ. ō
G.I. G.U. ō
N.M. Metab. ō Physical Status: I
Anesthetic history PREVIOUS GA s̄ problems Pre-anes. visit by: ———
Premedication NONE Time M. Result

MONITORS: ECG, BP, Precordial Steth, Esoph. TEMP, Pulse Ox, Capnograph, Foley, Nerve Stim., FeO2

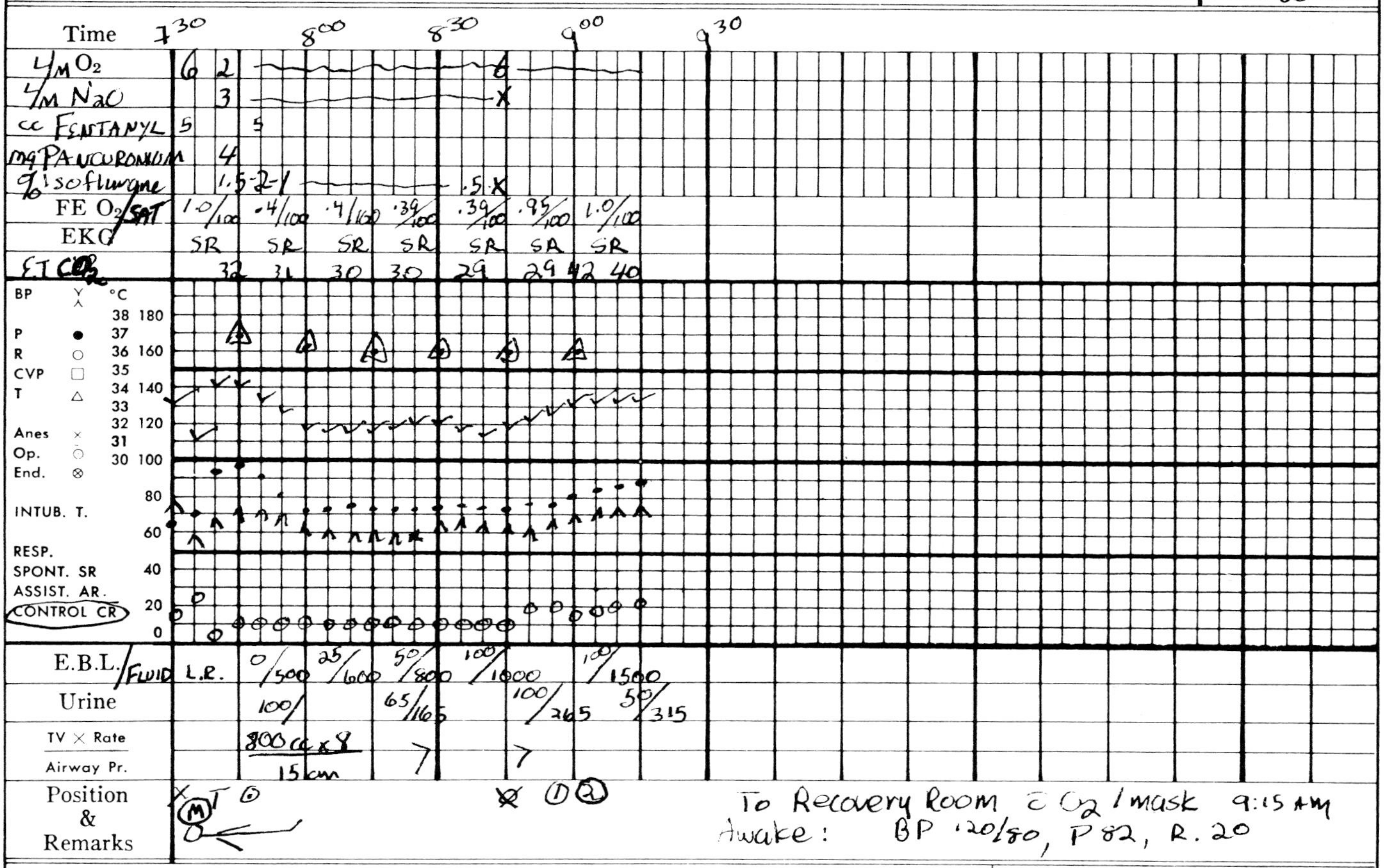

Time	7:30	8:00	8:30	9:00	9:30
L/M O_2	6, 2			6	
L/M N_2O	3			X	
cc FENTANYL	5, 5				
mg PANCURONIUM	4				
% isoflurane	1.5, 2, 1		.5 X		
FE O_2/SAT	1.0/100, .4/100	.4/100, .39/100	.39/100, .95/100	1.0/100	
EKG	SR, SR	SR, SR	SR, SA	SR	
ET CO_2	32, 31	30, 30	29, 29	42, 40	

BP ∨ ∧ / °C; P ●; R ○; CVP □; T △; Anes ×; Op. ○; End. ⊗; INTUB. T.; RESP. SPONT. SR; ASSIST. AR.; CONTROL CR
Scale: 38 180; 37; 36 160; 35; 34 140; 33; 32 120; 31; 30 100; 80; 60; 40; 20; 0

E.B.L./FLUID L.R.	0/500	25/600, 50/800	100/1000	100/1500	
Urine	100/	65/165	100/265	50/315	
TV × Rate	800 cc × 8	7	7		
Airway Pr.	15 cm				

Position & Remarks: ⓜ T ⓘ ⊗ ① ② To Recovery Room c̄ O_2/mask 9:15 AM. Awake: BP 120/80, P 82, R. 20

Remarks: Patient brought to OR, Monitors Applied. Preoxygenated. 7[40] Induction with Pentothal 300 mg, Succinylcholine 80 mg. (T) Trachea intubated with 8mm cuffed oral endotracheal tube using MAC 3, direct vision, atraumatic. Cuff inflated. Bilateral Breath Sounds. Taped at 22cm, Eyes protected.
① Neostigmine 2.5 mg + Robinul 0.6 mg
② suctioned + Extubated.
Noteworthy Events NONE
Agents: Primary ISOFLURANE Others N_2O, FENTANYL
Method Mech. Vent, SEMI-CLOSED Endotracheal 8 mm Relaxants Succ/PANC
Medications M. METHICILLIN 1gm IV 7:40
Total Fluids: 1500 cc LR
Anesthesiologists ———

BLOOD GASES	
TIME	NONE
FEO_2	
pH	
PCO_2	
PO_2	
HCO_3	
BE	
SAT	
Hg	
Hct	

Figure 1.5. The anesthesia record completed. Note the graphic representation of vital signs; indication of drugs and dosages as they are administered; documentation of P_ECO_2 and F_EO_2 concentrations; and running totals of fluids administered, blood loss, and urine output.

the risks. Catheterization provides the potential for trauma to the bladder and urethra and introduces another source of infection for the surgical patient.

Specialized and Intensive Monitoring

Invasive Hemodynamic Pressure Monitoring. Occasionally the patient's preexisting medical condition or the nature of the surgery requires that highly specialized and invasive monitoring be employed. Because of their potential complications, invasive monitors are reserved for situations in which conventional monitors do not provide adequate information. They are used for moment-to-moment control of patients at high risk for cardiovascular decompensation, in open-heart, major vascular, or intracranial surgery, and in procedures in which a large or rapid blood loss is anticipated.

Intra-arterial blood pressure monitoring provides beat-to-beat analysis of blood pressure and pulse characteristics. The tracing gives a good indication of the volume of each pulse and may help the observer draw conclusions about cardiac output and circulating volume as well as the effect of dysrhythmias. It is particularly useful when rapid pressure changes are expected and measurement needs to be taken more frequently than once a minute (the fastest cycle of the automated, noninvasive monitors). An indwelling cannula is inserted into a peripheral artery (usually the radial) and connected to a pressure transducer through noncompliant, small-bore tubing. The tubing is filled with heparinized saline and connected to a continual flushing system that provides a slow infusion of the heparinized solution to prevent clotting of the catheter or artery. Since the fluid in the tubing is noncompressible and the tubing itself noncompliant, the pressure exerted on the fluid column at the tip of the cannula is accurately transmitted to the the transducer. A wave form is generated by each arterial pulsation, and the systolic (peak), diastolic (nadir), and mean pressure digitally displayed. The cannula also provides ready access for blood sampling, making intraoperative determinations of arterial gases, pH, glucose, electrolytes, hematocrit, and other blood tests more convenient.

Transducers require special care, calibration, and "zeroing" in order to provide a valid pressure measurement. After the stopcock at the top of the transducer is opened to air, the transducer is positioned at the level of the patient's heart, and the electronics are adjusted to read zero. All pressure measurements must be made with the transducer at this reference level. Air bubbles in the tubing or transducer will "damp" the tracing and provide inaccurate readings.

Intra-arterial monitoring is not without complications. Clot can accumulate on the cannula tip, leading to thrombosis of the vessel, embolization, and even gangrene of the extremity. The frequency of this complication is minimized by the use of heparin flush, small cannulas, and limited duration of cannulation. When cannulation of the radial artery is anticipated, the patency of cross circulation from the ulnar artery is often assessed. This is done by a modified Allen test: after both the radial and ulnar arteries are occluded with the thumbs, the patient opens and closes the fist several times to blanch the hand. The hand is observed for flushing after the ulnar artery is released, but the radial still occluded. If the entire hand does not flush, the ulnar artery is not completely patent and the radial artery should not be cannulated since its potential obstruction might cause hand ischemia. Recent literature questions the efficacy of the Allen test in predicting whether distal ischemia may follow radial artery cannulation, but it is still frequently performed.

When large changes in intravascular fluid volume are expected, fluid replacement is more easily managed by monitoring the *central venous pressure* (CVP). CVP is the hydrostatic pressure exerted by the blood in the right atrium, and is an indirect measure of the amount of blood filling the right ventricle. In the normally functioning heart, the pressure required to fill the left ventricle is 4–5 torr higher than that for the right ventricle. While lower than the left heart filling pressures, the CVP still varies directly with these pressures. When blood volume is diminished or venous capacitance increased, less blood returns to the heart from the periphery, the ventricle is less well filled, and the CVP correspondingly low. Increased circulating blood volume or peripheral vasoconstriction will increase CVP. However, poor ventricular contraction or an impedance to ventricular outflow because of lung pathology will result in elevated CVP even with normal or diminished blood circulating volume.

Measuring CVP requires insertion (via internal or external jugular, subclavian, or cephalic vein) of a fluid-filled cannula into the right atrium or superior vena cava just above the atrium. The cannula may be connected to a water manometer or to a pressure transducer in a manner similar to that of the indwelling arterial cannula. Since intrathoracic pressures resulting from respiration are transmitted to the heart, measurements are taken at the end of expiration. The wave form generated with a transducer-monitoring system also provides information about atrial contraction and intracardiac valve function.

As mentioned above, when left heart failure occurs, or if there is valvular dysfunction, the CVP is not an adequate measure of circulating blood volume. In this situation a *pulmonary arterial catheter*, the Swan-Ganz, provides more accurate determinations of left heart filling pressures. The Swan-Ganz catheter is a long, multilumen catheter with an inflatable balloon on the tip. The catheter is inserted through an access sheath placed in the external or internal jugular or subclavian vein. When it has been threaded into the superior vena cava, the balloon is inflated with a small amount of air and the catheter advanced through the right heart into the pulmonary artery. The pressure wave from the distal port of the catheter is monitored throughout the entire time the catheter is being threaded into the pulmonary artery. The balloon allows the catheter to flow more easily through the heart along with the flow of blood. As the catheter is advanced within the pulmonary artery, the diameter of the vessels decreases and the balloon eventually becomes "wedged." In this position, if there is no abnormality in the pulmonary vasculature distal to the balloon, the pressure sensed at the tip of the catheter reflects that of the left atrium. This pressure is called the *pulmonary capillary occlusion pressure* (PCOP), the *pulmonary artery occlusion pressure* (PAOP) or, more commonly, the *wedge pressure*. During surgery and anesthesia, it is the changes in pulmonary artery pressures, wedge pressures, and cardiac output that provide the best information, allowing the anesthesiologist to optimize the patient's circulation with a combination of fluid administration, inotropic agents, and manipulations of peripheral resistance. Using right atrial pressure as a monitor of circulating volume is perfectly adequate in patients whose myocardial and valvular function is good, since differences in right and left heart outputs are not usually encountered. The pressure tracings displayed on the monitor are characteristic for each step of insertion and allow one to determine exactly when the catheter tip enters the right atrium, right ventricle, pulmonary artery, and the wedged position. When the catheter is correctly placed, deflating the balloon results in a normal pulmonary arterial pressure tracing while reinflating it brings the tracing back to the wedge configuration. Wedge pressures should be obtained only intermittently, with the balloon remaining deflated at all other times to prevent ischemia of the distal lung or trauma to the vessel wall.

In the absence of pulmonary arterial disease or pulmonary hypertension, the pulmonary arterial diastolic pressure (PADP) reflects the wedge and thus the left atrial pressure and can be used as a continuous monitor of left ventricular filling. The Swan-Ganz catheter also has a proximal port located in the right atrium, allowing right atrial pressures to be monitored continuously and its pressure wave displayed. This catheter also provides the user with the ability to measure cardiac output by the thermodilution technique. A measured amount of iced or room temperature saline is injected through the right atrial port while a thermistor sensor tip senses changes occurring in blood temperature. A portable computer connected to the catheter can then calculate the cardiac output as the integrated time versus temperature change curve, and provide a digital display.

Three additional services that may be provided by the pulmonary artery catheter are the continuous monitoring of blood temperature by the thermistor, the inclusion of a pacing port to allow a paced cardiac rhythm, and the ability to draw samples for measuring mixed venous oxygen saturation ($S\bar{V}O_2$). $S\bar{V}O_2$ provides the best available monitor of tissue perfusion and oxygen availability.

Pulmonary artery and right atrial pressure monitors are indispensable to anesthesiologists in many situations, but are not without their risks and complications. Insertion sites are another source of infection. Arrhythmias occur commonly when catheters or guide wires irritate the conduction system, and are very common with the insertion of pulmonary artery catheters. The risk of air embolism is always present when central catheters are in place, and thrombus formation is not uncommon. Pulmonary artery catheters have been reported to knot in the ventricle, even around chordae, and damage heart valves. Rupture of the pulmonary vessels has been reported, especially if the Swan-Ganz is advanced too far or one forgets to deflate the balloon. Finally, pneumothorax, hemothorax, or accidental carotid puncture occasionally occurs.

Transesophageal echocardiography (TEE) has been recently introduced into the operating room for detailed monitoring of volume status, valvular function, myocardial contractility, and early detection of myocardial ischemia. The probe is located at the tip of a gastroscope inserted through the patient's esophagus and is positioned behind the heart to provide a continuous picture of the heart displayed on a television monitor. Early ischemic events are often diagnosed by decreased contraction of affected segments of the left ventricular wall before ECG evidence becomes apparent. Volume status is easily assessed by the end-systolic diameter of the ventricle. With experience, the anesthesiologist can assess valvular efficiency and inotrophy. TEE is especially useful in diagnosing air or particulate matter entering the circulation.

Complications of TEE in the anesthetized patient are limited to trauma to the mouth or esophagus related to insertion of the gastroscope. The technology is expensive, but appears to be durable and very reliable in providing an accurate, comprehensive monitor of cardiac status.

Central Nervous System Monitoring. In patients with decreased intracranial compliance, further increases in *intracranial pressure* (ICP) can rapidly result in brainstem deformation and death. Since anesthetics and small changes in hemodynamic and ventilatory parameters can have profound effects on ICP, monitoring the pressure is often useful during anesthesia. This is accomplished by the neurosurgeon, who drills a small hole in the skull and inserts a cannula connected to a pressure transducer into one of the ventricles of the brain. Alternatively, a subdural or extradural transducer is implanted. A pressure tracing is displayed, and the mean pressure calculated and exhibited. The ventricular catheter has the advantage of allowing CSF to be withdrawn if necessary to reduce the pressure. Again, all of these methods are invasive and introduce the potential for infection.

Recently, the ability to monitor cerebral function by the *electroencephalogram* and its variations has been introduced into the operating room. The EEG is a complex wave generated by the electrical activity of the brain. The electrical potential is measured between small electrodes, either adhesive patches or needles that are applied to the scalp. The resulting voltage differences are displayed, allowing the user to compare the activities of the two hemispheres. Several different devices are available to process the EEG in various ways, the most common currently being the compressed spectral array (CSA). The CSA separates the EEG into component wave forms, and displays the information as a three-dimensional plot of frequency, amplitude, and time. EEG and processed EEG monitoring are most useful when a compromise of the cerebral circulation is anticipated, such as during cranial vascular surgery, carotid artery surgery, or cardiopulmonary bypass.

A more refined method of EEG monitoring measures the cortical response to sensory stimulation of a peripheral nerve. This is termed an *evoked potential response* and is obtained by applying repeated stimuli to a sensory nerve. The resulting cortical activity is averaged and displayed in a wave form that allows comparison of the latency and amplitude of the response over time. Alternatively, sections of the motor cortex may be stimulated and the peripheral motor response evaluated with a twitch recorder. A normal sensory or motor-evoked potential response is a good indication of normal transmission from peripheral nerve to brain. These monitors are most useful during spinal cord or vertebral column surgery, but can also be used to monitor cranial nerve and brainstem integrity when surgery places those structures at risk.

Intraoperative Fluid, Electrolyte, Blood, and Component Therapy

Venous Access. Intravenous catheters should be placed before the patient enters the operating room. Cannulation sites depend on the location of the surgical procedure and the patient's preexisting medical conditions (see EGS2, Chapter 5). Most anesthesiologists cannulate large veins on the dorsum of the nondominant hand or in the lower forearm with an 14–18 gauge plastic cannula. If significant blood loss is anticipated, several sites are cannulated with large-gauge catheters. Alternate sites include the cephalic or brachial veins, the external or internal jugular, the foot veins, or the subclavian veins. Cannulation of lower extremity veins in adults should be performed only as a last resort because of the possibility of superficial phlebitis. Femoral veins are used rarely, but reported complications are few if steps are taken to avoid infection. In infants, the scalp veins are often used, but these may be more fragile than those of the extremities. The only contraindication to any site is an infection in the area. Veins distal to an infected area should not be used nor should any distal to an arteriovenous fistula that has been established for hemodialysis. A distal intravenous infusion should not be started in patients who have had a lymph node dissection or surgery on vessels in the axilla because they may not have normal venous drainage from that arm. Before inducing anesthesia, the anesthesiologist must confirm that vascular access is adequate for rapid infusion of fluid, the cannula is firmly secured, and all connections are tight.

Fluid and Electrolyte Therapy. Intraoperative fluid therapy begins with an assessment of the volume status as the patient presents to the operating room. Despite recent evidence that a prolonged period of fasting is probably not necessary, most patients come to surgery having had no fluid intake for the previous 8–12 hours. Infants and small children will often have been administered clear liquids 4 hours before surgery. In both cases, at least part of that deficit is replaced with maintenance fluids. A preoperative "bowel prep," vomiting or nasogastric suction, fever, chronic or acute diuretic therapy, and chronic hypertension all contribute further to preoperative volume deficit. In most cases, some attempt at volume repletion should be made with a balanced isotonic solution (Ringer's lactate, normal saline, or Plasmalyte) before anesthesia is induced. Patients who are severely hypovolemic because of blood loss or bowel pathology demonstrate postural hypotension, even if they have been able to compensate by vasoconstriction. Generally, a normal heart rate and blood pressure indicate that circulating volume is adequate and that induction can proceed without undue concern about the vasodilation that follows administration of anesthetics. A detailed discussion of fluid and electrolyte therapy can be found in EGS2, Chapter 6. In normal adults, administration of glucose is not necessary and may even be detrimental. Whether infants need glucose is controversial, but the availability of rapid glucose determinations should allow the anesthesiologist to monitor glucose levels and plan fluid administration appropriately.

In replacing lost fluid and electrolytes, *preexisting conditions* and *insensible or unmeasurable losses* must be taken into account. Preexisting conditions such as inflammation, ascites, or pleural effusions continue intraoperatively. Insensible loss occurs through the respiratory tract, exposed surfaces (muscle, peritoneum, or pleura), perspiration, and the bowel. Several liters can be sequestered in the bowel if it is being traumatized or becomes ischemic. Respiratory insensible losses can be decreased by humidifying inspired gases and by using a low flow of gases so they are rebreathed after passing through the carbon dioxide absorber (a closed or semiclosed breathing circuit). Perspiration can be minimized by maintaining a normal body temperature and anesthesia deep enough to prevent sympathetic stimulation. Evaporation from exposed surfaces can be decreased somewhat by maintaining a lowered ambient temperature with high humidity.

Third space loss is that volume of fluid that enters the extravascular, extracellular space in response to the disease and the trauma of the surgical procedure. Formulas for fluid replacement during surgery take into account the site and nature of the procedure. For moderately traumatic surgery, such as that on the extremities or superficial structures, 2–5 mL/kg/hr are infused, and for more extensive surgery, requiring prolonged dissection and trauma to major organs, 5–10 mL/kg/hr are recommended. A balanced isotonic crystalloid solution most closely resembles the characteristics of fluid lost. Third space loss continues postoperatively, often for 2–3 days, and must be considered when calculating fluid requirements during this period. Unreplaced third space loss should be suspected when urine output and/or central pressures fall despite seemingly adequate volume infusions.

Colloid solutions such as albumin, hetastarch, and plasma may also be used to replace insensible and third space losses, but considerable controversy surrounds their use. They are expensive and expose the patient to the risk of infection if they have been prepared from donated blood. If crystalloid alone is used, the total volume infused can be 3–5 times greater than that of colloid. While most patients would not be harmed by a large, rapid fluid infusion, some patients could suffer cardiovascular, brain, or pulmonary consequences. Current recommendations are that colloid be considered to replace large, rapid fluid losses if (*a*) there is difficulty maintaining hemodynamic stability with crystalloid despite minimal external losses; (*b*) the risk of fluid deficit is high because of concomitant vasodilator therapy, preexisting cardiac or pulmonary pathology, or cerebral edema; (*c*) hemodynamic status cannot be monitored invasively; or (*d*) the colloid oncotic pressure is lower than 15 mm Hg. (See National Institutes of Health Consensus Conference: perioperative red cell transfusion. JAMA 1988;260(18):2700–2703).

Blood and Component Therapy. Surgical teams, including anesthesiologists, administer more than half the blood given to patients in the United States. Blood transfusions are given to maintain oxygen-carrying capacity when blood loss occurs. Unless blood loss is extensive, volume repletion is not an indication to transfuse, since volume repletion is adequately achieved with crystalloid and/or colloid solutions. Blood is usually replaced by component therapy: packed red blood cells are given to provide oxygen-carrying capacity, fresh frozen plasma is given to correct decreased levels of coagulation factors, and platelets are administered to correct low platelet concentrations or dysfunctioning platelets. Decisions about which components to transfuse would be much simpler if fresh whole blood were readily available, since fresh whole blood would replace exactly what is lost. Unfortunately, the tremendous cost and administrative difficulties of maintaining an adequate supply of such blood make the practice prohibitive. If packed cells are used to replace blood loss, they must be accompanied by crystalloid in a 3:1 ratio or by colloid in a 1:1 ratio to replenish the volume lost.

In determining when to transfuse, the major factor to consider is the lowest hemoglobin concentration or hematocrit that will maintain adequate tissue oxygenation in the patient. A 1988 National Institutes of Health consensus conference recommended that blood not be transfused when the hematocrit is 30% or higher, noting that patients with chronic anemia tolerate much lower levels without ill effect. The Food and Drug Administration recommended in 1989 that in patients with adequate circulating volume blood not be transfused until the hemoglobin falls below 7 g/dL. Patients with ischemic cardiovascular disease or pulmonary pathology precluding normal oxygen uptake need higher hemoglobin concentrations.

Despite the usual practice of transfusing fresh frozen plasma and platelets when 5–10 units of blood are given, it is recommended that these components not be given unless there is demonstrated clinical coagulopathy in the surgical field or laboratory tests prove a deficiency in coagulation factors of less than 50,000 platelets per high power field. It is evident from this brief discussion that the responsible practice of transfusion therapy requires a method of rapid assessment of hemoglobin, hematocrit, and coagulation function. Many operating rooms are equipped to provide these tests, and the recent appearance of small, hand-held prothrombin time (PT) and activated partial thromboplastin time (aPTT) analyzers has made the anesthesiologist's job much easier.

Complications. The major complications of blood or component administration include transfusion reactions, allergic reactions, electrolyte and acid-base abnormalities, dilutional coagulopathy, and infection. Major transfusion reactions are rare and usually due to errors in identifying patients. About 1 in 100 patients has an irregular antibody that should be detected in cross matching. The risk of an incompatible transfusion is 0.2% when ABO-Rh type specific blood is administered. The risk falls to 0.06% with an antibody screen and to 0.05% with a full cross match. A major hemolytic transfusion reaction (incidence 1:4000–1:6000) is diagnosed under anesthesia by sudden hypotension, hemoglobin in the urine, and a severe coagulopathy seen as uncontrollable bleeding in the surgical field and at sites of vascular cannulation. Treatment includes immediate discontinuation of the transfusion, hemodynamic support, maintenance of urine output by fluid administration and diuretic therapy, and administration of sodium bicarbonate to alkalinize the urine and prevent precipitation of acid hematin in the distal tubules of the kidney. If a coagulopathy is evident, it must be diagnosed accurately and treated appropriately, perhaps with the help of a hematologist.

Nonhemolytic transfusion reactions are febrile or allergic in nature and are caused by the presence of allergens or pyrogens in the transfused blood. Allergic reactions occur in about 3% of transfusions, rarely involving anaphylaxis. They are treated by antihistamines and fluid administration as needed. Anaphylactic shock requires intensive monitoring, hemodynamic support, epinephrine and steroid administration, and fluid replacement that may approach tens of liters in volume.

Banked blood preserved with citrate phosphate dextrose (CPD) undergoes significant chemical and hematologic changes that increase with the length of storage. Table 1.17 summarizes those changes, indicating the scope of electrolyte and acid-base abnormalities that must be compensated for when transfusing massive amounts. Most patients do not suffer biochemical effects from transfusion of up to 10 units of packed cells. Rapid electrolyte and blood gas determinations are available to detect any such effects. As can be seen from Table 1.17, there is a rapid decrease of platelet concentration and coagulation factors over time, increasing the risk of dilutional coagulopathy.

Infections currently attributed to transfusion of blood components include hepatitis, cytomegalovirus (CMV), and human immunodeficiency virus (HIV). Screening of donor blood eliminates most but not all of these, because of the long incubation period during which antigens or antibodies are not evident and because there are still hepatitis viruses that cannot be characterized as

Table 1.17.
Changes in CPD Blood with Storage

Test	Day of Storage			
	1	7	14	21
pH	7.1	7.0	7.0	6.9
PCO_2 (mm Hg)	48.0	80.0	110.0	140.0
Lactate (mEq/L)	41.0	101.0	145.0	179.0
Plasma bicarbonate (mEq/L)	18.0	15.0	12.0	11.0
Plasma potassium (mEq/L)	3.9	12.0	17.0	21.0
Plasma glucose (mg/100 mL)	345.0	312.0	181.0	231.0
Plasma hemoglobin (mg/100 mL)	1.7	7.8	13.0	19.0
Platelets (%)	10.0	0	0	0
Factors V and VII (%)	70.0	50.0	40.0	20.0

B or C. The risk of transfusion-associated hepatitis was estimated at 1:100 transfusions before the availability of a screening test for hepatitis C in 1990, and preliminary information indicates that much of that risk can be eliminated by screening for hepatitis C. In 1989, the risk of developing AIDS from a single transfusion was estimated as 1:40,000; further reductions are not anticipated soon. CMV is an almost normal flora in adults, causing no disease or symptoms. If transmitted to infants or immunocompromised patients, however, it can result in severe illness. Components transfused to this population are tested for CMV antibodies, thus eliminating most of the risk.

Retransfusion. From the preceding discussion, it is clear that exposure of the patient to transfusion of blood or blood products from other people must be minimized. The amount of donor blood transfused during most surgery can be markedly diminished by preoperative donation by the patient and by intraoperative and postoperative salvage and retransfusion of shed blood. Additionally, in most healthy patients acute intraoperative hemodilution can be safely tolerated and is accomplished by withdrawing one or two units of blood and replacing it with crystalloid or colloid solutions. At the end of the procedure, the patient's blood can be retransfused to bring hemoglobin levels back to normal.

Blood is salvaged intraoperatively and postoperatively by means of a suctioning apparatus that channels shed blood to a reservoir, where it is filtered and kept with heparinized saline until enough has been collected to warrant retransfusion. The blood is centrifuged and washed with saline, concentrated, and emptied into a transfusion bag. The result is a solution resembling packed red blood cells but with a hematocrit in the high 20s. Retransfusion of this blood has not been associated with major complications, as long as it is filtered on transfusion, although platelet counts may fall to <100,000 in the 2–3 days following surgery. Enough heparin is removed from the solution to prevent coagulopathy. Contraindications to intraoperative salvage include malignancies or infection in the surgical field.

Postoperative Recovery

Recovery from all but uncomplicated local anesthetics occurs in the PACU or recovery room under the supervision of specially trained nurses. An anesthesiologist and the surgeon are readily available to manage any complications that may occur. Immediate postoperative anesthetic problems include pulmonary and circulatory complications, renal dysfunction, bleeding abnormalities, hypothermia, pain, nausea, and vomiting.

Pulmonary Complications

Postoperative pulmonary problems are usually the result of the respiratory depressant effects of the inhaled or intravenous agents or of a residual neuromuscular blockade. Upper airway obstruction results from occlusion of the pharynx by the tongue or other soft tissue, and laryngeal obstruction occurs as a result of laryngospasm or injury. Laryngospasm is caused by irritation of the larynx and pharynx by secretions or upper airway manipulation. Signs of upper airway obstruction include flaring of the nares and suprasternal and intercostal retractions. Usually the obstruction is easily treated by neck extension and anterior displacement of the mandible. If these maneuvers are not successful, a nasopharyngeal or oropharyngeal airway should be inserted. If the obstruction still persists, positive pressure ventilation by mask or endotracheal tube may be necessary to prevent hypoventilation and hypoxemia.

Because cyanosis is a late symptom of decreasing oxygenation, most PACUs use pulse oximetry to detect early arterial desaturation. Besides airway obstruction and hypoventilation, reasons for hypoxemia in the recovery period include ventilation-perfusion abnormalities (atelectasis, remaining anesthetic effects), pulmonary vascular congestion and edema, and aspiration of gastric contents. Most patients demonstrate some degree of postoperative hypoxemia and benefit from supplemental oxygen therapy. To counteract the irritation induced by airway manipulation, the oxygen is usually heated and humidified. If the patient is to be discharged from the PACU without supplemental oxygen, pulse oximetry should be continued while the patient is breathing room air for at least 15 minutes.

Circulatory Complications

The most common circulatory complications in the immediate postanesthesia period include hypotension, hypertension, and cardiac arrhythmias. Hypovolemia is the most common cause of hypotension, usually because of either inadequate replacement of blood or "third space" loss that occurs as a result of surgery. Unrecognized postoperative hemorrhage is a serious complication that must remain foremost in the differential diagnosis of hypotension. If hypovolemia is the cause of hypotension, the treatment is fluid or blood resuscitation. Until the hypovolemia is corrected, elevation of the legs is helpful, and it may become necessary to provide pharmacological support with a pressor. Monitoring of volume status is the same in the recovery period as intraoperatively. Other complications include residual effects of anesthetics, acute myocardial ischemia or infarction, preexisting ventricular dysfunction, pulmonary embolus, and pneumothorax. If the hypotension is caused by myocardial dysfunction, it is helpful to follow pulmonary arterial and wedge pressures while treating it.

Hypertension in the postoperative period is often caused by pain, excitement, or delirium on emergence from anesthesia. If antihypertensive therapy has been withdrawn preoperatively, postoperative hypertension may be magnified. Volume overload, arterial hypoxemia, hypercarbia, acidosis, and hypothermia should also be suspected in the hypertensive patient. Treatment is based on the hypertension's etiology. When pain or excitement is the cause, hypertension should be treated only if it persists after adequate pain control has been achieved. If hypoxemia or hypercarbia is the cause, appropriate measures to restore adequate respiration and oxygenation should be instituted immediately. Volume, temperature, or acid-base status should be corrected as rapidly as possible. If pharmacologic therapy is instituted, there must be adequate monitoring of its effects.

Cardiac arrhythmias can be caused by hypoxemia, hypercarbia, electrolyte abnormalities, pain, excitement, or myocardial ischemia. The underlying cause should be determined before antiarrhythmic drugs are administered.

Virtually every patient in the PACU should be monitored with an ECG, frequent blood pressures, a pulse oximeter, and observation of respiration. Patients in whom large volume changes have occurred or are expected to occur should have their status assessed by urine outputs and, if indicated, central venous pressures. If these parameters are followed, sudden circulatory changes will be evident and easily correctable.

Renal Dysfunction

Oliguria is the result of either hemodynamic or mechanical compromise. Postoperative renal insufficiency is commonly seen in patients with preexisting renal disease, sepsis, massive trauma, major vascular or cardiac surgery, or pelvic pathology with intraoperative trauma to either the ureter or renal vessels. Because of the effects of aging on renal circulation and tubular function, geriatric patients are more likely to exhibit postoperative renal dysfunction. Patients who suffered prolonged hypotension during surgery or who required massive blood transfusion often exhibit intraoperative renal insufficiency continuing into the postoperative period. Patients at risk for postoperative renal dysfunction should be monitored with Foley catheter drainage of urine throughout the perioperative period. In patients with no predisposing factors, oliguria might be caused by an obstructed catheter or residual anesthetic or surgical effects, such as edema causing obstruction of a ureter. After ruling out a mechanical obstruction, the first treatment of developing oliguria in the PACU is optimizing the patient's volume status and cardiac output. Only then should diuretics be administered, because they further deplete the patient's intravascular volume and prevent the use of urine output as a monitor of volume status.

Other Complications

Postoperative *bleeding* is usually the result of inadequate hemostasis during surgery, and may relate to the fact that the blood pressure is higher in the PACU than it was under anesthesia. Coagulopathies may have been present preoperatively, or may develop because of massive transfusion of banked blood, intraoperative administration of anticoagulants, a transfusion reaction, or release of tissue substances that interfere with normal coagulation. After determining that the problem is not surgical hemostasis, laboratory tests should be performed to indicate which specific factor deficiencies need to be corrected.

Hypothermia occurs because operating rooms are cold and the patient's temperature-regulating mechanism is compromised during anesthesia. The anesthesiologist counters these effects by providing warm gases, warming intravenous fluids, using a heating blanket, and covering nonsterile parts of the body. Nonetheless, postoperative hypothermia is not uncommon, and is evident by shivering, continued somnolence, and prolonged action of muscle relaxants. Shivering is a problem because it causes hypertension, pain, and a marked increase in oxygen consumption. It should be treated aggressively by warming the patient and providing supplemental oxygen. In addition, small intravenous injections of benzodiazepines, Thorazine, or droperidol may be required.

Pain, the most common postoperative complication, is covered in the next section of this chapter. The most painful surgical procedures are upper abdominal, thoracic, and orthopedic. After pain, *nausea and vomiting* are the most common postoperative complications; they are often the result of treatment of pain with narcotics. Prolonged nausea and vomiting are the most frequent causes of unplanned admissions of patients scheduled for ambulatory surgery. These complications are more commonly seen in patients who have had abdominal or ophthalmological surgery and in patients with abdominal distention. Almost all anesthetic agents have been implicated. Agents used to treat nausea and vomiting all contribute to prolonged somnolence and cardiovascular instability.

Discharge Home

More than half of surgical procedures are currently being performed on patients who will be discharged home after recovery from anesthesia. It is usually required that the patient be accompanied by a responsible adult who will drive the patient home and be available should any assistance be required. In order to qualify for discharge, the patient should be awake and alert, ambulate without exhibiting weakness or postural hypotension, drink fluids without vomiting, and be able to urinate. In addition, the surgical site should be dry and dressed to ensure sterility. The patient should be instructed not to drive or operate machinery and not to drink alcohol or take any medication not prescribed by the surgeon or anesthesiologist.

About 5% of surgical outpatients are admitted postoperatively, usually because of intractable vomiting. Another common reason for unexpected admission is pain requiring narcotic injections. Far less frequent causes are urinary retention, surgical or anesthetic complications, or requirement for intensive treatment of concurrent medical conditions such as diabetes or hypertension.

Management of Postoperative Pain

Why Treat Postoperative Pain?

By blunting the reflexes that cause undesirable metabolic and motor responses, postoperative pain control may lead to improved patient outcome. Unlike patients who are in pain, patients who are comfortable can readily breathe deeply, cough, ambulate, and cooperate with physical and respiratory therapy. The metabolic responses to surgery, mediated by the autonomic nervous system, include increased production of ACTH, cortisol, catecholamines, renin, angiotensin II, and glucagon, with decreased production of insulin. The metabolic responses in turn produce such physiologic responses as tachycardia, hypertension, hyperglycemia, sodium and water retention, increased systemic vascular resistance, increased cardiac work, and increased myocardial oxygen consumption. The motor response to injury is characterized by splinting (involuntary local muscle contracture) and resistance to movement of the injured area. This resistance can result in the inability to take a deep breath leading to atelectasis, hypoxemia, and pneumonia, or it can result in the inability to move about, increasing the risk of deep vein thrombosis. Thus with good postoperative pain control, complications can be prevented, therapy facilitated, and recovery and discharge occur more quickly.

The most common method of providing postoperative analgesia is the systemic administration of opioid analgesics. A recent improvement in this technique, patient-controlled analgesia (PCA), allows the patient to control opioid administration. Nociceptive (pain-transmitting) impulses can be blocked by the administration of local anesthetics or occasionally by neurodestructive techniques such as the cryoprobe. Administration of local anesthetics and/or opioids by the subarachnoid or epidural route allows profound analgesia. However, there are risks and side effects associated with all of these modalities. The ability of the medical and nursing staff to recognize and treat these problems, the limitations of the particular hospital situation, and the needs of the local patient population must be considered when instituting any program of postoperative pain treatment.

Psychological Interventions

People differ in their reaction to pain. The suffering associated with pain may be reduced if an individual knows what to expect, is taught how to exercise some control over pain, and is reassured that help will be available. All patients deserve, consistent with age and mental status, a description of what will take place on the day of surgery, a description of sensations that will be experienced, and an explanation of the analgesic plan. The patient should be encouraged to ask for analgesia when needed and taught maneuvers that will minimize pain, such as how to cough or move in bed. The patient should be reassured that personnel will be available to treat their postoperative pain whenever it occurs.

Systemic Opioids

Postoperative pain is most commonly treated by the intermittent administration of opioid analgesics. The goal is to achieve an opioid blood level that provides analgesia without excessive sedation or respiratory depression. A number of opioid analgesics is available for use in the immediate postoperative period. The more commonly used opioids, doses by various routes, and timing of administration are summarized in Table 1.18. Systemic opioids have various side effects. All opioid agonists depress respiration. Significant respiratory depression is treated by administration of naloxone 0.04–0.4 mg i.v. Life-threatening respiratory depression may require endotracheal intubation and mechanical ventilation until the drug effect has subsided. Nausea and vomiting, the result of opioid stimulation of the chemoreceptor trigger zone (CTZ), can be treated by transdermal scopolamine, prochlorperazine 5–10 mg i.m., or changing to a different opioid. Opioids cause constipation by delay of intestinal transit, depression of small intestinal propulsive contractions, and decreased colonic peristalsis, resulting in increased water absorption and desiccation of feces. Biliary tract pressure is increased, which may result in biliary colic manifested by epigastric or chest pain. The biliary spasm may be reversed by naloxone or glucagon.

Table 1.18.
Systemic Opioids for Postoperative Pain: Suggested Adult Dose

Drug	Dose P.O. (mg)	I.M.	I.V.	Duration (hr)
Buprenorphine (Buprenex)		0.3–0.4	0.3–0.4	6
Butorphanol (Stadol)		1–4	0.5–2	3
Codeine	15–60	15–60		4
Hydrocodone (Vicodin)	5–10			6
Hydromorphone (Dilaudid)	3 (p.r.) 2 (p.o.)	1–2	1–2	4
Levorphanol (Levo-Dromoran)	2	2 (s.q.)[a]		6
Meperidine (Demerol)	100–200	75–100	25–50	3
Methadone	20	10	10	24 (p.o.) 4 (i.m., i.v., or s.q.)
Morphine	10–30	10	10	4
Oxycodone (Numorphan)	5			6

[a]s.q. indicates subcutaneous administration.

Patient-Controlled Analgesia

One of the disadvantages of systemic opioids by the oral, intramuscular, and subcutaneous routes is that the analgesia produced frequently is inadequate because of patient differences in rates of drug absorption and metabolism. For example, after i.m. meperidine, peak blood levels between individuals can vary three- to five-fold, and the time to reach peak blood level can vary three- to sevenfold. The blood level necessary to achieve analgesia also is variable; about a fourfold variation has been shown for meperidine. Furthermore, the therapeutic window is very small; a change in meperidine concentration as small as 0.05 μg/mL may be the difference between complete pain relief and no pain relief. The combination of unreliable drug delivery methods and variable therapeutic blood levels makes adequate opioid analgesia using traditional delivery methods very difficult. Added to these problems are the widespread misunderstanding of opioid pharmacology and an excessive concern for side effects. The result is poor postoperative analgesia for many patients.

In the 1970s the first patient-controlled analgesia devices became available. The device is programmed to deliver, on demand by the patient, a very small dose of drug through an intravenous cannula. For pain control, the patient pushes a button connected to the PCA device which then delivers the drug. A lockout interval begins, during which time any demands by the patient will not be honored. After the lockout interval is completed, the patient may demand another dose. The purpose of the lockout interval is to ensure the patient waits for the peak analgesic effect of one dose before receiving another dose. Most PCA devices allow for a slow continuous infusion of drug in addition to intermittent doses.

Numerous safety mechanisms exist on most PCA devices. One is an antisiphoning valve to prevent drugs from leaking out of a broken or improperly loaded syringe. One-way valves on Y-connectors in the tubing prevent the drug from traveling into secondary i.v. lines instead of into the patient. PCA tubing connected directly to the intravenous cannula also minimizes the amount of drug in the dead space of i.v. tubing. Locks on access doors and programming panels prevent tampering with the device. Microprocessor software is designed to eliminate many common programming errors, by requiring such precautions as minimum lockout intervals or limiting maximum PCA or continuous infusion doses. Alarms for line occlusion, low battery, empty syringe, and other malfunctions, are frequently included. A running total of the amount of drug administered is constantly updated, allowing the physician to determine the pattern and intensity of drug usage and hence the rate of decrease in the patient's postoperative pain.

To provide satisfactory postoperative analgesia using PCA therapy, the physician, nursing staff, and patient must be educated. The physician and nursing staff must understand the proper assembly and use of the PCA device, the pharmacology of the drug chosen, and the signs and treatment of side effects. The patient must be made to understand: (*a*) the proper mechanical use of the device; (*b*) that complete pain relief frequently is not achieved, but distressing pain can be avoided; and (*c*) that the device can be used to minimize the pain associated with ambulation, dressing changes, and physical therapy, if it is used before these maneuvers.

The ideal opioid for PCA would have a rapid onset and an intermediate duration of action. Drugs with a long duration of action—such as methadone and buprenorphine—are difficult to control, while drugs with a short duration of action—such as fentanyl and sufentanil—require the patient to administer doses very frequently, which may interfere with sleep. Mixed agonist-antagonist drugs have a maximum analgesic effect that is often not adequate for postoperative pain, and increasing doses beyond those achieving the "ceiling effect" produces only more side effects. In practice, the most commonly used drugs for PCA are morphine and meperidine.

A typical protocol for initiating PCA therapy is as follows. Upon arriving at the recovery room the patient receives a loading dose of opioid, the amount of which

Table 1.19.
PCA Therapy for Postoperative Pain: Suggested Drugs, Adult Doses, and Lockout Intervals

Drug	Dose (mg)	Lockout (min)
Morphine	0.5–3	5–20
Meperidine	5.0–30	5–15
Hydromorphone	0.1–0.6	5–15

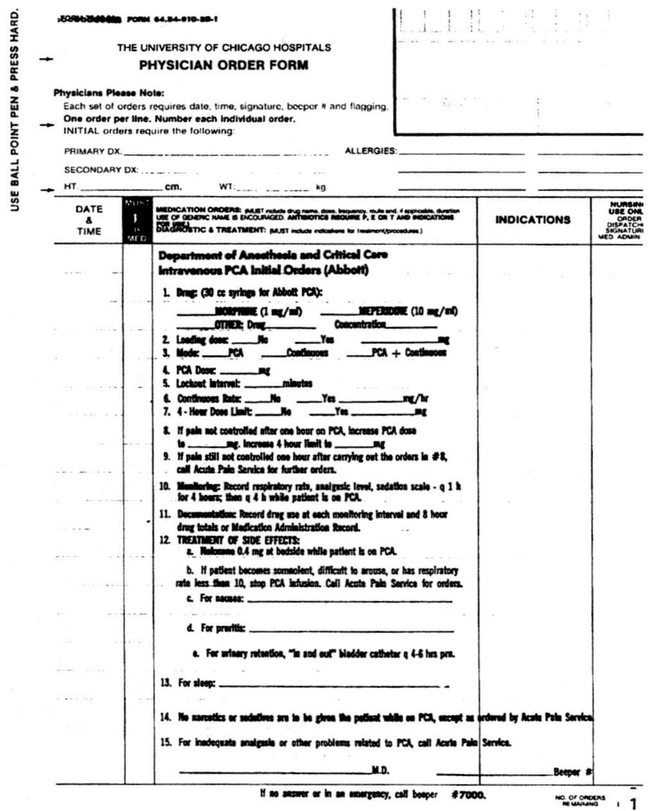

USE BALL POINT PEN & PRESS HARD.

FORM 64.94-010-98-1

THE UNIVERSITY OF CHICAGO HOSPITALS
PHYSICIAN ORDER FORM

Physicians Please Note:
Each set of orders requires date, time, signature, beeper # and flagging.
One order per line. Number each individual order.
INITIAL orders require the following:

PRIMARY DX: ______ ALLERGIES: ______
SECONDARY DX: ______
HT: ______ cm. WT: ______ kg

DATE & TIME	MUST 1 IF MED	MEDICATION ORDERS: (MUST include drug name, dose, frequency, route and, if applicable, duration. USE OF GENERIC NAME IS ENCOURAGED. ANTIBIOTICS REQUIRE P, E OR T AND INDICATIONS FOR USE.) DIAGNOSTIC & TREATMENT: (MUST include indications for treatment/procedures.)	INDICATIONS	NURSING USE ONLY ORDER DISPATCH SIGNATURE MED ADMIN

Department of Anesthesia and Critical Care
Intravenous PCA Initial Orders (Abbott)

1. Drug: (30 cc syringe for Abbott PCA):
   ______ MORPHINE (1 mg/ml) ______ MEPERIDINE (10 mg/ml)
   ______ OTHER: Drug ______ Concentration ______
2. Loading dose: ______ No ______ Yes ______ mg
3. Mode: ______ PCA ______ Continuous ______ PCA + Continuous
4. PCA Dose: ______ mg
5. Lockout interval: ______ minutes
6. Continuous Rate: ______ No ______ Yes ______ mg/hr
7. 4-Hour Dose Limit: ______ No ______ Yes ______ mg
8. If pain not controlled after one hour on PCA, increase PCA dose to ______ mg. Increase 4 hour limit to ______ mg
9. If pain still not controlled one hour after carrying out the orders in #8, call Acute Pain Service for further orders.
10. Monitoring: Record respiratory rate, analgesic level, sedation scale - q 1 h for 4 hours; then q 4 h while patient is on PCA.
11. Documentation: Record drug use at each monitoring interval and 8 hour drug totals or Medication Administration Record.
12. TREATMENT OF SIDE EFFECTS:
    a. Naloxone 0.4 mg at bedside while patient is on PCA.
    b. If patient becomes somnolent, difficult to arouse, or has respiratory rate less than 10, stop PCA infusion. Call Acute Pain Service for orders.
    c. For nausea: ______
    d. For pruritis: ______
    e. For urinary retention, "in and out" bladder catheter q 4-6 hrs prn.
13. For sleep: ______
14. No narcotics or sedatives are to be given the patient while on PCA, except as ordered by Acute Pain Service.
15. For inadequate analgesia or other problems related to PCA, call Acute Pain Service.

______ M.D. ______ Beeper #

If no answer or in an emergency, call beeper #7000.

NO. OF ORDERS REMAINING 1

Figure 1.6. Standard orders for postoperative PCA at the University of Chicago.

depends on such factors as the individual patient, the type of anesthetic given, and the amount of narcotic given intraoperatively. A typical loading dose for morphine is 0.1 mg/kg while for meperidine it is 1 mg/kg, given over 15–30 minutes until adequate analgesia is achieved. The patient assumes control of the PCA device when sufficiently recovered from anesthesia. If the dose is inadequate, as evidenced by inadequate analgesia after frequent administration, it is increased by about 50%. If the dose is excessive, as evidenced by sedation or dizziness, it is decreased by about 50%. A continuous infusion of morphine 1 mg/hr or meperidine 10 mg/hr is sometimes used to decrease the frequency with which the patient needs to demand doses, thereby improving sleep. However, continuous infusion should be used with caution in the elderly and in patients with renal or hepatic insufficiency or cardiac failure. Typical morphine consumption on PCA is 1–2 mg/hr; for meperidine it is 10–20 mg/hr. Therapy is continued until patients are able to tolerate opioids orally or analgesia is not needed. With orthopedic patients PCA therapy is often continued until physical therapy has begun. Suggested dose and lockout intervals for three narcotics commonly used for PCA therapy are summarized in Table 1.19.

Whenever opioids are given, resuscitation equipment and naloxone should be readily available. Also, whenever narcotics are given, the side effects of pruritus, constipation, nausea, vomiting, and urinary retention should be expected and treated. Pruritus is best treated with diphenhydramine, 25–30 mg i.m. or i.v.; nausea and vomiting with prochlorperazine 10 mg i.m.; and urinary retention with a single straight bladder catheterization. If the patient is still in retention after straight catheterization, a Foley catheter may be used for 12–24 hours. A set of standard orders for PCA facilitates remembering to order treatment for these side effects, and is illustrated in Figure 1.6. Excessive sedation is treated by decreasing the dose and stopping any continuous infusion of narcotic. If respiratory depression is present, it may be necessary to give naloxone, 0.1–0.4 mg i.v., intubate, and provide ventilatory support. For patients on PCA therapy, all orders for narcotics, sleeping pills, and other sedatives should be written by the same individual or service. A single source of orders minimizes unnecessary and potentially hazardous duplication of these orders.

Complications related to PCA therapy are extremely rare, and are minimized by training the medical and nursing staff, understanding the pharmacology of the opioid used, educating the patient, selecting the patient carefully, and using a dilute opioid solution such as morphine 1 mg/mL or meperidine 10 mg/mL, unless a more concentrated solution is needed in an individual situation because of tolerance or other factors.

Epidural and Spinal Analgesia

The widespread use of epidural and spinal analgesia for postoperative pain control is recent. The epidural or subarachnoid infusion of local anesthetics produces profound analgesia at the price of variable degree of sensory, motor, and sympathetic blockade, depending on the drug and technique employed. The discovery of opioid receptors in the late 1970s led to the use of subarachnoid opioids for postoperative analgesia. Subarachnoid opioids produce reliable analgesia without sensory, motor, or sympathetic blockade; however, profound respiratory depression may occur as late as 24 hours after injection. Various combinations of local anesthetics and opioids have been used in an effort to minimize the side effects associated with each agent, but the ideal agent or technique has yet to be found.

Epidural Analgesia. Epidural analgesic agents may be administered by intermittent techniques or by continuous infusion. Regardless of the method employed, best results are obtained when the agent is deposited at the vertebral level approximating the middle of the spinal segments affected by the surgery. The epidural catheter should be inserted with normal sterile technique and securely fixed with tape. An occlusive dressing is used when contamination by fluid or incontinence is a problem. Depending on the site of surgery, the catheter may then be draped across the back toward the neck or brought along the flank to the lateral position. Often the anesthesiologist inserts the catheter before surgery, uses it to inject opioids and/or local anesthetics during surgery, and then leaves it in for postoperative analgesia.

To minimize the frequency of redosing and tachyphylaxis, long-acting local anesthetics, such as bupivacaine 0.125–0.25%, are most commonly used for continuous infusion in the postoperative period or during labor. The concentration of 0.125–0.25% bupivacaine provides sensory analgesia with a minimum of motor blockade. Sympathetic blockade may occur with epidural administration of local anesthetics, and would be dangerous in a patient with cardiac disease or hypovolemia. On the other hand, sympathetic blockade causes vasodilation and improved tissue blood flow, which is advantageous in vascular surgery or in patients at risk for thromboembolism.

Opioids are also used for epidural analgesia. Usually a loading dose is given (morphine 2–3 mg, meperidine 5–10 mg, or fentanyl 0.05–0.1 mg). Analgesia is maintained with either intermittent reinjection of the same dose when the patient becomes aware of pain or continuous infusion (at a rate of 0.5 mg/hr morphine, 20 mg/hr meperidine, or 0.075 mg/hr fentanyl usually with 0.125% bupivacaine). The greatest risk associated with epidural opioids is respiratory depression, which may occur early (within 1 hour) because of vascular uptake of drug or late (up to 24 hours) because of diffusion of opioid from the spinal cord to the brain. Highly lipid soluble opioids such as fentanyl and sufentanil are associated with early respiratory depression, while the less lipid soluble agents such as morphine are associated with late respiratory depression.

Side effects occurring with epidural opioids include pruritus, nausea and vomiting, and urinary retention. Pruritus is highly variable, nonsegmental, and most commonly seen with morphine. The mechanism is unknown. Benadryl 25 mg i.m. or naloxone 0.04–0.1 mg i.v. usually helps. It is possible to titrate naloxone to minimize side effects while retaining analgesia. Nausea and vomiting, less commonly seen, are probably related to stimulation of the chemoreceptor trigger zone in the medulla. They have been successfully treated with prochlorperazine 5–10 mg i.m.; droperidol 0.625–1.25 mg i.v.; metoclopramide 5–10 mg i.v.; or transdermal scopolamine patches. Urinary retention is seen occasionally. The cause is poorly understood but may be related to inhibition of the micturition reflex. Usually, intermittent bladder catheterization is sufficient, but an indwelling catheter may be used as well.

Combinations of local anesthetics and opioids are being used epidurally more often because low concentrations of both agents provide analgesia with minimum side effects. In a healthy adult patient, a combination of 0.1% bupivacaine with 0.05 mg/mL morphine, 1 mg/mL meperidine, or 0.005 mg/mL fentanyl is infused at a rate of 5–7 mL/hr through a thoracic epidural catheter or 8–12 mL/hr through a lumbar epidural catheter.

Spinal Analgesia. While both opioids and local anesthetics may be given by the intrathecal route, there are several drawbacks to this technique. Headache occasionally occurs after lumbar puncture, but the recent introduction of fine-bore catheters has reduced the incidence of this complication. Pruritus, nausea and vomiting, urinary retention, and respiratory depression are more commonly seen when opioids are given intrathecally rather than epidurally. When local anesthetics are used, motor blockade may limit postoperative ambulation as well as physical and respiratory therapy. As with epidural analgesia, a catheter may be placed in the subarachnoid space before surgery and used to supplement the anesthetic in the operating room as well as to provide postoperative analgesia.

Monitoring

Patients who receive local anesthetics intraspinally must be monitored for side effects of sympathetic blockade, hypotension, systemic toxicity, seizures, cardiac arrhythmias, motor blockade, and urinary retention. Patients who receive opioids intraspinally must be monitored for side effects of nausea and vomiting, pruritus, urinary retention, respiratory depression, and sedation. A variety of protocols and devices has evolved to monitor these side effects. Patients have been monitored in intensive care settings and on general units with such devices as motion sensors, strain gauges, impedance monitors, pulse oximeters, and expired CO_2 monitors. However, no monitoring technique or protocol has been shown to be superior to any other. It appears that the safe and effective use of these analgesic techniques requires that the patient be monitored on a regular basis by trained personnel capable of recognizing and treating complications (see protocol in Figure 1.7). In addition, physicians must be available on a 24-hour basis to respond to problems as they arise.

Other Techniques

Nonsteroidal Anti-inflammatory Drugs. Although there has been increasing use of nonsteroidal anti-inflammatory drugs (NSAIDs) for pain control, their exact role has not yet been defined. NSAIDs appear to produce analgesia during tissue injury by inhibiting the release of prostaglandins, which sensitize peripheral nociceptors. When the nociceptive impulse delivered to the central nervous system is increased, the perception of pain is increased. Prostaglandins may also exert hyperalgesic effects in the central nervous system. Although it would appear worthwhile to administer NSAIDs before surgery, several side effects may limit their usefulness. NSAIDs inhibit platelet function, which may interfere with hemostasis. Also, prostaglandins may themselves be necessary for wound healing. The antipyretic activity of NSAIDs may mask the febrile response to infection and thus delay its treatment. Renal insufficiency and failure are also associated with the

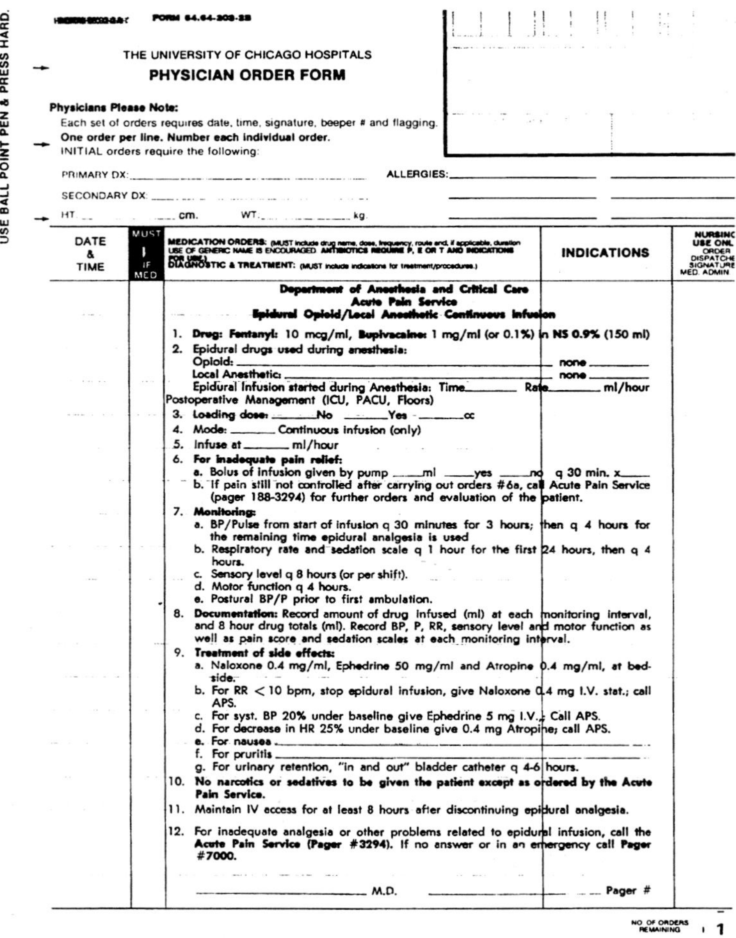

USE BALL POINT PEN & PRESS HARD.

FORM 84.84-208-28

THE UNIVERSITY OF CHICAGO HOSPITALS
PHYSICIAN ORDER FORM

Physicians Please Note:
Each set of orders requires date, time, signature, beeper # and flagging.
One order per line. Number each individual order.
INITIAL orders require the following:

PRIMARY DX: ______ ALLERGIES: ______
SECONDARY DX: ______
HT ______ cm. WT ______ kg.

DATE & TIME	MUST ✓ IF MED	MEDICATION ORDERS: (MUST include drug name, dose, frequency, route and, if applicable, duration. USE OF GENERIC NAME IS ENCOURAGED. ANTIBIOTICS REQUIRE P, E OR T AND INDICATIONS FOR USE.) DIAGNOSTIC & TREATMENT: (MUST include indications for treatment/procedures.)	INDICATIONS	NURSING USE ONLY ORDER DISPATCHED SIGNATURE MED. ADMIN.

Department of Anesthesia and Critical Care
Acute Pain Service
Epidural Opioid/Local Anesthetic Continuous Infusion

1. **Drug: Fentanyl:** 10 mcg/ml, **Bupivacaine:** 1 mg/ml (or 0.1%) in **NS 0.9%** (150 ml)
2. Epidural drugs used during anesthesia:
   Opioid: ______ none ______
   Local Anesthetic: ______ none ______
   Epidural Infusion started during Anesthesia: Time ______ Rate ______ ml/hour

Postoperative Management (ICU, PACU, Floors)

3. Loading dose: ______ No ______ Yes ______ cc
4. Mode: ______ Continuous infusion (only)
5. Infuse at ______ ml/hour
6. **For inadequate pain relief:**
   a. Bolus of infusion given by pump ______ ml ______ yes ______ no q 30 min. x ______
   b. If pain still not controlled after carrying out orders #6a, call Acute Pain Service (pager 188-3294) for further orders and evaluation of the patient.
7. **Monitoring:**
   a. BP/Pulse from start of infusion q 30 minutes for 3 hours; then q 4 hours for the remaining time epidural analgesia is used
   b. Respiratory rate and sedation scale q 1 hour for the first 24 hours, then q 4 hours.
   c. Sensory level q 8 hours (or per shift).
   d. Motor function q 4 hours.
   e. Postural BP/P prior to first ambulation.
8. **Documentation:** Record amount of drug infused (ml) at each monitoring interval, and 8 hour drug totals (ml). Record BP, P, RR, sensory level and motor function as well as pain score and sedation scales at each monitoring interval.
9. **Treatment of side effects:**
   a. Naloxone 0.4 mg/ml, Ephedrine 50 mg/ml and Atropine 0.4 mg/ml, at bedside.
   b. For RR < 10 bpm, stop epidural infusion, give Naloxone 0.4 mg I.V. stat.; call APS.
   c. For syst. BP 20% under baseline give Ephedrine 5 mg I.V.; Call APS.
   d. For decrease in HR 25% under baseline give 0.4 mg Atropine; call APS.
   e. For nausea ______
   f. For pruritis ______
   g. For urinary retention, "in and out" bladder catheter q 4-6 hours.
10. **No narcotics or sedatives to be given the patient except as ordered by the Acute Pain Service.**
11. Maintain IV access for at least 8 hours after discontinuing epidural analgesia.
12. For inadequate analgesia or other problems related to epidural infusion, call the **Acute Pain Service (Pager #3294).** If no answer or in an emergency call **Pager #7000.**

______ M.D. ______ Pager #

NO. OF ORDERS REMAINING 1

Figure 1.7. Standard orders for postoperative epidural narcotic analgesia at the University of Chicago.

use of these compounds. While a few parenteral forms of NSAIDs are becoming available, most NSAIDs can be delivered only orally or rectally, which is not possible in many surgical situations.

Peripheral Neural Blockade. Regional anesthetic techniques for control of postoperative pain involve the use of local anesthetic agents to interrupt the transmission of nociceptive impulses to the central nervous system. In addition to analgesia, most neural blockade techniques produce complete sensory and motor blockade. If analgesia is desired for more than a few hours, a repeat block or an infusion technique becomes necessary. Patients receiving neural blockades must be monitored for side effects, such as toxicity of the local anesthetic agent from either peripheral absorption or intravascular injection, unexpected spinal or epidural blockade, and circulatory depression because of sympathectomy. An anesthetized area of the body may not be adequately protected by the patient and therefore must be shielded from injury. If a lower extremity is anesthetized, ambulation is delayed. Pneumothorax may occur in intercostal blocks, interpleural blocks, and occasionally with brachial plexus blocks. Neural blockade for postoperative pain control requires an increased level of nursing surveillance, care, and perhaps help with ambulation; the availability of such care, often on a special "step-down" unit, should be determined before undertaking these procedures.

A variety of techniques exists for peripheral blockade of postoperative pain. The surgical wound itself may be infiltrated or simply washed with local anesthetics before suturing. Brachial plexus blockade may be used for upper extremity injury. Lumbar plexus, femoral, and sciatic nerve blocks have been used for lower extremity procedures. Intercostal nerve blocks have been used for chest wall and abdominal wall pain. Interpleural blockade has been used for the control of pain in a variety of abdominal surgical procedures and in painful conditions of the chest wall such as rib fractures and mastectomy. It is not as useful for control of pain after thoracotomy. These techniques may be performed intermittently or continuously, using a catheter to infuse local anesthetic.

Although the blocks described frequently require specialized techniques or personnel that may not be available at many medical centers, there are many single injection regional blocks that can be performed by the surgeon at the time of surgery. These blocks frequently are effective and have an acceptably low incidence of complications, but unfortunately they are under utilized. Inguinal, iliohypogastric, and dorsal penile nerve blocks have been used successfully for a variety of surgical procedures in the inguinal and genital regions. Direct infiltration and even topical application of local anesthetics to a surgical wound can be used for pain control in many situations.

Cryoanalgesia. Cryoanalgesia has been used most frequently for the control of chest wall pain following thoracotomy. The technique involves placing a cryoprobe either percutaneously or under direct vision at surgery on the nerve to be disrupted. Using nitrous oxide or liquid nitrogen, the tip of the probe is cooled to approximately −60°C. Applying the probe to the nerve causes an ice ball to form around the nerve, which results in axonal degeneration but spares the nerve sheath architecture. The nerve grows back at the rate of 1–3 mm per day without the scarring, neuritis, or neuromas occasionally seen with surgical sectioning of the nerve or with chemical neurolysis. The analgesia usually lasts from a few weeks to a few months. There are several disadvantages to the technique. Analgesia is frequently incomplete, with residual pain in areas not affected by the blocks such as the shoulder, the midback, and chest tube sites. Cryogenic lesions of surrounding tissue or full thickness skin destruction may occur. The equipment needed for cryoanalgesia is expensive, and the usefulness of this technique must be considered before undertaking such an investment.

Transcutaneous Electrical Nerve Stimulation. In transcutaneous electric nerve stimulation (TENS), analgesia is provided by means of a weak electrical current that is transmitted through the skin surface to a painful area. The mechanism of analgesia has not been fully explained but is probably due to inhibition of pain transmission at the spinal or central level by the barrage of impulses generated by non-nociceptive receptor stimulation. TENS has been used successfully to control pain after knee, hip, and low back operations; it is not as effective after herniorrhaphy and thoracic procedures.

Developing Techniques. Various nonnarcotic, nonlocal anesthetic techniques are under investigation. These include intrathecal and epidural administration of such drugs as ketamine, clonidine, and calcitonin, as well as systemic administration of tricyclic antidepressants. While the safety and efficacy of these techniques have not been established, this field has grown so rapidly in the past decade that one should expect new treatments to be available soon.

Appendix

Patient Factors Influencing Anesthesia

To maintain homeostasis during surgery, the anesthesiologist must not only support respiration and circulation, but also must interfere with the patient's stress response by blocking pain, manage endocrine responses using anesthetics and other drugs, and oversee the patient's medical conditions. Even the healthiest patient exhibits a complex physiological response to stress, even though the stress may not be consciously perceived. Preexisting medical conditions alter that response to the extent that it may become life threatening. Every patient responds uniquely to the drugs administered and to the attempts to control the physiologic state during and after surgery. This section describes the effects of commonly occurring medical conditions on the surgical patient. It also identifies the information required by the anesthesiologist and explains its importance in both clinical decision making and patient outcome.

Cardiovascular System

Anesthesia almost always depresses normal cardiovascular function. Consequently, when cardiovascular disease of any type is present the anesthesiologist must have a thorough knowledge of the patient's degree of dysfunction and of the probable effects of surgery and anesthesia.

Hypertension. Preexisting hypertension makes intraoperative blood pressure control difficult. In the normal patient, intraoperative hypertension is a sign of sympathetic stimulation because of inadequate analgesia or anesthesia; it is most effectively treated by increasing depth of anesthesia with volatile agents, narcotics, or intravenous anesthetics. The patient with preexisting hypertension that is not controlled on a stable medication regimen may exhibit wide swings in blood pressure as a result of varying levels of stimulation, of anesthetic administered, or of attempts to control hemodynamic status with volume restriction or infusion. A controlled hypertensive responds much like a normal patient, as long as medication is continued throughout the perioperative period.

Techniques to control intraoperative hypertension are determined by the cause. If "light" anesthesia or pain is considered to be the cause, anesthesia is the treatment. Only where the level of anesthesia is appropriate, in the best judgment of the anesthesiologist, should β blockers or vasodilators be used. If there is strong suspicion of fluid overload as a contributing cause, intravenous diuretic therapy often is indicated, provided the continuing surgical procedure will not result in significant fluid loss of its own.

A rare but very dangerous cause of intraoperative hypertension is the interaction of monoamine oxidase (MAO) inhibitors or tricyclic antidepressants with catecholamines or catecholamine-like drugs (such as ephedrine). MAO inhibitors and tricyclics interfere with the metabolism of catechols and may allow dangerously high concentrations at the sympathetic nerve ending. Despite this potential danger, the most recent recom-

Table 1A.1.
Impact of Antihypertensive Drugs on the Perioperative Period

Class of Drug (Examples)	Potential Problems
Diuretics	Hypovolemia
	Vasodilation
	Decreased urine output if omitted
	Electrolyte abnormalities (usually K^+)
Drugs that deplete neurotransmitters (reserpine, guanethidine)	Denervation sensitivity to direct acting pressors
	Abnormal response to indirect acting pressors
	Reserpine decreases MAC[a] by 20–30%
	Bradycardia
	Orthostatic hypotension
False neurotransmitters (methyldopa)	Decrease MAC if centrally acting
	Abnormal response to indirect acting pressors
	Bradycardia
	Orthostatic hypotension
β-receptor blocking agents	Additive hypotension and bradycardia with anesthetics
	Possible bronchiolar constriction
	Rebound hypertension and tachycardia on withdrawal
α_1 receptor blocking agents (prazosin)	Additive hypotension with anesthetics
	Decreased MAC
α_2 receptor agonists (clonidine)	Rebound hypertension and tachycardia on withdrawal
	Additive hypotension with anesthetics
	Decrease MAC
Arteriolar vasodilators (hydralazine)	Postural hypotension
	Decreased response to pressors
Calcium channel blocking agents	Hypotension, decreased contractility and conduction delays additive to anesthetics
	Decrease MAC about 25%
	Potentiate neuromuscular blocking agents
Angiotensin converting enzyme inhibitors	Hypotension with many anesthetics
	Hyponatremia

[a]MAC is discussed in the section on pharmacology of inhalation agents. Simply put, it is a measure of anesthetic potency. If MAC is decreased by another drug, that drug has an additive or potentiating effect on anesthesia.

mendation is to continue the drugs throughout the perioperative period in order to prevent dangerous withdrawal phenomena, and to make every effort to avoid sympathetic stimulation or exogenous catechol administration intraoperatively.

Table 1A.1 lists potential perioperative problems in the patient on an antihypertensive medication regimen. Despite these potential drug interactions, the majority of data indicates that all antihypertensive medication, with the possible exception of diuretics, should be continued through the immediate preoperative period. When propranolol and clonidine first became commonly used for hypertension control, there was concern that their depressive effects on the cardiovascular system would preclude safe administration of anesthetics, but it soon became evident that there was worse danger of rebound hypertension and tachycardia upon their abrupt withdrawal.

A plan for dealing with hyper- and hypotension intraoperatively should be formulated long before intervention is required, and the anesthetic and monitoring techniques should be carefully chosen, taking into consideration any possible interactions. In the chronic hypertensive patient, even one on a medication regimen, there are end-organ manifestations of the disease. Cardiovascular manifestations include ischemic disease, left ventricular dysfunction, aortic stenosis, and central and peripheral vascular insufficiency. Renal vascular disease leads to chronic renal insufficiency. Carotid and cerebrovascular disease lead to focal cerebral ischemia, altered autoregulation, and stroke. For appropriate evaluation, therefore, each hypertensive patient needs a preoperative ECG, chest x-ray, serum electrolytes, blood urea nitrogen (BUN) and creatinine, CBC, and an assessment of neurological function. Preoperatively, a careful history and physical examination should help determine the presence of angina, the degree of dyspnea on exertion, and the degree of congestive failure. If the ECG is abnormal, as it often is, further evaluation is required to determine the contractile state of the myocardium and the myocardial oxygen supply/demand status. Sometimes a dipyridamole-thallium scan or angiography will be indicated, but recently the ready availability of echocardiography has replaced these more invasive procedures in many patients.

The anesthesiologist should determine the range of blood pressures and heart rates for which the hypertensive patient is asymptomatic and then set limits (usually within about 10–20% of this range) at which intervention during surgery becomes necessary. Finally, early planning of monitoring in consultation with the surgeon facilitates maintenance of blood volume and myocardial and tissue oxygenation throughout surgery.

Table 1A.2.
Clues to Ischemic Heart Disease

History	Chest pain with arm or neck radiation, especially if relieved by nitroglycerin
	Dyspnea on exertion, exposure to cold, straining or after eating
	Orthopnea
	Paroxysmal nocturnal dyspnea
	Nocturnal coughing
	Peripheral or pulmonary edema
	History or ECG evidence of MI
	Cardiomegaly
	Family history of CAD at patient's age
Concurrent disease	Carotid bruit
	Unexplained tachycardia
	Diabetes
	Hyperlipidemia
	Hypertension
	Left ventricular hypertrophy on ECG
	Peripheral vascular disease
	Aortic disease

Ischemic Heart Disease. Myocardial infarction (MI) is the leading cause of mortality in the elderly undergoing surgery. The anesthesiologist must administer just enough anesthetic to achieve anesthesia without causing undue cardiovascular depression or allowing a significant stress response in the patient, either of which can upset the myocardial oxygen supply/demand ratio and cause ischemic damage. Until proven otherwise, the patient presenting with any of the complaints listed in Table 1A.2 is considered to suffer ischemic heart disease, even if the ECG is normal. The anesthesiologist must take a preoperative history and conduct a physical examination. Tests should include an ECG, chest x-ray, and other tests of myocardial oxygenation as indicated. Echocardiography is very helpful in evaluating regional myocardial function. If surgery is so emergent as to preclude more of an evaluation, the patient is treated as though ischemic heart disease is present.

Surgery in the face of a recent MI or acute coronary vascular insufficiency carries a mortality rate of 1.7%–27%, depending on the nature of the surgery, the time from infarction, and the perioperative management. Preoperative optimization of myocardial oxygenation with medication, angioplasty, or even coronary artery bypass graft (CABG) surgery, reduces the morbidity and mortality significantly. Patients who have undergone successful CABG surgery have a much reduced incidence and severity of perioperative morbidity from subsequent surgery. Delay for 6 months after an MI greatly reduces mortality from subsequent surgery.

Patients at risk for ischemic episodes during anesthesia are carefully monitored (with some combination of ECG, ST segment trending, PA and wedge pressures, cardiac output, and transesophageal echocardiography) and managed to maintain the correct myocardial oxygen supply/demand ratio for tissue oxygenation. Because myocardial perfusion occurs mainly during diastole, maintaining a slow heart rate is paramount. Patients with a history of myocardial ischemia are usually treated with agents to lower the heart rate and contractility, as well as with drugs to reduce peripheral and coronary vascular resistance. Such drugs are continued throughout the perioperative period. As with hypertensive patients, a range of acceptable values is determined for the patient preoperatively, and a plan formulated to maintain those values intraoperatively. Because the most likely time for reinfarction in patients is 48–72 hours postoperatively, monitoring for ischemia with some or all of the above methods is begun before anesthesia is induced and continues long into the postoperative period.

Congestive Heart Failure. The failing heart presents various problems at the time of surgery. It cannot easily maintain an adequate output during surgery and anesthesia, yet pharmacologic agents used to treat congestive heart failure (CHF) impact on anesthetics and other drugs used during surgery. Pulmonary hypertension and pulmonary edema seriously interfere with both oxygenation and uptake of inhaled anesthetic agents. Because pharmacokinetics are usually abnormal, dosage and timing of drug administration must be carefully titrated.

The goal of preoperative preparation of patients with CHF is to maximize their cardiac output without compromising myocardial oxygenation so that vital organ perfusion continues despite reduced blood circulation. As with any other chronic medical problem, a stable therapeutic regimen should be in effect before elective surgery; medications should be continued throughout the perioperative period, even though dosages may need to be modified. The patient's optimal ranges of blood pressure, heart rate, cardiac output, and peripheral resistance should be determined before surgery, along with the means that will be used to maintain them. In cases of severe CHF, the patient may be admitted to the intensive care unit the day before surgery, so that a pulmonary arterial catheter can be inserted and a Starling curve calculated to correlate the effect on cardiac output of changes in pulmonary artery, wedge, and right ventricular pressures, and systemic vascular resistance.

An additional difficulty that patients with CHF present is that they are usually taking digoxin, a drug with a very narrow therapeutic window. Too little drug results in a less than optimal therapeutic effect, while too much results in toxicity. Most patients with CHF also take diuretics to control their blood volume and so are at risk for both hypovolemia (relative and absolute) and electrolyte imbalance. It is recommended that digitalized patients not be anesthetized for elective surgery if their serum potassium falls below 3.5 mg/dL. Instead, total body K^+ should be returned to normal with therapy over 48–72 hours while the hazards of hyperkalemia are not overlooked. Table 1A.3 lists the arrhythmias often associated with digoxin and hypokalemia, which are also indicators of digoxin toxicity.

Choice of anesthetic technique and agents depends on the patient's blood volume, pulmonary vascular resistance, optimal filling pressures, state of myocardial oxygenation, and the ability of the heart to increase out-

Table 1A.3.
Arrhythmias Associated with Digitalization and Hypokalemia

Atrial	Sinus bradycardia
	Rapid atrial rate with 2:1 or 3:1 block
	Atrial premature contractions
	SA block
Junctional	AV node block often with atrial tachycardia
	Junctional tachycardia
Ventricular	Ventricular premature contractions
	Ventricular tachycardia
	Ventricular fibrillation

put on demand. Most anesthetics and sedatives, including local anesthetic agents, vasodilate and/or depress myocardial contractility. Patients on chronic diuretic therapy compensate for depleted blood volume by peripheral vasoconstriction and become hypotensive when anesthetized and vasodilated. Therefore, these patients should receive carefully monitored prophylactic fluid administration before receiving any vasodilating drugs. The circulation should be monitored (usually with a pulmonary artery catheter) before the first drug is administered. If surgery can be performed using a regional anesthetic, the myocardial depression caused by most anesthetics and adjuncts may be avoided. However, CHF patients have reduced clearance of local anesthetics resulting in higher blood levels and increased risk of toxicity, which requires altering the original dose and the timing of repeat injections. Patients with severe CHF may not be able to maintain adequate ventilation when lying supine on the operating table unless their respiration is assisted or controlled. They are thus not candidates for major regional anesthesia unless it is used in combination with general anesthesia and mechanical ventilation.

To provide intraoperative support of cardiac output, either dopamine, dobutamine, or amrinone in continuous infusion can be administered. Tachycardia is not tolerated in these patients and heart rate cannot easily be controlled with β blockers or Ca^{++} channel entry blockers because of the myocardial depression they may cause. Increased peripheral vascular resistance must also be avoided, because the failing heart cannot contract against an increased load.

Valvular Heart Disease. Each patient with valvular disease must be carefully evaluated preoperatively to determine the status of the heart, lungs, and peripheral perfusion. Valvular disease can cause profound disruption of rate and rhythm, contractility, pulmonary and peripheral vascular resistance, and preload and myocardial oxygenation. While the prevalence of rheumatic valve disease is declining, congenital bicuspid aortic stenosis, mitral valve prolapse, hypertropic cardiomyopathy (idiopathic hypertropic subaortic stenosis), and calcific mitral insufficiency are all increasing. Endocarditis or an MI can result in acute valvular insufficiency. A diseased valve is an ideal colonizing spot for circulating bacteria. Therefore, regardless of the lesion, antibiotic prophylaxis for *Staphylococcus* must be started before surgery and continued through the first postoperative day. Despite the potential for intraoperative and postoperative bleeding, anticoagulation may be judged essential to prevent fatal embolic phenomena. In this situation, regional anesthesia is contraindicated, as are blind needle sticks such those for central venous access in the internal jugular or subclavian veins.

Stenosis. Stenotic lesions require maintaining preload, contractility, rate, and rhythm within a narrow range. Atrial kick is helpful in mitral stenosis, so maintenance of sinus rhythm is desirable. Coronary vessel perfusion in the patient with aortic stenosis requires maintaining peripheral resistance (especially diastolic blood pressure) within a narrow range in order to allow flow across the stenosis.

Insufficiency. Patients with valvular insufficiencies often benefit from reduced pulmonary or peripheral vascular resistance. The easier the forward flow, the less blood regurgitates across an incompetent valve. When valves are both stenotic and insufficient, the anesthesiologist must treat what is felt to be the most hemodynamically significant lesion, yet be ready to alter strategy should that choice prove incorrect.

Mitral Valve Prolapse. Mitral valve prolapse (MVP) is the most commonly encountered valve lesion, occurring in about 6% of otherwise normal people. It is more prevalent in females and is commonly seen in association with other chest skeletal anomalies, von Wilebrand's syndrome, autonomic dysfunction, and migraine anxiety syndrome. Signs and symptoms of MVP include palpitations, dyspnea, atypical chest pain, dizziness, and syncope. Episodes of supraventricular or ventricular tachycardia occur in up to 50% of patients with MVP, while 25% suffer episodes of bradycardia. Sudden death occurs in about 1–2% of patients with MVP, probably because of ventricular fibrillation. The presence of an unexplained murmur with any one of the listed symptoms signals the possibility of MVP and requires further investigation. Patients with MVP are at increased risk for morbidity from intraoperative and postoperative dysrhythmias, and probably benefit from prophylactic antibiotics.

Idiopathic Hypertrophic Subaortic Stenosis. Idiopathic hypertrophic subaortic stenosis (IHSS) is an obstruction of the left ventricular outflow track by hypertrophied septum muscle. Stenosis occurs when contraction of the ventricle approaches its maximum in mid to late systole. Mitral regurgitation may occur as well. As the disease progresses, the left ventricle hypertrophies because of the pressure gradient across the stenosis. Arrhythmias are common because the conduction system is involved in the septal hypertrophy. Obstruction to the forward flow of blood is minimized by maintaining approximately the same peripheral blood pressure and ventricular volume that the patient functions with in everyday life, and by preventing an increased left ventricular contractile force. Patients with IHSS usually are treated with β-adrenergic blocking agents and/or Ca^{++} channel blockers, a therapy that should be continued throughout the perioperative period. Inhalation anesthetics reduce myocardial contractility and help maintain cardiac output during surgery.

Intravenous Drug Abuse. The chronic intravenous drug abuser who presents for surgery may have bacterial endocarditis with resultant valvular lesions. Preoperative anticoagulation and antibiotic prophylaxis should be utilized. Other commonly encountered medical problems in i.v. drug abusers include pulmonary fibrosis and hypertension, renal and hepatic insufficiency, hepatitis, and AIDS. Virtually every drug abuser, whether addicted or not, exhibits tolerance to sedatives, narcotics, and anesthetics. Patients who abuse cocaine or other "uppers" may exhibit increased sensitivity to adrenergic agonists and vasoconstrictors.

Disorders of Rhythm. Dysrhythmias in the surgical patient may be benign, an indication of more serious disorders, or life threatening. Because pharmacologic intervention requires drugs with serious side effects, it is critical that physicians distinguish between dysrhythmias that require intervention and those that do not.

Tachycardia. Sinus tachycardia is associated with several conditions, most of which could be corrected or stabilized before surgery. Tachyarrhythmia in an otherwise normal patient is rare and usually is related to stress. A patient with sinus tachycardia should be evaluated for hypervolemia, hypovolemia, hypoxemia, hypercarbia, hyperthermia, drug toxicity, catecholamine-secreting tumors, thyrotoxicosis, and autonomic dysfunction. Atrial fibrillation or flutter with a rapid ventricular rate is usually a sign of serious cardiac dysfunction, such as ischemia or CHF, and the patient will benefit from stabilization before anything but the most emergent surgery is considered.

Bradycardia. Except in aerobically fit sports enthusiasts, bradycardia usually implies a profound conduction system disorder. An unexplained history of dizziness or syncope requires a cardiac evaluation. Patients with temporary or permanent complete atrioventricular (AV) block benefit from preoperative placement of a pacemaker. An incomplete AV block progresses to a complete heart block only rarely. As a precaution, however, many anesthesiologists place an intravenous access sheath in a central vein preoperatively in case a temporary pacemaker is needed.

Pacemakers. Surgical patients with a pacemaker already in place and working generally present little problem to the anesthesiologist. It is important, however, to be aware of the original rhythm problem, the patient's current condition and drug therapy, the exact type of pacemaker in place (the chamber sensed, the chamber paced, the sensing pattern, and the default rhythm), and what to do if it malfunctions because of radio frequency. The default rhythm is that to which the pacemaker resorts when there is a problem with its normal function. Radio frequency from cautery or other instruments has been reported to inhibit firing, especially of demand pacemakers. Should this occur, the pacemaker must immediately be converted to a fixed rate pacer or reprogrammed, neither of which is difficult to accomplish if the necessary equipment, such as a programmer, is available. To avoid this problem altogether, bipolar rather than unipolar cautery should be used. To prevent cautery current from traversing the pacemaker wires, the grounding pad should be placed so that the pacemaker wires are not between it and the operative site.

Ventricular Ectopy. Ventricular ectopy on the preoperative ECG presents a difficult problem. Because certain patterns of premature ventricular contractions (PVCs) have been associated with increased perioperative risk, the current recommendation is that PVCs be further assessed if they occur more frequently than 3 per minute, if they occur in couplets or runs of more than 2, or if they are multifocal. They may be a symptom of drug toxicity, electrolyte abnormality, or ischemia, all of which should be stabilized preoperatively. The next step in such an assessment is usually a 24-hour monitoring sequence for better diagnosis. Many drugs are currently in use to treat PVCs. The medication is begun preoperatively and generally continued during the perioperative period. The greatest risk from PVCs is the potential for tachyarrhythmia and decreased cardiac output.

Respiratory System

The preoperative preparation of the patient should identify the characteristics and consequences of pulmonary disease. While a simple history and physical examination should suffice in most patients, often further investigation is required in order to determine the degree of alteration in volumes, flow patterns, oxygenation, and CO_2 excretion. Table 1A.4 lists important aspects of the preoperative evaluation of the respiratory system that could indicate the need for further workup and a plan for perioperative therapy. If pathology is suspected, a chest x-ray should be obtained to determine the baseline state of the patient's lungs and heart and to establish that there is no reversible condition that should be treated before surgery and anesthesia. In all patients with preexisting pulmonary disease, the goals of preoperative testing and therapy should include those listed in Table 1A.5.

Infectious Diseases. Most infectious diseases of the lungs are reversible to some extent. Chronic bronchitis and bronchiectasis can be improved with antibiotics and measures to improve sputum clearance. Elective surgery should not be undertaken in a patient with acute lower respiratory infections, even if only a local anesthetic is planned. General anesthetics and surgery itself have been shown to result in a temporary interruption of normal immune responses, decreased ciliary clearance of secretions and debris in the respiratory tract, and increased tenacity of secretions. Patients with pneumonia or acute bronchitis are at risk for worsened condition, reactive airway with bronchospasm and laryngospasm, thick sputum obstructing airways, and prolonged hypoxemia. Frequently they require mechanical ventilation in the recovery period. Uncomplicated viral upper respiratory infections probably do not

Table 1A.4.
Preoperative Evaluation of the Respiratory System

History	Dyspnea (with what degree of exertion?)
	Coughing (sputum production?)
	Recent respiratory infection
	Hemoptysis
	Wheezing, use of drugs for asthma
	Pulmonary complications from previous surgery
	Neuromuscular disease
	Smoking
	Age
Examination	Breathing frequency and pattern
	Body habitus (chest wall anatomy, obesity)
	Upper airway evaluation
	Auscultation of lungs
Laboratory	Electrolytes
	Chest x-ray
	Arterial blood gases
	Pulmonary function tests

Table 1A.5.
Preparing the Patient with Pulmonary Disease for Surgery and Anesthesia

- Control infections
  - Eradicate acute infections
  - Suppress chronic infections with antibiotic treatment
- Treat bronchospasm
  - Institute treatment with bronchodilating drugs
  - Document optimal treatment
    - Obtain blood levels of drug
    - Document relief with pulmonary function testing
- Improve sputum clearance
  - Institute pharmacologic therapy
  - Treat with incentive spirometry, postural drainage, or other therapies
  - Prepare patient for postoperative therapy
- Optimize right ventricular performance
  - Treat congestive heart failure
- Institute measures to prevent pulmonary embolism
  - Administer anticoagulants
  - Institute sequential compression of lower extremities
  - Arrange for early mobility
- Encourage reduction or cessation of smoking

markedly increase the risk for surgery and anesthesia if they are not accompanied by bacterial infection and fever. Many physicians, however, would postpone the procedure until the acute phase of the infection has passed, since manipulation of the airway and generalized immunosuppression can lead to a worsening of the infection or bacterial superinfection.

Approximately one-third of American adults smoke cigarettes. Smoking results in increased airway irritability, sputum production, decreased oxygen-carrying capacity, and obstructive airway disease. Cessation 2–3 months before surgery allows for maximal reversal of these effects. Sputum production and airway hyperreactivity will not diminish appreciably unless the patient quits smoking more than a few weeks before surgery. However, carboxyhemoglobin levels will revert to normal within a day or so with corresponding improvement in oxygen delivery to tissues.

Chronic Obstructive Pulmonary Diseases. Chronic obstructive pulmonary diseases make the patient susceptible to bronchospasm and laryngospasm with airway manipulation. In addition to preoperative control of chronic infection and sputum mobilization, preparation of the patient with severe symptoms should include an assessment of expiratory flow patterns with pulmonary function testing, a chest x-ray to determine the extent of bullae formation, and testing of blood gases on room air to determine the patient's baseline.

For these patients the course of surgery usually is uneventful, as most anesthetic agents have a relaxing effect on bronchiolar smooth muscle. Postoperatively, however, these patients must be monitored as they assume spontaneous respiration and manage their secretions in the presence of continued sedation, narcotic suppression of respiratory drive, and pain-induced immobility. While it may seem that regional anesthesia would be preferable to general anesthesia with intubation and prolonged sedation, often it is not. The supine (or any other) position decreases chest compliance and a high level of motor blockade diminishes the contribution of intercostal and abdominal muscles to expiration. Also, during regional anesthesia the patient might cough; the anesthesiologist could do nothing to control that cough short of inducing complete muscle relaxation, which would require intubation and ventilation.

Asthma. Asthmatic patients should be in remission at the time of surgery and anesthesia, but even so present an increased risk of bronchospasm on manipulation of the airway, intubation, and whenever surgical stimulation results in an autonomic response. Asthma is controlled in the perioperative period by maintaining a therapeutic level of the patient's usual medication, by avoiding drugs with histamine-releasing or bronchoconstricting effects, and by using a stress-free anesthetic. Many patients use inhalers to control their attacks, and these can be used just before induction and on emergence, as well as during anesthesia. It is important that the patient's preoperative history include information about current or recent use of oral or inhaled steroid preparations both perioperatively and postoperatively so that steroid coverage can be maintained (see the section on adrenal insufficiency).

Nervous System

Patients with preexisting neurological conditions present varied problems during surgery, most of which can be anticipated if assessment and preparation are complete. Increased intracranial pressure and cerebrovascular insufficiency are perhaps the most difficult to manage, and acute or chronic spinal cord disorders present many dilemmas. Chronic neurological conditions present less of a management problem, but usually coexist with other factors associated with debilitation that the anesthesiologist must consider preoperatively.

Table 1A.6.
Signs and Symptoms of Increased ICP

Headache
Neck rigidity
Projectile vomiting
Blurred vision
Somnolence
Coma
Papilledema
Absent arterial pulsation in disc
Systolic hypertension
Bradycardia
Respiratory irregularity
Noncardiogenic pulmonary edema

Increased Intracranial Pressure. The most commonly occurring conditions associated with increased intracranial pressure include tumor, trauma, hydrocephalus, and intracranial bleeding. Increased ICP usually accompanies hepatic failure, severe hyperglycemia with or without ketoacidosis, acute hyponatremia or water intoxication, myxedema coma, and eclampsia. Preoperative management is the same regardless of whether the surgical procedure is designed to relieve the intracranial hypertension. The most common methods of reducing ICP are diuresis to decrease cellular water content, steroids to decrease cellular water and stabilize the blood-brain barrier, and acute hyperventilation to decrease intracranial volume by cerebral vasoconstriction. Diuresis and steroids provide chronic treatment, while hyperventilation is effective only for 24–36 hours.

Hyperventilation is used in only the most extreme cases, since it requires endotracheal intubation and mechanical ventilation in the intensive care unit.

Patients with increasing ICP are at risk for profound brainstem damage and death caused by herniation of the cerebellar tonsils through the foramen magnum. Most anesthetic drugs—as well as glucose, fluid, and blood pressure alterations—exacerbate the condition. Spinal fluid drainage, intentional or not, may also result in herniation if an acute loss of CSF pressure occurs. Signs and symptoms of increased ICP that may be observed preoperatively are listed in Table 1A.6.

When a patient presents for anesthesia with increased ICP, management consists of reducing the impact of surgical stimulation that further increases intracranial hypertension. If responsive, the patient is asked to hyperventilate voluntarily before induction of anesthesia. All of the i.v. induction agents except ketamine profoundly decrease cerebral blood flow and metabolism, and so are particularly useful in this situation. Intravenous lidocaine (1–1.5 mg/kg) is very effective 1–2 minutes before intubation to prevent the increased cerebral blood flow associated with this very stimulating event.

Anesthesia should be tailored to prevent sympathetic response to surgical stimulation, hypercarbia, and increased venous pressure that may be associated with coughing on the endotracheal tube or "fighting" the ventilator. It is generally accepted now that inhalation agents in moderate concentrations do not cause further intracranial hypertension when used in conjunction with hyperventilation ($Pa{CO_2} \leq 25$).

Cerebrovascular Insufficiency. Cerebrovascular insufficiency may be acute, chronic, or intermittent. Elderly patients with carotid artery disease and flow impairment frequently present for unrelated surgical procedures, their only finding being an asymptomatic carotid bruit. Carotid disease that is neither symptomatic nor marked by ulcerated plaques need not be corrected before elective surgery; but even if carotid disease has been "corrected," it is safe to assume that significant intracerebral vascular disease remains.

If a patient presents with suspected cerebrovascular insufficiency, measures that should be taken to prevent an ischemic episode intraoperatively include administering anticoagulants and cerebral vasodilators, manipulating cerebral perfusion pressure, avoiding cerebral vasoconstriction by maintaining $Pa{CO_2}$ in the normal range, and using anesthetics known to decrease cerebral metabolic rate such as the i.v. agents and isoflurane. As with cardiovascular disorders, in cerebrovascular disorders the acceptable range of intraoperative values is chosen preoperatively when the patient is awake and asymptomatic.

Surgical patients who have previously suffered a cerebrovascular accident may suffer from a wide variety of related problems that require special attention and preparation. Bedridden patients are often cachectic and hypovolemic; they have skin breakdown, bony demineralization, and autonomic dysfunction. Cachexia leads to poor wound healing, infection, and hypoproteinemia-induced edema. It can be corrected by a period of preoperative nutritional support. Skin and bony abnormalities place the patient at risk for pressure sores and fractures during and after surgery. Hypovolemia and autonomic dysfunction make it difficult to manage intraoperative and postoperative blood volume changes without further risk to the central nervous system. Chronic denervation leads to life-threatening hyperkalemia in response to depolarizing muscle relaxants. Renal function is frequently compromised, leading to altered pharmacokinetics of anesthetic drugs and adjuncts. In the bedridden patient, postoperative respiratory and thromboembolic complications are frequent. Methods like incentive spirometry and chest physical therapy must be used to prevent atelectasis and congestion. Thromboembolism must be prevented using physical therapy, anticoagulation, pneumatic stockings, and frequent position changes. Finally, the conscious stroke victim may suffer from debilitating depression, which can impede recovery and threaten survival.

Chronic Neuromuscular Disease. Patients with chronic demyelinating diseases, whether bedridden or not, present many of the same problems as stroke patients. Many are treated with steroids or adrenocorticotropic hormone (ACTH) and require perioperative dosages large enough to cover possible acute stress-induced adrenal insufficiency (see adrenal insufficiency). The anesthesiologist should prepare the patient

Table 1A.7.
Causes of Acute Onet of Seizures

Drug intoxication (alcohol, cocaine, amphetamines)
Drug withdrawal (alcohol, narcotics, sedatives, hypnotics, tranquilizers)
Acute hypoxia
Hyponatremia
Hypocalcemia
Hypercalcemia
Neoplasm
Infection
Fever
Uremia
Trauma
Cerebrovascular insufficiency
Cerebrovascular accidents

to expect a postoperative relapse or worsening of symptoms, because these frequently occur despite the best medical management.

Spinal Cord Injury. Acute cord injury, whether caused by compression, trauma, or vascular insufficiency, may leave the patient without sympathetic, motor, and/or sensory function below the level of the lesion. Usually the patient presents for surgery to relieve compression, hoping to reverse but more often to prevent further injury. The patient is often maximally vasodilated and unable to compensate for position and blood volume changes. The patient is at great risk for further cord injury and loss of function while being positioned and during episodes of intraoperative hypotension. Thus, assessment and management of blood volume status is an important part of anesthetic management.

The chronic paraplegic or quadriplegic patient may present with any or all of the conditions previously discussed in debilitated patients. Additionally, patients with high cord lesions (T6 or above) are at risk for sudden severe hypertension and tachycardia with ventricular ectopy caused by autonomic hyperreflexia, which occurs with almost any stimulus below the level of intact cord, including a distended bladder. The frequency and severity of such episodes can be reduced during surgery by complete sensory deafferentation of the surgical site and of the viscera using local, regional, or general anesthesia. Renal, cardiovascular, and psychological dysfunction often are encountered in the cord-injured patient and should be assessed carefully and optimized before surgery.

Epilepsy. The chronic epileptic patient is of concern because of drug therapy. Most anticonvulsants interact with anesthetics because of their effect on the central nervous system and because of the activity they induce in the hepatic microsomal enzyme system, which also metabolizes most anesthetic drugs. If there is an acute onset of seizures during surgery, their cause must be found and treated (see Table 1A.7 for some common causes). Whether acute or chronic, however, they should be controlled as well as possible before surgery, and the medication regimen should be continued throughout surgery.

Table 1A.8.
Medical Conditions Commonly Associated with Diabetes Mellitus

Atherosclerotic disease	Aortic Carotid Cerebrovascular Peripheral
Myocardial ischemia	Silent Angina Myocardial infarction
Microvascular disease	Neurovascular Renal Coronary Retinal
Autonomic dysfunction	Gastroparesis Hypo- and hypervolemia Inadequate baroceptor responses Inadequate sweating Sexual dysfunction
Altered response to infection	
Altered wound healing	

Endocrine Disorders

While virtually every endocrine disorder can affect the patient during the perioperative period, the three most common are diabetes mellitus, adrenal disease, and thyroid disorders.

Diabetes Mellitus. The two types of diabetes mellitus, insulin-dependent (IDDM, Type 1) and non-insulin-dependent (NIDDM, Type 2), have different consequences and treatments. In either type, chronic tight control of blood glucose levels delays onset of complications. Hypertension, myocardial ischemia and dysfunction, renal insufficiency, cerebrovascular insufficiency, peripheral vascular insufficiency, and peripheral neuropathy are all frequently associated with diabetes in the adult, and occasionally in children and are of concern in the perioperative period (see Table 1A.8). Tight control of blood glucose during surgery may increase wound healing and decrease infection rate in Type 1 patients. There is no evidence that it confers any benefit to Type 2 patients except during pregnancy and possibly during cerebral ischemic episodes. Extreme hyperglycemia should be avoided because it can cause cerebral edema, osmotic diuresis, and ketoacidosis in Type 1 patients, and hyperosmolar nonketotic coma in Type 2 patients. Hypoglycemia, on the other hand, can cause hypotension and seizures in either type of diabetic.

In order to control intraoperative glucose levels, it is necessary to have at hand a means of measuring blood glucose. A recommended regimen is to begin with half the usual morning dose of subcutaneous insulin, run a drip of dextrose 5% in water (D_5W) at about 125 mL/hr/

70 kg, and use a sliding scale of regular insulin injections during and after surgery. Blood glucose should be monitored hourly. An alternative plan is to administer a continuous intravenous drip of insulin (at a rate in units/hr = plasma glucose in mg/dL / 150) and a separate drip of 5% glucose, regulated according to hourly blood glucose determinations. A safe blood glucose range is 100–200 mg/dL. Type 2 diabetics usually tolerate a much higher level without side effects, but are at risk for hyperosmolarity as the glucose level approaches 600 mg/dL. It is important to recognize that in the hyperglycemic patient urine output may not be a reliable monitor of blood volume status.

Adrenal Disease

Cushing's Syndrome. The most common cause of Cushing's syndrome is exogenous administration of steroids, which causes the adrenal glands to atrophy because they are not called upon to function. Other causes include (*a*) increased ACTH production secondary to pituitary microadenoma and (*b*) ectopic production of ACTH by tumors of the lung, pancreas, or thymus. Adrenal adenoma or carcinoma accounts for less than 10–20% of noniatrogenic Cushing's disease. Preoperative preparation of the Cushing's patient requires evaluation and control of fluid status, hypertension, and hyperglycemia. If the adrenal glands or the ACTH-secreting tumor are being removed, mineralocorticoid as well as glucocorticoid replacement are commonly begun at the time of tumor removal and continued until the patient can be weaned from them in the postoperative period. If the surgery is for other reasons, a bolus dose of steroid is given on the day of surgery to prevent stress-induced adrenal insufficiency with cardiovascular collapse caused by hypovolemia or inadequate response of blood vessels to vasoconstrictive stimuli (see below).

Adrenal Insufficiency. Primary adrenal insufficiency, or Addison's disease, usually is caused by an autoimmune process that results in destruction of adrenocortical cells. Secondary adrenal insufficiency can be caused by tumor, hemorrhage into the gland, or withdrawal of steroid or ACTH therapy. In addition to a deficiency in steroid hormones, mineralocorticoid deficiency results in electrolyte abnormalities. Addisonian patients usually suffer from hypovolemia, hyponatremia, and hyperkalemia, but do not have severe difficulties unless stressed by infection, injury, or surgery. Addisonian crisis can be prevented or is treated by prompt administration of steroids at a dose equal to 300 mg of hydrocortisone in a 24-hour period and should be given the day of surgery. This dosage has been used because it has been thought to approximate the maximum output of the adrenal glands during a 24-hour period. Recently, however, it has been reported that doses equalling 100 mg per day of hydrocortisone hemisuccinate or hydrocortisone phosphate also prevent addisonian crisis. The steroids can be tapered starting the next day. Patients with mineralocorticoid deficiency are likely to present with hyperkalemic alkalosis, hyponatremia, and hypovolemia. Dysrhythmias in the untreated patient are the result of hyperkalemia.

Pheochromocytoma. While pheochromocytoma is a rare cause of hypertension, 60% of patients with pheochromocytoma who die in the hospital are previously undiagnosed and die during surgery unrelated to their tumor. Inducing anesthesia in the undiagnosed patient can lead to severe hypertension and death. Occasionally, the only clue to pheochromocytoma is a history of unexplained severe hypertension or tachycardia during a previous anesthetic. The signs and symptoms of pheochromocytoma include the presence of unexplained episodic hypertension, tachycardia, flushing, sweating, or headache. Recognizing this disorder can be lifesaving. The patient with a known pheochromocytoma can be well prepared preoperatively with α and occasionally β blockade. The goal of preoperative preparation is control of intermittent hypertension and tachycardia, and normalization of the circulating blood volume and red cell mass. Electrolytes, BUN, and creatinine should be normal before surgery proceeds.

Perioperative mortality from resection of pheochromocytoma has fallen from 40–60% to 0–3% with the introduction of preoperative α-adrenergic blockade. Prazosin or phenoxybenzamine counteract the vasoconstriction induced by surges of catecholamines, as well as restore normal blood volume, control blood pressure, and reduce symptoms. Patients with tachycardia or dysrhythmias also benefit from β blockade but only after α receptors have been blocked. Most patients require a stabilization period of at least 2 weeks before surgery. Surgery can proceed when they no longer experience episodic symptoms. No particular anesthetic technique has been shown to result in a better patient outcome than any other. A smooth perioperative course depends first on preparation and then on monitoring and immediate correction of intraoperative blood volume, blood pressure, and rhythm changes.

Thyroid Disorders

Hyperthyroidism. Hyperthyroidism in surgical patients usually is caused by diffuse multinodular enlargement of the gland (Graves' disease), but can also be caused by pregnancy, thyroiditis, choriocarcinoma, or pituitary adenoma that secretes thyroid-stimulating hormone. In all but the most urgent cases, hyperthyroid patients are treated to reduce all symptoms, especially cardiac, before surgery. Treatment is usually with propylthiouracil or methimazole and 6 weeks may be required before symptoms resolve. Currently, the trend is to treat hyperthyroidism with only iodine and propranolol, with symptoms expected to normalize in 7–14 days. However, this therapy may not normalize cardiac function. All medications should be continued throughout the perioperative period. Table 1A.9 contrasts the signs and symptoms of hyper- and hypothyroidism, and should alert students to suggested routes for preoperative investigation.

If surgery is urgent in the untreated hyperthyroid patient, cardiac symptoms can be stabilized by administering β blockers to control heart rate and hypertension, as

Table 1A.9.
Signs and Symptoms of Thyroid Dysfunction

Hyperthyroid	Hypothyroid
Weight loss	Weight gain
Diarrhea	Slow gastric emptying
Warm, moist skin	Dry "thick" skin
Muscle weakness, wasting	Fatigue, weakness
Menstrual abnormalities	
Nervousness	Slow mentation
Jitteriness, tremor	Slow movement
Heat intolerance	Cold intolerance
Tachycardia	Bradycardia
Cardiomegaly	Cardiomegaly
Atrial fibrillation	
Mitral valve prolapse	
Papillary muscle dysfunction	
Dyspnea, orthopnea	Dyspnea, orthopnea
Congestive failure	Congestive failure
	Impaired free water clearance
	Pericardial and pleural effusions
Anemia, thrombocytopenia	
Increased alkaline phosphatase	
Hypercalcemia	
Bone loss	
	Decreased MAC for anesthetics

well as by monitoring of pulmonary artery and wedge pressure. There is risk, however, of further reducing ventricular function. Attention to intravascular volume status is necessary throughout the perioperative period, especially since most anesthetics cause vasodilation. A "thyroid storm," as evidenced by a sudden onset of fever, severe hypertension, tachycardia, and disorders of consciousness, should be treated immediately with β blockers and iodine, to block the peripheral actions of thyroid hormone. At the same time, a search for precipitating stress such as infection should begin, since successful treatment of thyroid storm depends on controlling both the cause and the effects.

No one anesthetic technique has proved superior in avoiding intraoperative problems in patients with either pheochromocytoma or hyperthyroidism. Of importance are the preoperative preparation, continuation of therapy throughout the operative period, and anticipation of possible problems resulting from hypovolemia or electrolyte, rhythm, or blood pressure abnormalities.

Hypothyroidism. Most hypothyroid patients who come to surgery have been treated with thyroid hormone replacement and have stable cardiovascular systems. Occasionally, untreated myxedematous patients present for emergent procedures and must be managed acutely. T3 hormone can be given intravenously, but must be carefully titrated to avoid myocardial ischemia. Volume and electrolyte status should be carefully monitored, and special measures taken to keep the patient warm. Hypothyroid patients have excessive responses to anesthetics, sedatives, narcotics, and muscle relaxants. Because postoperative ventilatory depression is frequent, the patient and family should be prepared for the possibility of prolonged sleepiness, intubation, and mechanical ventilation after anesthesia.

Table 1A.10.
Manifestations of Renal Failure

Decreased excretion of water and electrolytes
  Edema, pleural and pericardial effusions
  Hyperkalemia
Anemia
Coagulopathy
Neuropathies
  Peripheral
  Autonomic
Hypertension
Atherosclerosis with vascular disease
Pericarditis
Congestive heart failure

Renal Disease

As renal tubular function diminishes, patients become uremic and may present to surgery with varying degrees of renal failure. Chronic hemodialysis reverses many of the effects of uremia. Diabetes and chronic hypertension are the two most frequent causes of chronic renal failure; they must be managed concurrently. Table 1A.10 lists alterations to be expected in patients with renal failure, and suggests steps to take in their preoperative evaluation and preparation.

Cardiovascular stability is difficult to achieve in patients with renal disease because of anesthetic-induced depression, surgical-stress-induced catecholamine activity, and the large shifts in blood volume that occur during surgery. Remaining renal function is preserved only by maintaining renal perfusion close to baseline. Because renal excretion is so important in eliminating the intravenous agents and muscle relaxants, doses of anesthetics must be carefully tailored based on remaining renal function to avoid prolonged postoperative depression. Urine output should be carefully monitored in patients with partial renal function. If diuretics are used or if the patient is hyperglycemic, however, urine output does not reflect the patient's volume status and invasive monitoring becomes necessary.

If patients with chronic renal failure come to surgery immediately after dialysis, they present with a low circulating blood volume. The anesthesiologist is concerned both with maintaining the patency of the vascular access site for hemodialysis and with the protection of other organ systems. Frequently, immediate postoperative dialysis is required because of the blood or fluid needed to maintain intraoperative homeostasis or to correct electrolyte abnormalities. This dialysis may be accomplished in the PACU.

Gastrointestinal System

This section will discuss the patient presenting to surgery with a full stomach, bowel obstruction, morbid obesity, or hepatic failure.

Full Stomach. Patients with more than 25 mL of gastric content with a pH of less than 2.5 have been shown to be at increased risk for pulmonary aspiration syndrome. Preoperative treatment and special induction techniques can reduce this risk to near zero; a high level of suspicion at the time of the preoperative evaluation is often lifesaving. Table 1.2 (in the main body of the chapter) summarizes the conditions that would lead to suspicion of a patient with a full stomach.

The preoperative preparation of the patient with a full stomach, designed to reduce the volume and increase the pH of the gastric contents, is discussed in the section on premedication. Induction of anesthesia must proceed with extreme caution even after pharmacologic preparation, because once the protective airway reflexes are abolished there is no way aspiration can be prevented if regurgitation occurs. The risk of aspiration is not eliminated by inserting a nasogastric tube to suction the stomach or by using a regional anesthetic technique. It is always possible for the patient to lose consciousness or control of the airway should things not go as planned.

Bowel Obstruction. Patients presenting for surgery with bowel obstruction are often critically ill, and little time can be spared for preoperative preparation. Bowel obstruction rapidly leads to perforation, peritonitis, and septic shock, especially in the elderly or chronically ill patient. These patients are assumed to be hypovolemic, to have electrolyte abnormalities, and to have full stomachs not completely drained by nasogastric suction. If the obstruction has been protracted, abdominal distention and pain will interfere with lung expansion; there can be an accompanying atelectasis and pleural effusion that interfere with efficient oxygenation. The profound hypovolemia usually accompanying this condition must be reversed before anesthesia can be induced safely. Even in the elderly patient with cardiovascular disease, several liters of crystalloid solution can be infused rapidly if filling pressures are monitored. Preoperative monitoring of urinary output is a useful guide to the adequacy of volume replacement.

The most life-threatening manifestation of bowel obstruction is septic shock, which occurs when the integrity of the bowel mucosa is lost allowing Gram-negative bacteremia to ensue. Septic shock usually presents as a hyperdynamic state with hypotension and high fever. When the patient is hypovolemic, as is usually the case with a bowel obstruction or perforation, the hyperdynamic state may not be evidenced until fluid resuscitation has occurred. Gram-negative bacteremia results in a 47% mortality rate.

Early in septic shock, bacterial endotoxin activates mediators that act on smooth muscle causing vasodilation and myocardial depression. These effects are impossible to reverse, thus making the management of septic shock particularly difficult. The heart tries to compensate by increasing both rate and contractility, but if blood volume is low this compensation will not be adequate and blood pressure will fall. Because of inadequate tissue perfusion, the patient becomes acidotic and thus unable to respond to catecholamines or other agents used to support the cardiovascular system.

Initial treatment consists of antibiotics and volume expansion. Fluid is infused rapidly, guided by careful hemodynamic and urine output monitoring and frequent determinations of pH, blood lactate, and mixed venous O_2 saturations to assess tissue perfusion. Antibodies to bind endotoxin have been used experimentally. Vasoconstrictors should be used only when volume has been restored and systemic vascular resistance continues to remain low. Myocardial contractility is improved with low-dose dopamine, dobutamine, amrinone, or epinephrine, which may be added to the volume restoration to increase cardiac output. High-dose corticosteroid therapy has been shown to be ineffective. Patients in septic shock often develop coagulopathies that are treated before and during surgery.

Controversy exists whether fluid resuscitation should be carried out with crystalloid or colloid solutions. Colloid solutions include albumin, plasma, and hetastarch (Hespan). Proponents of crystalloid therapy cite the lower cost, decreased exposure to blood donors, less lung water accumulation, and no difference in outcome between the two. Resuscitation with crystalloid solutions requires 3–4 times as much volume, resulting in postresuscitation edema that may require a longer period of intensive care. Patients with bowel obstruction and septic shock require a period of postoperative ventilation regardless of the resuscitation fluid therapy. As in any critical illness, red cell transfusions should be used to maintain adequate oxygen-carrying capacity. While there is controversy over the optimal hematocrit, most critical care specialists agree that a hemoglobin level of over 10 g/dL blood is usually necessary.

Morbid Obesity. Morbid obesity, defined as being twice the ideal body weight, increases the risk of anesthesia and surgery 2–3 times. Many of the pulmonary and cardiovascular problems stem from the fact that pulmonary compliance is mechanically reduced by the mass of fat on the chest wall and in the abdomen. Functional residual capacity also is diminished in these patients. The increased work of breathing results in an increased oxygen cost at the same time oxygenation is reduced because of ventilation-perfusion abnormalities due to incomplete expansion. These problems are magnified when the patient lies down. The high circulating blood volume and cardiac output are secondary to the large tissue mass that must be perfused. Pulmonary and systemic hypertension are caused in part by the high blood volume and relative hypoxemia, but also by hyperlipidemia and other risk factors for cardiovascular disease. Polycythemia results from chronic hypoxemia. Sleep apnea, occurring initially because of mechanical obstruction to the upper airway, may become central over time, increasing the respiratory depressant effects of anesthetics, sedatives, and narcotics. Table 1A.11 lists the medical problems common in morbidly obese patients; the preoperative evaluation should search for possible sources of increased risk.

Table 1A.11.
Conditions Associated with Morbid Obesity

Pulmonary
Increased work of breathing
Restrictive lung disease
Hypoxemia
Pulmonary hypertension
Periodic alveolar hypoventilation (sleep apnea)
Pickwickian syndrome
Cardiovascular
Increased circulating blood volume
Increased cardiac output
Systemic hypertension
Biventricular failure
Ischemic heart disease
Other
Diabetes mellitus
Hyperlipidemia
Polycythemia
Liver failure
Increased gastric volume and acidity
Psychological problems
Anatomy: difficult airway, i.v. access, BP measurement, etc.

These cardiovascular and respiratory abnormalities may eventually result in the Pickwickian syndrome, which consists of chronic alveolar hypoventilation, hypoxemia, hypercarbia, congestive heart failure, and daytime somnolence. Pickwickian patients, representing 5–10% of all morbidly obese patients, may develop acute pulmonary edema and die of dysrhythmias when they lie down. They are thus at great risk of death during surgery. Even the most "normal" morbidly obese patient needs supplemental oxygen from the time of lying down on the operating table until several days postoperatively. These patients also should be considered to have a full stomach, no matter how long they have fasted, because of high intra-abdominal pressure. As in all patients, diabetes and hypertension should be treated carefully. The status of myocardial oxygenation should be assessed before surgery and perioperative management should proceed as though the patient were at risk from congestive failure and myocardial ischemia. Because the most prevalent cause of perioperative morbidity in this population is thromboembolic, the patient must be encouraged to resume activity early in the postoperative period. Low-dose anticoagulation regimes are also frequently employed. Postoperative ventilatory support can be avoided if there has been appropriate preoperative preparation and if the nursing staff is attentive. Because morbidly obese patients often suffer from depression and a poor self-image, their psychological state also should be attended to during this time. Their contribution to their own recovery is essential.

Liver Failure. Preoperative evaluation should begin with an examination of hepatic function that includes bilirubin, enzymes, and coagulation profile. A thorough evaluation of the cardiovascular and respiratory systems is essential. The physiological consequences of hepatic failure are summarized in Table 1A.12.

Table 1A.12.
Conditions Associated with Liver Disease

Hepatic dysfunction
Hyperbilirubinemia
Altered drug metabolism and excretion
Coagulopathy
Hypoglycemia
Electrolyte abnormalities
Portal hypertension
Ascites
Variceal bleeding
Cardiopulmonary
Peripheral vasodilation
Decreased sensitivity to catecholamines
Increased circulating blood volume
Intrapulmonary and extrapulmonary shunting
Increased cardiac output
Cardiomyopathy
Renal insufficiency
Hepatic encephalopathy

Not much can be done to improve the overall condition of the patient in end-stage liver failure, but if surgery is required the preoperative preparation should correct any fluid, electrolyte, and coagulation abnormalities. The presence of ascites usually is associated with hypoproteinemia and hypoxemia, both of which can be treated. Esophageal varices are cause for concern even if they are not actively bleeding, especially if the surgery is to reduce portal hypertension: temporary occlusion of the portal vein or vena cava often results in resumption of active bleeding requiring major blood transfusions. The coagulopathy of liver failure can be treated with fresh frozen plasma and platelet transfusions. Support of the cardiovascular system requires monitored blood volume resuscitation to maintain urine output and tissue oxygenation. Hypoglycemia is an ongoing concern, even in the early stages of liver disease, requiring that blood glucose levels be checked often before and during surgery. Because hepatic encephalopathy is accompanied by increased intracranial pressure, appropriate precautions must be taken to avoid further increases in intracranial pressure.

The chronic alcoholic patient, whether or not in hepatic failure, requires special consideration. Such a patient is suffering from a severe multisystem disease that includes cardiomyopathy, nutritional deficiencies, peripheral and central nervous system abnormalities, and often pulmonary dysfunction as well. Alcoholic cardiomyopathy manifests as cardiomegaly and congestive heart failure, and often is not amenable to treatment. The patient with a failing heart, no matter what the cause, should be prepared and managed as discussed above in the section on cardiac diseases. Nutritional deficiency often results in megaloblastic anemia, and red cell mass may be severely deficient. Alcoholics often are cigarette smokers and so suffer from chronic lung disease. If they are cirrhotic, intrapulmonary shunting with hypoxemia may occur. Finally, because acute alcohol withdrawal may occur during surgery, prophylactic treatment with benzodiazepines may be warranted when a history of recent intake or past delirium tremens indicates the possibility of withdrawal during the perioperative period.

Hematologic Disorders

Anemia and Polycythemia. Both anemia and polycythemia need to be corrected preoperatively, but controversy exists as to what optimum hemoglobin and hematocrit levels should be. Patients with chronic anemia due to hematologic disease or renal failure do well with a hemoglobin level in the range of 6–8 g/dL, and there is no evidence that transfusing them up to a more normal level improves their perioperative course. On the other hand, if the anemia is acute or if the patient is unable to compensate with increased cardiac output, the reduction in oxygen-carrying capacity that results from hemoglobin of less than 8 g/dL can be detrimental. A preoperative hemoglobin level of at least 10 g/dL has historical been suggested as a cutoff point for elective surgery, but conclusive data showing that this practice results in a better patient outcome are lacking, and many anesthesiologists now allow patients to come to surgery with hematocrits of 20% if they are otherwise normal. Current practice is to individualize therapy after the cause of anemia is discovered and the level of compensation assessed. Polycythemia, whatever the cause, reduces blood flow to tissues and places the patient at increased risk for thromboembolism. It is easily managed preoperatively by phlebotomy, with the blood being stored should the patient require transfusion at a later time.

Sickle Cell Hemoglobinopathies. Hemoglobin S (Hb S) causes erythrocytes to distort and aggregate when in an environment of decreased oxygen. Patients with sickle cell trait (Hb A-S) are probably not at increased risk during anesthesia and surgery, because their cells do not sickle until the hemoglobin saturation falls below 20%. Patients with sickle cell disease (Hb S-S) and sickle cell-thalassemia disease (Hb S-C) are anemic because of failure of the bone marrow to keep up with erythrocyte destruction. They suffer from hemolytic crises and organ infarctions because of circulatory obstruction. Sickling occurs with decreased arterial oxygen content, with acidosis, hypothermia, and blood stasis. It occurs in proportion to the level of Hb S. Preoperative preparation of patients with sickle cell disease or sickle-thalassemia requires hemoglobin electrophoresis to determine the level of Hb S. Exchange transfusions usually are carried out until the proportion of Hb S to normal red blood cells is less than 40%, but data linking this practice to a better outcome are lacking. Intraoperative management includes keeping the patient oxygenated, warm, and hydrated. Measures to avoid venous stasis include elevating the legs and using sequential compression boots. Postoperatively, patients with sickle cell hemoglobinopathies should be given supplemental oxygen until they demonstrate prolonged normal oxygen saturation on room air.

Coagulopathies. Specific coagulopathies should be corrected preoperatively with replacement of the deficient factors. Platelet dysfunction is associated with many chronic medical conditions, as well as with aspirin or other anti-inflammatory agents. It is generally agreed that only about 30–50,000 functioning platelets/mm^3 are necessary for normal coagulation, but obtaining a platelet count does not assess their function. If there is suspicion of platelet abnormality, a bleeding time or specific tests for platelet function should be obtained, with platelet transfusions administered as necessary. Patients with chronic liver failure and uremia often lack many coagulation factors; they are best evaluated by obtaining a prothrombin time (PT) and partial thromboplastin time (PTT). They are also likely to have dysfunctioning platelets, although their numbers may be normal. Fresh frozen plasma and platelet transfusions usually restore coagulation function to a level that will allow surgical hemostasis.

SUGGESTED READINGS

Firestone LL, Lebowitz PW, Cook CE. Clinical procedures of the Massachusetts General Hospital. 3rd ed. Boston: Little, Brown, 1988.

Levine RD. Anesthesiology: a manual for medical students. Philadelphia: JB Lippincott, 1984.

Liu PL, ed. Principles and procedures in anesthesiology. Philadelphia: JB Lippincott, 1992.

Mulroy MF. Regional anesthesia: an illustrated procedural guide. Boston: Little, Brown, 1989.

Roizen MF. Anesthetic implications of concurrent diseases. In: Miller RM, ed. Anesthesia. 3rd ed. New York: Churchill Livingstone, 1989:255–358.

Roizen MF. Routine preoperative evaluation. In: Miller RM, ed. Anesthesia. 3rd ed. New York: Churchill Livingstone, 1989:225–254.

Schweitzer M. Monitoring under anesthesia. In: DeKornfeld TJ, ed. Anesthesiology: a concise textbook. New York: Medical Examination Publishing, 1986.

Scott DB. Acute pain management. In: Cousins MJ, Bridenbaugh PO, eds. Neural blockade in clinical anesthesia and the management of pain. 2nd ed. Philadelphia: JB Lippincott, 1988:861–883.

Skills

1. Perform a preoperative evaluation for a healthy patient undergoing an uncomplicated surgery, including the following: history, pertinent physical examination, assessment, laboratory data required, and preoperative medication.
2. Given a list of several surgical procedures, indicate whether local, regional, general, or any combination of anesthetics would be appropriate.
3. Obtain informed consent from patients for general, regional, and local anesthetics.
4. Demonstrate ability to start large-bore i.v.s in surgical patients.
5. Interpret an anesthetic record on a surgical procedure that you have witnessed.

6. Demonstrate ability to manage the airway in an unconscious patient using oropharyngeal or nasopharyngeal airways and a mask.
7. Demonstrate ability to interpret data from the following operating room monitors: ECG, arterial line tracing, capnograph, CVP, pulmonary arterial line.

Study Questions

1. Why is it important to schedule a visit with the anesthesiologist as early as possible after surgery is scheduled?
2. If a patient is scheduled for local anesthesia for anything more than a "lump or bump," why is an empty stomach, laboratory workup, and an i.v. necessary?
3. Who is at risk for aspiration pneumonitis in the perioperative period, and how can that risk be minimized?
4. What do the following contribute to general anesthesia: short-acting barbiturates, depolarizing relaxants, inhalational agents, narcotics, muscle relaxants?
5. What monitoring is required by the American Society of Anesthesiologists for every patient under the care of an anesthesiologist in the operating room?
6. List several ways to use narcotics in the treatment of acute pain.
7. Calculate the maximum value of 1% Xylocaine that can be given to a 60-kg woman undergoing removal of a large lipoma of the thigh.
8. What is the rationale for stabilizing the treatment of hypertension in the preoperative period? Of CHF? Of ischemic heart disease?
9. Describe an appropriate workup and preoperative treatment regimen for a patient with severe chronic obstructive lung disease.
10. Describe measures taken before and during anesthesia to reduce the possibility of brainstem ischemia in patients with severely increased intracranial pressure.
11. Describe two ways of treating diabetes during the perioperative period.
12. Why is the morbidly obese patient at increased risk from surgery and anesthesia?

2

Pediatric Surgery: Surgical Diseases of Children

Mary Alice Helikson, M.D.
Philip J. Wolfson, M.D.

ASSUMPTIONS

The student has a working knowledge of human embryology.

The student understands the physiologic differences between neonates, children, and adults.

The student is sensitive to the emotional needs of pediatric patients and is able to communicate effectively with the patients and their families.

OBJECTIVES

PERIOPERATIVE MANAGEMENT OF THE PEDIATRIC SURGICAL PATIENT

1. Compare the intracellular and extracellular fluid compartments in children and adults. Calculate daily fluid and electrolyte requirements for children based on preexisting deficits, maintenance requirements, and abnormal ongoing losses.
2. Compare the indications for enteral versus parenteral nutrition in pediatric surgical patients, and explain how each type of nutritional support may be provided.
3. Define respiratory failure and describe how it may be managed with supplemental oxygen, different types of ventilators, and extracorporeal membrane oxygenation (ECMO).
4. Outline the appropriate preoperative preparations for children, and list the important components of their operating room environment.
5. Discuss the emotional needs of children undergoing operations. Describe various pain control measures that may be provided postoperatively.

NEONATAL SURGICAL CONDITIONS

1. Explain the pathophysiology of congenital diaphragmatic hernias and relate it to the clinical presentation, appropriate management, and mortality rate of patients.
2. Illustrate the different anatomical configurations of esophageal atresia and tracheoesophageal fistula, and describe how they are diagnosed and treated.
3. List the clinical manifestations of congenital intestinal obstruction. Describe the common causes of congenital obstruction at each level of the intestinal tract.
4. Describe the various types of anorectal malformations and relate their anatomy to treatment and prognosis.
5. Discuss the etiology, clinical presentation, and treatment of necrotizing enterocolitis.
6. Discuss the management of an infant with jaundice, particularly as it relates to biliary atresia.
7. Compare omphalocele and gastroschisis in terms of embryology, appearance, associated anomalies, and management.
8. List the pros, cons, and contraindications to neonatal circumcision.

SURGICAL CONDITIONS IN THE OLDER CHILD

1. Describe the anatomical differences between an inguinal hernia, communicating hydrocele, and noncommunicating hydrocele, and discuss the rationale for the treatment of each.
2. Discuss the proper timing for repair of umbilical hernias.
3. Discuss the management of a boy with an undescended testicle, including the optimal age and reasons for orchidopexy.
4. Describe the typical patient with pyloric stenosis, the optimal techniques for demonstration of the "olive," and the proper management of the condition.
5. Compare the presentations of acute inflammatory conditions of the abdomen in young children and adults.

6. Describe the clinical manifestations of nonperforated and perforated appendicitis in children.
7. Describe the typical patient with intussusception, the importance of early recognition, and the treatment.
8. Discuss the three common complications of a Meckel's diverticulum.
9. List the common causes and characteristics of gastrointestinal bleeding in the neonate, the young child, and the adolescent.
10. Describe the symptomatology and potential complications of gastroesophageal reflux in infants and children, and outline the diagnostic workup and indications for surgery.
11. Contrast hemangiomas and vascular malformations in terms of appearance, natural history, and treatment.

TUMORS

1. List the common malignancies of childhood and their relative incidence.
2. Describe the treatment options for chronic venous access in children.
3. For each of the following pediatric tumors, discuss the age of presentation, clinical manifestations, diagnostic workup, approach to treatment, and prognosis: (*a*) neuroblastoma, (*b*) Wilms' tumor, (*c*) hepatic tumors, (*d*) rhabdomyosarcoma, (*e*) sacrococcygeal teratoma, and (*f*) lymphoma.

TRAUMA

1. List the major differences between pediatric and adult trauma.
2. In order of priority, outline the principal steps in the resuscitation of the severely injured child.
3. Discuss the management of the pediatric accident victim with injuries to the (*a*) head, (*b*) chest, (*c*) abdomen, and (*d*) urinary system.
4. Outline those characteristics of the pediatric trauma victim that raise the possibility of child abuse.
5. Describe the treatment of the pediatric burn patient, with emphasis on fluid resuscitation and care of the burn wound.
6. Outline the management plan for a child who may have aspirated or ingested a foreign object.

The principles involved in managing infants and children with surgical diseases are in many ways similar to those for adults; however, important differences must be kept in mind. Many of the congenital anomalies that are dealt with surgically in children have no counterpart in older individuals and indeed would be lethal if not corrected promptly in early childhood. Functionally, young children are not merely small adults; their unique metabolic needs and often limited reserves demand special attention in order to maintain their physiological processes well within the narrow range of normality. On the other hand, children have a tremendous capacity for repair and regeneration and usually lack many of the preexisting chronic illnesses that so often afflict their elders. If handled skillfully, these young individuals have the ability to recover rapidly from even major surgical procedures and subsequently to live long and productive lives. Finally, pediatric surgical patients and their parents have special emotional needs. The physician must be attentive to these needs during what is frequently a very trying time for the entire family.

Perioperative Management of the Pediatric Surgical Patient

Fluids and Electrolytes

Fluid and electrolyte management of pediatric patients must be extremely precise if these patients are to maintain homeostasis. Compared to adults, infants and children have greater metabolic demands and a much more rapid turnover of body water and electrolytes. Furthermore, because the neonatal kidney has a limited ability to concentrate urine and also must excrete a relatively fixed quantity of sodium, it is unable to conserve sodium and water effectively when these supplies are limited, or to excrete sodium sufficiently when it is present in excess. In addition, relatively small amounts of fluids and electrolytes can make big differences in children, to whom the actual quantities given are miniscule compared to those given adults. Although children's needs may be first estimated according to standard formulas, frequent readjustments must be made based on careful monitoring of the patient's condition.

Neonates have approximately 75% of their weight as total body water (TBW), a significantly higher proportion than the adult pool of 55–60% (Fig. 2.1). This higher TBW is attributed to the larger quantity of extracellular fluid (ECF) in children; ECF makes up 40% of weight for infants and 20% of weight for adults. Extremely premature infants have even more TBW, as much as 80% of their weight, of which 50% is ECF. At birth the ECF is even more expanded, and during the first week of life approximately 5% of weight is lost as this surplus water is excreted.

In calculating fluid and electrolyte requirements for children who are unable to receive enteral feeds, the following quantities must be considered:

1. Replacement of preexisting deficits
2. Maintenance requirements
3. Replacement of ongoing abnormal losses

Preexisting Deficits. Children with acute surgical illnesses may have significant fluid and electrolyte deficits from poor oral intake, vomiting, diarrhea, peritonitis, sepsis, burns, or hemorrhage. Intravascular volume must be rapidly restored in order to maintain adequate tissue perfusion for normal organ function, particularly if the child requires an urgent operation. Table 2.1 indicates various degrees of dehydration, describes their clinical signs, and estimates the quantities of fluid necessary for correction. Since most surgical diseases produce isotonic dehydration, these deficits are usually

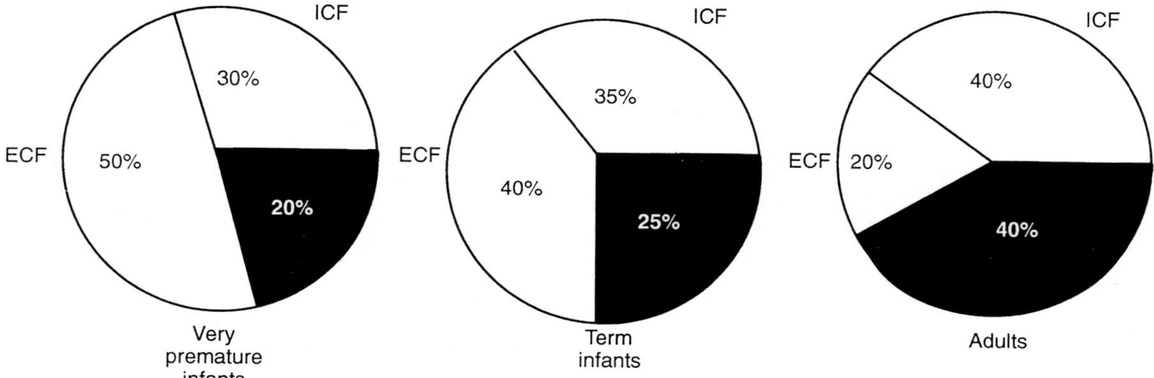

Figure 2.1. Body fluid compartments in very premature infants, term infants, and adults. Unshaded areas represent percentage of body weight as total body water. ECF, extracellular fluid; ICF, intracellular fluid.

Table 2.1.
Intravenous Replacement of Preexisting Deficits

Degree of Dehydration % of Weight Loss	Clinical Findings	Fluid Required for Correction (mL/kg)
Mild—5	Irritability, dry mucous membranes, oliguria	50
Moderate—8	Increased severity of above, decreased skin turgor, sunken eyes, fever, tachycardia	80
Severe—12	Lethargy, hypotonia, hypotension, poor capillary refill, uremia, acidosis	120

corrected with a balanced salt solution. Lactated Ringer's solution is often preferred, because its electrolyte constituents closely resemble those of plasma. Although pediatricians often aim to correct dehydration over 24 hours, rehydration should proceed much more rapidly if the child requires an urgent operation and/or is in shock. Fluid boluses may be infused in 20 mL/kg aliquots every 10 to 20 minutes as necessary, while the patient is closely monitored for signs of improvement.

In patients with severe sodium deficits, hyponatremia may be reversed with additional sodium equal to the deficit in mEq measured in the serum, multiplied by the calculated ECF, as follows:

$$\text{Na needed (mEq)} = (138 - \text{measured serum Na}) \text{ (mEq)} \times (0.35 \text{ weight}) \text{ (kg)}$$

Potassium deficits may be replaced by adding up to 40 mEq of KCl to each liter of intravenous fluids (instead of the usual 20 mEq/L—see below).

Children who are significantly anemic or are actively bleeding may require blood transfusions. Although a hemoglobin level of 10 g/dL is usually adequate for children, neonates require levels closer to 15 g/dL. Component therapy is preferred. Packed red cells may be administered in pediatric "units" of 10 mL/kg, which is roughly equivalent to a standard unit in an adult. Total blood volume is 0.85 mL/kg in infants. With massive transfusions, platelets and fresh frozen plasma (to restore clotting factors) are needed as well.

Maintenance Requirements. Maintenance fluids and electrolytes are those quantities that must be provided to compensate for renal excretion and for insensible losses through the skin and lungs. The amount of water required can be calculated from the following formula:

100 mL/kg/day (or 4 mL/kg/hr) up to 10 kg
+ 50 mL/kg/day (or 2 mL/kg/hr) from 11 kg to 20 kg
+ 20 mL/kg/day (or 1 mL/kg/hr) over 20 kg
= total maintenance requirement

Exceptions to the above formula include the following conditions: (*a*) in premature infants, in whom evaporation from the very thin skin permits water losses of up to twice the standard maintenance calculations; (*b*) during the first few days of life, when the need to eliminate surplus ECF lowers the maintenance requirement to 65–100 mL/kg/day; and (*c*) during fever and various disease states (such as sepsis), when the metabolic rate is elevated and fluid needs are increased.

Daily requirements for electrolytes are:

sodium, 3 mEq/kg/day
potassium, 2 mEq/kg/day

In addition, a minimal quantity of glucose must be provided as substrate for oxidation in order to provide for some protein sparing and to avoid hypoglycemia. These constituents can all be provided by

D5% in 0.25 normal saline + 20 mEq/liter KCl

at the infusion rate as calculated above.

Abnormal Ongoing Losses. Abnormal losses include measurable as well as immeasurable "third-space" fluid losses. Measurable losses refer to abnormal external drainage and in the surgical patient usually arise from the gastrointestinal tract or from various drainage tubes. These losses are most accurately replaced on a volume-for-volume basis. Ideally, the electrolyte content of the particular fluid to be replaced can be analyzed directly. Alternatively, gastric drainage can be approximated as D5% in 0.5 normal saline + 10 mEq/liter KCl. Alimentary tract losses distal to the pylorus can be replaced with lactated Ringer's solution. Third-space losses refer to those fluids and electrolytes that are pathologically sequestered within the body and are neither in equilibrium nor available to the intravascular space. In children with surgical diseases, such fluid can accumulate in the gastrointestinal tract from obstruction and inflammation, in body cavities as ascites and pleural effusions, and diffusely as edema from the leaky capillary syndrome that accompanies shock. Operative manipulation can produce edema in the tissues from the direct trauma itself.

Third-space losses cannot be directly measured, and their intravenous replacement must therefore be approximated. Sequestered fluid is almost always isotonic, and its replacement may be given as balanced salt solution. One method to provide for the expected regional fluid loss from operative trauma is to run the intravenous fluids at 1 1/2 to 2 times maintenance for the first 24 hours postoperatively, depending on the magnitude of the operation.

The adequacy of intravenous fluid therapy can only be determined by observing the response of the patient. Useful parameters are level of activity, color, skin turgor and temperature, heart rate, and blood pressure. Most helpful is the urine output, which should exceed 1–2 mL/kg/hour. Children receiving fluids solely as intravenous infusions should have serum electrolytes every other day measured at least.

Nutrition

The well-nourished child who will be eating within a few days of his or her operation does not need nutritional support other than the basic fluids and electrolytes as outlined above. On the other hand, the ability to provide total parenteral nutrition (TPN) indefinitely for any sized patient allows survival for many children who otherwise would succumb during the perioperative period. Because of their limited nutritional reserves, small children, and especially preterm infants, have much greater energy needs than adults. Severe consequences of malnutrition can thus develop very rapidly, including lack of growth, impaired organ function, immunological incompetence, and the inability to heal wounds.

Enteral Nutrition. The provision of nutrients through the intestinal tract is ideal. Compared with TPN, enteral feeding is more physiological, less prone to complications, and far less costly. Maternal breast milk is the standard for infants and may be collected and frozen for later use in surgical patients. Commercially available cow's milk formulas, such as Enfamil and Similac, contain nutritional constituents similar to those of breast milk. Soy-based formulas, such as Isomil, are used for infants with milk protein allergy or lactose intolerance. More elemental formulas, like Pregestimil, contain nutrients in their simplest forms and are indicated when normal absorption is impaired, as in the short bowel syndrome. Infants should receive at least 150 mL/kg/day of these formulas in order to obtain 100–110 cal/kg/day.

If a baby is unable to suck but has an otherwise functional intestinal tract, a small nasogastric tube may be inserted for gavage feedings. A child who requires prolonged tube feedings (such as from an inability to swallow due to neurological disease) is better off with a surgically placed gastrostomy tube, since nasogastric tubes are irritating, easily displaced, and can promote aspiration.

Parenteral Nutrition. A majority of children with major surgical disorders require TPN while the gastrointestinal tract is temporarily nonfunctional. All nutrient requirements are supplied intravenously by the administration of carbohydrates, proteins, fats, electrolytes, trace elements, and vitamins. Intravenous nutrition may be infused either through a peripheral or a central vein. Peripheral alimentation is preferred because surgical insertion of a catheter is not required and potential complications are fewer. Glucose can be given up to a concentration of 12.5%, and the remainder of the required calories is largely supplied as emulsified fat. When peripheral veins are scarce, central TPN is used either through the superior or inferior vena cava. These vessels are accessed either by a cutdown procedure in the neck or groin, or percutaneously, usually through the subclavian vein. A silicone catheter with a subcutaneous cuff is preferred, since it is minimally thrombogenic and tends to resist infection. Concentrations of up to 25% glucose can be infused centrally.

The nutritional needs of each child on TPN are calculated daily, and the appropriate solution is prepared (see Table 2.2). TPN is infused at maintenance fluid rates and must be administered by an infusion pump. Concentrations are gradually increased over several days until daily requirements are achieved. All children receiving TPN are monitored closely. Weights are recorded daily. Urine is monitored for glucose, and blood is analyzed periodically for glucose, electrolytes, lipids, bilirubin, and liver enzymes.

Complications of TPN may be mechanical, septic, and metabolic. Mechanical complications are most common with centrally placed catheters, and include malposition, venous thrombosis, pneumothorax, and hemothorax. Infection of central venous catheters is a major hazard, and scrupulous surgical and nursing techniques must be followed. Bacterial contamination may be treated with antibiotics, and the catheter can often be preserved. Fungal contamination of central catheters necessitates their removal.

Metabolic complications include hyperglycemia, hypoglycemia, hyperlipidemia, and electrolyte imbalances. Liver damage may occur in any patient on TPN, but preterm infants are most susceptible. Its cause is not known, but it is probably multifactorial. Initially, cholestasis can be identified by a rise in serum bilirubin and alkaline phosphatase levels. Although hepatic injury is usually reversed when the TPN is discontinued, fibrosis and cirrhosis may subsequently develop.

Table 2.2.
Total Parenteral Nutrition Requirements[a]

Component	Neonate	6 months–10 years	>10 years
Calories (kcal/kg/day)	90–120	60–105	40–75
Fluid (mL/kg/day)	120–180	120–150	50–75
Dextrose (mg/kg/min)	4–6	7–8	7–8
Protein (gm/kg/day)	2–3	1.5–2.5	0.8–2.0
Fat (gm/kg/day)	0.5–0.3	1.0–4.0	1.0–4.0
Sodium (mEq/kg/day)	3–4	3–4	3–4
Potassium (mEq/kg/day)	2–3	2–3	1–2
Calcium (mg/kg/day)	80–120	40–80	40–60 (600/day)
Phosphate (mg/kg/day)	25–40	25–40	25–40
Magnesium (mEq/kg/day)	0.25–1.0	0.5	0.5
Zinc (μg/kg/day)	300	100	3 mg/day
Copper (μg/kg/day)	20	20	1.2 mg/day
Chromium (μg/kg/day)	0.2	0.2	12 mg/day
Manganese (μg/kg/day)	6	6	0.3 mg/day
Selenium (μg/kg/day)	2	2	10–20/day

Respiratory Management

Respiratory failure, the inability to maintain adequate gas exchange through the lungs, is quite common in surgically ill children. It frequently results from hyaline membrane disease, meconium aspiration, congenital diaphragmatic hernia, sepsis, pneumonia, pneumothorax, or the direct effects of surgical trauma. Infants have high oxygen requirements and very narrow and easily obstructed air passages. They depend almost exclusively on their diaphragms rather than on accessory chest wall muscles for air movement. Infants thus have a very narrow safety margin concerning respiration, and any distress must be managed urgently. Signs of respiratory failure include agitation, nasal flaring, tachycardia, chest wall retraction, grunting, and cyanosis. Evaluation should include a physical examination, chest x-ray, and arterial blood gas analysis.

Airway maintenance is crucial, and suctioning should be frequent in order to clear mucus, vomitus, or blood. Supplemental oxygen may be administered by nasal prongs, a face mask, or a hood. Endotracheal intubation provides the most secure airway, is always necessary when prolonged mechanical ventilation is to be used, and may facilitate pulmonary suctioning and physical therapy. The size of the tube to be inserted may be estimated from the diameter of the child's external nares or little finger. In general, term neonates use a 3-mm French tube, 5-year-olds a 5-mm tube, and adolescents a 7-mm tube. For children below 8 years of age the tubes are uncuffed and should be sufficiently small to allow an air leak around the cricoid in order to prevent subglottic stenosis.

Mechanical ventilation is usually indicated when the P_{O_2} falls below 60 mm Hg in spite of supplemental oxygen, or the P_{CO_2} rises above 60 mm Hg. The two varieties of positive pressure ventilators used are volume and pressure ventilators. Volume ventilators deliver a preset tidal volume regardless of the pulmonary compliance and are used in most patients beyond the newborn period. Pressure ventilators deliver breaths up to a preset pressure and are preferred for infants, in whom the very low volumes involved and mandatory air leak would prevent accurate delivery of a preset volume.

The ventilator should be adjusted to its lowest possible settings consistent with adequate gas exchange, as monitored by frequent blood gas determinations. Initial settings are generally a tidal volume of 10 mL/kg for volume ventilators, an inspiratory pressure of 18–25 cm of H_2O for pressure ventilators, and for both a positive end-expiratory pressure (PEEP) of 3–5 cm of H_2O and a rate (for infants) of 25–40 breaths/min. Oxygen levels must not be excessive, particularly in preterm neonates who are at great risk for pulmonary toxicity that can lead to chronic fibrosis, known as bronchopulmonary dysplasia, and retinal damage to the eye.

Pneumothoraces are very common in children receiving positive pressure ventilation and should be suspected whenever there is sudden deterioration in the respiratory status. A chest x-ray or transillumination confirms the diagnosis. Although definitive treatment is the placement of an intercostal drainage tube, expeditious needle aspiration provides immediate relief if the child is in severe distress.

High frequency ventilation is a recent innovation in which very low tidal volumes are directed down the trachea at extremely rapid rates (150–2500 breaths/min). Although its mechanism of action is unclear, high frequency ventilation allows adequate gas exchange to occur at lower airway pressures than with conventional rates, producing less trauma to the lungs when very high ventilatory settings are needed.

Extracorporeal membrane oxygenation (ECMO) is a form of prolonged cardiopulmonary bypass in which gas exchange occurs in an external circuit containing the patient's flowing blood (Fig. 2.2). ECMO can provide complete respiratory support, independently of the lungs, allowing them to rest and recover while organ function is well maintained. ECMO is reserved for the most desperately ill babies, since it requires cannu-

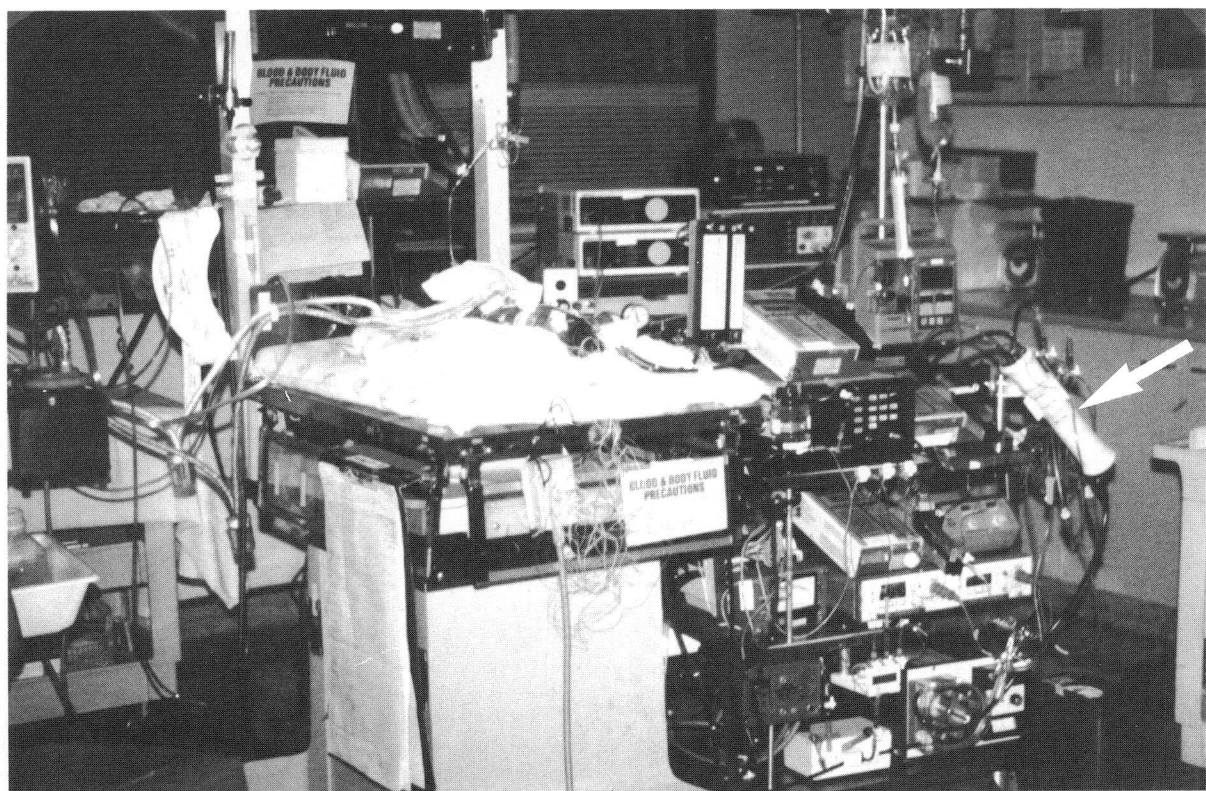

Figure 2.2. Newborn infant on ECMO. Arrow indicates membrane lung.

lation of major vessels and systemic heparinization. Nevertheless, the survival rate in newborn infants treated with ECMO is over 80%. Results are not yet as encouraging in older children and adults, and clinical trials continue.

Operative Care and Monitoring

The ability to perform major surgery successfully on preterm infants is a recent development, largely the result of increased understanding of neonatal physiology and advances in ventilatory technology. Even extremely preterm neonates can be safely brought through surgery, provided the anesthesiologist is knowledgeable and attentive to their special needs and the surgeon handles the fragile tissues with the utmost gentleness and skill. General anesthesia is used for almost all children who undergo operations. Exceptions are high-risk babies with chronic cardiopulmonary disease having operations below the umbilicus (e.g., inguinal hernia repair), in whom spinal or caudal anesthesia may be employed.

A thorough history and physical examination is a prerequisite to any operation. Traditionally, a CBC and urinalysis have been required, although these tests may not be necessary in healthy children. Other studies, such as serum electrolytes, coagulation parameters, arterial blood gas determinations, electrocardiograms (ECGs), and x-rays, are obtained preoperatively only when indicated.

Children should be in the best possible condition at the time of their operation. There are enough inherent risks in surgery to warrant minimizing any others when possible. A child with an upper respiratory infection should have elective surgery postponed until the infection is resolved. A patient in shock should be resuscitated as completely as possible before even an urgent operation. Children having elective operations should not ingest any solids or milk for 12 hours before surgery. Older children may have clear liquids until 6 to 8 hours preoperatively, and infants up to 6 months of age are allowed clear liquids until 4 hours before surgery.

Technological advances have greatly facilitated the ability to monitor small patients noninvasively. Blood pressure determinations by cuff with the Dinamapp are highly accurate, even in shock states, and can be performed automatically at preset intervals. Pulse oximetry has revolutionized the monitoring process, both in and out of the operating room. Hypoxia can occur suddenly, particularly in the tiny infant covered with drapes, as the endotracheal tube becomes blocked, slips out of the trachea, or migrates down a mainstem bronchus. These complications must be recognized and corrected promptly in order to avert disaster. The pulse oximeter provides continuous measurement of the percentage of oxygen saturation of hemoglobin by assessing the differential light absorption of oxygenated and reduced hemoglobin, using a light shined through the distal part of an extremity. Any reduction below 98–100% calls for immediate investigation as to the cause.

Since the advent of the Dinamapp and pulse oximeter, indwelling arterial catheters are used less often than previously but are still very helpful in cases of cardiopulmonary instability. Blood pressure measurement is continuous, and arterial blood gas determinations can be made frequently. The umbilical artery is a reliable, accessible site for the placement of these catheters in neonates.

Central venous pressures are an estimate of the adequacy of blood volume in relation to left ventricular function, and can help guide intravenous fluid requirements. In the presence of preexisting cardiopulmonary disease, Swan-Ganz catheters, which more accurately reflect left-sided heart pressures, are more reliable. However, since they are cumbersome to insert in small individuals and have relatively high complication rates, they are used less frequently in pediatric than in adult patients. Urethral catheters should be inserted in any unstable patient as well as before any lengthy operative procedure, in order to continually monitor urine output.

Infants can rapidly become hypothermic in the operating room, which may lead to peripheral vasoconstriction, acidosis, and even death. Premature infants have a surface area up to 10 times that of adults per unit weight. They have little subcutaneous fat to act as insulation. Anesthesia abolishes their muscular activity and causes vasodilation, which augment heat loss. Also, they may have exposed body cavities. Children can be kept warm by adequately heating the operating room, using radiant heaters and warming mattresses, covering the extremities and head, and warming all prep solutions and intravenous fluids. Body temperature must be monitored continuously during all operations.

Term infants less than 3 months of age and even older premature babies have immature respiratory centers and are prone to apneic spells following general anesthesia. Elective operations should therefore be delayed in these infants. If they must undergo emergency procedures that cannot be postponed, these infants must have close postoperative monitoring for 24 hours or longer.

Emotional Support and Pain Management

Even the most routine operation for the surgeon is often a major traumatic event in the lives of patients and their families. It can be particularly difficult for patients between the ages of 1 and 4 years, when they are knowledgeable enough to be afraid, yet unable to understand the bewildering events going on around them. Older children and adolescents are particularly fearful of physical injury and mutilation. Parents are often devastated at the prospect of their child having to undergo an operation, with the dread of general anesthesia often superseding their fear of the operative procedure itself. Guilt and misinformation are common.

Much can be done to alleviate the anxieties of both children and parents. The approach must be individualized, depending on the age of the child and the temperament of the patient and family. Honest and open explanations are best, with the child included in the discussions and provided with ample opportunity for questions. Videos and booklets, a tour of the clinical facility, and an opportunity to play with the medical equipment (for example, using it on dolls, depending on the patient's age) can transform an alien, hostile setting into a familiar and friendly one. Even when procedures must be unpleasant or painful, children are better off knowing what to expect rather than having their vivid imaginations fantasizing the worst. An excellent relationship with parents and a clear understanding on their part of the upcoming events is most important, since parents often transmit their own feelings to their children. Informed parents can also do much to prepare children at home.

Separation from parents should be minimized. Preoperative workups can often be done before a hospital admission, and children should be discharged postoperatively as soon as medically indicated. Many operations can be performed on an outpatient basis, beginning at 3 months of age for term babies, and at approximately 60 weeks after conception for premature infants. Parents can remain with their children until the last possible moment before they enter the operating room, and may be present in the recovery room when their children awaken.

Premedications are often given to allay anxiety. They are administered orally, since an injection would defeat their purpose. In the operating room, younger children are induced for anesthesia with a face mask (which can be scented), and older children can choose between mask or intravenous induction.

Postoperative pain is all too often inadequately managed, because of exaggerated concerns about the potential for narcotic addiction or respiratory depression. Long-acting local anesthetics can be given during general anesthesia to effectively limit postoperative pain for hours. Narcotics, such as morphine (0.1 mg/kg) or meperidine (1 mg/kg), can be given through existing intravenous catheters to patients over 6 months of age, in order to avoid the pain of intramuscular injections. Since apnea is a concern in children under 6 months of age, narcotics should be given to these individuals only in the closely monitored setting of a critical care unit. For children over 10 years of age, patient-controlled analgesia, in which the patient can trigger the infusion of medication within preset limits, has been demonstrated to provide superior pain relief with less total narcotic than with traditional pain control methods. Acetaminophen (10 mg/kg) with or without codeine (1 mg/kg) can be prescribed orally or rectally for lesser degrees of pain.

Neonatal Surgical Conditions

Congenital Diaphragmatic Hernia

Congenital diaphragmatic hernias (CDHs) are among the most urgent of all neonatal surgical conditions. Although many advances have been made in the treatment of affected infants, the mortality rate remains disappointingly high, and certain aspects of CDH

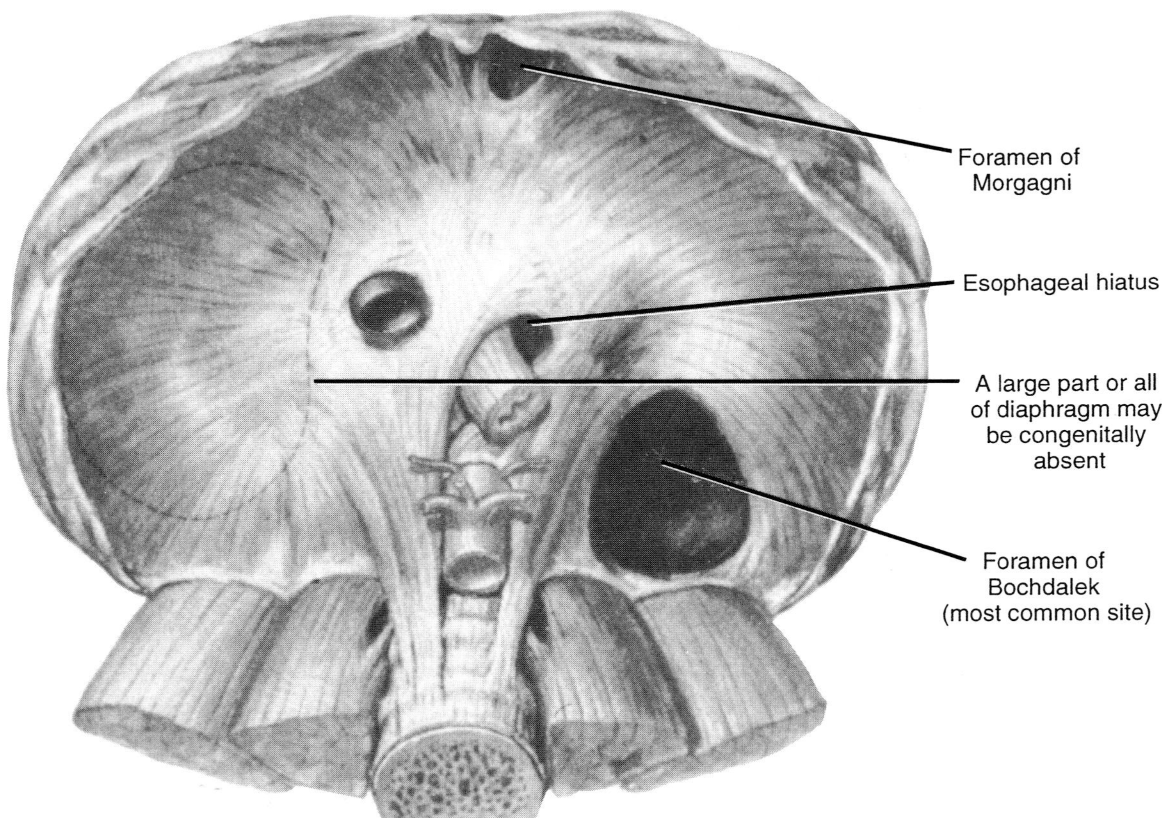

Figure 2.3. Locations of congenital herniations in the diaphragm. Posterolateral (Bochdalek) hernias are much more common than retrosternal (Morgagni) hernias.

management are still controversial. CDHs of Bochdalek, by far the most common type, consist of a defect in the posterolateral diaphragm, and occur on the left side 85% of the time. Morgagni hernias, which are retrosternal defects, do not often present as an emergency in the newborn period (Fig. 2.3).

Embryologically, the extruded midgut normally returns to the abdominal cavity between the ninth and 10th weeks of gestation. If the posterolateral pleuroperitoneal canal has not yet closed, the viscera can pass through it and into the chest. The stomach, intestine, liver, and spleen may all be involved. The developing lungs are compressed in utero, resulting in varying degrees of pulmonary hypoplasia, most severe on the ipsilateral side. The pulmonary arterioles are particularly immature, with abnormally thick, muscular walls.

Pathophysiology. At the time of birth these babies may have respiratory distress due to (*a*) mechanical compression of the lungs by the herniated viscera, (*b*) pulmonary hypoplasia, and (*c*) persistent pulmonary hypertension (PPHN). Pulmonary vascular resistance remains abnormally high following birth, because of the paucity of pulmonary arterioles and their thick walls. The ensuing right-to-left shunting of blood across the foramen ovale and ductus arteriosus produces hypoxemia, as desaturated blood enters the systemic circulation. Hypoxia, hypercarbia, and acidosis are all potent stimuli for further pulmonary arteriolar vasoconstriction, increasing vascular resistance still further and thus setting up a vicious cycle. Much medical intervention in patient CDH involves attempting to reverse PPHN.

Clinical Presentation. Symptoms, often severe but occasionally mild or absent, include dyspnea and cyanosis, diminished breath sounds on the side of the hernia, and a shift of the heart to the opposite side. The abdomen is characteristically scaphoid. The diagnosis is confirmed by chest x-ray revealing air-filled loops of bowel in the chest with mediastinal deviation (Fig. 2.4).

Treatment. Until recently, immediate surgical intervention was thought mandatory. Evidence has shown, however, that time is well spent resuscitating and, if possible, stabilizing these babies preoperatively. The duration of this preoperative effort varies with the baby and is not fully agreed upon. Oxygen is administered and mechanical ventilation performed through an endotracheal tube. Positive pressure breathing through a face mask is contraindicated, since some gas will be directed into the esophagus and further distend the herniated bowel. A nasogastric tube is placed to minimize gastric distention. The babies are hyperventilated to reverse hypoxia and induce alkalosis, in order to relax the constricted pulmonary arterioles. Pharmacological agents (such as tolazoline) have been used as pulmo-

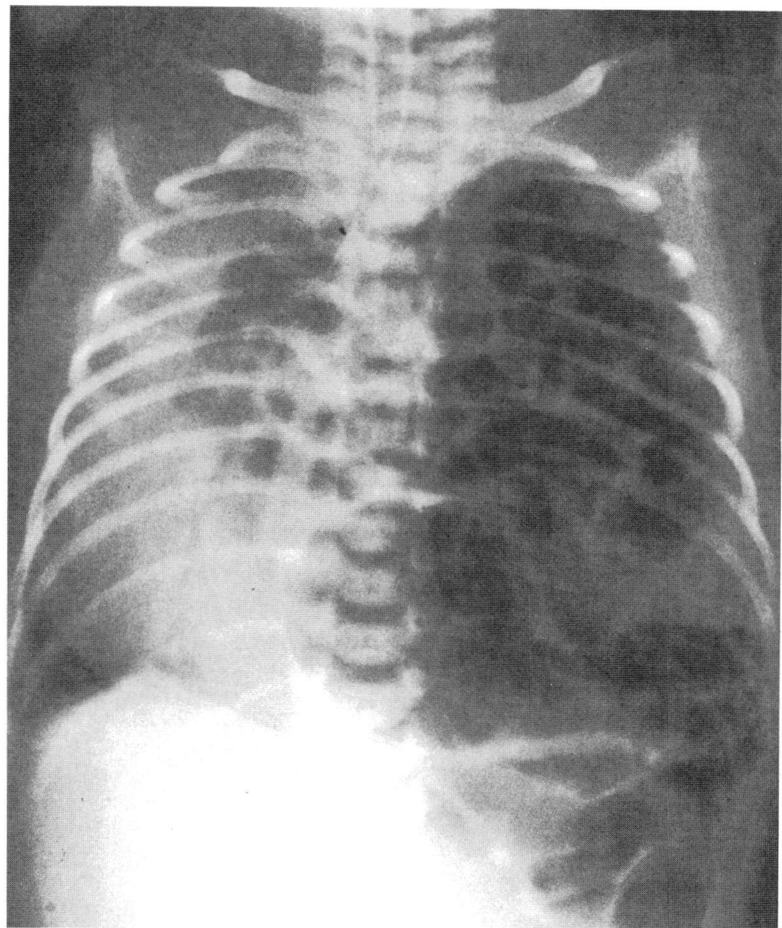

Figure 2.4. Congenital diaphragmatic hernia in a neonate. Intestinal loops are in left chest with mediastinal displacement to the right.

nary artery vasodilators, but improved survival with their use is unproven.

The surgical approach is usually through the abdomen. The viscera are reduced and the diaphragmatic defect closed. If the opening is too large to suture primarily, a prosthetic patch is used. Postoperatively, intensive ventilatory support is continued, with very slow weaning.

Recent innovations in treating severe CDH babies include high frequency ventilation (HFV) and ECMO. HFV may achieve better gas exchange with lower airway pressures than does conventional ventilation. ECMO has been used in extremely unstable babies both pre- and postoperatively. Bleeding from operative sites because of the systemic heparinization required is a major hazard.

The mortality rate of infants presenting with a CDH within 24 hours of birth has been 50%. Most survivors have little disability, as the lungs continue to grow and develop. In selected centers using ECMO, the mortality rate has been reduced to between 30% and 40%, although the numbers involved are still small.

CDH is increasingly being diagnosed in utero by antenatal ultrasound, and delivery can then be performed in a hospital prepared to care for these babies. Antenatal in utero repair of CDHs have been performed in animals in an attempt to prevent the development of pulmonary hypoplasia, but limited experience in humans is thus far disappointing.

Esophageal Atresia and Tracheoesophageal Fistula

Esophageal atresia (EA) is a congenital interruption in the continuity of the upper and lower portions of the esophagus (Fig. 2.5**A**). A tracheoesophageal fistula (TEF) is an abnormal communication between the trachea and esophagus (Fig. 2.5**E**). Although either condition may occur alone, they more frequently appear together (Figs. 2.5**B**, 2.5**C**, 2.5**D**). By far the most common pattern is type C (85%), in which the upper esophagus ends blindly and the lower portion communicates with the trachea. The overall incidence of these anomalies is 1:3000–4000 live births.

The embryological events that produce EA and TEFs are not completely known, but somehow the septation process that normally divides the foregut into trachea and esophagus by the seventh week of gestation is incomplete. In addition, the more rapidly growing

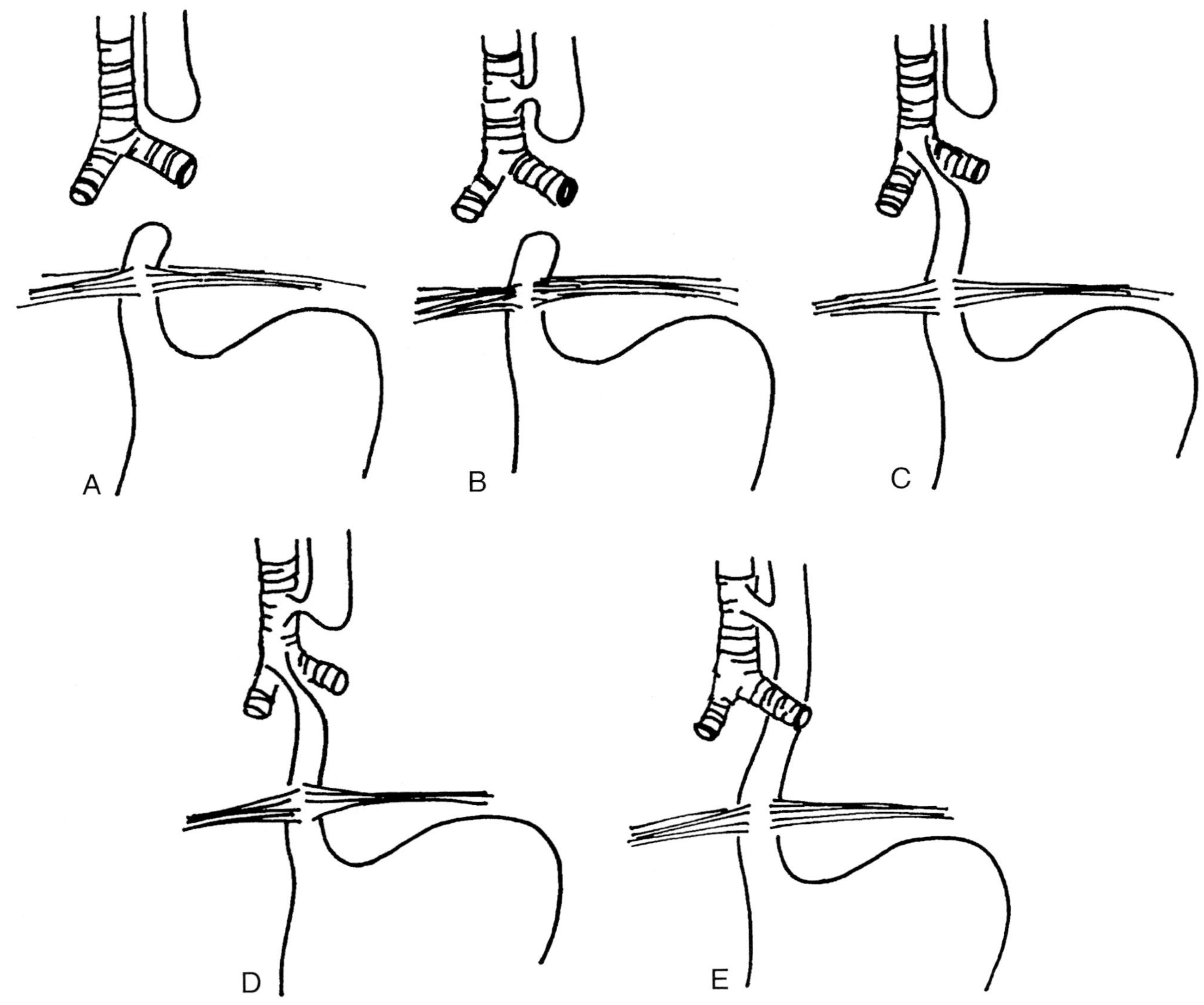

Figure 2.5 A–E. Anatomical patterns of esophageal atresia and tracheoesophageal fistula. See text.

trachea may partition the upper and lower esophagus into discontinuous segments. EA and TEFs are often found with other abnormalities, termed the VACTER association (Vertebral, Anal, Cardiac, Tracheal, Esophageal, Radial or Renal), and the presence of an anomaly of any of these structures should prompt a search for others.

Clinical Manifestations. An infant with EA with or without a TEF will immediately choke and regurgitate with feeding, as the blind-ending upper esophageal pouch rapidly fills. An alert nurse will initially notice excessive drooling, since even saliva cannot be swallowed. An attempt to pass a nasogastric tube will encounter resistance, and an x-ray will confirm the tip to be in the upper mediastinum. Air seen in the abdomen assures the presence of a TEF. An isolated EA will be associated with no gas in the gastrointestinal tract, since air cannot be swallowed. Contrast material may be given carefully to outline the upper esophageal pouch, but is not strictly necessary.

A patient with an isolated TEF, the so-called "H" type fistula, may not present until after the neonatal period, since the esophagus is patent. The patient develops recurrent aspiration pneumonias, and the diagnosis is established by endoscopy and/or a contrast swallow.

Treatment. Immediate measures must be taken to prevent aspiration. The baby should be placed upright to minimize reflux of gastric contents from the fistula into the trachea. The nasogastric tube in the upper pouch is placed to suction in order to keep it empty of oral secretions. Intravenous fluids and broad-spectrum antibiotics are administered.

Most neonates with EA and TEFs can undergo primary repair, with division of the fistula and anastomosis of the upper and lower esophageal segments through a right thoracotomy. If the infant is extremely premature or ill with other major anomalies and cannot

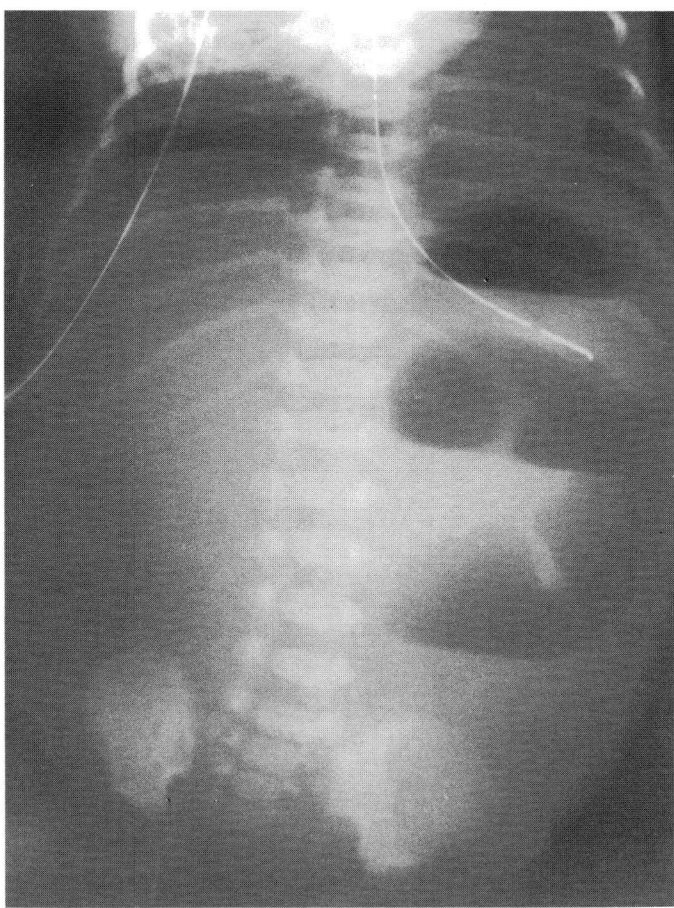

Figure 2.6. Newborn infant with complete jejunal obstruction from atresia. Air is visualized in stomach and proximal jejunum only.

tolerate a lengthy procedure, or if the gap between upper and lower esophageal segments is long, a staged repair is necessary. A gastrostomy is first performed to keep the stomach empty and prevent aspiration of gastric contents, and subsequent ligation of the TEF then permits safe gastrostomy feeding. Upper and lower esophageal segments may take several months to grow sufficiently close to be approximated. Only in rare instances should a colon or gastric interposition be necessary to bridge the gap.

Postoperative complications may include an anastomotic leak, stricture, recurrent TEF, and gastroesophageal reflux. Reflux is particularly common and may require a subsequent fundoplication. Most neonates with EA and TEFs recover well, with mortality limited to those who are extremely premature or have other major anomalies.

Congenital Gastrointestinal Obstruction

Congenital gastrointestinal obstruction refers to an obstruction that is present at birth. The site of the obstruction may be anywhere from stomach to anus, and it can result from a wide variety of causes. These disorders should be managed with some urgency because the obstructed neonate can rapidly develop fluid and electrolyte derangements, may aspirate vomitus, and can acquire sepsis from perforation of the distended bowel or necrosis from an underlying midgut volvulus.

Four clinical manifestations of congenital obstruction, which may occur variably, are:

1. Polyhydramnios. The fetus swallows 50% of amniotic fluid daily, which is largely absorbed in the upper intestinal tract. A high obstruction allows this fluid to back up and accumulate in excessive quantities.
2. Bilious vomiting. Nonbilious vomiting is common in infants; bilious vomiting is much more often pathological.
3. Abdominal distention. Distention develops within 24 hours of birth in distal obstructions, as swallowed air accumulates above the blockage.
4. Failure to pass meconium. Within 24 hours of birth, 95% of babies pass meconium. A delay may signify obstruction.

If obstruction is suspected following a careful history and physical examination, plain x-rays are performed, as swallowed air is an excellent contrast material. If a few dilated loops of bowel with air-fluid levels and no distal air can be seen (Fig. 2.6), complete, proximal obstruction is diagnosed and no further imaging studies are needed. If the obstruction appears to be partial or is questionable, with some distal air visualized, an upper gastrointestinal contrast study is most useful. If many distended loops of bowel are seen, suggesting a distal obstruction (Fig. 2.7), a barium enema is indicated.

Initial management should always include nasogastric tube decompression, intravenous hydration, and prophylactic antibiotics. The need for and timing of surgery then depends on the nature of the obstruction and the overall condition of the baby.

Duodenal Obstruction. Duodenal obstruction is commonly caused by: (*a*) atresia, (*b*) annular pancreas, and (*c*) malrotation. Most such obstructions are distal to the ampulla, so the vomiting is bilious. Duodenal atresia may take several forms, including complete separation of the proximal and distal duodenal segments, stenosis, or a web across the lumen. Embryologically, the duodenal epithelium overgrows and transiently occludes its lumen. It is believed that failure of subsequent complete recanalization is responsible for the various forms of atresia. Duodenal atresia is strongly associated with Down's syndrome. Annular pancreas is produced when the ventral pancreatic bud fails to rotate around and become incorporated into the dorsal bud; the two instead fuse around the duodenum, occluding it partially or completely. Rotation of the intestine normally occurs embryologically after the midgut (the duodenum to the transverse colon) has returned to the abdominal cavity from the yolk sac. The vertical midgut rotates 270° in a counterclockwise direction, placing the cecum in the right lower quadrant and the duodenojejunal junction in the left upper quadrant. Subsequently, the ascending and descending colon is fixed retroperitoneally by fibrous attachments that arise

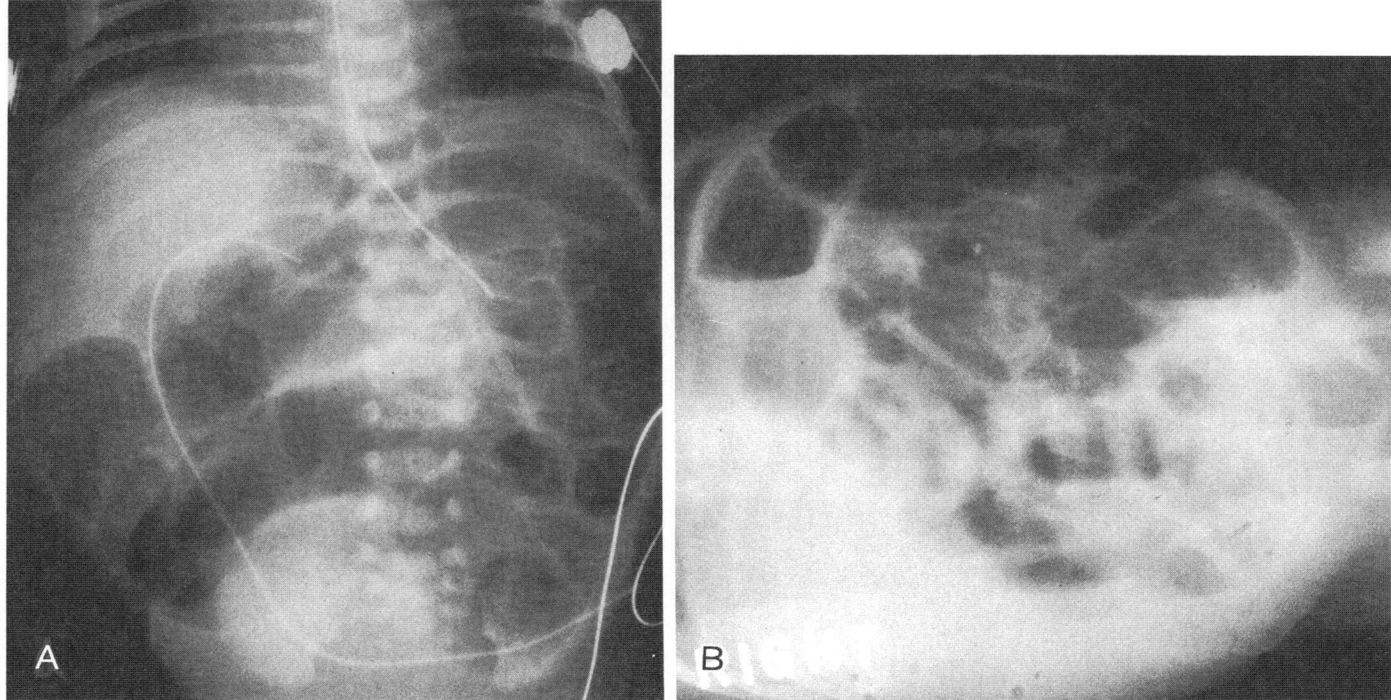

Figure 2.7. **A**, Supine and **B**, decubitus radiographs of a 3-day-old boy with low congenital intestinal obstruction. Multiple dilated bowel loops with air fluid levels are present.

from the lateral abdominal walls. In malrotation, this process is incomplete. The cecum is located either high in the right abdomen, or remains completely in the left abdomen, and the duodenojejunal junction is located to the right of the midline. This configuration allows the intestine, which is suspended between these closely fixed points, to twist as a midgut volvulus (Figs. 2.8**A** and 2.8**B**). Midgut volvulus may occur at any age where there is congenital malrotation, but is most common in the first month. It is the most dangerous form of duodenal obstruction, for if not corrected early, before signs of peritonitis develop, the entire midgut will undergo necrosis. Ladd's bands may also obstruct the duodenum in association with malrotation. The peritoneal attachments from the lateral abdominal wall, which normally fix the cecum retroperitoneally, now cross over the duodenum to reach the high, malrotated cecum, and may cause partial or complete obstruction by compression (Fig. 2.8**C**).

The diagnosis of complete duodenal obstruction at birth is established by visualizing a "double bubble" on x-ray, as air is present in the stomach and in the proximal, dilated duodenum, but none is seen distally (Fig. 2.9). If the obstruction is incomplete, some air will be noted below.

Duodenal obstruction demands expeditious surgery, unless midgut volvulus has been ruled out. For atresia and annular pancreas the obstruction is bypassed, as the proximal duodenal segment is anastomosed to the distal duodenum or to a loop of jejunum (Fig. 2.10). Gastrojejunostomies are poorly tolerated in infants, as marginal ulcers and the blind loop syndrome (in the duodenal sweep) can develop. In malrotation, the volvulus is untwisted, Ladd's bands are cut, and the duodenum and cecum are widely separated from each other.

Jejunoileal Obstruction. Congenital obstruction of the small intestine can be caused by: (*a*) atresia, (*b*) meconium ileus, and (*c*) intestinal duplication. Atresia of the small intestine, as of the duodenum, may range from a web across the lumen to complete separation of the intestinal segments. The atresias may also be multiple, and occasionally a considerable length of small bowel is lost. Unlike duodenal atresia, the etiology is believed to be from in utero vascular accidents, such as a localized twist or intussusception. Since there are no intraluminal bacteria antenatally, the resulting necrosis produces localized atrophy rather than bacterial peritonitis.

Meconium ileus is due to the impaction of sticky, inspissated meconium in the distal ileum, the narrowest portion of the intestinal tract. It occurs in 10% of patients with cystic fibrosis, from the abnormally viscid enzymes secreted by the exocrine pancreatic and intestinal glands. The diagnosis should be suspected if there is a family history of cystic fibrosis, which is an autosomal recessive disorder. X-rays often demonstrate a peculiar foamy appearance of the dilated air-filled bowel loops and a lack of air fluid levels, as the thick meconium is mixed with air and fails to layer out. Calcification on abdominal x-ray indicates that an antenatal perforation has occurred.

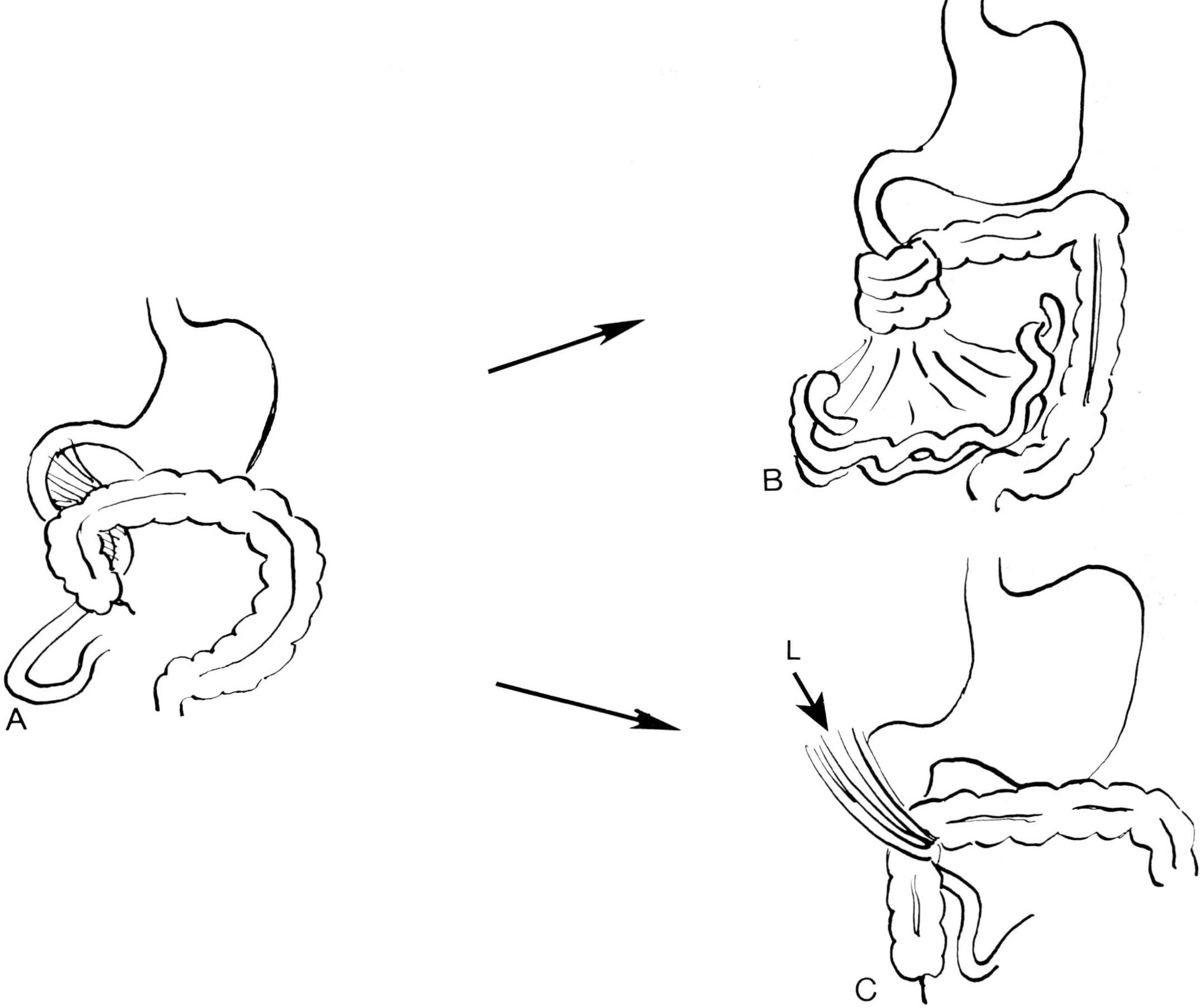

Figure 2.8. **A**, Congenital malrotation of intestine with high cecum and right-sided duodenojejunal junction forming a narrow pedicle. **B**, The midgut has twisted as a volvulus. **C**, Ladd's bands can also obstruct the duodenum in malrotation. L, Ladd's bands.

Duplications are endothelial-lined cystic or tubular structures adjacent to any portion of the alimentary tract on the mesenteric side, and share a common wall with the normal bowel. When these structures do not communicate with the adjacent intestine, mucous secretions accumulate within the duplication, which distends, impinging on the neighboring intestine. Obstructive symptoms may appear in the neonatal period or later on.

Atresias and duplications are managed surgically by resection and end-to-end anastomosis. Meconium ileus can frequently be treated nonoperatively with gastrografin enemas. Gastrografin is a radiopaque fluid with a very high osmolarity that causes fluid to be drawn into the bowel lumen. The sticky meconium is hydrated, and may be spontaneously evacuated. Intravenous fluids must be infused during the procedure, in order to avoid systemic hypovolemia. If the obstruction persists or if there is evidence of perforation, surgery is mandatory.

Colon Obstruction. Congenital colon obstruction may be due to: (*a*) Hirschsprung's disease, (*b*) the neonatal small left colon syndrome (*c*) a meconium plug, and, rarely, (*d*) atresia.

Hirschsprung's disease is a disorder in which ganglion cells are absent from the wall of the distal intestinal tract. Embryologically, these cells migrate from the esophagus to the anus; in Hirschsprung's disease they are arrested in their descent. The transition zone is most often at the rectosigmoid colon but can occur any-

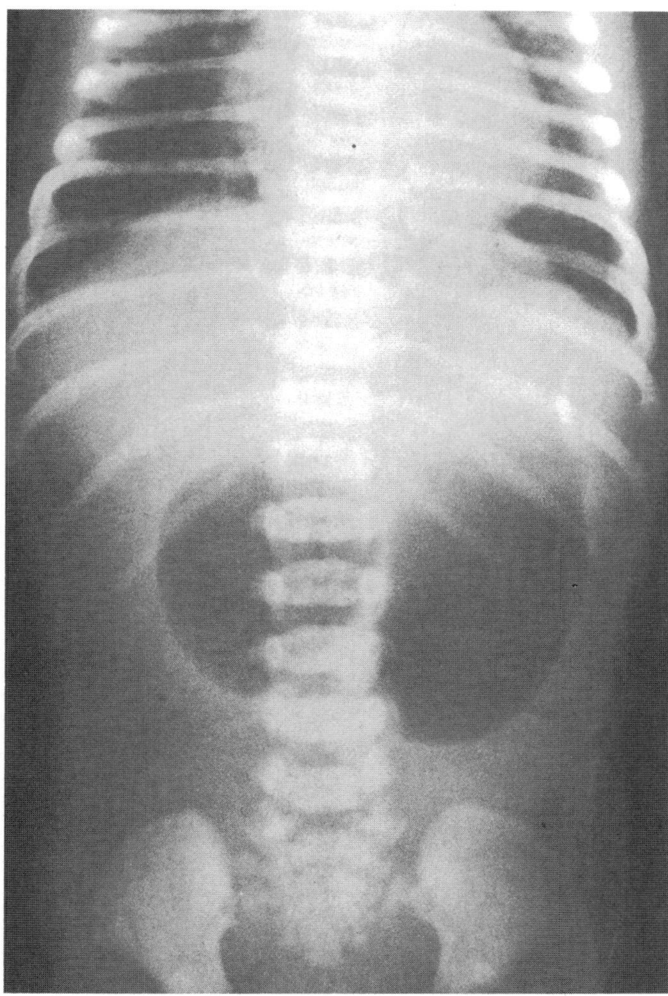

Figure 2.9. "Double bubble" sign in a neonate with duodenal atresia. Air is visualized in stomach and proximal, dilated duodenum only.

where, with the entire colon or even the small intestine being aganglionic. This aganglionic bowel does not undergo normal peristalsis, producing a functional obstruction at the transition zone. The obstruction may present in the neonate as a complete, low, congenital obstruction, or in older children as chronic constipation. Boys are four times as frequently affected as girls. A barium enema usually demonstrates the transition zone, as contrast flows from normal caliber, aganglionic bowel into dilated, ganglionic intestine more proximally (Fig. 2.11). A rectal biopsy will confirm the absence of ganglion cells.

Surgical treatment for Hirschsprung's disease is usually staged. A temporary colostomy is brought out above the transition zone. Several months later, when the proximal bowel is no longer dilated, a pull-through procedure is performed, in which the ganglionic bowel is brought down and anastomosed to the anal canal. The aganglionic segment may be removed in its entirety (Swenson procedure, Fig. 2.12**A**) or its mucosa stripped and the proximal intestine brought down within the outer muscular sleeve (Soave procedure, Fig. 2.12**B**). Alternatively, the ganglionic bowel may be brought behind and anastomosed to the aganglionic rectum that is left in situ (Duhamel procedure, Fig. 2.12**C**).

Occasionally, patients with Hirschsprung's disease may develop a poorly understood enterocolitis, with dehydration, peritonitis, and sepsis. Treatment must be prompt with intravenous fluids, antibiotics, and colonic irrigations. The mortality rate is high.

Neonates with colonic obstruction may have the meconium plug or small left colon syndromes. Both of these disorders are functional and are cured by the dilation of the left colon following a barium enema. The small left colon syndrome is most common in infants of diabetic mothers. Babies are usually normal after treatment, although a sweat chloride test should be performed to rule out cystic fibrosis.

Anorectal Malformations

Anorectal malformations represent a spectrum of disorders in which the rectum fails to reach its normal perineal termination. When the rectum ends above the levator muscles the malformations are classified as high, and when the rectum passes through these muscles they are classified as low. High lesions are more frequent in males and low ones in females. Although the rectum may end blindly in both the high and low varieties, it much more often terminates in an anterior fistulous communication. In males with high anomalies, the fistula communicates with the urethra or bladder (Fig. 2.13**A**); in females it connects with the interposed vagina (Fig. 2.13**B**). In both sexes with low malformations, the fistula drains externally, anterior to the normal anal site (Figs. 2.13**C** and 2.13**D**). Since anorectal malformations are part of the VACTER complex, associated abnormalities, particularly urinary anomalies, frequently occur as well.

Clinical Manifestations. The diagnosis of an imperforate anus is usually obvious on inspection. Either no perineal opening exists (Fig. 2.14) or a fistula may be visible. In males the external fistula is usually a small opening in the perineum anterior to the normal anal location; it sometimes is located as far forward as the scrotal raphe. Females may also have an external fistula draining into the anterior perineum, or else into the posterior vulva behind the hymen. A single perineal orifice in a female signifies a cloaca, where the rectum, vagina, and urethra all open into a common chamber. This high anomaly is complex.

The management of babies with high and low anorectal malformations differs considerably, and it is important to distinguish between them. The presence of an external fistula always signifies a low lesion. In the absence of a visible fistula, most lesions are high. If the level of the rectal termination is not clear, an "invertogram" may be performed. The baby is held upside down, and if on lateral x-ray air in the rectum rises to within 1 cm of the perineal skin, the lesion is low; if not, it is probably high. Recently, computed tomography (CT) and magnetic resonance imaging (MRI) have

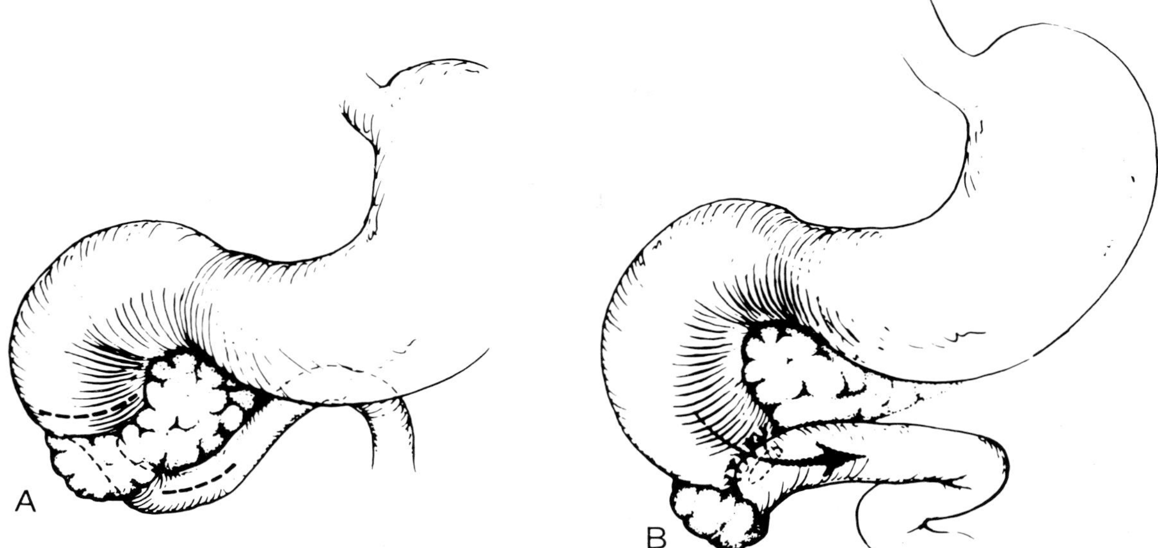

Figure 2.10A, B. Duodenoduodenostomy for annular pancreas.

been used to identify the level of the rectum more precisely.

Treatment. Continence normally depends on the coordinated actions of external sphincter, internal sphincter, and levator muscles. Since the levators are most important, infants with low lesions in whom the bowel descends normally within the levator sling have an excellent functional outlook. A fistula only slightly anterior to the normal anal location can often function as a normal anus and is left alone. Otherwise, a perineal anoplasty can be done to establish an adequate communication between the rectum and the perineum, at the center of the external sphincter. This operation may be done in the newborn period or later, if the external fistula can be dilated sufficiently to permit the passage of stool.

All infants with high anorectal malformations require an initial colostomy. At 6 months to 1 year of age, a pull-through procedure is performed, in which the rectum is mobilized, brought through the center of the levator sling, and anastomosed to the perineum. Although various types of pull-throughs have been described, the Pena operation, in which all the muscles are divided posteriorly in the midline, has recently gained favor because of the excellent visualization that is obtained.

The functional prognosis for these children is mixed. Those with low lesions achieve excellent continence. Individuals with high anomalies often have difficulty with toilet training, and over 50% ultimately have at least occasional soiling. In these cases, daily enemas may help considerably to keep the rectum empty and the perineum clean.

Necrotizing Enterocolitis

Necrotizing enterocolitis (NEC) is a type of hemorrhagic necrosis of the intestinal mucosa that can progress to infarction of the entire bowel wall. It occurs exclusively in the newborn period, mainly in premature infants but occasionally in term babies who have other debilitating illnesses. It is the most frequent indication for emergency surgery in neonates. The etiology of NEC is multifactorial, including: (*a*) ischemic damage to the intestinal mucosa, from hypoxia or low flow states; (*b*) bacterial invasion of the damaged bowel wall; and (*c*) the presence of food in the lumen as a substrate for the bacteria. NEC is rare in unfed babies. The bacteria that produce NEC are polymicrobial, including Gram-positive and Gram-negative aerobes, as well as anaerobes. The ileocecal region is most frequently affected, but any portion of the gastrointestinal tract may be involved.

Clinical Manifestations. Clinical signs of NEC are nonspecific initially and consist of lethargy, refusal to feed, fever, and apneic spells. Gastrointestinal manifestations follow, including vomiting, bloody diarrhea, and abdominal distention and tenderness. Full-blown sepsis may supervene.

Abdominal x-rays demonstrate an ileus pattern, with diffusely dilated intestinal loops. The hallmark of NEC is visualization of gas within the bowel wall, pneumatosis intestinalis. The gas is produced by proliferating bacteria and is seen in 80% of infants with NEC. It appears as a lucent halo around the bowel wall (Fig. 2.15). Air may be evident in the portal vein as well. Laboratory findings are nonspecific, but are consistent with a systemic infection. Positive blood cultures, leukocytosis or leukopenia, thrombocytopenia, and acidosis may be present.

Treatment. Most infants with NEC will recover with expeditious medical treatment. The goals are to maximize perfusion of the intestine and treat the infection. Fluid resuscitation is performed to restore intravascular volume, a nasogastric tube is inserted to decompress the intestinal tract, and broad-spectrum antibiotics are administered. Careful monitoring is essential.

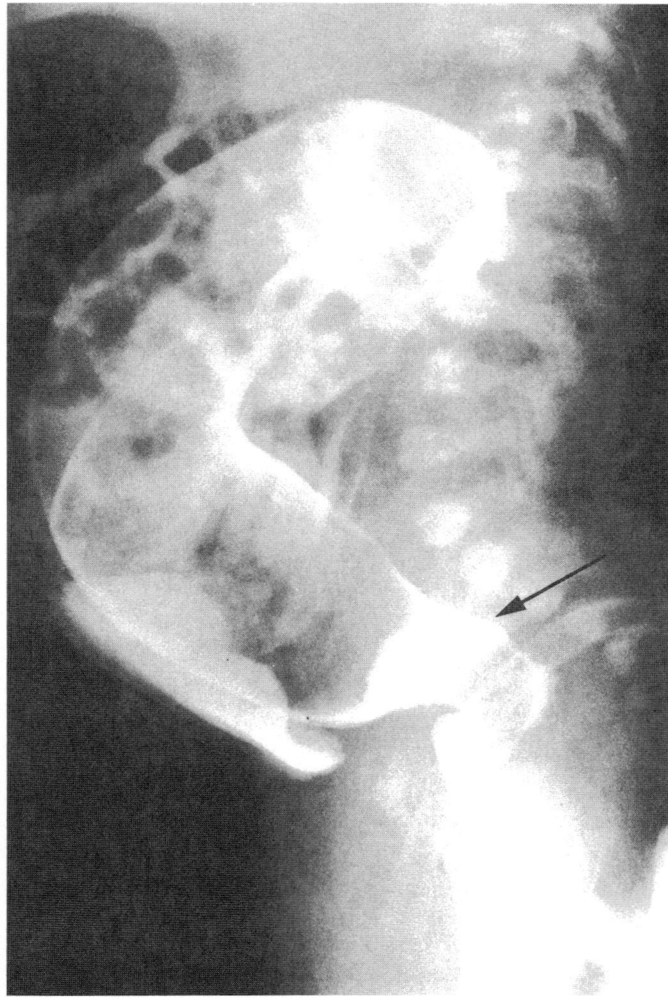

Figure 2.11. One-week-old boy with Hirschsprung's disease. Barium enema demonstrates transition zone (arrow) between distal, aganglionic rectum and dilated proximal bowel.

Indications for surgery are intestinal perforation or full-thickness necrosis. Perforation is readily identified by the presence of free air on abdominal x-ray. Gangrene without perforation may be difficult to diagnose but is suggested by the presence of a tensely distended abdomen, erythema of the abdominal wall, marked thrombocytopenia, or clinical deterioration in spite of vigorous medical therapy. In these circumstances, a small needle can be inserted into the abdomen and fluid aspirated. If it is dark brown or contains bacteria on Gram's stain, laparotomy is indicated. At surgery the entire intestine is inspected, cultures are taken, and all areas of necrosis are resected. The ends are exteriorized as stomas, since an anastomosis in this setting of acute infection carries a prohibitive risk of leakage.

Postoperatively, the same vigorous medical treatment is pursued as preoperatively. Enteral feeding is not resumed until approximately 2 weeks following clinical improvement and quantities are increased only gradually as the mucosa slowly regenerates. The stomas are preferentially closed months later, when the child is thriving, unless malabsorption requires that it be done sooner.

Approximately 15% of babies with NEC will subsequently develop intestinal obstruction from late stricture formation; surgical repair is necessary. The survival rate of babies with NEC is 80% overall; infants who require surgery have survival rates of 50% to 70%.

Prevention. Since NEC is rare in unfed babies, withholding enteral feeds in high-risk infants may be preventive, although long-term TPN has its own hazards. Breast milk may be partially protective as compared with formula, possibly because of its immunoglobulin content.

Neonatal Jaundice: Biliary Atresia and Choledochal Cyst

Neonatal jaundice is usually due to physiological unconjugated hyperbilirubinemia and is most often self-limited. An elevated direct bilirubin level in excess of 2 mg/dL for 2 weeks demands further investigation. Biliary atresia is a sclerotic obliteration of the extrahepatic biliary ducts, occurring at about the time of birth. Usually the entire ductal system, but occasionally only a portion, is affected. The intrahepatic ducts are also involved to some extent in the disease process, since they are not dilated as they are in extrahepatic obstruction. The cause is not known, but a viral etiology is currently favored. It is conjectured that biliary atresia, neonatal hepatitis, and possibly choledochal cysts (dilation of the extrahepatic ductal system with distal obstruction) represent a spectrum of the same disease. Alternatively, choledochal cysts may be produced by a weakening of the common bile duct wall by refluxed pancreatic enzymes, which promotes cystic dilation (Fig. 2.16).

Clinical Manifestations. An infant with biliary atresia presents with progressively increasing jaundice, usually discovered when the patient is several weeks of age. The stools become light colored and the liver is palpably enlarged. Laboratory investigations reveal an elevated serum bilirubin, most of which is conjugated. Liver enzymes and alkaline phosphatase levels are only mildly or moderately raised. The urine contains bile, but no urobilinogen, a finding consistent with obstructive jaundice.

Choledochal cysts may present at any age, but 50% of them appear in early infancy. In infants, clinical findings are similar to those for biliary atresia. In older patients, the liver is not usually enlarged and the cyst itself may be palpable.

Diagnosis. Biliary atresia must be diagnosed early, since the prognosis worsens rapidly with increasing age at operation. Neonatal cholestatic jaundice can be caused by a wide variety of infectious and metabolic disorders, such as TORCH (Toxoplasmosis, Other infections, Rubella, Cytomegalovirus infection, and Herpes simplex) infections, α-1-antitrypsin deficiency, galactosemia, TPN, hypoxic injury to the liver, or neonatal hepatitis. Most of these conditions are easily ruled

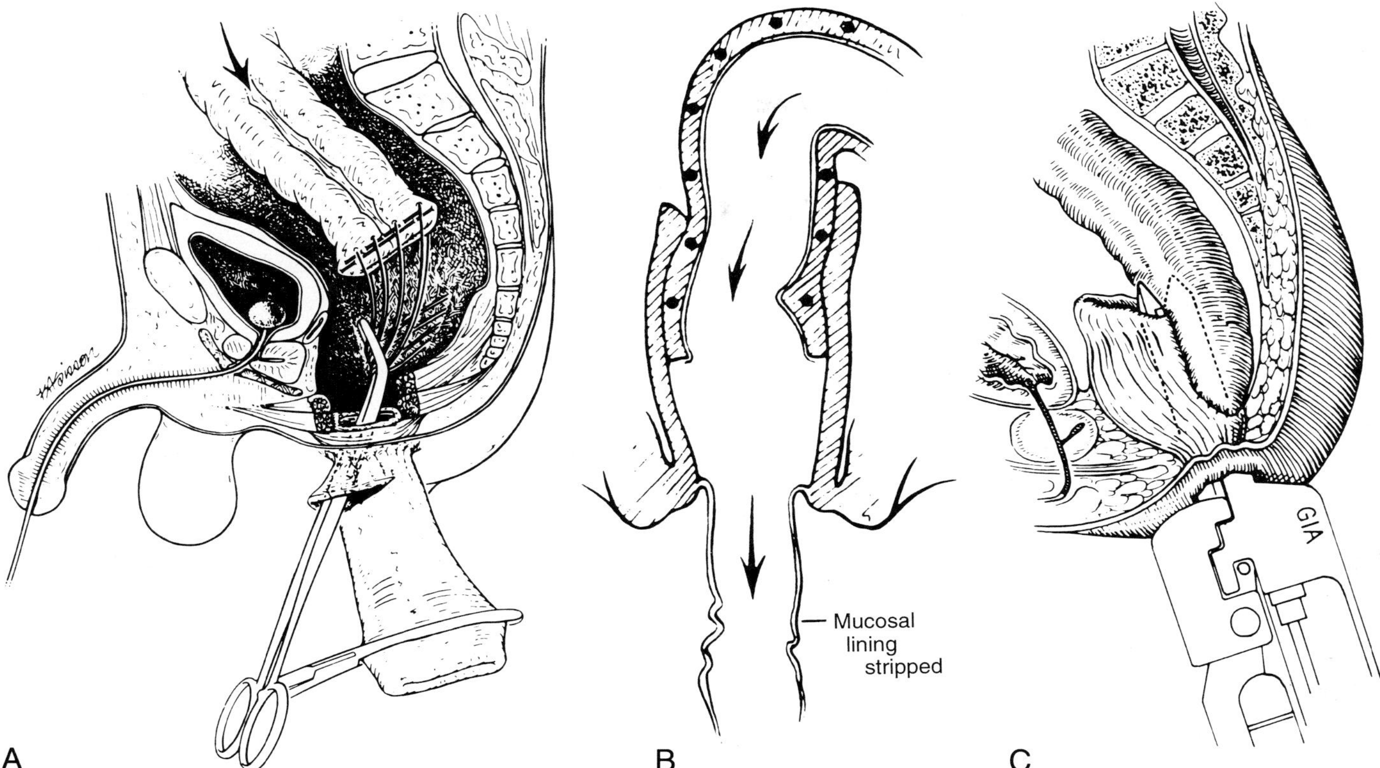

Figure 2.12. Pull-through operations for Hirschsprung's disease. **A**, Swenson procedure: the aganglionic intestine is resected completely and the ganglionic bowel brought down and anastomosed to the anal canal. **B**, Soave procedure: the mucosa from the aganglionic intestine is stripped and removed; the ganglionic bowel is pulled down to the anal canal within the remaining outer muscular sleeve. **C**, Duhamel procedure: the aganglionic rectum is left in place, and the ganglionic intestine brought behind it and anastomosed side-to-side.

out by screening tests and the overall clinical setting. The exception is neonatal hepatitis, usually a self-limited disorder, which is often difficult to distinguish from biliary atresia.

No single nonoperative study diagnoses biliary atresia with certainty. Ultrasonography can detect dilation of the bile ducts and identify a choledochal cyst. Hepatic scintiscans (such as the DISIDA scan), following pretreatment with phenobarbital to promote hepatic excretion, can be useful. The appearance of radionuclide in the intestine is proof of patency of the bile ducts and rules out biliary atresia. Percutaneous liver biopsy may be helpful as well. If biliary atresia is still suspected, a laparotomy is performed. The hilum of the liver is inspected and an operative cholangiogram is performed if possible. If patency of the bile ducts is demonstrated, neonatal hepatitis is presumed and the operation is terminated.

Treatment. The Kasai portoenterostomy operation for biliary atresia is based on the fact that although they are not visible, microscopically patent hepatic ductules are present in the porta hepatis. This fibrous-appearing tissue is cut across and anastomosed to the intestinal tract for drainage. This procedure has many variations to prevent reflux of bowel contents to the liver, which predisposes to ascending cholangitis. A nonfunctional Roux-en-Y loop of bowel can be used and is often temporarily exteriorized as an abdominal stoma. A one-way nipple valve has also been constructed in the intestinal conduit to be anastomosed to the porta.

Choledochal cysts are best excised, with anastomosis of a nonfunctional bowel loop to the (usually dilated) proximal hepatic ducts.

Results. The success of the Kasai operation depends on the age of the patient (bile will drain in 90% of patients before 60 days of age but only occasionally after 90 days of age), the diameter of the microscopic hepatic ductules (good drainage if they are over 150 microns), and the absence of advanced hepatic fibrosis. Recurrent postoperative cholangitis is common and prophylactic antibiotics are given. Portal hypertension and bleeding esophageal varices are also frequent sequela. The overall mortality rate of these patients is approximately 50%, usually due to progressive cirrhosis. If these children are not operated upon, the mortality rate is 100% by 2 years. The outlook for individuals undergoing resections for choledochal cysts is excellent.

Liver transplantation is now an option for children who develop progressive hepatic failure despite the Kasai operation. Because infant liver donors are in short supply, reduced segments from adult donors have recently been used. The survival rate among liver recipients is approximately 75%.

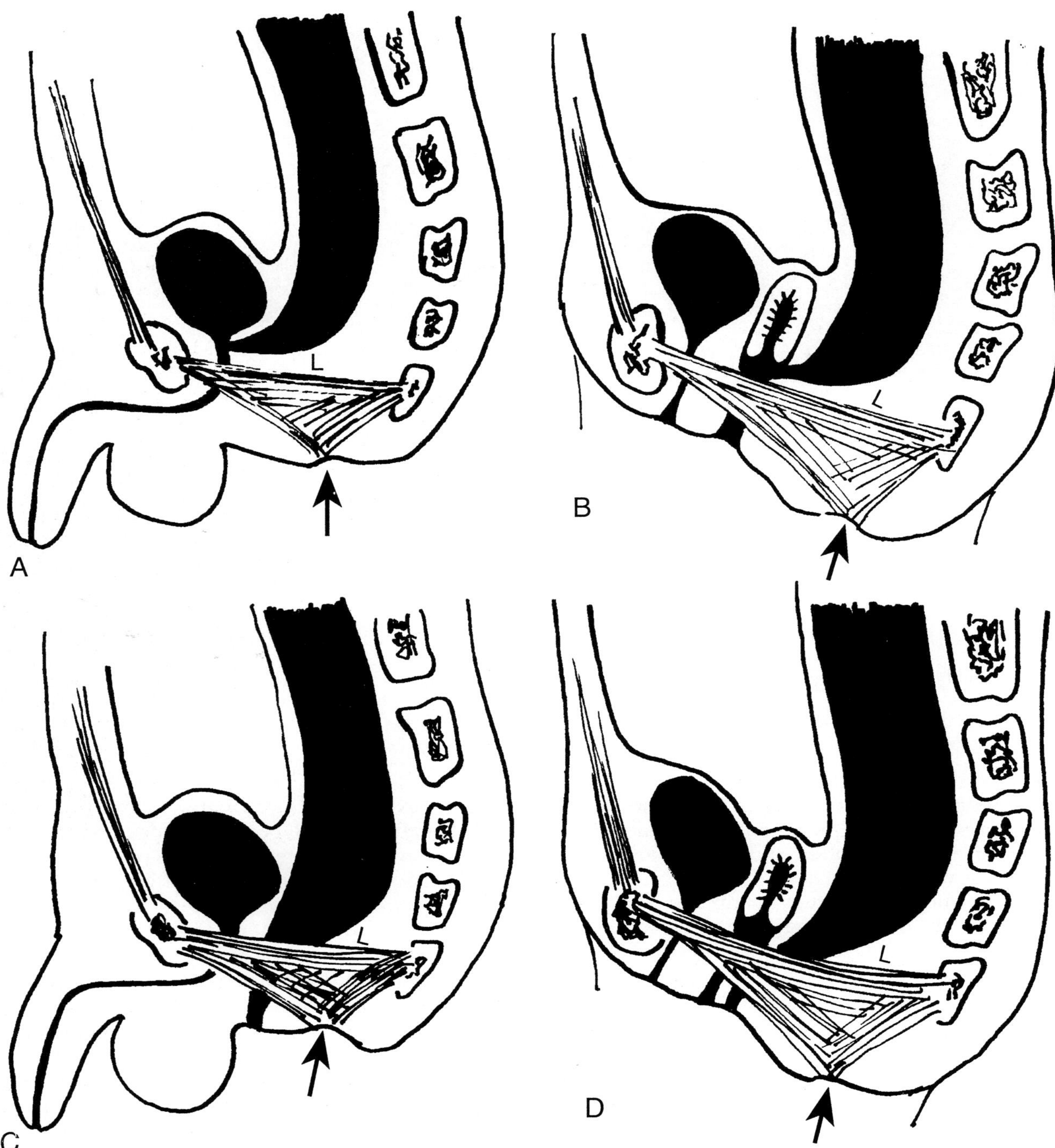

Figure 2.13. Types of congenital anorectal malformations. **A**, Male with high defect and rectourethral fistula. **B**, Female with high rectovaginal fistula. **C**, Male with low defect and anoperineal fistula. **D**, Female with anovulvar fistula. L, levator muscles; arrow, normal anal location at external sphincter.

Abdominal Wall Defects: Omphalocele and Gastroschisis

Omphalocele and gastroschisis are both congenital defects of the abdominal wall, through which the abdominal contents protrude externally to a varying degree. Infants with an omphalocele have an opening in the center of the abdomen, and the exteriorized viscera are covered by a translucent membrane (Fig. 2.17). The umbilical vessels insert onto the center of the sac. In gastroschisis, the abdominal wall opening is to the side of the umbilical cord, usually on the right (Fig. 2.18). The exposed viscera have no sac covering them and are usually thickened and edematous from the irritating effects of chronic exposure to amniotic fluid.

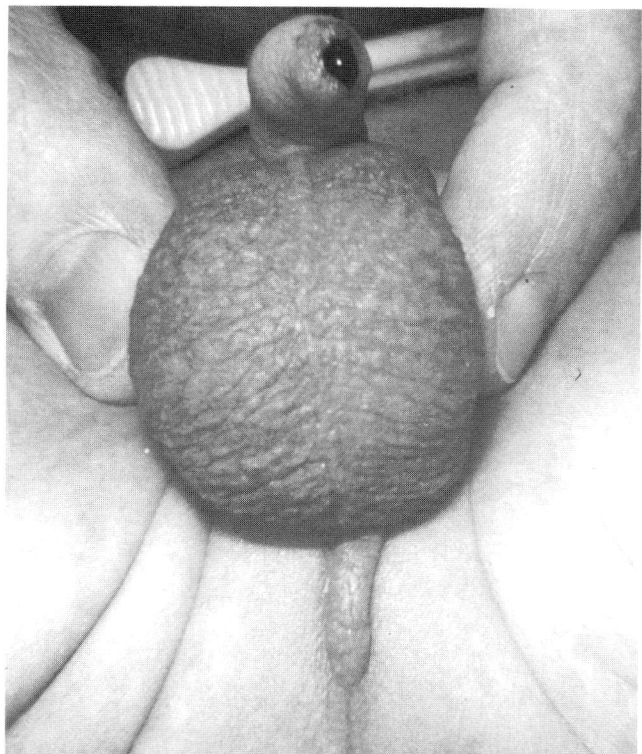

Figure 2.14. Newborn male with high anorectal malformation and rectourethral fistula. The perineal opening is absent and meconium is visualized at the urethral meatus.

Babies with omphaloceles have a very high incidence of associated multisystem anomalies, including chromosomal defects. In contrast, the only associated disorder noted with increased frequency in infants with gastroschisis is intestinal atresia. These atresias are produced by compression of the exteriorized bowel against the rim of the abdominal wall in utero.

Embryology. The abdominal wall is formed by four folds, the cephalic, caudal, and two lateral folds, each of which converge ventrally to form a large umbilical ring. This ring surrounds the umbilical vessels and yolk sac and eventually contracts to close the abdominal wall. Between the fifth and tenth weeks of gestation, the rapidly growing intestine is extruded into the yolk sac and then returns to the abdominal cavity where it undergoes rotation. An omphalocele is produced by failure of the lateral folds to close, with the viscera remaining in the yolk sac. Gastroschisis probably arises from antenatal perforation of the developing abdominal wall within the umbilical ring. It characteristically occurs at the area where one of the paired umbilical veins undergoes atrophy, a relative point of weakness.

Management. Infants born with an omphalocele or gastroschisis are at immediate risk for fluid and heat loss, as well as for the development of infection. The abdomen should be covered with sterile gauze soaked in warm saline and wrapped in plastic. Intravenous fluids and broad-spectrum antibiotics are administered,

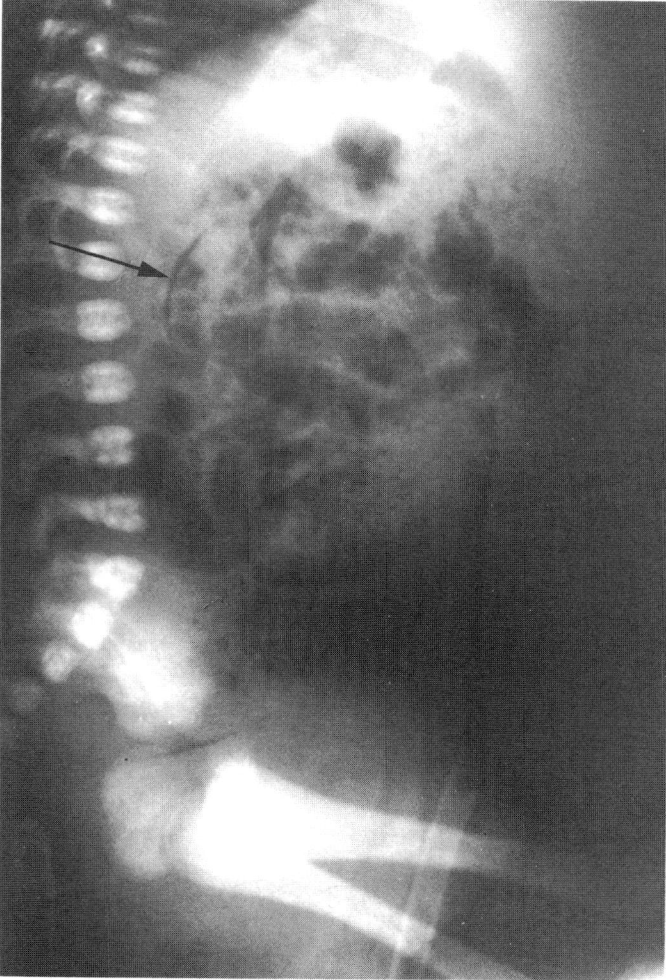

Figure 2.15. Premature neonate with necrotizing enterocolitis and pneumatosis intestinalis. Arrow indicates intramural air.

and a nasogastric tube placed to suction in order to prevent further intestinal distention. Infants with gastroschisis are at risk for the abdominal organs to become constricted where they exit from the abdominal wall. The viscera must not hang down to the side with the baby supine; they can be kept on top of the abdomen or the baby can be turned on its side. Cyanosis of the viscera mandates immediate enlargement of the defect at the bedside.

At surgery, the abdominal opening is enlarged in order to permit the organs to be placed into the peritoneal cavity, which is then closed. At times, the abdomen has not grown sufficiently large to accommodate the viscera. Closure with undue tension is hazardous and can compromise respiration, impair venous return through the inferior vena cava, and cause necrosis of the bowel. If necessary, a prosthetic sheet (made, for example, of Gore-Tex) is sutured around the edges of the abdominal defect, covering the organs as a silo (Fig. 2.19). Manual compression is applied daily in order to gradually replace the viscera and expand the abdominal cavity, un-

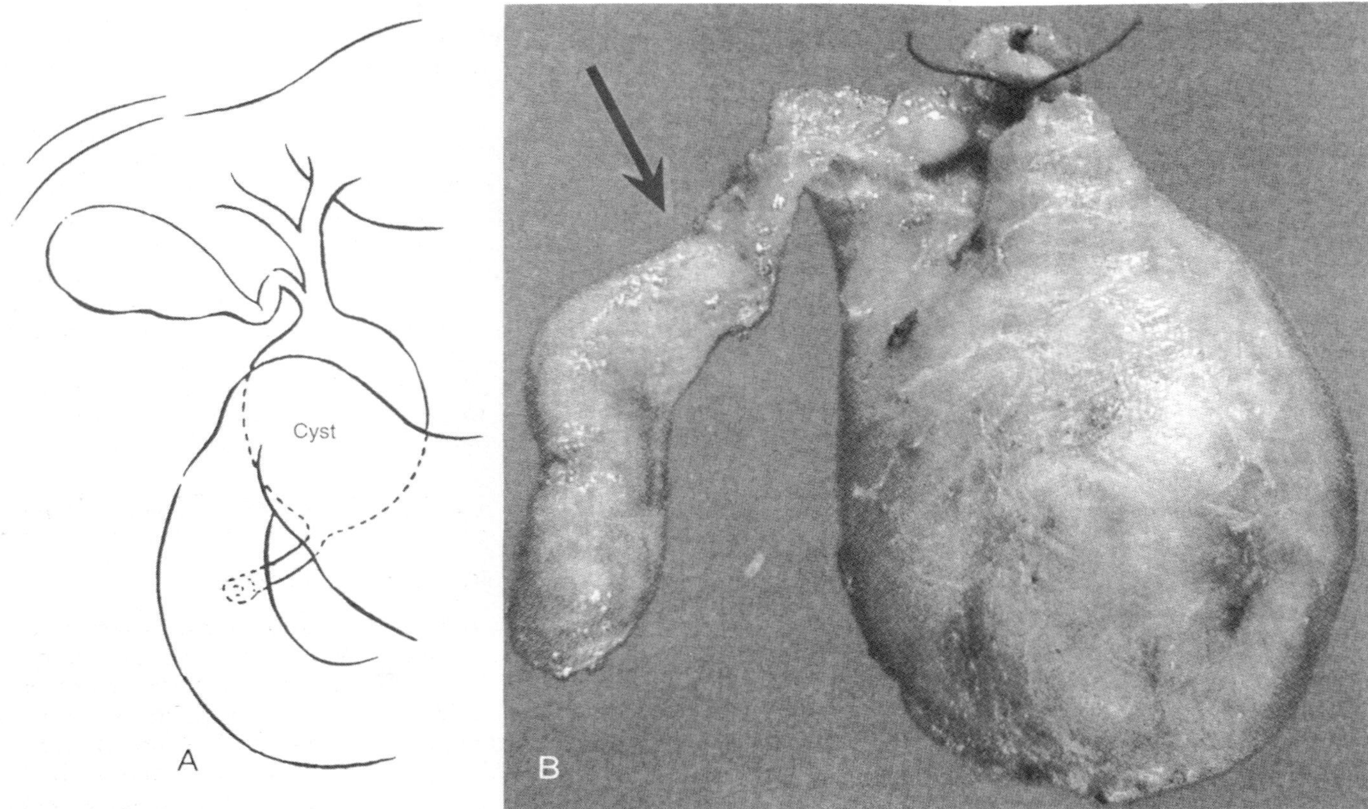

Figure 2.16. Choledochal cyst. A, Diagrammatic representation. B, Operative specimen. (Arrow, gallbladder.)

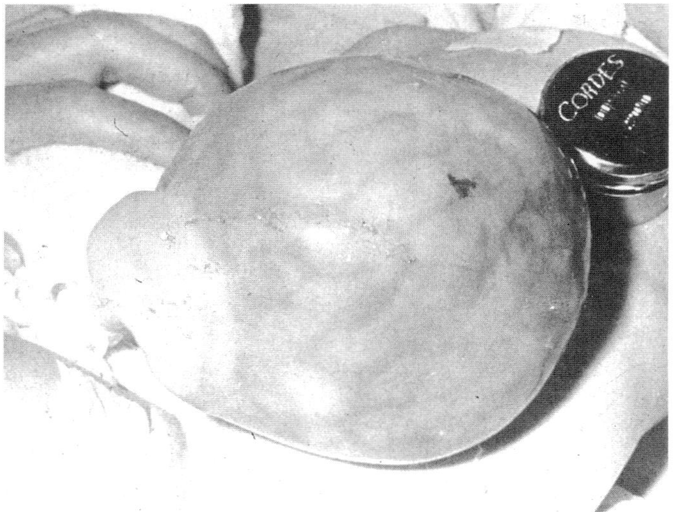

Figure 2.17. Large omphalocele containing visible loops of intestine. Umbilical cord arises from the sac.

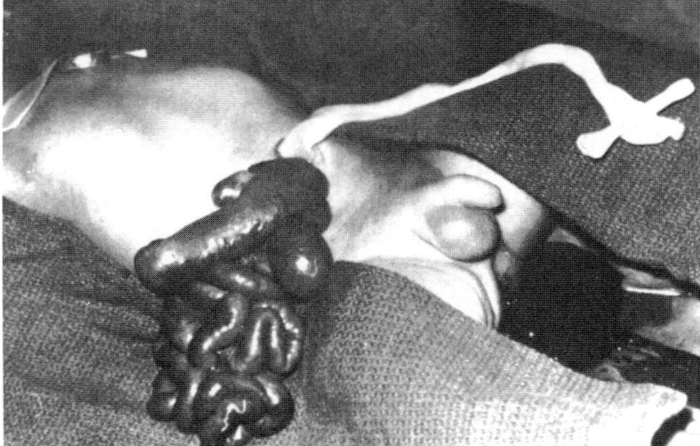

Figure 2.18. Gastroschisis, with exteriorized intestine uncovered by any sac (abdominal wall defect is to the side of the umbilicus).

til the prosthesis can be removed and the abdomen closed.

On occasion, infants with omphaloceles have such severe, life-threatening anomalies or poor prognoses that surgery is not desirable. The sac can be painted with alcohol or povidone iodine, and as it dries an eschar will form that will contract and epithelialize. This process requires several weeks.

Atresias associated with gastroschisis may be repaired at the original operation or deferred until the edema and inflammation subside. The malrotation that is present in babies with abdominal wall defects is rarely clinically significant. The appendix is often removed, because if appendicitis develops later in life its abnormal location will make early diagnosis difficult.

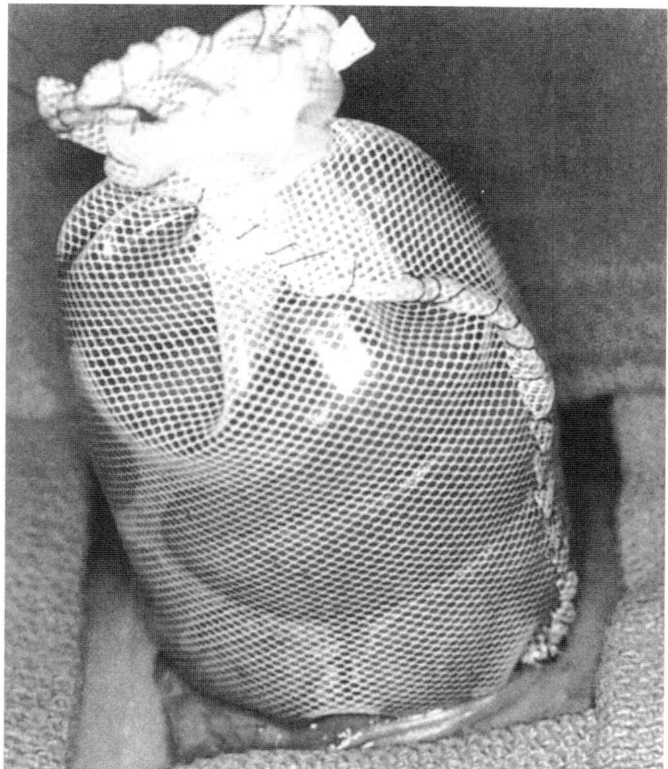

Figure 2.19. Giant omphalocele with defect temporarily closed with prosthetic silo of reinforced silastic.

Infants with gastroschisis may develop prolonged intestinal dysfunction due to the chronic inflammation, and TPN may be necessary for several weeks until the ileus resolves.

Circumcision

Circumcision is among the oldest of surgical procedures known, and is by far the most frequently performed operation on males in the United States. In contrast to the 90% of boys who undergo neonatal circumcision in this country, in Canada 40% and Australia only 15% of boys undergo routine circumcision. The operation is rarely performed in Europe. Circumcision remains controversial even within the medical profession. In 1989 the American Academy of Pediatrics acknowledged the lack of unanimity about the subject of circumcision, noting that the decision should properly be made by the parents, after the benefits and risks have been explained.

The prepuce, or foreskin, completely covers the glans except for a small opening at the urethral meatus. Its undersurface is fused with the glans at birth, and it is not until older childhood that the foreskin is fully retractable. True phimosis refers to the inability to pull back the foreskin because of fibrotic scarring at the preputial orifice, and not to these congenital physiological adhesions.

Neonatal circumcision has advantages and disadvantages. Among the advantages are that it will prevent the development of phimosis, paraphimosis (the inability to pull the foreskin back over the glans once it has been retracted), and posthitis (infection of the foreskin). Also, recent evidence shows that circumcision lowers the incidence of urinary tract infections in boys during the first year of life by 10-fold. Circumcision prevents cancer of the penis, although this malignancy is uncommon and may also be prevented by proper hygiene. Disadvantages include the fact that in the vast majority of males it will be a medically unnecessary procedure, it is painful, and it carries a definite (although very low) risk of technical complications. Contraindications to circumcision include serious illness of the baby, as well as genital anomalies such as hypospadias, in which the foreskin will be needed for eventual operative correction.

Surgical Conditions in the Older Child

Inguinal Hernia and Hydrocele

Inguinal hernias and hydroceles are extremely common in children, and their repair is the most frequent operation performed by pediatric surgeons. Hernias occur in 3% of children overall, with the incidence rising to 30% in very premature infants. Boys are affected six times as frequently as girls. Inguinal hernias in children are virtually all indirect, with the hernia sac emerging from the internal inguinal ring. Direct hernias, in which the defect is in the floor of the inguinal canal, are rare in young individuals.

Embryology. At 3 months of gestation the processus vaginalis forms as an outpouching of the peritoneum and passes through the internal inguinal ring. This processus then migrates down the inguinal canal into the scrotum, preceding the testicle, and comes to lie within the spermatic cord. The processus usually becomes obliterated around the time of birth, except for the most distal portion, which wraps itself around the testicle as the tunica vaginalis.

Continued patency of part or all of the processus vaginalis accounts for the development of hernias and hydroceles. If the processus remains widely open proximally, in continuity with the peritoneal cavity, intra-abdominal contents may protrude a variable distance into it, forming an inguinal hernia (Fig. 2.20**B**). If the processus remains open but is too narrow to admit any viscera, only peritoneal fluid may enter. Usually, this fluid surrounds the testicle within the widened tunica vaginalis, forming a communicating hydrocele (Fig. 2.20**C**). Less often, if the distal processus obliterates, the fluid accumulates above the testicle as a hydrocele of the spermatic cord (Fig. 2.20**D**). Finally, with obliteration of the proximal processus, fluid may remain trapped distally in the tunica vaginalis, producing a noncommunicating hydrocele (Fig. 2.20**E**).

In girls, the round ligament is a vestigial structure analogous to the spermatic cord, and it has the same relationship with the processus vaginalis. The ovary

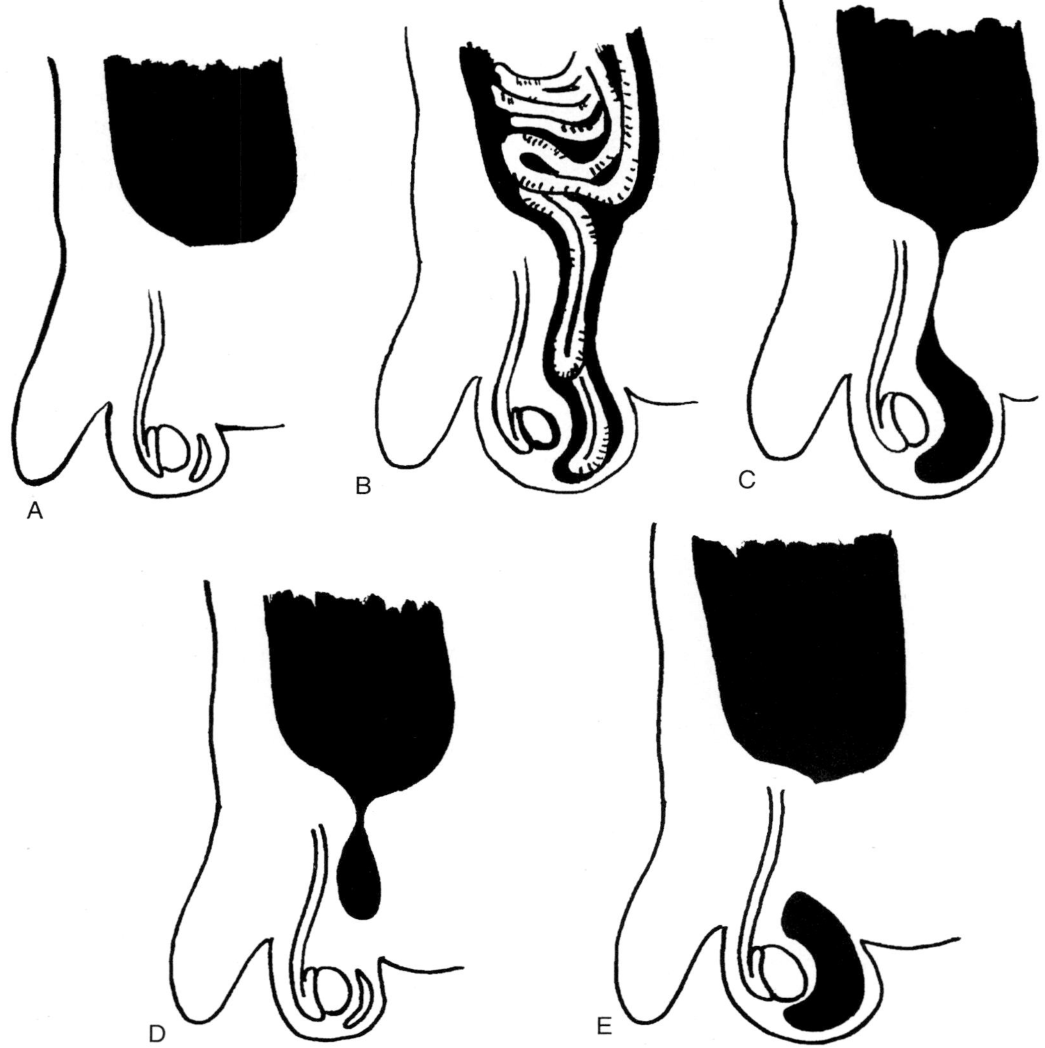

Figure 2.20. Hernia and hydrocele. **A**, Normal. **B**, Inguinal hernia. **C**, Communicating scrotal hydrocele. **D**, Hydrocele of cord. **E**, Noncommunicating hydrocele.

and Fallopian tube, rather than the intestine, are most likely to protrude through a patent processus.

Clinical Manifestations. Approximately half of all inguinal hernias appear before an infant is 1 year of age. They occur twice as often on the right side as on the left, since the right testicle descends later embryologically, and its processus is therefore less likely to have closed. Of inguinal hernias, 10% are bilateral. An inguinal hernia usually presents as an intermittent bulge in the groin or scrotum, brought on by crying or straining. On examination, it is palpable as a firm mass that completely disappears with digital pressure (Fig. 2.21). If not apparent, a hernia may be brought out by applying suprapubic pressure in infants or by asking older children to jump up and down or strain. Indirect evidence of an inguinal hernia consists of a palpable thickening of the spermatic cord where it crosses the pubic tubercle. A hydrocele usually appears as diffuse swelling of the hemiscrotum (Fig. 2.22). If it communicates, it will fluctuate in size throughout the day as it fills and empties. Noncommunicating hydroceles remain fairly constant in size but may gradually regress as fluid is absorbed.

Usually, one can differentiate a hernia from a hydrocele on examination. A hydrocele is more mobile, is not reducible, and does not extend upward toward the internal ring. A hydrocele of the cord may be particularly difficult to distinguish from an incarcerated hernia, since both present as irreducible masses above the testis. Hydroceles produce no symptoms, whereas incarcerated hernias cause pain and may produce intestinal obstruction. Transillumination is not particularly useful, since air-filled bowel transmits light as readily as does fluid.

Treatment. All inguinal hernias in children should be repaired. They never resolve and are at risk for incarceration and strangulation. The operation consists of a high ligation of the sac at the internal ring, which effec-

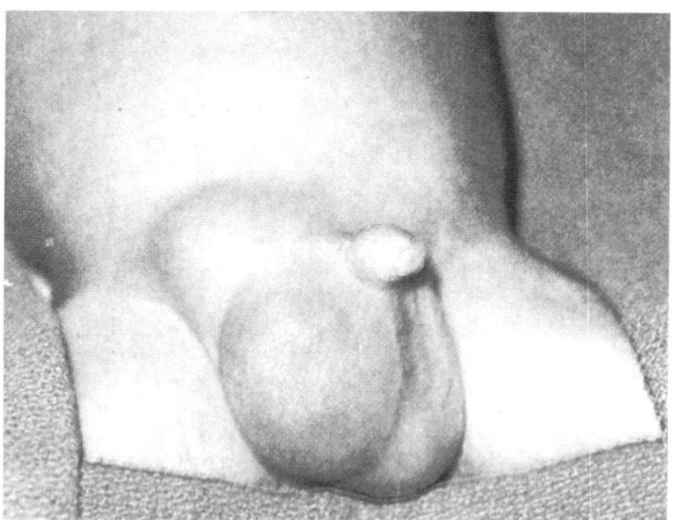

Figure 2.21. Right inguinal hernia in a 5-month-old boy.

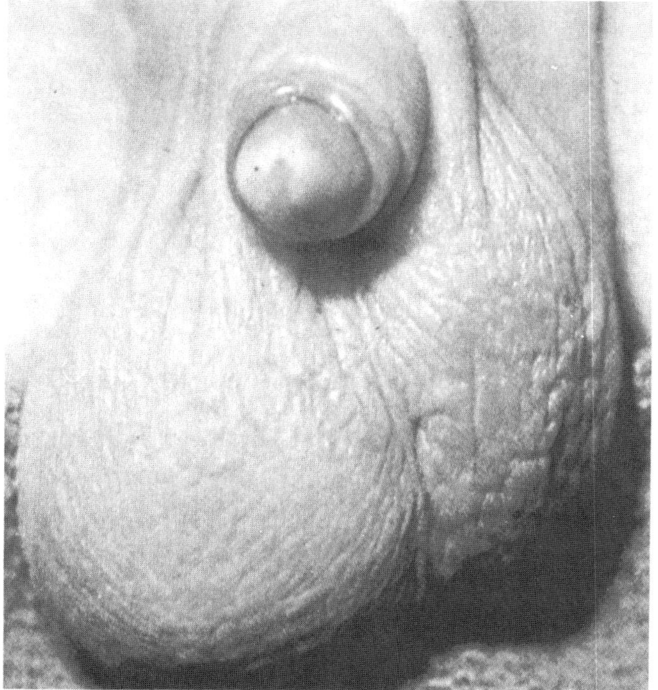

Figure 2.22. Right scrotal hydrocele in a 9-month-old boy.

tively obliterates the patent processus. Repair of the floor of the inguinal canal, as in adults, is unnecessary. The operation is generally performed on an outpatient basis. Some pediatric surgeons prefer to operate on all inguinal hernias whenever they are diagnosed. However, in the absence of symptoms, many recommend a delay until 3 months of age for term infants and longer for premature infants. The very young are at risk for postanesthesia apnea, and when surgery is necessary these infants must be monitored postoperatively in the hospital overnight.

An incarcerated hernia is an emergency, not only because of the risk of strangulation of the hernial contents, but also because the testicle may become ischemic. An incarcerated hernia in a child can almost always be reduced. Pressure is applied bimanually, and the hernia is pushed back through the internal ring. If necessary, meperidine (1–2 mg/kg IM) is administered for sedation (infants must then be monitored for apnea). Following successful reduction, surgery is delayed for 48 hours until edema of the sac subsides. Only rarely will necrotic viscera be reducible. If reduction fails, surgery is performed without delay.

A child with one inguinal hernia has an increased risk of developing another one on the contralateral side. Opinion is divided about exploring the asymptomatic side at the time of unilateral hernia repair. Many surgeons recommend exploration where there is a greater likelihood of bilaterality, such as in premature boys and in all girls (in whom there is also no danger of damaging the vas or spermatic vessels during surgery).

Unlike hernias, hydroceles may resolve within the first year of life. After that year, a hydrocele that persists or develops should be repaired, because the narrow sac can widen and turn into a hernia.

Umbilical Hernia

Umbilical hernias are caused by failure of complete contraction of the umbilical ring. They are especially frequent in blacks, in whom the incidence approaches 50%. Unlike inguinal hernias, most umbilical hernias resolve spontaneously, and the risk of incarceration is extremely low. The diagnosis is apparent by the presence of a bulge within the umbilicus. The enlarged fascial defect is readily palpable.

Surgery is usually recommended when the hernia persists in the child beyond 4 years of age. Parents are often quite anxious about these very visible protrusions, and if the fascial defect remains larger than 1.5 cm by the time the child is 2 years of age, spontaneous closure is unlikely and repair may be undertaken. Girls especially should have an umbilical hernia corrected before pregnancy, a time when the increased intra-abdominal pressure could lead to complications.

Cryptorchidism

A cryptorchid testis is one that has not descended into the scrotum, an event that normally takes place between the seventh and ninth months of gestation. The incidence of cryptorchidism at the time of birth is 3% in term infants and up to 30% in preterm infants. Most initially cryptorchid testes undergo spontaneous descent within the first year.

Ultrastructural studies reveal that by the second year of a child's life cryptorchid testes already have histological abnormalities. Previously, it was thought that if these testes were surgically placed into the scrotum, where it is 2°C below body temperature, they would function normally. Now, however, cryptorchid testes are considered to be abnormal initially. If they remain cryptorchid they will never produce sperm, whereas if

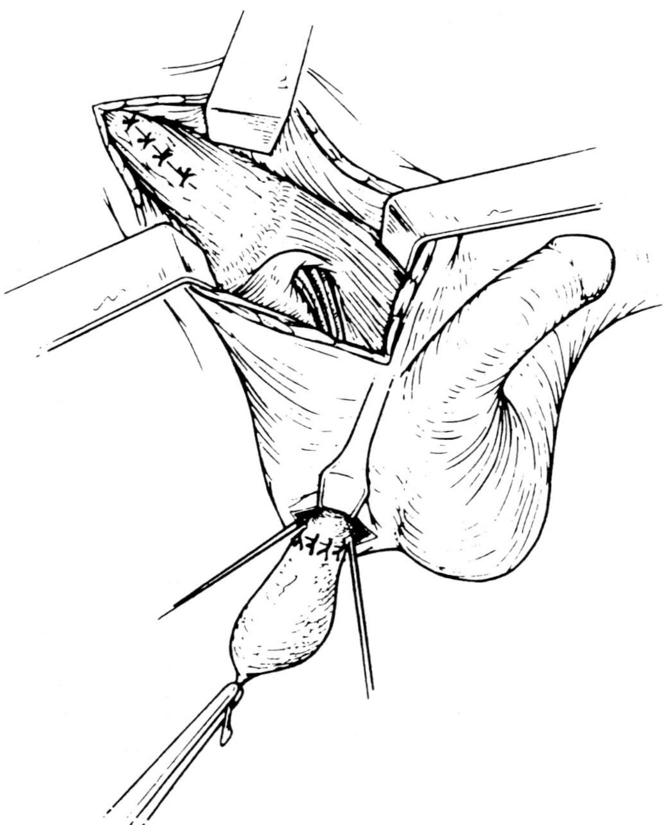

Figure 2.23. Orchidopexy for cryptorchidism, in which the undescended testicle is brought down and implanted into the scrotum between the dartos layer and the skin.

they are placed in their normal environment early in the child's life, their potential for sperm production is maximized. Evidence even suggests that if a cryptorchid testis is left undescended it may adversely affect spermatogenesis of the opposite, normally descended testicle.

The incidence of subsequent testicular malignancy in children with cryptorchid testes is 10 to 40 times that of the general population, beginning in young adulthood. Although it is not believed that early orchidopexy lowers this risk to normal, it does facilitate the early detection of testicular tumors on physical examination.

Cryptorchid testes are almost all associated with a patent processus vaginalis. This predisposition to inguinal hernia development is corrected at the time of orchidopexy. Other problems encountered by boys with cryptorchidism include an increased risk of torsion, more vulnerability to trauma, and psychological concerns about having only one testicle in the scrotum.

Clinical Manifestations. A cryptorchid testicle is absent in the scrotum and may or may not be palpable in the groin. It must be differentiated from the much more common retractile testis that is pulled up transiently by an active cremasteric reflex. If the testicle can be manipulated into the scrotum without tension, even if it does not remain there, the parents can be assured that there is no abnormality and that observation alone is indicated.

A testicle that is not palpable at all may be totally absent or located above the internal ring. Ultrasonography as well as CT and MRI scanning have been advocated as imaging modalities. Failure of these studies to visualize a testicle is not sufficient proof of its absence, however; operative exploration is still needed. Recently, laparoscopy has been used to search intra-abdominally, but the technique is not yet in widespread use. In infants with bilateral nonpalpable testes, a human chorionic gonadotropin (HCG) stimulation test may be performed. If the serum testosterone level fails to rise markedly in response to HCG administration, no testicular tissue exists.

Treatment. Hormonal treatment with HCG, and more recently with luteinizing hormone-releasing hormone (LHRH), has been advocated as initial treatment of cryptorchidism, but the results are conflicting. Hormonal therapy may rationally be attempted in boys with bilateral cryptorchidism, in whom it is more plausible that there is an underlying hormonal deficiency responsible for the undescended testes.

Orchidopexy is recommended for all boys whose testes remain undescended and is performed when the patient is between 1 and 2 years of age (Fig. 2.23). If orchidopexy has not been undertaken by late puberty, orchiectomy is indicated.

Results. Following early successful orchidopexy for unilateral cryptorchidism, 80% to 90% of boys will subsequently be fertile. Only 50% of boys with bilateral cryptorchidism will be fertile following bilateral orchidopexy. In contrast, testosterone production by the testes is unaffected by their location, and secondary sexual characteristics develop normally in all these boys.

Pyloric Stenosis

Pyloric stenosis is a progressive hypertrophy of the musculature of the pylorus in infancy, leading to gastric outlet obstruction. It is a common disorder, occurring in 1 in 500 infants. It affects males four times as frequently as females, and it has a familial component. The etiology of pyloric stenosis is not known. One hypothesis is that there is abnormal development of the ganglion cells in the wall of the pylorus. Another proposal is that milk curds propelled against the pylorus produce submucosal edema that initially blocks the gastric outlet, leading to subsequent work hypertrophy of the muscular pylorus.

Clinical Manifestations. An infant with pyloric stenosis typically presents at 2 weeks to 2 months of age with nonbilious vomiting after feeding. The vomiting, which may be projectile, becomes progressively worse until little is held down. The infant remains hungry between vomiting episodes and sucks vigorously. Stool frequency and urinary output diminish as less oral intake is retained.

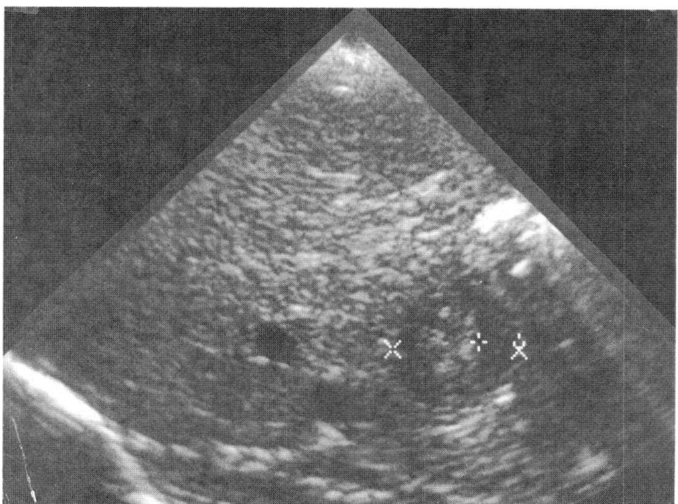

Figure 2.24. Pyloric stenosis seen on ultrasonography. Markers demonstrate thickened wall of pylorus on cross section.

On examination the infant may appear irritable and dehydrated to a variable degree. Peristaltic waves are sometimes seen moving across the abdomen. The hallmark of pyloric stenosis is the palpable "olive," a hard, round, moveable mass in the epigastrium. With experience and patience, an examiner can feel this mass in most children with pyloric stenosis. It is helpful to empty the infant's stomach with a tube or to examine the infant immediately after it has vomited, and crucial that its abdominal muscles be relaxed. The infant can be given Pedialyte or a pacifier coated with sugar during the examination. When an olive is identified, no imaging studies are necessary.

In the absence of a palpable olive, ultrasonography is highly accurate in diagnosing pyloric stenosis, as the length, diameter, and wall thickness of the pylorus are all increased (Fig. 2.24). If this study is equivocal, a barium swallow is obtained, which will demonstrate a narrowed, elongated pyloric channel.

Treatment. Before the infant undergoes surgery, it must be rehydrated. These infants have been vomiting gastric contents and may have a hypochloremic, hypokalemic, metabolic alkalosis. Depending on the extent of the dehydration and alkalosis, D5% 1/2 or D5% normal saline with up to 40 mEq/liter KCl is administered at 1 1/2 to 2 times the maintenance rate. When urine output is 1–2 mL/kg/hour and serum electrolytes are normal, operative correction may proceed. The operation performed is a pyloromyotomy. Through a small laparotomy, a longitudinal incision is made along the hypertrophic pylorus. The cut muscle edges are spread apart down to the mucosa, without entering the lumen.

Feeding is initiated 12 hours postoperatively and increased gradually over the next 24 hours. It is not uncommon for the infant to have transient vomiting caused by a chronically overdistended stomach. The infant is discharged in 1–3 days, and there are no sequela.

Acute Abdomen

Few terms in medicine convey as much sense of urgency and drama as "the acute abdomen." Indeed, one is usually confronted with an acutely ill patient about whom a rapid decision must be made regarding the need for an emergency operation, often with a limited data base. Older children and adolescents with acute abdominal conditions present in much the same manner as adults. Infants and young children, however, respond quite differently, and it is challenging to distinguish those with an immediate need for abdominal surgery from the large number of children who fill pediatricians' offices.

Young children tend to have a uniform response to illness. Whether they are suffering from streptococcal pharyngitis, lobar pneumonia, viral gastroenteritis, or appendicitis, they frequently develop fever, vomiting, and a "stomachache." They also have a limited ability to express their symptoms or to cooperate during an examination. Their omentum is not fully developed and therefore not capable of walling off inflammatory processes in the abdomen. These processes can rapidly progress to diffuse peritonitis. For all these reasons, the inflamed appendix is usually perforated by the time the condition is correctly diagnosed in children under 5 years of age. It is imperative that young children with unexplained abdominal pain be evaluated and followed very carefully.

The examination begins with the overall appearance of the child, such as whether the child "looks sick" and how he or she moves around. A child with crampy abdominal pain is fussy and intermittently draws the knees up and cries. In contrast, a child with diffuse peritonitis lies quietly on the side in the fetal position, breathing shallowly and avoiding any unnecessary motion. Involuntary guarding is the single most useful sign in differentiating a surgical abdomen from other disorders. Since young children frequently cry and tense their abdominal muscles when being examined, it is important to establish trust and be extremely patient. Serial examinations over time by the same observer can be most useful.

The pelvis is relatively shallow in small children, and a digital rectal examination may provide important information. Intra-abdominal contents may be palpated, and purulent material, which drains into the dependent cul-de-sac, may be felt as a fluctuant, tender mass against the anterior rectal wall.

The child's age and sex as well as the results of the history and physical examination are all important in attempting to ascertain the precise cause of a surgical abdomen. However, it is far more important to determine whether a patient needs an operation than to diagnose the exact etiology of the abdominal condition preoperatively.

Appendicitis. Acute appendicitis is the most common condition requiring emergency surgery in childhood. It occurs in 7% of the population at some time in their lives. It is rare in the newborn period, after which its incidence increases progressively, peaking in adolescents and young adults. Appendicitis is caused by obstruction of the base of the appendix by a fecalith or lymphoid hyperplasia. Mucosal secretions distend the appendix and increase intraluminal pressure, leading to bacterial overgrowth and impairment of perfusion. If timely intervention does not occur, perforation takes place in 36 to 48 hours.

Clinical Manifestations. The initial symptom is almost always pain, classically periumbilical and diffuse at the onset, and then localizing to the right lower quadrant. The distention of the appendix transmits poorly localized visceral pain, which is referred to the T10 dermatome, the central portion of the abdomen. As the inflammation progresses to involve the serosa, the surrounding parietal peritoneum transmits well-localized somatic pain at the site of the appendix, which is usually the right lower abdomen. Anorexia, nausea, and vomiting are common. If a child is truly hungry, the diagnosis of acute appendicitis is questionable.

The patient's temperature is typically normal or mildly elevated. High fever suggests a ruptured appendix or some other diagnosis. Abdominal examination will usually reveal diminished bowel sounds and signs of localized peritonitis, with involuntary guarding, tenderness, and rebound in the right lower quadrant. Rectal examination may be normal, but often elicits tenderness on the right side if the inflamed appendix extends into the pelvis.

Children with ruptured appendicitis are usually quite ill, with high fever and localized or generalized peritonitis. They frequently have a tender rectal examination, and a mass may be palpable either abdominally or rectally.

Laboratory studies should always include a complete blood count (CBC) and urinalysis. The white blood count (WBC) is usually elevated and/or shifted to the left. Many white cells in the urine suggest a urinary infection, although a few white cells or red cells are consistent with an inflamed appendix in contiguity with the urinary tract. Abdominal x-rays are obtained only in patients in whom the diagnosis of appendicitis is questionable or in the very young, in whom the diagnosis is always difficult. The only pathognomonic sign of appendicitis is a calcified fecalith that can be visualized in only 5% of cases. Radiographic findings are usually less specific, such as mild distention of small bowel loops and obliteration of the right psoas shadow.

The classic presentation of appendicitis is by no means universal, and in many children the diagnosis will be equivocal. Observation with repeated examinations is most helpful, because the positive findings will worsen if the patient has appendicitis. Ultrasonography is over 90% accurate in identifying an acutely inflamed appendix by visualizing a noncompressible, tubular structure at the point of maximal tenderness. It is particularly helpful in adolescent females to rule out such entities as an ovarian cyst, adnexal torsion, and pelvic inflammatory disease. A barium enema may be useful in atypical cases, demonstrating a mass effect or spasm of the cecum and terminal ileum. Laparoscopy has been proposed as a diagnostic aid for appendicitis, but anesthesia is required; in children it is probably no more invasive to make a small incision and actually remove the appendix.

Treatment. Following rapid intravenous hydration and the administration of broad-spectrum antibiotics, appendectomy is indicated for all children with appendicitis. If the appendix is not ruptured, the antibiotics may be discontinued within 24 hours; for perforated appendicitis, a full 7- to 10-day course is warranted. Recovery from nonruptured appendicitis is rapid, and children are discharged in several days. Perforated appendicitis has a high incidence of complications, particularly intra-abdominal abscesses and wound infections. Intra-abdominal abscesses can often be drained percutaneously, under ultrasound guidance. Wound infections are opened and drained.

Intussusception. Intussusception is a telescoping of one portion of the intestine into another. Most frequently it is ileocolic, as the distal ileum invaginates and travels a variable distance around the colon. Intussusception is an emergency condition, because the involved intestine usually becomes strangulated.

Children between 6 months and 2 years of age are most commonly affected. Rarely, a pathological lead point is found as the causative factor, such as a Meckel's diverticulum, a polyp, a lymphoma, or a hematoma. Mostly, intussusception is idiopathic, although hypertrophy of Peyer's patches in the submucosa has been hypothesized to act as the lead point in many of these cases.

Clinical Manifestations. Intussusception sometimes follows a viral illness. It is characterized by intermittent bouts of colicky abdominal pain in which the child cries and draws the knees to the chest. Between these episodes the child is initially well but becomes increasingly lethargic. Vomiting is frequent, eventually becoming bilious as intestinal obstruction develops. Blood and mucus may be passed rectally as "currant jelly stools" resulting from congestion and ischemia of the intestinal mucosa.

On examination these children may be irritable and/or somnolent, as well as dehydrated. A tender, sausage-shaped mass can often be palpated in the right upper abdomen. Digital rectal examination may yield blood and mucus. Abdominal x-rays appear normal early on, although eventually dilated small intestinal loops consistent with obstruction will develop. Unfortunately, the diagnosis can be difficult because many of the aforementioned symptoms and signs may be absent. If intussusception is suspected, a barium enema is mandatory. Ileocolic intussusception will appear as a filling defect in the colon, at which point the flow of barium stops (Fig. 2.25).

Treatment. The hydrostatic pressure of the barium enema can be used to reduce the intussusception and will be successful in the majority of children. The child is then admitted for 24 hours of observation. Surgery must be performed promptly if barium reduction fails. Following expeditious hydration, the intussusception is manually reduced and the appendix removed. If the in-

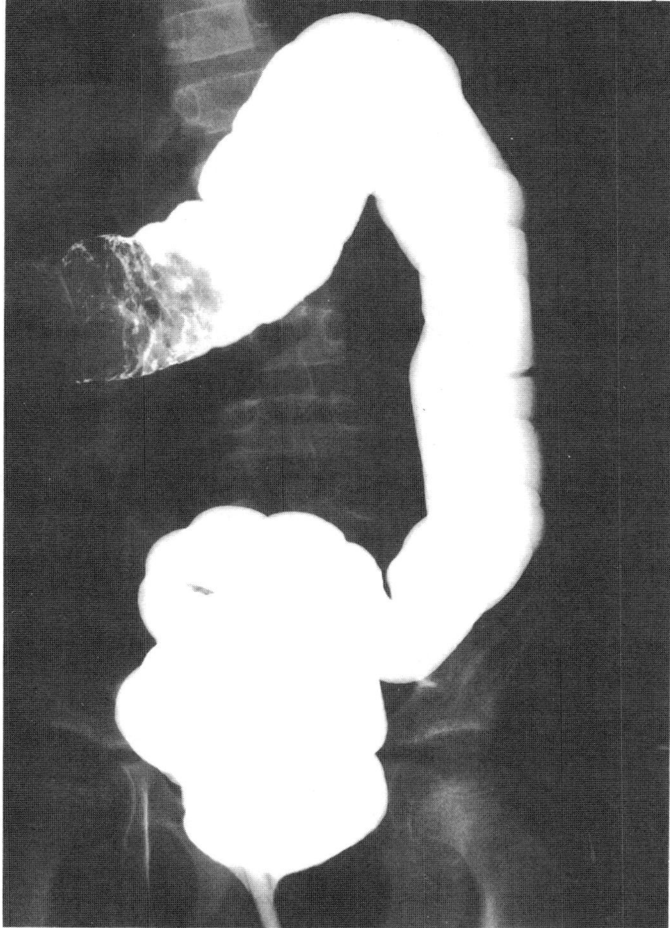

Figure 2.25. Ileocolic intussusception. Barium enema outlines filling defect in transverse colon.

testine is necrotic or a pathological lead point is identified, that segment of intestine is resected.

Recurrent intussusception occurs in 5% of children, regardless of whether the reduction was accomplished by barium or at surgery. Ileoileal intussusception and intussusception occurring in older children are much more likely to be associated with a pathological lead point. In these instances, barium reduction is rarely successful.

Meckel's Diverticulum. A Meckel's diverticulum is present in 2% of the population and is located in the ileum within 100 cm of the ileocecal valve. It contains heterotopic tissue in 50% of symptomatic patients, most often being lined with gastric mucosa.

Embryologically the yolk sac communicates with the intestine through the vitelline (omphalomesenteric) duct. This structure normally involutes between the fifth and seventh weeks of gestation. If it remains completely open, intestinal contents will drain from the umbilicus following cord separation after birth and form a vitelline fistula. Much more commonly, only the intestinal side of the vitelline duct remains patent and forms a Meckel's diverticulum. The distal end may lie freely or be attached to the undersurface of the umbilicus by a fibrous band.

Although most Meckel's diverticula remain asymptomatic, they may be complicated by bleeding, obstruction, and inflammation. Bleeding results from peptic ulceration adjacent to the ectopic gastric mucosa of the diverticulum. It usually occurs in children under 5 years of age. The resulting rectal bleeding is painless, dark red, and may be massive. Contrast x-rays rarely visualize the diverticulum, whereas technetium pertechnetate scans, which demonstrate increased uptake in gastric tissue, are positive in 50% of cases. Treatment is by surgical resection of the Meckel's diverticulum along with the adjacent ulcer.

A Meckel's diverticulum can cause intestinal obstruction by acting as the lead point of an intussusception, or by allowing the intestine to twist around it as a volvulus when the diverticulum is fixed to the anterior abdominal wall. A barium enema is rarely successful in reducing intussusception associated with a lead point, and surgical intervention is necessary.

Meckel's diverticulitis occurs in somewhat older children. Appendicitis is almost always misdiagnosed preoperatively, as their manifestations are so similar. Whenever a normal appendix is found at laparotomy for presumptive appendicitis, the distal ileum must be inspected for the possibility of Meckel's diverticulitis.

The management of a patient in whom an asymptomatic Meckel's diverticulum is found incidentally at surgery is controversial. The lifelong risk of a Meckel's diverticulum producing disease is approximately 4%. The risk is greater in young individuals, if there is heterotopic tissue within the diverticulum, and possibly if it is greater than 2 cm in length, has a narrow neck, or is tethered to the anterior abdominal wall. These factors should all be considered in deciding whether to resect a Meckel's diverticulum in the asymptomatic patient.

Gastrointestinal Bleeding

Gastrointestinal (GI) bleeding may occur throughout infancy and childhood, and is usually quite frightening to parents. Fortunately, most GI bleeding in children is mild and can be managed easily and safely. The sources of bleeding in a given child may be ascertained by the child's age, level of bleeding (upper or lower), color and amount of blood, and associated findings. If the bleeding is massive and the child hemodynamically unstable, rapid resuscitation is required, with insertion of large-bore intravenous catheters, fluid administration and blood transfusions, and prompt investigations as to the cause of the hemorrhage. For smaller amounts of bleeding, which are much more common, outpatient evaluation is appropriate.

In neonates, the site of bleeding is often never found. Swallowed maternal blood is passed as black stools and identified by determining the relative quantities of adult and fetal hemoglobin in the blood. An anal fissure produces small amounts of bright red blood and is visualized by inspection. Stress ulceration, midgut volvulus, necrotizing enterocolitis, and clotting disorders can produce bleeding in infants, and are usually recognized by the overall clinical setting. Other causes of neonatal GI bleeding include formula intolerance, duplications (containing acid-secreting heterotopic gastric tissue), and hemangiomas.

Young children may bleed from many of the causes listed above, as well as from esophageal varices, intussusception, infectious diarrhea, Meckel's diverticula, and polyps. Juvenile polyps are common in this age group and are actually hamartomas, with no malignant potential. They are found mostly in the left colon and typically present with bright to dark red rectal bleeding that coats the stools. Juvenile polyps may be removed endoscopically or observed, since they frequently autoamputate. Anal fissures are often caused by hard stool and are characterized by bright red blood and pain on defecation. Treatment with stool softeners and local ointments is usually effective.

Older children may have GI hemorrhage from peptic ulcerations and inflammatory bowel disease in addition to many of the conditions above. Peutz-Jegher's polyps and familial polyposis may also be seen. The Peutz-Jegher's syndrome is an autosomal dominant disorder characterized by multiple hamartomatous polyps in the gastrointestinal tract, especially in the small intestine, as well as melanin spots on the lips and buccal mucosa. Intussusceptions, usually transient, and recurrent gastrointestinal bleeding are common. Surgery is reserved for persistent intussusception and serious bleeding. Familial polyposis, also an autosomal dominant disease, consists of numerous adenomatous polyps in the colon. It usually presents in the second decade of life with abdominal pain and rectal bleeding. Malignant transformation is inevitable in adulthood, and a prophylactic colectomy should be performed by 15 years of age.

The evaluation of a child with GI bleeding will depend on its specific characteristics. Appropriate studies may include hemoglobin levels, coagulation tests, nasogastric aspiration, contrast studies, upper and lower endoscopy, a Meckel's technetium scan, and angiography. Treatment will vary with the etiology and amount of bleeding.

Gastroesophageal Reflux

Gastroesophageal reflux (GER) is extremely common in infants because the lower esophageal sphincter is relatively incompetent in the first few months of life. It is usually of minor consequence and is responsible for the occasional regurgitations and wet burps common in infants. In some infants the vomiting is severe and may even mimic pyloric stenosis. Medical management is usually effective for uncomplicated reflux, with upright positioning, thickening the feeds, and possibly administering metoclopramide. Children generally outgrow reflux by 1 year of age.

Some children have significant complications of GER that make them more likely to require surgical intervention. These complications include:

1. Failure to thrive
2. Aspiration causing recurrent pneumonia or wheezing
3. Apnea, probably due to reflux-induced laryngospasm or a vagal reflex (may be one cause of SIDS)
4. Peptic esophagitis, which can lead to stricture formation (more common in older children)

Evaluation of a child with possibly significant GER is initiated with a barium swallow. Obstructive lesions must be ruled out, and if massive GER is observed, no further diagnostic studies may be necessary. If GER is suspected clinically but not documented by barium x-ray, the more sensitive pH probe study or a nuclear scintiscan of the esophagus is indicated. Endoscopy is useful to demonstrate esophagitis, but is much less often used in children than in adults.

Surgery is indicated if medical management fails to control the complications of GER, or sooner for life-threatening complications, such as apnea. Many operative procedures have been devised, but the Nissen fundoplication, in which the gastric fundus is wrapped 360° around the lower esophagus, is performed most commonly in children. Complications include the gas bloat syndrome, in which patients become distended after feeding because they cannot burp, and the inability to vomit. These problems are usually outgrown.

Certain groups of individuals have a much higher incidence of intractable GER than the general population. These are children with chronic neurological and psychomotor disturbances, and those who have had esophageal atresia or a diaphragmatic hernia. Surgery is more likely to be necessary in these patients.

Neck Masses

Neck masses are very frequently found in children, and in most instances can be accurately diagnosed by the history and physical examination alone. These masses seldom carry the same ominous import as they do in adults, but certain malignancies can occur. Surgical excision may be required for definitive treatment, and occasionally for diagnosis.

Midline Neck Masses. Embryologically, the thyroid gland descends from the base of the tongue. The thyroglossal duct, along the path of descent, normally becomes obliterated. Persistence of this structure can result in the formation of a thyroglossal duct cyst. Characteristically, this cyst appears between 2 to 10 years of age as a firm, round, midline neck mass (Fig. 2.26). It rises with swallowing and protrusion of the tongue. Infection is a frequent complication.

A dermoid cyst probably arises from trapped epithelial elements, and may also present as a midline neck mass. It is usually more superficially located than a thyroglossal duct cyst. An ectopic thyroid, arrested in its antenatal descent, may occur as a midline neck mass and may represent the patient's only thyroid tissue. Finally, enlarged lymph nodes may appear in the midline of the neck.

Evaluation of a child with a midline neck mass should include an ultrasound or a thyroid scan to be certain that there is a normally located thyroid gland. If so, the mass may be safely excised. A thyroglossal duct cyst must be removed together with its tract and the

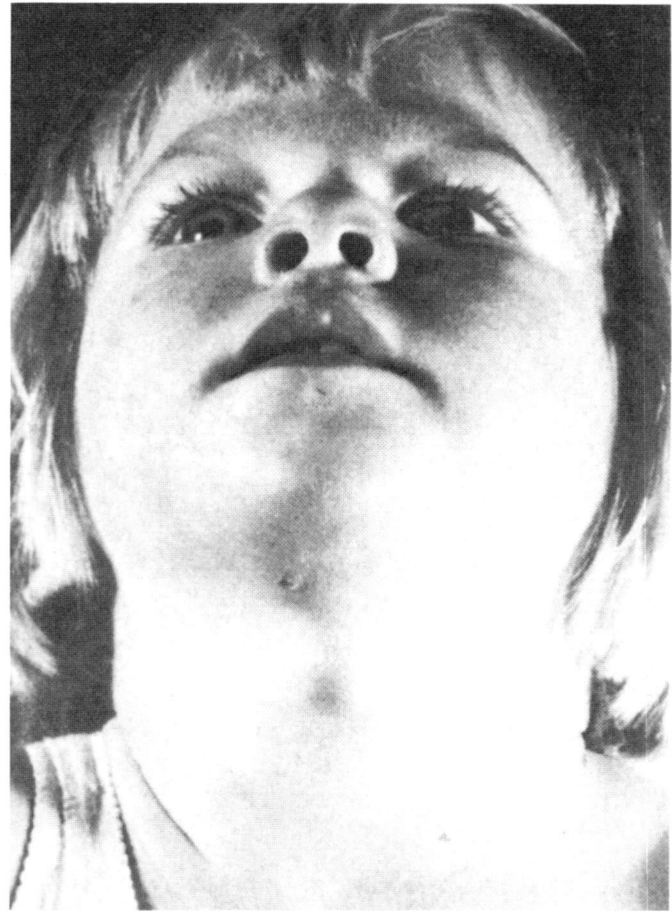

Figure 2.26. Thyroglossal duct cyst in a 5-year-old girl.

center of the hyoid bone, in order to prevent recurrence. An ectopic thyroid may be divided and placed on both sides of the neck, or it may be excised and thyroid replacement then given.

Thyroid nodules are usually recognized by their location. Although uncommon in children, their occurrence may be due to the same abnormalities as those in adults. A thyroid nodule in a child is more likely to be malignant, however, and lobectomy with biopsy is always indicated.

Lateral Neck Masses

Lymphadenopathy. Acute cervical lymphadenitis occurs predominantly in very young children as a result of a staphylococcal or streptococcal infection, usually following an upper respiratory infection. The child is febrile and the neck swelling shows classic signs of inflammation, including erythema, warmth, tenderness, and induration. Antibiotics may be curative, but if an abscess develops, incision and drainage are necessary.

Chronic lymphadenopathy is extremely common in the cervical region and usually represents nonspecific benign hyperplasia. Other causes of enlarged cervical lymph nodes are infections with atypical mycobacteria, cat scratch disease, and, rarely, lymphoma. The latter is suggested if the nodes are hard, fixed, or continue to grow, and if the patient has systemic symptoms such as fever, malaise, and weight loss. Open biopsy of enlarged cervical lymph nodes is indicated if they are greater than 2 cm in diameter and persist for 6 weeks, or sooner if malignancy is suspected based on the above findings.

Cystic Hygroma. Cystic hygromas, or lymphangiomas, are congenital malformations of the lymphatic vessels characterized by multiloculated cystic masses lined with endothelium and filled with lymph. They may occur anywhere but are most common in the posterior triangle of the neck, followed by the axilla. They may be present at birth and almost always appear within the first 2 years of age. Cystic hygromas can usually be diagnosed on physical examination as soft, compressible masses, with ill-defined borders. They may become infected and rarely regress. Resection is indicated.

Branchial Cysts and Sinuses. Branchial cleft cysts and sinuses arise from failure of complete closure and resorption of the various branchial clefts and arches. Sinuses present as small cutaneous openings that frequently drain clear fluid. Cysts occur as subcutaneous masses and are less complete abnormalities than sinuses, in that external closure has occurred. Skin tags and collections of cartilage may also occur. Remnants of the second branchial cleft are by far the most common and are located along the anterior border of the sternomastoid muscle. Remnants of the first cleft are found near the ear or the angle of the mandible. These clefts and sinuses may become infected. Removal is required once any infection has been controlled.

Hemangioma

Vascular tumors are extremely common in childhood and may be found in up to 10% of 1-year-old children. Terminology used to describe them is variable and confusing. Generally, hemangiomas are considered to be benign vascular tumors characterized initially by cellular proliferation, followed in many cases by involution. In contrast, vascular malformations are congenital structural errors of morphogenesis that are not proliferative and grow with the child.

Most hemangiomas appear within the first few weeks after birth, grow rapidly during the first year, and then slowly regress over the next several years. They are commonly located in the head and neck but may be found anywhere. Hemangiomas can be superficial or deep and may involve the viscera. Superficial lesions, often termed "capillary" hemangiomas, are firm, bright red, and raised; they are considered to be the most likely to regress spontaneously (Figs. 2.27**A** and 2.27**B**). Deep lesions, sometimes called "cavernous" hemangiomas, are softer and may have a blue discoloration; they may be less likely to resolve spontaneously.

Most hemangiomas should be left alone, since the majority will resolve spontaneously in early childhood. Indications for treatment include significant facial distortion; interference with function, as occurs with le-

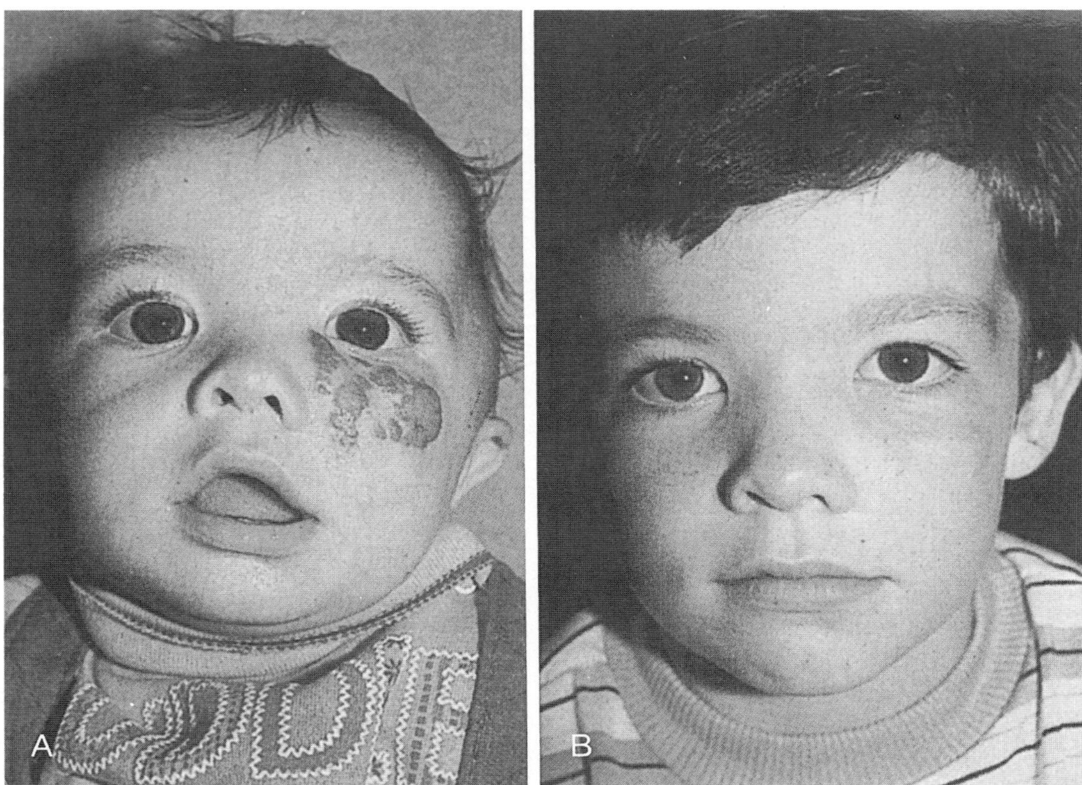

Figure 2.27. **A**, Superficial hemangioma in an infant boy. **B**, Regression by 5 years of age.

sions in the eyelid or airway; thrombocytopenia from platelet trapping; and congestive heart failure. Management may then include steroids (by intralesional injection or systemically), radiation, embolization, or surgical excision, depending on the location and characteristics of the hemangioma.

Vascular malformations are much less frequent than hemangiomas and tend to remain stable over time. The port wine stain is seen at birth as a deep purple, nonraised lesion, usually on the face. It never regresses and is treated with cosmetic coverage or laser ablation.

Another vascular malformation is the congenital arteriovenous fistula. These anomalies are most common in the extremities and central nervous system. In the extremities, they are usually multiple and cause heart failure and hypertrophy of the involved limb. Treatment is not completely satisfactory and consists of elastic compression, ligation of the involved vessels, or embolization.

Tumors in Children

Few ordeals are more devastating for young people and their families than childhood cancer. Cancer ranks second behind trauma as the leading cause of death in children, and it accounts for 11% of deaths among children in the United States. Fortunately, the outlook for children with malignancies has improved markedly in the past two decades, largely as a result of multi-institutional clinical trials. Modern treatment for many of the common pediatric tumors increasingly relies on a multidisciplinary approach using surgery, chemotherapy, and radiotherapy, as well as sophisticated diagnostic imaging.

The frequency distribution of malignant neoplasms in children differs markedly from that of adults. Leukemia (30%), central nervous system tumors (20%), and lymphoma (12%) predominate. Neuroblastoma and Wilms' tumors each account for 5–10% of pediatric cancers, followed by malignancies of the liver, bone, and other soft tissues.

Cancer therapy, potent as it is, often has major side effects. Chemotherapy predominantly affects rapidly dividing cells and may produce myelosuppression, nausea, vomiting, diarrhea, alopecia, skin rashes, and abnormalities of the liver and kidney. Radiation may damage normal tissues within the irradiated field, including bone, lung, liver, and kidney. Patients receiving combined chemotherapy and radiotherapy are at particular risk for the development of a second malignancy.

Children with cancers who are receiving multimodal therapy may benefit greatly from the placement of a long-term central venous catheter. These lifelines can be used for the administration of chemotherapy and intravenous nutrition, as well as for blood sampling. Hickman and Broviac catheters have a subcutaneous cuff and external tubing. Catheters with implanted subcutaneous reservoirs are often preferred, as they are completely internalized. These ports are then painlessly accessed percutaneously, using a special needle. General anesthesia is usually required for the insertion of all these devices.

Neuroblastoma

Neuroblastoma is the most common extracranial solid tumor of childhood. It has the unique ability to undergo maturation to a benign form, ganglioneuroma, and spontaneously disappear more frequently than any other human malignancy. Tiny neuroblastomas are found in 1% of infants who die from other causes, a number which represents 100 times the incidence of the tumor actually found to be clinically significant. Unfortunately, despite these unusual biological features and modern therapeutic capabilities, most children with neuroblastoma have a poor outlook.

Neuroblastoma is derived from embryonal neural crest tissue and can arise anywhere in the sympathetic nervous system. Of these tumors, 75% originate in the abdomen and 50% in the adrenal medulla. Other sites include the posterior mediastinum and neck. Most children with neuroblastoma excrete catecholamines and their breakdown products in the urine.

Clinical Manifestations. The majority of neuroblastomas present in the first 2 years of life, and 80% are found by the time a patient is 8 years of age. An abdominal mass is the presenting feature in most children. Tumors of the mediastinum may produce respiratory distress, cause Horner's syndrome from involvement of the stellate ganglion, or be noted incidentally on a chest x-ray. Paraplegia can occur from extension through the intervertebral foramina with compression of the spinal cord. Cerebellar ataxia may be seen, the cause of which is unknown. Systemic symptoms are very common, including fever, weight loss, failure to thrive, anemia, and hypertension. Most children already have metastases at the time of diagnosis. The most common sites are bone, bone marrow, liver, lymph nodes, lung, and subcutaneous tissue.

Investigations of a child with a suspected neuroblastoma include ultrasonography, CT and MRI scans, a bone scan, bone marrow aspiration, and measurement of urinary catecholamines. Myelography must be performed if neurological symptoms suggest intraspinal extension. Several staging systems have been proposed for neuroblastoma that specify the extent of disease and the completeness of surgical resection.

Treatment. Therapy must be individualized, depending on the child's age, tumor location, and extent of disease. Surgical resection is the mainstay of treatment when possible and is currently the only method of cure. In instances where tumor recurrence is likely or there is residual cancer, postoperative radiation and multiagent chemotherapy are usually indicated. For advanced disease with an unresectable tumor, chemotherapy may be given initially to shrink the lesion and permit subsequent resection. Bone marrow transplantation rescue has been used following massive chemotherapy and total body irradiation, with prolonged relapse-free survival. Cures have not yet been reported, and transplantation takes a tremendous toll on the child, the family, and the staff. Immunotherapy is being evaluated as well.

Prognosis. The overall survival rate is 40% but depends greatly on the age of the patient (younger ones do better) and the extent of the disease. The survival rate for patients less than 1 year is 75%, but only 20% for those over 2 years. For localized disease completely resected, the survival rate is 100% but falls to less than 20% for metastatic disease. A special situation exists for infants less than 1 year of age with metastases limited to the liver, bone marrow, and skin, in whom the survival rate is over 80%, even with little or no treatment.

In Japan, a screening program has been developed for neuroblastoma, in which the urine of all infants at 6 months of age is measured for catecholamine products. The survival rate is over 75% for tumors detected in screened infants, compared to 23% for neoplasms diagnosed in unscreened infants.

Wilms' Tumor

Wilms' tumor is an embryonal neoplasm of the kidney and is often associated with other anomalies, such as hypospadias, hemihypertrophy, and aniridia (congenital absence of the iris). This tumor may occur bilaterally. In contrast to neuroblastoma, Wilms' tumor is a neoplasm for which the survival has improved from 10% to 80% in several decades.

Clinical Manifestations. Most children with Wilms' tumors are 1 to 5 years of age. They usually present with an asymptomatic abdominal mass. Occasionally there is abdominal pain, hematuria, or hypertension, but systemic manifestations such as fever, anorexia, and weight loss are much more characteristic of neuroblastoma.

Metastases, which are much less common than in patients with neuroblastoma, may occur in regional lymph nodes, in the abdomen by tumor rupture, and in the lungs. Wilms' tumors may also extend through the renal vein and into the inferior vena cava. Involvement of bone is very rare.

Investigations should include ultrasonography and CT scans of the abdomen and chest (Fig. 2.28) in an attempt to determine the extent of the disease.

Treatment. Surgery is indicated to resect the involved kidney and to determine the stage of disease. If the tumor is unresectable, chemotherapy is administered to shrink it before resection is attempted. All patients receive chemotherapy with actinomycin D and vincristine. In patients who have unfavorable histology (10%), residual tumor, or metastatic disease, doxorubicin and radiotherapy are usually added. Patients with bilateral Wilms' tumors undergo bilateral partial nephrectomies and chemotherapy.

The prognosis for Wilms' tumors depends on the stage, size, histological grade, and age of the patient (as with neuroblastomas, younger children do better). The long-term survival rate for patients with localized tu-

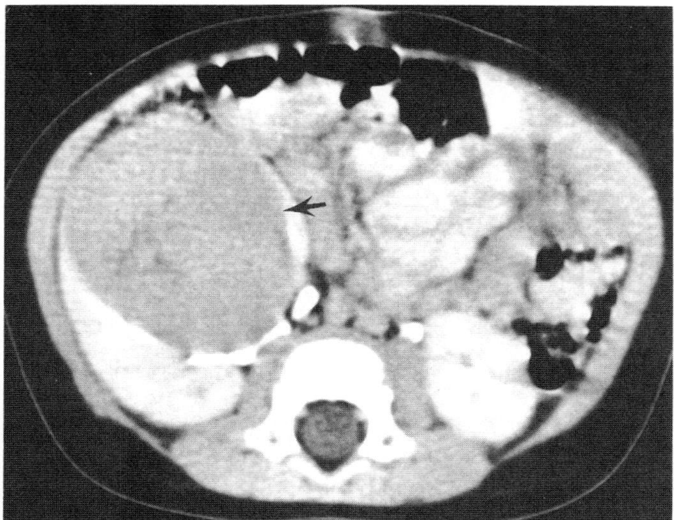

Figure 2.28. Large Wilms' tumor of right kidney (arrow) seen on contrast-enhanced CT scan.

mors is over 90%, and for those with even extensive disease and unfavorable histology it is over 50%.

Neonates may have renal tumors resembling Wilms' tumors, termed mesoblastic nephromas. These growths are always benign, and resection alone is curative.

Teratomas

Teratomas are a bizarre group of neoplasms that originate early in embryonic cell division and can manifest at any age. It is unclear whether they arise from germ cells or from other totipotential embryonic cells. The time-honored requirement that a teratoma must contain all three germinal layers has been replaced by Willis's definition that it be "composed of multiple tissues of kinds foreign to the parts in which it arises." Teratomas frequently occur in the gonads or near the midline of the body, locations where undifferentiated cells might be found. Teratomas contain a very wide variety of tissue types of varying degrees of differentiation and may be benign or malignant. Benign teratomas produce symptoms by compressing adjacent organs or by twisting. Malignant teratomas may invade and metastasize.

The most common locations for teratomas in children are the sacrococcygeal region and the ovary. Other frequent sites are the neck, anterior mediastinum, retroperitoneum, testicle, and central nervous system. Operative resection is usually curative for benign teratomas. Patients with malignant teratomas usually undergo resection and receive chemotherapy, but recurrences and metastases are common.

Sacrococcygeal Teratoma. A sacrococcygeal teratoma is the most common tumor found in neonates and can be quite massive (Fig. 2.29). It arises from the coccyx and usually has an external component covered with skin. It may also have a significant internal portion extending in front of the sacrum and entering the pelvis. Rarely, the entire tumor is internal, with no visible abnormality.

Sacrococcygeal teratomas occur predominantly (75%) in females. Resection should be prompt, because the incidence of malignancy is only 10% in neonates but increases to over 50% in patients 2 months of age. The coccyx must also be removed. The outlook for cure as well as for normal function in patients with benign sacrococcygeal teratomas is excellent. Survival of patients following malignant transformation is unlikely.

Sacrococcygeal teratomas are increasingly diagnosed in utero. Delivery by cesarean section is recommended, as rupture of the tumor with exsanguination can occur during vaginal delivery.

Hepatic Tumors.

Tumors of the liver are the third most common abdominal malignancy in childhood, following neuroblastomas and Wilms' tumors. Approximately three-quarters of hepatic neoplasms in children are malignant. Patients with liver tumors usually present with an abdominal mass, often associated with discomfort, anorexia, weight loss, and occasionally, jaundice.

Hemangiomas are the most frequent benign tumor of the liver in children. These dilated vascular spaces may be solitary or multiple and are sometimes accompanied by cutaneous hemangiomas. They may produce congestive heart failure and platelet trapping. If asymptomatic, hepatic hemangiomas are best left alone; many will spontaneously regress. Symptomatic lesions can be treated with steroids, embolization, ligation of the hepatic arteries, or surgical resection. Digitalis and diuretics may be beneficial for heart failure.

The most common malignant tumors of the liver are hepatoblastoma and hepatocellular carcinoma. Hepatoblastoma is more common and is found in children under 3 years of age. Serum α-fetoprotein levels are usually elevated. Hepatocellular carcinoma usually occurs in older children, is more invasive, and is more often multicentric. Resection is the treatment of choice and may follow a course of chemotherapy if the tumor is initially unresectable. The survival rate for patients with hepatoblastoma is over 50%, but the rate for those with hepatocellular carcinoma is substantially less. Liver transplantation is being evaluated for unresectable hepatoblastomas without metastases, with mixed results.

Rhabdomyosarcoma

Rhabdomyosarcoma is the most common soft tissue sarcoma in children, accounting for 4% to 8% of pediatric malignancies. Rhabdomyosarcomas are a diverse group of tumors derived from primitive mesenchymal cells and may appear anywhere in the body. The embryonal type, found mostly in infants and young children, tends to occur in the genitourinary tract, head and neck, and orbit. The alveolar type occurs in older children and usually involves the trunk and extremities. These tumors invade locally and metastasize by lymphatic and hematogenous spread. The presenting

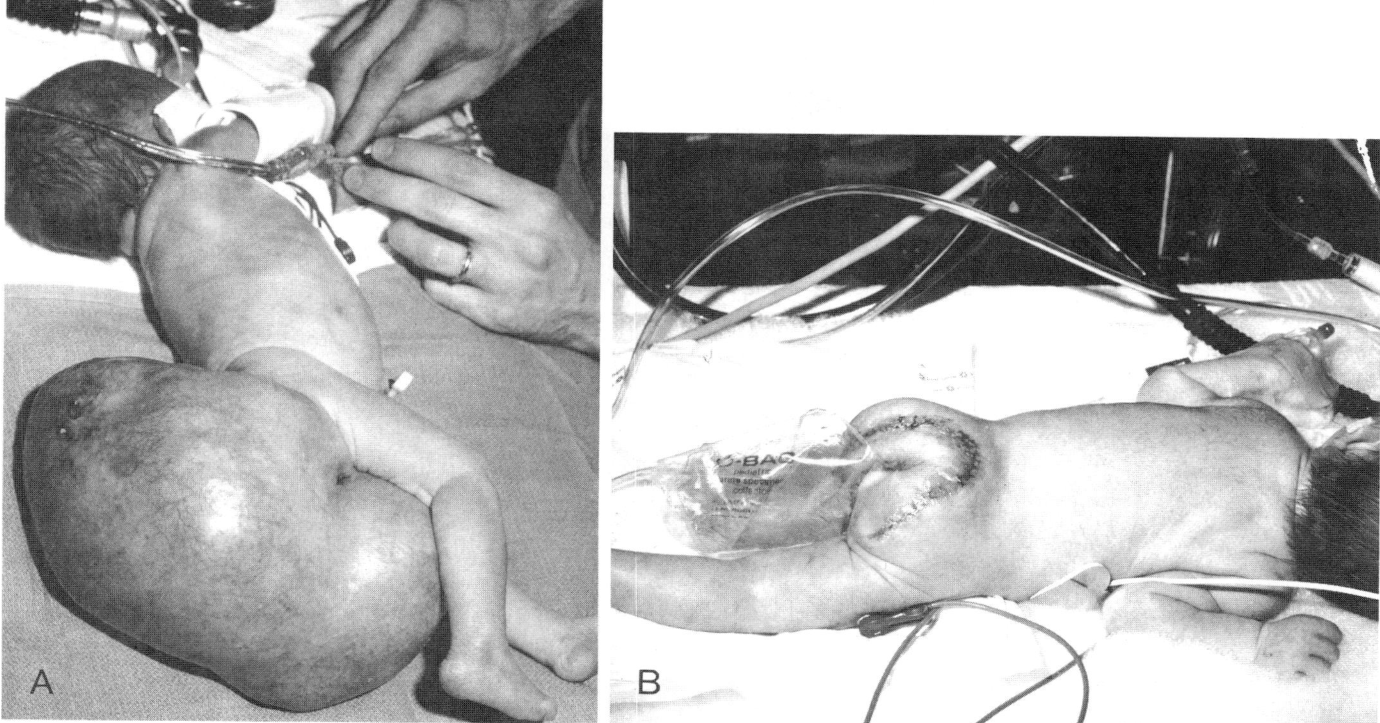

Figure 2.29. **A**, Sacrococcygeal teratoma in a newborn infant displacing the anus anteriorly. **B**, Same infant postoperatively.

symptoms vary widely, depending on the site of disease, but often consist of an asymptomatic mass. Diagnosis is established by biopsy, usually following imaging studies.

Multimodal therapy has been increasingly successful for rhabdomyosarcoma. Although wide local resection is optimal for early lesions, radical mutilating surgery is performed much less frequently than previously, with more reliance on ancillary therapy. Some tumors, such as those of the orbit, may be treated successfully with chemotherapy and radiotherapy alone. Vincristine, actinomycin D, and cyclophosphamide have been the most effective chemotherapeutic agents. Overall, the survival rate of patients is 70% (in contrast to 20% 20 years ago) and ranges from 83% for patients with localized disease completely resected, to 20% for children with distant metastases.

Lymphoma

Lymphomas are malignancies of lymphoid tissue. Hodgkin's disease tends to occur in older children and usually presents with enlargement of superficial lymph nodes, most often cervical. Non-Hodgkin's lymphoma is found earlier in childhood in a wide variety of locations and is often disseminated at the time of presentation. Biopsy is always necessary to establish the diagnosis, but surgical excision is not the definitive treatment for most individuals with lymphoma. A staging laparotomy is recommended for many Hodgkin's disease patients with disease above the diaphragm, in order to identify most accurately the presence of any intra-abdominal spread. This procedure alters the stage and influences therapy in approximately one-third of patients. Laparotomy for staging in non-Hodgkin's lymphoma patients is not indicated, as disseminated disease is presumed and chemotherapy is always administered.

Trauma

Trauma is the most common cause of death in children and accounts for more fatalities than all other causes combined. In addition to the 13,000 children killed each year by accidents in the United States, over 50,000 are permanently disabled, and 2 million are temporarily incapacitated and require emergency room evaluation. The automobile is responsible for 50% of accidental deaths in children. Burns, drowning, poisoning, falls, athletic injuries, firearms, and child abuse are also significant causes of death and injury. The most effective means for reducing deaths and disability from childhood trauma is by prevention, since accidents from all these causes can be drastically reduced through education and legislation.

The treatment that young trauma victims receive often determines whether they survive and in what capacity. It is essential that children with major injuries be transported to centers that are fully equipped to deal with their complex needs. It has been amply demonstrated that many preventable deaths can be avoided by care at specialized trauma centers.

Important differences between adult and pediatric trauma patients include:

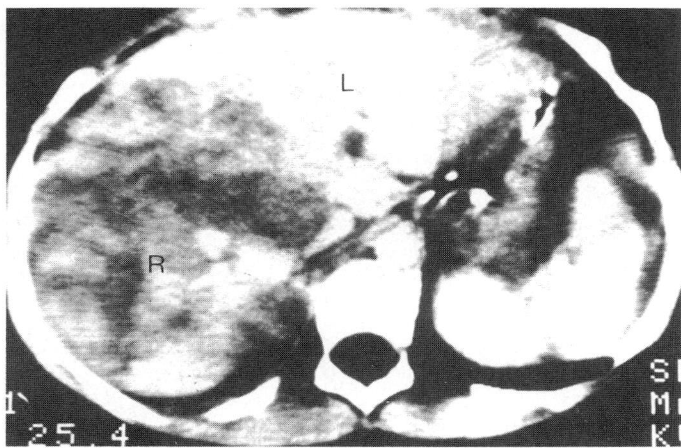

Figure 2.30. Seven-year-old girl with intrahepatic hemorrhage from automobile accident. Contrast-enhanced CT scan reveals inhomogeneity with irregular areas of low attenuation in right lobe of liver (R). Left lobe is normal (L).

1. Blunt trauma predominates in children. As a result, multisystem involvement is frequent, and the extent of internal damage is not always obvious.
2. Blood pressure may be a poor guide as to the level of shock. Children can very effectively compensate for hypovolemia by increasing their peripheral resistance. Hypotension develops only following loss of 25% of blood volume.
3. Head injuries occur more often in pediatric trauma because the head is relatively large and poorly stabilized.
4. Children are at greater risk for hypothermia because of their proportionately larger body surface area.
5. The young skeleton is quite flexible and more readily transmits applied forces. Children may therefore sustain major visceral damage in the absence of overlying fractures.
6. Injury to the epiphyseal growth plate can result in growth inhibition and deformity.
7. Gastric dilation is more common from aerophagia and may compromise respiration, promote aspiration, or simulate peritonitis.
8. Psychologically, the pain and fear that accompany trauma can have longer lasting adverse effects on children.

The ABC's of resuscitation, centering on the airway, breathing, and the circulation, in which priority is given to life-threatening conditions, are similar to those for adults. (See Chapter 14, Trauma and Burns, in EGS2.) They include the following principles:

1. The airway must be maintained. Any obstruction such as blood, vomitus, or the tongue is cleared. A plastic airway or endotracheal tube can be inserted. The neck must be immobilized until a cervical spine injury is ruled out.
2. Breathing is supported by positive pressure ventilation if necessary. A tension pneumothorax should be decompressed immediately by needle aspiration, after which a chest tube is placed.
3. The circulation must be supported. External bleeding is controlled by direct pressure. Large-bore intravenous catheters are inserted percutaneously if possible, or by cutdown if necessary. Blood samples are sent for a CBC, an amylase level, and type and cross matching. Ringer's lactate may be administered rapidly in 20 mL/kg boluses. Failure of the patient to respond hemodynamically to three such infusions is an indication to transfuse packed red blood cells and consider surgical intervention.
4. A history is taken and a more thorough physical examination is performed, including a rectal examination.
5. A nasogastric tube is inserted to decompress the stomach; a Foley catheter is placed to obtain urine for analysis and monitor output; chest tubes are placed if necessary; and monitor leads (ECG, pulse oximeter, temperature probe) are connected.
6. Unstable fractures are splinted and open wounds are covered.
7. Imaging studies are obtained as indicated. X-rays are usually taken of the cervical spine and chest. Films may also include the remainder of the spine, head, abdomen, and extremities. A CT scan of the head is obtained if there is any alteration of consciousness. An abdominal CT scan, intravenous pyelogram (IVP), or cystogram is indicated for suspected intra-abdominal or urinary tract injuries.
8. A decision must be made as to whether an urgent operation is needed, or if the patient should be transported to a suitable facility for further supportive care and monitoring.

Head

Head injuries are the major cause of death in children from trauma, although, compared with adults, children also have an enhanced ability to recover from severe head trauma. Any localized intracranial hematoma identified by CT scan must be promptly drained. More commonly, a cerebral contusion occurs which will result in a diffuse edema that can impair brain perfusion by raising intracranial pressure. This elevated pressure is controlled by hyperventilation to produce hypocapnia (which limits cerebral vasodilation), by fluid restriction and diuretics (only after the patient is fluid resuscitated), and possibly by steroids and barbiturates. Continuous intracranial pressure monitoring is helpful. (See Chapter 8, Neurosurgery.)

Chest

Most injuries to the chest can be managed nonoperatively with chest tube drainage, transfusions, and observation. Indications for surgery are massive, continued blood loss or uncontrolled air leaks through chest tubes; pericardial tamponade; and suspected injury to the esophagus, diaphragm, and great vessels. Pericardiocentesis can be lifesaving for pericardial tamponade, but should always be followed by operative repair of the underlying cardiac injury. Pulmonary contusions are very common in children following blunt trauma and appear as focal or diffuse alveolar infiltrates on chest x-ray. Treatment is nonspecific, with respiratory support as needed. (See Chapter 6, Diseases of the Heart, Great Vessels, and Thoracic Cavity.)

Abdomen

Abdominal surgery following trauma is always required for a child with a distended, tense abdomen or free intraperitoneal air on x-ray, as these findings indicate either massive intra-abdominal bleeding or a perforated viscus. In the absence of these findings, if abdominal injury is suspected, a CT scan is indicated (Fig. 2.30). A laparotomy is not always necessary even for moderate intra-abdominal bleeding; if the child can be stabilized with transfusions (up to 40 mL/kg), close observation with bed rest in a critical care unit is preferred. Diagnostic peritoneal lavage is not used as often as in adults, since CT scans not only identify the source of intraperitoneal bleeding but evaluate the retroperitoneum and kidneys as well. Every effort should be made to salvage a ruptured spleen, whether surgery is required or not, since children are particularly susceptible to overwhelming postsplenectomy sepsis.

Urinary Tract

Trauma to the urinary tract usually produces hematuria, which is an indication to perform an IVP or CT scan. Most injuries are minor and resolve with observation. Surgical repair is necessary if there is any extravasation of urine from the kidneys or bladder, and for injuries of the major renal vessels.

The presence of gross blood at the urethral meatus is a contraindication to the insertion of a Foley catheter during resuscitation, as a urethral injury is likely. A urethrogram should be obtained before catheter placement.

Child Abuse

The incidence of child abuse is unknown but seems to be increasing. In young trauma victims, intentional injury should be suspected if there is a discrepancy between the history and physical findings, if there has been a prolonged delay from the time of injury until presentation for medical care, if there is a history of recurrent trauma, or if the parents respond inappropriately to the child or to medical advice. The child is often overly fearful or withdrawn. The types of injuries vary widely, but may include sharply demarcated burns in unusual areas; long bone fractures in children under 3 years of age; trauma in genital or perianal areas; evidence of previous injuries such as old scars or healed fractures; and bizarre injuries such as bites, cigarette burns, and rope marks.

The physician must not only treat the child medically but admit him or her to the hospital for protection and must contact the proper authorities.

Burns

Following the automobile, burns are the second most common cause of accidental death in children. One-third of burn injuries are due to child abuse. Major burns produce a most profound physiological insult to the child. The burned individual rapidly develops severe hypovolemia from evaporative loss through the damaged skin barrier and from the seepage of plasma into the tissues through leaky capillaries. There is a marked hypermetabolic state and multiple organ failure frequently supervenes. Infection is a constant threat. Children with significant burns should be cared for in a specialized burn center. (See Chapter 14, Trauma and Burns, in EGS2)

Burns are classified according to their depth:

First degree—involves epidermis only and produces erythema, as in sunburn.
Second degree—involves partial thickness of dermis and is characterized by blister formation; extremely painful.
Third degree—necrosis of full-thickness dermis; skin is leathery with no sensation.

In calculating the percentage of body burns in children, the "rule of nines" used for adults does not apply. The Lund and Browder chart (Fig. 2.31) may be used, and should include all second- and third-degree burns. Hospital admission is advised if a second-degree burn involves more than 10% of body surface area, or a third-degree burn covers more than 2%. Inpatient care is also recommended for significant burns of the hands, feet, face, or perineum, and in children under 2 years of age.

Treatment. Minor burns are treated by debridement, cleansing, silver sulfadiazine antimicrobial cream, and occlusive dressings. Intact blisters are generally left alone. The wound should then be washed and dressed once or twice a day at home. Scrupulous care is necessary, as infection can convert a partial-thickness injury into full-thickness necrosis.

Major burns are treated with full-scale resuscitative efforts as for other pediatric trauma. In addition, the burns are cleansed and dressed. Bronchoscopy and pulmonary support may be needed for inhalational injuries. Analgesia should be provided. If the burned, leathery skin constricts and impairs distal perfusion to an extremity or limits respiration, emergency escharotomy is necessary at the bedside.

Fluid resuscitation should always be adjusted to the responses of the patient. However, several formulas provide initial guidelines. The Parkland formula is as follows:

Ringer's lactate at 4 mL/kg/% burn for 24 hours, with half being given in the first 8 hours
Colloid is usually started after 24 hours, when capillary integrity is improved.
Enteral fluids and nutrition are administered as soon as the ileus resolves.

Estimation of Size of Burn by Percent

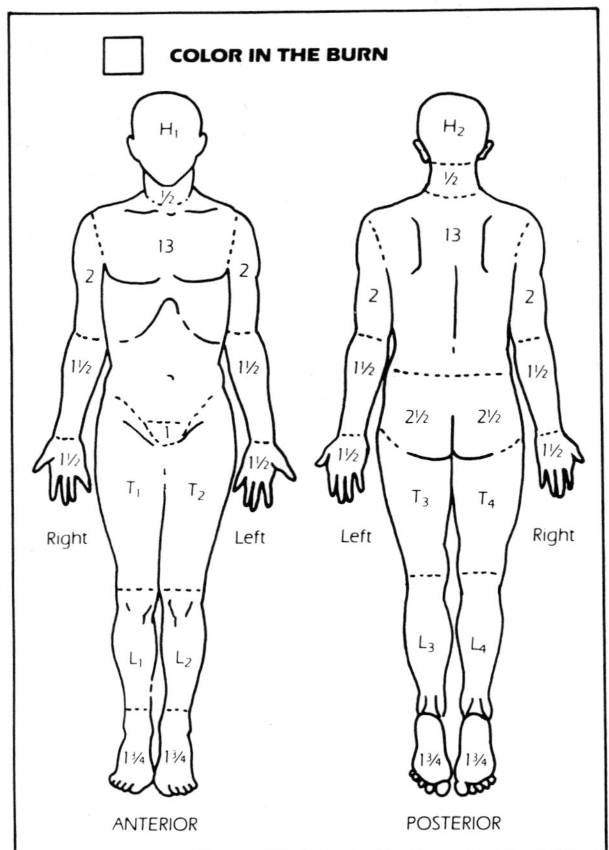

CALCULATE EXTENT BURN

	ANTERIOR	POSTERIOR
Head	H_1 ____	H_2 ____
Neck	____	____
Rt. Arm	____	____
Rt. Forearm	____	____
Rt. Hand	____	____
Lt. Arm	____	____
Lt. Forearm	____	____
Lt. Hand	____	____
Trunk	____	____
Buttock	(R) ____	(L) ____
Perineum	____	____
Rt. Thigh	T_1 ____	T_4 ____
Rt. Leg	L_1 ____	L_4 ____
Rt. Foot	____	____
Lt. Thigh	T_2 ____	T_3 ____
Lt. Leg	L_2 ____	L_3 ____
Lt. Foot	____	____
SUBTOTAL	____	____

% TOTAL AREA BURNED ____ %

CIRCLE AGE FACTOR

	PERCENT OF AREAS AFFECTED BY GROWTH AGE					
	0-1	1-4	5-9	10-14	15	Adult
H (1 or 2) = ½ of the Head	9½	8½	6½	5½	4½	3½
T (1, 2, 3, or 4) = ½ of a Thigh	2¾	3¼	4	4¼	4½	4¾
L (1, 2, 3, or 4) = ½ of a Leg	2½	2½	2¾	3	3¼	3½

Figure 2.31. Modified Lund and Browder chart.

Full-thickness burns are often surgically excised and covered within several days of injury, in order to restore normal physiology and prevent infection. Coverage may be provided with partial-thickness autografts or, temporarily, with pigskin. For large burns, multiple staged excisions are necessary.

Rehabilitation may be prolonged, and often includes a compressive, elastic garment that is worn for months in order to limit hypertrophy of the burn scar. Psychological problems are common and must be fully addressed.

Foreign Body Aspiration and Ingestion

Young children place into their mouths all manner of objects, some of which are aspirated or ingested.

Aspiration. An aspirated object that completely obstructs the larynx will rapidly lead to suffocation unless it is coughed out or promptly removed. A smaller object that passes through the larynx usually lodges in a main bronchus. Complete obstruction will cause atelectasis as air is absorbed distally, and pneumonia often results. In contrast, partial obstruction of a bronchus produces

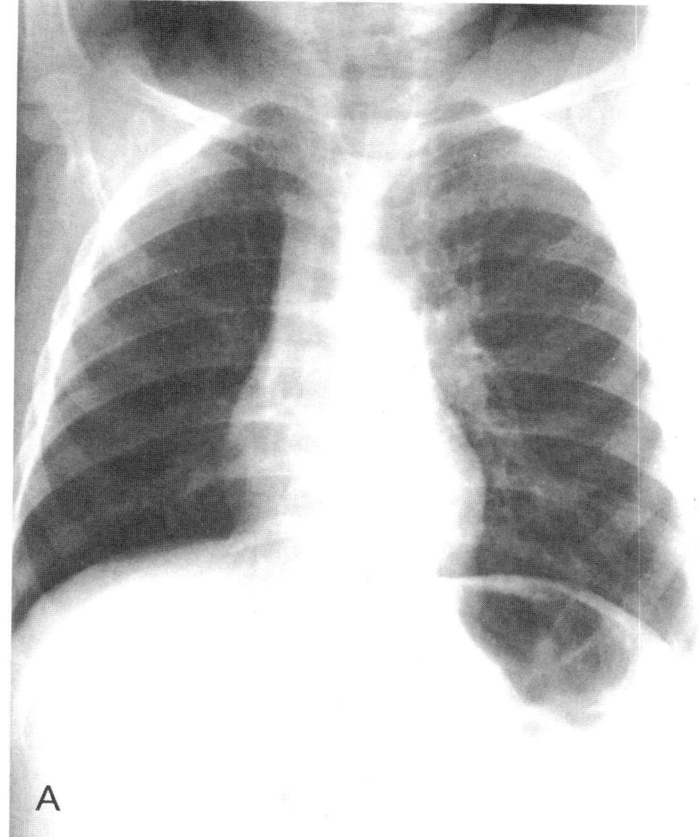

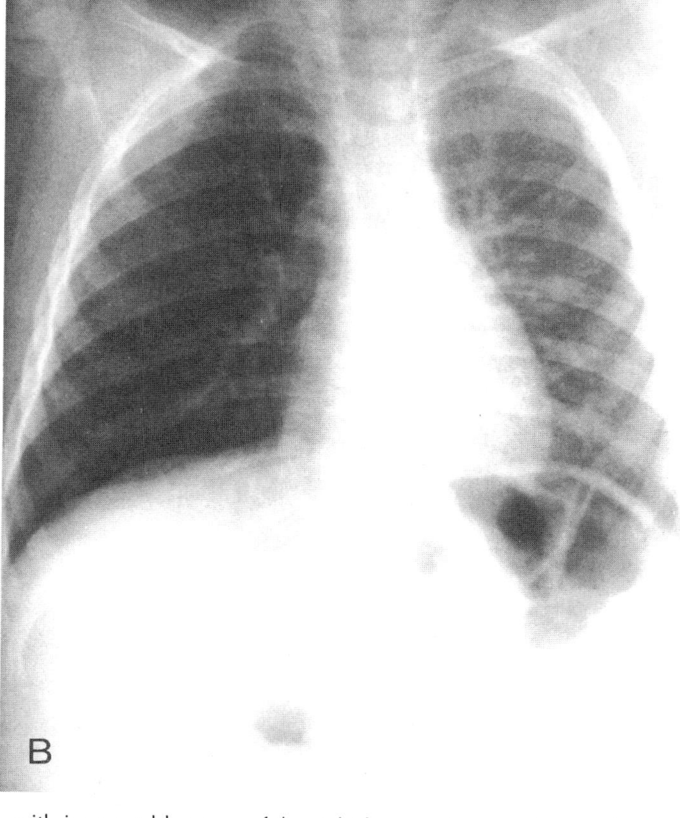

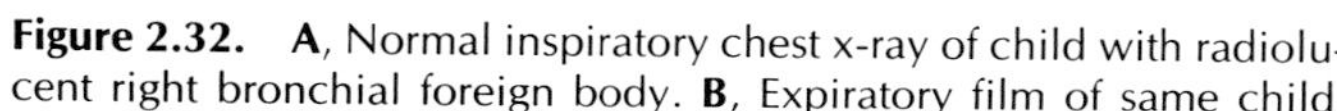
Figure 2.32. **A**, Normal inspiratory chest x-ray of child with radiolucent right bronchial foreign body. **B**, Expiratory film of same child, with increased lucency of the right lung and mediastinal shift to the left.

hyperinflation distally through a ball valve effect, as the airway collapses around the object during expiration and excessive air is trapped.

Clinical Manifestations. Choking and coughing may or may not occur. Once these symptoms subside, the patient frequently evidences unilateral wheezing and/or decreased air entry on the affected side. A chest x-ray will rarely reveal a radiopaque foreign body but often demonstrates hyperaeration of the involved lung or lobe. Expiratory films and fluoroscopy are very helpful, as expiration exaggerates the hyperinflation and produces a mediastinal shift in the opposite direction (Figs. 2.32**A** and 2.32**B**). Other x-ray findings consistent with foreign body aspiration are persistent atelectasis and recurrent or nonresolving pneumonia.

Treatment. If there is any suspicion of foreign body aspiration, rigid bronchoscopy is performed under general anesthesia. When identified, the object is removed.

Ingestion. Most foreign objects that are swallowed and reach the stomach will pass unimpeded through the gastrointestinal tract (Fig. 2.33). Parents are instructed to strain all stools, and weekly x-rays are taken. If a sharp object remains in the same position for a week, or a blunt object for a month, endoscopic or operative removal is considered. Symptoms of obstruction, perforation, or bleeding are definite indications for intervention. If a swallowed object is seen to be lodged in the esophagus on x-ray, there is a significant risk of perforation. Accordingly, extraction by rigid endoscopy is necessary.

An exception to the above recommendations concerns swallowed alkaline disc batteries, which can leak and cause local necrosis. If they pass beyond the esophagus, expectant observation is still warranted, but if they fail to progress for a week, in spite of purgatives and enemas, their removal may be indicated.

Caustic substances may be ingested accidentally by young children, or purposely by adolescents in a suicide attempt. Strong alkali (such as lye), which penetrates tissues deeply and produces liquefaction necrosis, predominantly injures the esophagus. In contrast, acid, which causes a surface coagulation necrosis that tends to limit deeper penetration of the esophagus, more frequently damages the stomach. All patients who have potentially ingested corrosive substances require prompt evaluation. For severe injuries, airway control and fluid resuscitation may be necessary. Rarely, emergency surgery is required for peritonitis or mediastinitis, which are indicative of full-thickness necrosis. Otherwise, endoscopy is indicated to assess the degree of injury. Although controversial, significant

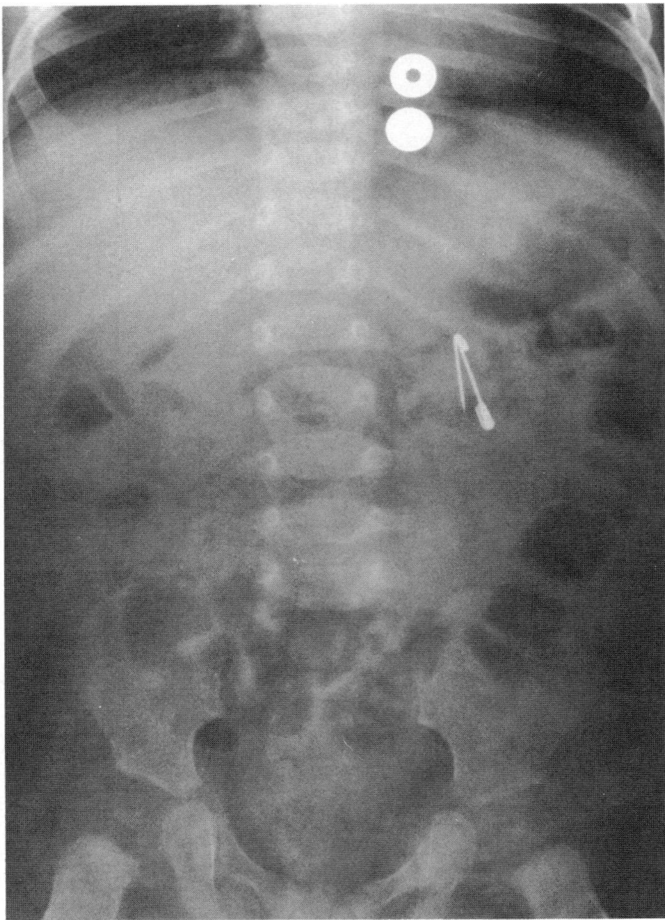

Figure 2.33. Abdominal radiograph of infant with swallowed sharp foreign body that passed uneventfully.

esophageal burns are usually treated with steroids and antibiotics, and sometimes with the passage of an intraluminal stent, in order to prevent subsequent stricture formation. When they occur, most strictures can be successfully managed with repeated dilations. Strictures resistant to dilation are treated surgically by esophageal replacement with either a stomach or colon interposition. Patients who have sustained caustic strictures to the esophagus are at increased risk for the late development of esophageal carcinoma.

SUGGESTED READING

Filston HC. Pediatric surgery. In: Sabiston DC, ed. Textbook of surgery. Philadelphia: WB Saunders, 1986:1253–1298.

Guzzetta PC, Anderson KD, Altman RP. Pediatric surgery. In: Schwartz SI, Shires SI, eds. Principles of surgery. New York: McGraw Hill, 1989:1687–1728.

Greene MG, ed. The Harriet Lane handbook. 12th ed. St. Louis: Mosby Year Book, 1991.

Holder TN, Ashcraft KW, eds. Pediatric surgery. 2nd ed. Philadelphia: WB Saunders, 1991.

Leape LL. Patient care in pediatric surgery. Boston: Little, Brown, 1987.

Raffensperger JG, ed. Swenson's pediatric surgery. 5th ed. Norwalk: Appleton & Lange, 1990.

Welch KJ, Randolph JG, Ravitch MM, et al. Pediatric surgery. 4th ed. Chicago: Year Book Medical Publishers, 1986.

Neonatal Surgical Conditions

Grosfeld JL, Weber TR. Managing alimentary tract obstruction in the newborn. Drug Therapy Hosp 1981;47–57.

Karrer FM, Lilly JR, Stewart BA, Hall RJ. Biliary atresia registry, 1976 to 1989. J Pediatr Surg 1990;25(10):1076–1081.

Pena A. Atlas of surgical management of anorectal malformations. New York: Springer-Verlag, 1990.

Tagge DU, Tagge EP, Drongowski RA, et al. A long-term experience with biliary atresia: reassessment of prognostic factors. Ann Surg 1991;214:590–598.

Surgical Conditions in the Older Child

Hadziselimovic F, Herzog B. Cryptorchidism. Pediatr Surg Int 1987;2: 132–141.

Mulliken JB, Young AE. Vascular birthmarks: hemangiomas and malformations. Philadelphia: WB Saunders, 1988.

Tumors in Children

Donaldson, SS. Rhabdomyosarcoma: contemporary status and future directions. Arch Surg 1989;124:1015–1020.

Grosfeld JL. Neuroblastoma: a 1990 overview. Pediatr Surg Int 1991;6: 9–13.

Kobrinsky NL, Talgoy M, Shuckett B, Gritter HL. Wilms' tumor. Pediatr Ann 1988;17(4)238–250.

Kushner BH, Cheung NV. Neuroblastoma. Pediatr Ann 1988;17(4): 269–284.

Malogolowkin MH, Ortega JA. Rhabdomyosarcoma of childhood. Pediatr Ann 1988;17(4):251–268.

Smith EI, Castleberry RP. Neuroblastoma. Curr Prob Surg 1990;27(9): 575–620.

Trauma in Children

Advanced trauma life support program: instructor manual. Chicago: American College of Surgeons 1988;215–233.

Coren CV. Burn injuries in children. Pediatr Ann 1987;16(4):328–339.

Lund CC, Browder ND. The estimation of areas of burns. Surg Gynecol Obstet 1944;78:463.

Rumack BH, Rumack CM. Disk battery ingestion (Editorial). JAMA 1983;249(18):2509–2511.

Skills

1. Demonstrate the ability to perform an abdominal examination on a young child with:
   a. Acute abdominal pain.
   b. Blunt trauma.
   c. Abdominal distention.
   d. Projectile nonbilious vomiting.
   e. An abdominal mass.
2. Demonstrate the ability to perform a groin examination, correctly identifying an inguinal hernia, a communicating hydrocele, and an undescended testis.
3. Demonstrate the ability to examine a newborn infant for surgically correctable congenital anomalies.
4. Calculate:

a. Daily maintenance requirements for a 3-kg infant and a 15-kg child.
b. Resuscitation fluid requirements for a hypovolemic 15-kg child and a 55-kg adolescent.

5. Describe the steps you would follow to replace a gastrostomy tube.

Study Questions

1. What is the blood volume of a 3.5-kg infant?
2. Write intravenous fluid orders for:
   a. An 8-year-old, 30-kg girl with ruptured appendicitis, who is 10% dehydrated and is scheduled to undergo surgery in 1 hour.
   b. A well-hydrated, 10-kg toddler following operative reduction of an intussusception, who will be NPO for the next 24 hours.
3. How should postoperative pain be treated in:
   a. A 1-month-old boy following pyloromyotomy?
   b. An 18-month-old toddler after operative reduction of intussusception?
   c. A 15-year-old girl who has undergone an appendectomy?
4. Outline the management of a newborn term infant with severe respiratory distress, a scaphoid abdomen, and a chest x-ray demonstrating intestinal loops in the left chest.
5. A 12-hour-old baby has bilious vomiting and a distended abdomen and has not passed meconium. What are the possible causes, and how would you work up such an infant?
6. A 4-month-old boy has a right inguinal mass. How would you differentiate a hernia from a hydrocele, and how would that distinction affect the treatment?
7. What would be your recommendations to the parents of a 2-month-old boy with an empty right scrotum, and the right testicle palpable in the groin?
8. An 8-month-old girl with severe psychomotor retardation from hypoxic encephalopathy has persistent nonbilious vomiting after feeds. How would you evaluate this child, and what would be the indications for operative correction of her gastroesophageal reflux?
9. What is the differential diagnosis of a 2-year-old girl with a large, asymptomatic left flank mass, and how should she be evaluated?
10. A 4-year-old boy who has been involved in an automobile accident is unconscious and has a distended abdomen. What are the appropriate steps, on order of priority, in caring for this child?

3 Ophthalmology: Diseases of the Eye

Alan S. Crandall, Jr., M.D.,
Richard L. Anderson, M.D., Irving Raber, M.D.,
Gregory S. Doren, M.D., Michael P. Teske, M.D.,
Robert P. Liss, M.D., George L. White, Jr., Ph.D.,
and William M. McLeish, M.D.

ASSUMPTIONS

The student is familiar with the anatomy and physiology of the eye, eyelids, and orbit.

The student is able to perform a basic, complete eye examination.

The student understands local and systemic effects of commonly used ocular and systemic drugs on the eye.

The student is familiar with light physics and optics.

OBJECTIVES

DISEASES OF THE CORNEA

1. Understand the anatomy and function of the cornea and precorneal tear film.
2. Understand the use of the slitlamp to examine the cornea and its value in determining the anatomic site of pathology within the cornea and anterior segment.
3. Describe indications for corneal transplantation and what the surgery entails.
4. Describe two surgical methods of correcting aphakia.
5. Explain recurrent erosion syndrome, its associated conditions, and a strategy for clinical management.
6. Understand the evaluation and management of a corneal infiltrate.
7. Understand the various types of refractive surgery.
8. Define pterygia and describe their clinical management.
9. Identify three surgical methods for treating corneal surface disorders.

DISEASES OF THE ANTERIOR CHAMBER

1. Define glaucoma and its various categories.
2. Describe the pathophysiology of the different types of glaucoma and their presenting signs and symptoms.
3. Describe basic glaucoma treatment and the different therapies for the various kinds of glaucoma.
4. Discuss the indications for surgical rather than medical therapy for glaucoma.

DISEASES OF THE LENS

1. Understand how the basic anatomy of the lens relates to the formation of the different types of cataract.
2. Understand how the anatomic location of the cataract determines its effect on visual function.
3. Be able to select those patients who would benefit most from cataract surgery.
4. Describe the various techniques of cataract surgery and the risks associated with them.
5. List the advantages and disadvantages of the various types of optical correction after cataract surgery.

DISEASES OF THE RETINA AND VITREOUS

1. Describe the signs and symptoms of retinal tears and detachments.
2. Discuss the principles and techniques involved in the treatment of retinal tears and detachment.
3. List the major indications for vitreous surgery, the goals involved, and the potential complications.
4. Describe the management of penetrating eye injuries, with or without retained intraocular foreign bodies.
5. List the major indications, goals, and potential complications for laser photocoagulation surgery involving the posterior segment of the eye.

DISEASES OF THE NASOLACRIMAL SYSTEM, EYELIDS, AND ORBIT

1. List the indications for nasolacrimal duct probing in infants.
2. Explain the differences between a dacryocystorhinostomy and a Jones tube procedure and give the indications for each.
3. List the indications for tarsorrhaphy.
4. Describe the importance of ptosis as a finding on physical examination.
5. Describe and contrast the most frequent lesions causing proptosis in children and adults.
6. List the indications for removal of an eye.

DISEASES OF THE EXTRAOCULAR MUSCLES

1. Describe the anatomy and function of the extraocular muscles.
2. Describe the innervation of the extraocular muscles and how it relates to strabismus.
3. Discuss the relationship between hyperopia, accommodation, and strabismus.
4. Describe the concept of single binocular vision and how it relates to the treatment of congenital esotropia.
5. Describe the fundamentals, goals, and possible complications of strabismus surgery.

OCULAR DISORDERS

1. List the common causes of "red eye," especially those conditions that are threatening to loss of sight.
2. Discuss the significance of visual field defects, papillary disorders, hypertensive retinopathy, retinal vein occlusion and emboli, third and sixth nerve palsies, and diplopia.

Diseases of the Cornea

Anatomy and Function of the Cornea

The cornea is a clear, avascular structure that provides structural integrity to the anterior segment of the eye and serves as a major refractive component. Comprising about one-sixth of the outer wall of the eye, the cornea is similar in structure to neighboring sclera. Corneal collagen is more uniformly oriented, however, and the cornea itself dehydrated: these two factors contribute to maintenance of corneal clarity. The cornea and overlying tear film provide two-thirds of the refractive component of the eye, while the lens accounts for the remainder.

The precorneal tear film, crucial to the health of the eye, is produced by the lacrimal gland and specialized glands in the conjunctiva and eyelids. The tear film is composed of three layers: the superficial layer, produced by the meibomian glands, is oily and helps prevent evaporation; the middle one, produced by the lacrimal gland, is watery and comprises the bulk of tear film; the innermost layer, produced by goblet cells, is mucoid and contributes to even spreading of the tear film. Deficiencies in any of these layers can lead to optical disturbances and compromise the health of the eye.

The cornea is composed of five layers. In anterior to posterior order, these include the epithelium, Bowman's membrane, stroma, Descemet's membrane, and endothelium. The epithelium is a nonkeratinized, stratified squamous cell layer forming a smooth surface over the cornea. It can be damaged easily by minor trauma resulting in corneal abrasions. If the epithelium basement membrane is damaged, adhesion of epithelium is compromised and recurrent abrasions may result. Because the cornea is supplied by numerous nerve endings, these abrasions can be extremely painful. Supporting the epithelium is Bowman's membrane, consisting of randomly dispersed collagen firmly anchored into corneal stroma. While epithelium regenerates without scarring, Bowman's membrane does not. The next layer, stroma, accounts for 90% of normal corneal thickness. Its three main constituents—collagen-producing fibroblasts, collagen lamellae, and mucopolysaccharide ground substance—combine to produce a tough, elastic protective coat. Posterior to corneal stroma is Descemet's membrane, the basement membrane for the fifth layer, endothelium. Corneal endothelium, derived from neuroectoderm, is a functionally complex monolayer of hexagonal cells that do not regenerate. The main function of this layer is to keep the cornea in a partially dehydrated state and therefore preserve its clarity. It accomplishes this function by maintaining a tight barrier between corneal stroma and aqueous humor, and by pumping water out of corneal stroma. The cell density of this layer decreases with age, and, even though remaining cells enlarge to accommodate lower cell counts, corneal clarity is compromised when the endothelial cell count falls to 400–700 cells/mm^2. As the cell count falls, corneal stromal edema increases followed by corneal epithelial edema. These developments lead to loss of vision and breakdown in corneal epithelium.

The cornea metabolizes glucose primarily by means of glycolysis, receiving 90% of this substrate from aqueous humor. Oxygen is delivered to corneal epithelium from the tear film and the environment. Corneal tissue posterior to and including corneal stroma receives oxygen from the aqueous humor. Given its proximity to glucose-rich aqueous humor and oxygen-rich air, the cornea is able to function well even though it is avascular. The tear film provides added immunological protection in the form of enzymes and immunoglobulins.

Examination of the cornea involves observation of the tissue itself as well as measurements of its shape (Fig. 3.1). The slitlamp is the most important instrument for evaluating the cornea, because it allows creation of an optical cross-section of the cornea, permitting direct visualization of any pathology. Examination is facilitated by the use of a topical anesthetic. By adjusting the light beam and the incident angle of observation, different areas within the cornea can be highlighted. Fluorescein stain is instilled to detect areas of corneal abrasion; in such areas it glows strongly under a cobalt

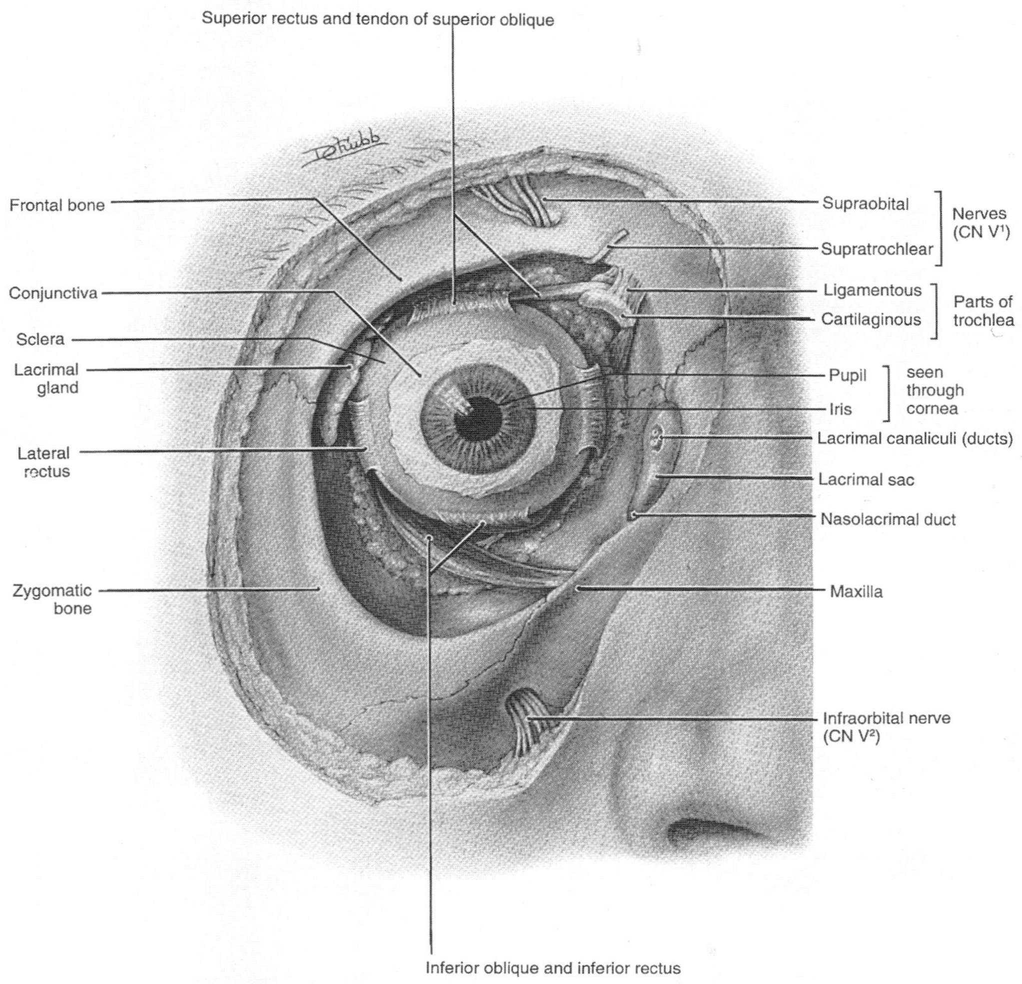

Figure 3.1. Orbital cavity, dissected from the front.

blue light. Even a simple penlight can give useful information, however. An irregular corneal surface can be detected by an irregular light reflex from any point source of light.

The curvature of the cornea and, therefore, its refractive ability is measured with a variety of instruments. The most common quantifiable method uses a keratometer to measure the radius of curvature of the central cornea. These measurements are important in guiding refractive procedures and predicting appropriate intraocular lens (IOL) power. More expensive and newer machines provide a topographical analysis of the corneal surface much the same way that topographical maps represent the earth's surface. These too are helpful for refractive procedures. The quality of the refracting surface of the cornea can be assessed with the keratometer and a keratoscope. The latter projects a Placido's disk—concentric rings that show surface topography, analogous to elevation lines on topographical maps. These measurements are helpful in postoperative care of cornea patients, especially in suture removal.

The endothelial cell layer of the cornea is visualized and photographed using specular microscopy. This technique provides information regarding the quality and quantity of the endothelial cells that are responsible for maintaining the relatively dehydrated state of the cornea, thus ensuring its clarity.

Principles of Corneal Surgery

Corneal surgery is performed for three main reasons: (*a*) to produce a clear visual pathway (as in a cornea transplant for a corneal scar), (*b*) to maintain the integrity of the globe (as in a lamellar cornea transplant for a perforation), and (*c*) to affect inherent corneal structure

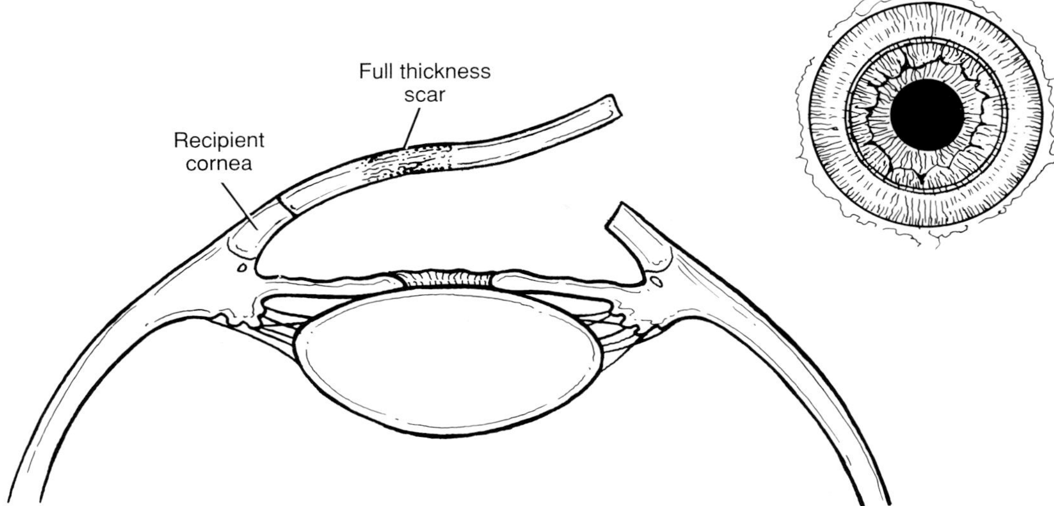

Figure 3.2. Penetrating keratoplasty.

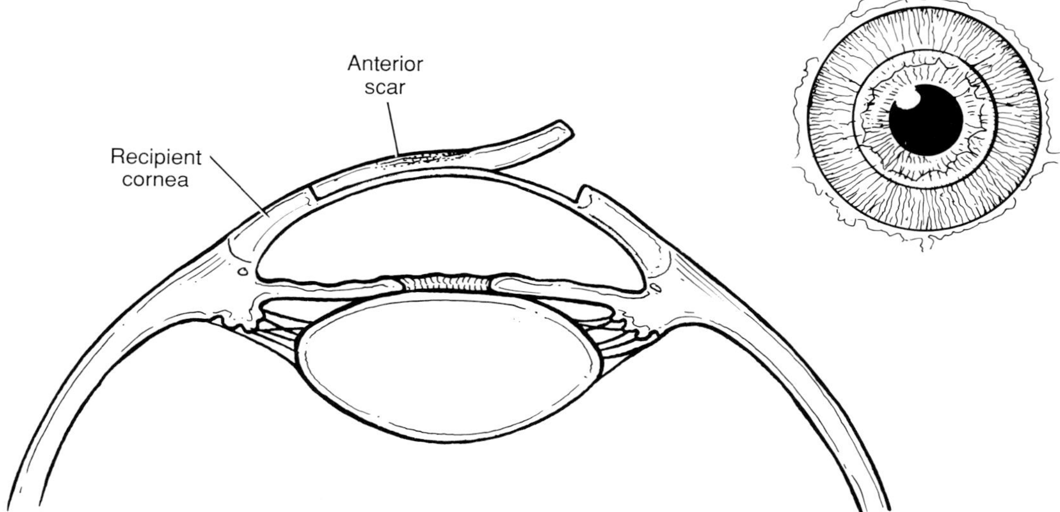

Figure 3.3. Lamellar keratoplasty.

to produce refractive or functional changes (as in radial keratotomy to reduce myopia). Much of corneal surgery's recent success has been due to such technological advances as the operating microscope, finer and better suture materials, improved instrumentation, and better tissue preservation.

For patients to have good vision after surgery, it is important to maintain a smooth corneal surface and clear corneal substance. Care must be taken to approximate wounds carefully without torque, to make sure sutures are placed at equal depths within tissue, and to place an ideal tension on the suture. Various devices have been developed to help determine correct tissue tension, although most surgeons find experience and practice the best aids.

Much corneal surgery arises from diseases that fail to respond to nonsurgical treatment. Examples include keratoconus initially treated with a contact lens, infectious keratitis treated with intensive fortified antibiotics, or herpes simplex keratitis treated with antivirals. Other cornea problems, such as aphakic bullous keratopathy with diffuse corneal edema, are surgical diseases from the outset. Our discussion will involve only those diseases of the cornea that are treated primarily with corneal surgery. It is important for the student to realize, however, that many medical interventions typically precede the necessary surgery.

Corneal Transplantation

Corneal transplantation is the most frequently performed tissue transplant in the United States, comprising approximately 30,000 procedures a year. The success of this procedure has been facilitated by several factors, including improved means of tissue preserva-

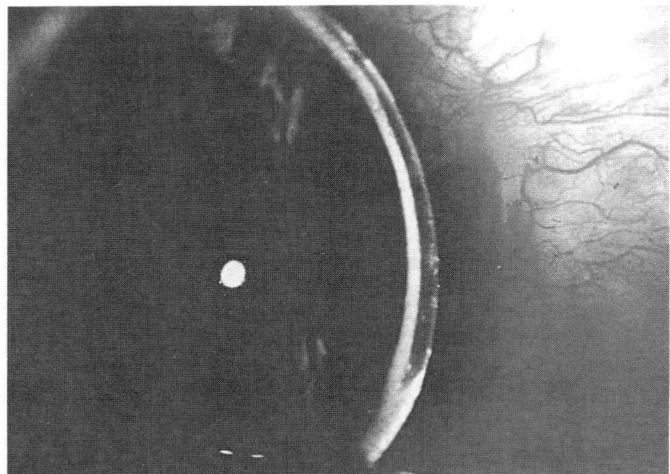

Figure 3.4. Slitlamp photo of lamellar keratoplasty. Note the residual opacification in the host bed.

Table 3.1.
Indications for Penetrating Keratoplasty

Indication	Percent
Pseudophakic bullous keratopathy	22.9
Fuch's dystrophy	16.3
Keratoconus	15.1
Aphakic bullous keratopathy	14.4
Regraft	10.1
Virus	4.4
Other	16.8
Total	100.0

tion and the nationwide network of eye banks that have increased the availability of corneal tissue. Corneal transplantation involves replacing full-thickness cornea (penetrating keratoplasty, Fig. 3.2) or partial-thickness cornea (lamellar keratoplasty, Fig. 3.3). The location of the corneal opacity determines the procedure. For full-thickness corneal lesions, only a full-thickness penetrating keratoplasty will suffice. For anteriorly placed corneal lesions, a lamellar keratoplasty can be performed. Often a full-thickness procedure is performed even though a partial-thickness procedure would do, because in most patients undergoing the partial-thickness procedure, scarring causes the development of a fine haze that interferes with vision (Fig. 3.4).

Corneal transplantation is performed for a variety of reasons: (*a*) to improve vision by creating a clear visual pathway, (*b*) to maintain the integrity of a structurally compromised globe, (*c*) to replace diseased corneal tissue that is unresponsive to medical treatment, and (*d*) to improve surface disorders and eliminate pain. Common indications for corneal transplantation are listed in Table 3.1.

Indications

Pseudophakic and Aphakic Bullous Keratopathy. Pseudophakic bullous keratopathy, or permanent corneal clouding after intraocular lens implant surgery, is the most common indication for corneal transplantation in the United States. All cataract surgery results in some loss of endothelial cells; in some patients this loss brings them under the critical number of remaining cells required to maintain corneal clarity. Depending on the degree of endothelial damage, the cornea may become cloudy immediately following the surgery or, more characteristically, months to years after the surgery. Aphakic bullous keratopathy refers to corneal opacification following cataract surgery without an IOL implant.

Intraocular lens implants following cataract surgery became popular in the late 1970s. Early lens design resulted in a high incidence of corneal edema and problems such as glaucoma and hyphema manifesting years later. Sometimes these lenses can be replaced with better designed implants before the cornea becomes permanently hazy. Once the cornea becomes opacified, visual rehabilitation requires a penetrating keratoplasty combined with IOL exchange. Although the incidence of pseudophakic bullous keratopathy is less than 1%, the sheer number of cataract surgeries performed in the United States annually makes this keratopathy the most common indication for corneal transplantation. As advances in cataract surgery produce less trauma to the eye, the incidence of pseudophakic bullous keratopathy is expected to decrease.

Patients with pseudophakic bullous keratopathy first notice diminution in vision as the cornea imbibes fluid. During the early stages of corneal edema, the patient complains of hazy, blurred vision that is worse on awakening and gradually clears as the day goes on. With the lids closed during sleep, fluid cannot evaporate from the corneal surface; after the eyes are open, the imbibed fluid evaporates with resultant decrease in corneal haze. Hypertonic saline drops and ointment promote corneal deturgescence, as does the use of a hair dryer on low heat setting held at arm's length and directed toward the eyes. As the cornea becomes more edematous, small blisters form in the corneal epithelium that tend to break down, causing severe ocular pain and irritation.

A penetrating keratoplasty will alleviate any discomfort from corneal epithelial breakdown as well as improve visual acuity. For patients who are poor candidates for corneal transplant, other procedures that can be tried include bandage contact lenses (extended-wear lenses that can remain in the eye), corneal surface scarification (with multiple fine-needle punctures or a diathermy probe), or conjunctival flaps. For a flap, a thin layer of healthy intact conjunctiva is mobilized and pulled down over the corneal surface as a "hood" flap and sutured into place (Figs. 3.5 and 3.6). A conjunctival flap can also be used to treat corneal infections unresponsive to antimicrobic therapy. Applying the flap over the infected cornea apparently stimulates the body's immune system to eradicate infection. If there is

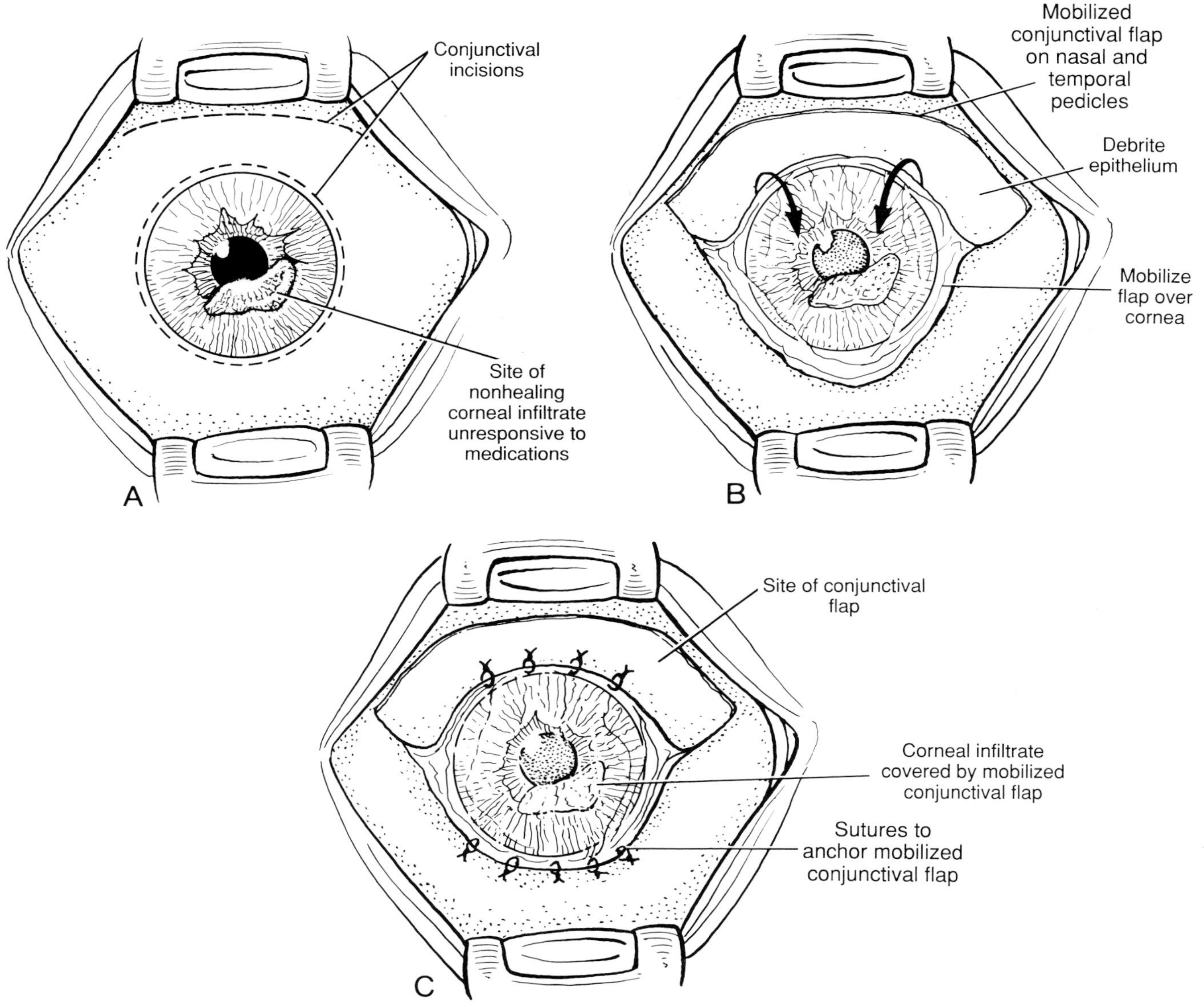

Conjunctival incisions
Site of nonhealing corneal infiltrate unresponsive to medications
A

Mobilized conjunctival flap on nasal and temporal pedicles
Debrite epithelium
Mobilize flap over cornea
B

Site of conjunctival flap
Corneal infiltrate covered by mobilized conjunctival flap
Sutures to anchor mobilized conjunctival flap
C

Figure 3.5. Conjunctival flap.

good visual potential, a penetrating keratoplasty may be performed later through the flap after the inflamed corneal stroma has become scarified.

Keratoconus. Keratoconus is a progressive dystrophy of the cornea in which the central cornea becomes thinner than normal with a subsequent forward bulge. The bulge takes on a conoid shape, resulting in visual distortion and decreased visual acuity. It tends to be bilateral, although one eye may be much more involved than the other. Most cases are sporadic but 10% are hereditary. Keratoconus has a higher incidence in such systemic disorders as Down's syndrome, atopy (Type I allergic reaction), and Marfan's syndrome. Eye rubbing may play a role in the development of keratoconus, and there is ongoing debate over whether contact lens wear may be a cause.

The disease tends to progress through adolescence and stabilize in young adulthood, although worsening

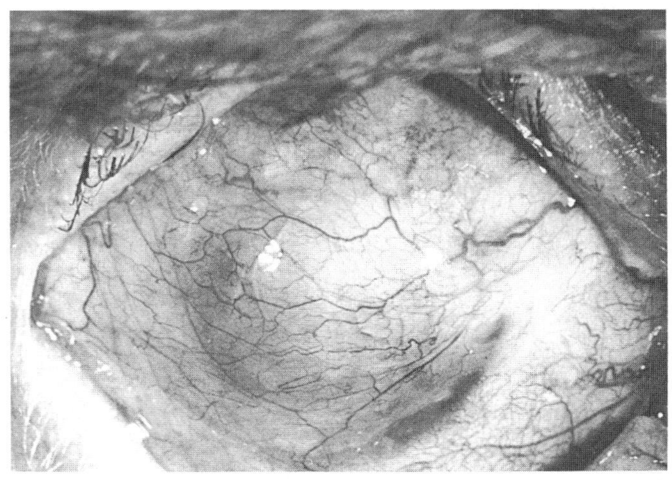

Figure 3.6. Well-healed conjunctival flap.

may occur at any age. Most patients can achieve excellent vision with rigid gas-permeable contact lenses, which ameliorate associated irregular astigmatism. Surgery is indicated in patients who cannot be fit with contact lenses because of steep or irregularly shaped corneas or in those who have central corneal scarring.

Penetrating keratoplasty is the procedure of choice for keratoconus, with a success rate of 80–90%. Some surgeons have achieved good results using epikeratophakia to flatten the cones of patients who have small, central cones and little scarring who are contact lens intolerant. This procedure uses a donor cornea that is frozen before being lathed commercially into a tissue contact lens. Epikeratophakia is advantageous because the globe does not have to be entered (reducing the risk of endophthalmitis) and immunologic rejection of the lens has never been reported. Visual results tend to be poorer than with penetrating keratoplasty, however. Occasionally, a patient's cornea has thinned to such a degree that penetrating keratoplasty is not possible: too little tissue is left in which to sew the donor button. In these patients, a lamellar keratoplasty is performed to "bulk up" the recipient cornea. After this procedure heals, a penetrating keratoplasty can be performed.

Some patients experience an acute rupture of Descemet's membrane with sudden inflow of aqueous humor into the corneal stroma. This is referred to as acute hydrops and usually is accompanied by acute pain and decreased vision. When the hydrops heals, the cornea frequently flattens, and, if the scarring does not involve the visual axis, patients who previously failed with a rigid contact lens can now be fitted with one. Most patients with acute hydrops, however, ultimately go on to penetrating keratoplasty, which is best deferred until after all the corneal edema has resolved.

Corneal Dystrophies. Corneal dystrophies are inherited conditions that manifest with variable findings according to the anatomic layer affected. They are bilateral and largely autosomal dominant with variable penetrance.

Superficial corneal dystrophies include map-dot-fingerprint dystrophy (Cogan's microcystic dystrophy). Abnormalities in the corneal epithelium result in changes in the epithelium basement membrane that manifest as fine map, dot, or fingerprint lines on slitlamp examination of the cornea. Patients with this condition may be asymptomatic, but spontaneous episodes of recurrent corneal erosion can occur. Conservative treatment includes topical lubricants, hypertonic saline drops and/or ointment, and bandage contact lenses. If these measures do not help the epithelium adhere to its underlying basement membrane, debridement to the epithelium in the involved area paradoxically may help achieve stability. A procedure called anterior stromal puncture is gaining acceptance. This procedure uses a fine needle to make small puncture marks just beyond Bowman's membrane into corneal stroma. These small scars allow the overlying epithelium to achieve better adhesion to its basement membrane. Even when the punctures are made within the visual axis, visual deficits are rare, although patients may complain of changes in the quality of their vision.

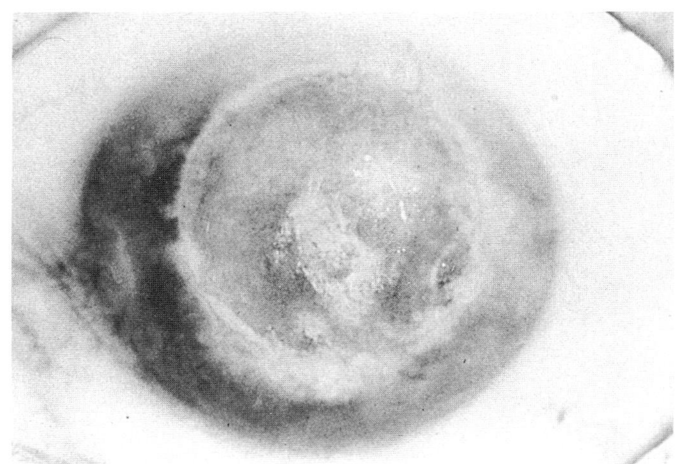

Figure 3.7. Recurrent lattice dystrophy in a penetrating keratoplasty.

Corneal stromal dystrophies are many, but the three classic ones are granular, lattice, and macular dystrophies. Granular dystrophy is characterized by hyaline material deposits into corneal stroma, producing a "bread crumb" appearance with intervening clear areas of cornea. It progresses slowly leading to gradually worsening vision. Symptoms often do not start until midlife. Treatment with penetrating keratoplasty offers a good prognosis. Lattice dystrophy results from amyloid deposits within corneal stroma giving the appearance of fine, refractile lines forming a web. This pattern is often best seen in retroillumination. Recurrent erosions are common and may lead to stromal haze and decreased vision. The treatment of choice is penetrating keratoplasty. Recurrences of lattice dystrophy in the corneal graft are common, but may take years to develop (Fig. 3.7). Macular dystrophy tends to be more severe than granular or lattice dystrophy, and unlike them has an autosomal recessive inheritance pattern. Mucopolysaccharide deposits tend to spread diffusely through corneal stroma leading to decreased vision at an early age. These deposits reach the periphery with no clear cornea between them. Penetrating keratoplasty is performed to improve vision.

Posterior dystrophies include Fuchs' endothelial dystrophy, a common, autosomal dominantly inherited disorder characterized by the early development of endothelial dysfunction associated with decreased endothelial cell counts. Most commonly found in postmenopausal women, this disorder manifests on slitlamp examination as endothelial excrescences (corneal guttae) often associated with pigment. The amount of corneal edema depends on the severity of the disease (Fig. 3.8). As the disease progresses, epithelial breakdown may occur, eventually producing subepithelial scarring. Symptoms of blurred vision and irritation usually do not manifest until the fifth or sixth decade. In the early stages of the disease, topical hypertonic saline may be

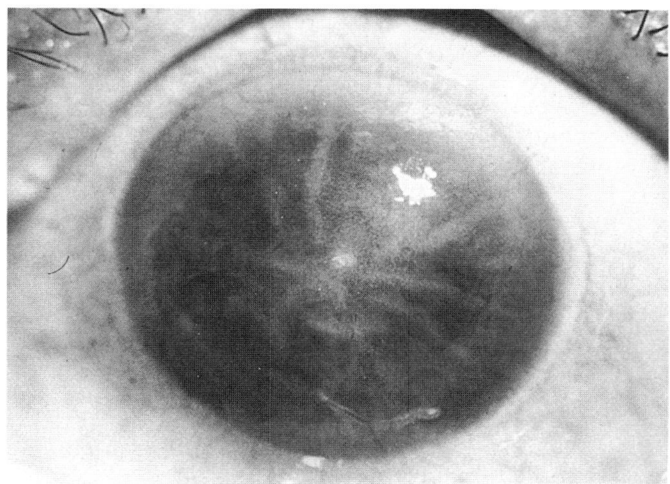

Figure 3.8. Corneal edema secondary to Fuch's dystrophy.

used to dehydrate the cornea, and bandage contact lenses may be inserted to neutralize corneal astigmatism. In later stages, corneal transplantation is the only alternative for improving visual acuity.

Infectious Keratitis. Infectious keratitis is usually caused by bacteria, rarely by fungi or parasites. Infectious corneal infiltrates are associated with contact lenses, especially extended-wear soft contact lenses. Symptoms include pain, redness, purulent discharge, decreased vision, and photophobia. After appropriate cultures and smears are obtained by scraping the involved cornea under topical anesthesia, treatment is with broad-spectrum, fortified topical antibiotics. (Fortified antibiotics are more concentrated than the usual ones and need to be specially formulated by a pharmacist). Most such "corneal ulcers" are successfully treated with medication. If a patient fails to respond to initial treatment, cultures are repeated looking for more unusual organisms. Occasionally, a corneal biopsy is needed to identify the offending microbial agent. For patients who do not respond to medical therapy, corneal transplantation is required to excise the infected tissue.

Corneal transplantation technique is modified slightly because of the infected nature of the case. The size of the graft is determined by the size of the corneal infiltrate. If the corneal infiltrate is not totally excised, the residual organisms will reinfect the graft and possibly the inside of the eye. After excising the infected cornea, the surgical tray is replaced with a new sterile tray of instruments that are used on the donor cornea to finish the surgery. The host corneal tissue button is sent not only to microbiology but also to pathology to check for organisms at the wound edge, just as one would look for evidence of tumor cells at the edge of a tumor resection. Fortified antibiotics are used topically after surgery, and the surgeon may choose to use intraocular and/or intravenous antibiotics. While preservation of a clear graft is desirable, the overriding concern is elimination of the infectious process. Immune-system-suppressing topical steroids are consequently use with caution, if at all.

The most common cases requiring cornea transplantation because of infection are (*a*) fungal or amoebic infectious keratitis and (*b*) severe bacterial keratitis that has led to corneal perforation. If an infected cornea perforates, cyanoacrylate tissue adhesive can be used to seal the perforation and allow the underlying tissue to heal, once the acute infectious process has been eradicated.

Sterile corneal ulceration may occur in association with such connective tissue disorders as rheumatoid arthritis, systemic lupus erythematosus, and Wegener's granulomatosis. The sterile infiltrates usually occur in the corneal periphery and frequently respond to topical or anti-inflammatory therapy. If they go on to perforate, cyanoacrylate tissue adhesive can be used. A bandage contact lens is placed over the cornea to protect against mechanical irritation from lid movement that can dislodge the adhesive. If successfully applied, the glue allows the corneal stroma to fill in beneath it. The glue usually spontaneously dislodges in a few months, following which the bandage contact lens is removed. The use of tissue adhesive is limited by the size of the corneal perforation. If the perforation is greater than 2–3 mm, it cannot be sealed by glue and requires a "patch" graft, which involves plugging the hole in the cornea with a piece of donor corneal tissue.

Technique

Donor Tissue. A cornea donor may be any deceased person under 75 years of age who has no transmittable disease or history of eye disease. Patients from whom cornea tissue would be refused include those who test human immunodeficiency virus (HIV) positive, those who have had previous intraocular surgery, and those with hepatitis, rabies, sepsis, Jakob-Creutzfeldt disease, or glaucoma. The quality of donor tissue depends on age of donor, time between death and tissue harvest, and time between death, processing, and preservation. While younger donors and speed of harvest, processing, and preservation are preferred, many older donors can have excellent corneal quality as documented by endothelial cell counts. Both the Eye Bank and the surgeon assess the quality of the tissue. Tissue typing is not performed, since rejection is unusual.

Donor cornea and a thin rim of surrounding sclera are preserved in solutions containing nutritional, preservative, and antibiotic solutions. Even though the risk of transplanting contaminated tissue is rare, cultures of the donor corneal rims should taken at the time of preservation and also at the time of surgery. Currently, donor tissue may be preserved for 5–7 days following donor death. Cryopreservation allows corneal preservation for many years but is neither practical nor economical.

Full-Thickness Transplant. Corneal transplantation may be performed using an eyelid block and either local retrobulbar injection or general anesthesia. A lid speculum is placed in the conjunctival sac avoiding pressure on the globe itself. Usually, a small stainless steel ring

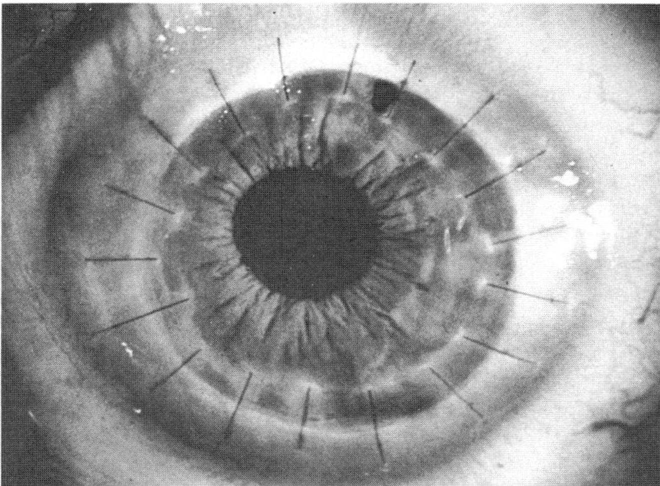

Figure 3.9. Clear penetrating keratoplasty with intact interrupted sutures.

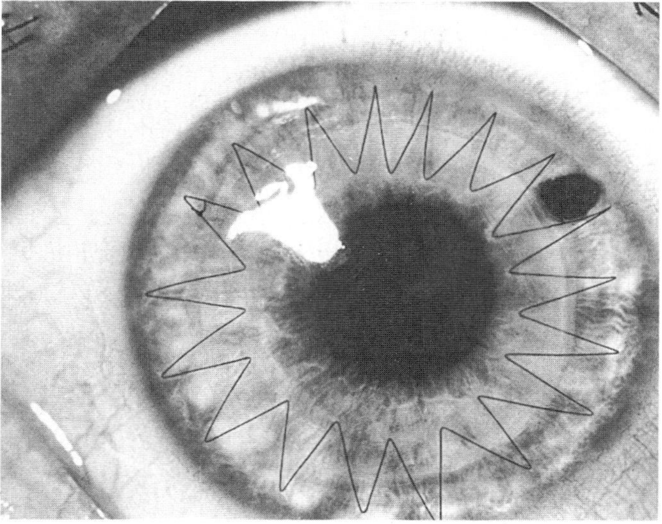

Figure 3.10. Clear penetrating keratoplasty with intact running sutures. Note peripheral iridectomy at 2 o'clock position.

called Flieringa's ring is sewn to the sclera to support the globe when the eye is open. Since the eye is an elastic structure, it tends to collapse when the cornea is removed, especially in children.

A corneal trephine (a circular blade) of appropriate size is centered on the cornea and a partial-thickness (80%) cut made in the host. The donor cornea is prepared using a separate trephine with the endothelial side of the corneal button up. This cut is about 1/2 mm larger in diameter than the host trephination to lessen the likelihood of postoperative complications and to make closing the eye technically easier. After the donor cornea is punched, it is placed on a protected Teflon block and covered by its preservative solution. Great care is taken to avoid trauma to the donor cornea that could cause endothelial cell loss leading to graft failure.

After the donor cornea is prepared, the host eye is entered with a sharp blade. The host button is cut out with curved corneal scissors, and further intraocular surgery is performed as needed. Such surgery might include removal and replacement of intraocular lenses, placement of a secondary IOL in a previously aphakic eye, removal of prolapsed vitreous humor from the anterior chamber of the eye, resection of scar tissue, or cataract extraction and primary IOL implant.

Once these other procedures are completed, the donor cornea is brought to the operative field and sewn into place. Various suturing methods are used, depending on surgeon preference (Figs. 3.9 and 3.10). The ultimate goal is to achieve a perfectly replaced cornea with no induced astigmatism. After the cornea is sewn to the recipient bed and the anterior chamber is reformed with balanced salt solution, the wound is inspected to make sure it is secure. The supporting ring is removed, antibiotics and steroids are administered if necessary, and a pressure patch with shield is applied.

The postoperative management of a penetrating keratoplasty patient includes the use of topical steroids, topical antibiotics, and topical lubricants. If there is elevated intraocular pressure, topical and/or systemic antiglaucoma medications are used. Because topical antibiotics are potentially epithelial toxic, they are gradually withdrawn over a period of several weeks. Topical steroids need to be used for several months to reduce intraocular inflammation and prevent immunologic graft rejection.

Visual rehabilitation following penetrating keratoplasty takes much longer than that following other anterior segment surgical procedures. Avascular, clear corneal wounds heal much more slowly than limbal wounds, taking up to one year or longer for visual recovery to be complete. If patients obtain good visual acuity with a stable refraction and not too much astigmatism, sutures are best left in place, since removing them can result in large astigmatic errors. It is important to warn the patient about the potential for erosion and exposure of disintegrating sutures, which can be a source of irritation and infection. It must be emphasized to all patients to seek prompt ophthalmic evaluation should they experience any pain, redness, irritation, or discharge suggestive of suture exposure.

Intraoperative complications include damage to adjacent anterior segment structures such as the iris or lens. Bleeding from the iris or anterior chamber angle may occur when removing poorly designed or poorly positioned intraocular lenses. The most feared intraoperative complication is expulsive hemorrhage, the forceful expulsion of intraocular contents secondary to acute choroidal hemorrhage. This rare complication is more common in elderly patients, those with glaucoma, and those with previous eye surgery. The most important priority is to get the eye closed. Secondary surgical intervention can be performed several days later, after the ocular status has stabilized.

Postoperative complications include rejection, endophthalmitis, persistent epithelial defects, infectious keratitis, elevated intraocular pressure, retinal detachment, and epithelial downgrowth. The incidence of rejection is approximately 10–20% for good prognosis cases such as corneal scars, keratoconus, and certain corneal dystrophies. Most rejection episodes occur 3–12 months after surgery, with the incidence higher in younger patients, presumably because of their more active immune systems. If caught early, rejection episodes can often be aborted by the intensive use of steroids, topically in the form of drops or ointment, subconjunctivally by injection, or parenterally by mouth. Patients who have undergone penetrating keratoplasty are instructed to seek prompt ophthalmic evaluation at the first signs of rejection, such as conjunctival injection, pain, irritation, light sensitivity, and decreased vision. Rejection in its early stages is often not noticed by patients but is observed during a routine follow-up visit. Permanently rejected corneas become cloudy. They may be retransplanted, although with each subsequent transplant the chance of rejection increases.

The prognosis of corneal transplants depends primarily on the underlying disease for which the transplant is being done. Favorable prognostic factors include the lack of preoperative inflammation, avascularity of the diseased cornea, normal intraocular pressure, and healthy ocular surface and adnexa. Poor indicators include active inflammation, surface disorders such as dry eyes syndrome, lid abnormalities, corneal vascularity, glaucoma, and chemical burns. The results of penetrating keratoplasty in children are not as good as in adults because of such factors as associated other congenital ocular abnormalities, difficulty with follow-up, and amblyopia. Some disorders such as certain corneal dystrophies and herpes simplex keratitis tend to recur in corneal transplants. All the stromal dystrophies have been known to recur in a transplant, although it may take years for such recurrence to become apparent, and the recurrence may differ from the characteristic appearance of the primary dystrophy.

While the prognosis for a clear corneal transplant is fairly good, in some cases astigmatism and anisometropia (significant difference in refractive error between the eye that has had surgery and the one that has not) often preclude full visual rehabilitation of the eye that has had surgery. Contact lenses are helpful in neutralizing the astigmatism or anisometropia. Unfortunately, some patients are contact lens intolerant, particularly the elderly who have difficulty handling or tolerating the lenses. Astigmatic keratorefractive surgery is sometimes required to remedy excessive astigmatic or anisometropic refractive errors. Visual results following penetrating keratoplasty depend not only upon the clarity and regularity of the transplanted corneal button, but upon the healthy function of the retina and optic nerve.

Partial-Thickness Transplants. A lamellar corneal transplant is useful for patients with anterior corneal disease, as in some scars or inherited dystrophies. This procedure obviates the need to enter the eye, thereby virtually eliminating the risk of endophthalmitis. In addition, the recipient corneal endothelium is left intact, thereby eliminating the risk of immunologic endothelial rejection. The procedure is also useful in serving as a patch graft in patients with acute corneal perforations that require immediate surgical closure.

The surgical procedure of lamellar keratoplasty is technically more demanding than that of penetrating keratoplasty. A corneal trephine is used to make a partial-thickness incision into the host cornea, following which a lamellar dissection is carried across the outlying trephination. The lamellar dissection is deep enough to remove the anterior stromal opacification while leaving a posterior bed of clear corneal stroma for the corneal donor. Donor tissue also requires precise lamellar dissection and is best performed from an intact donor globe.

Postoperative management is similar to that of penetrating keratoplasty, although fewer topical steroids are used. Healing of lamellar grafts tends to be quicker. The major drawback of lamellar keratoplasty is the difficulty in achieving a smooth lamellar bed, which increases the potential for interface scarring that may restrict vision. However, in select patients with anterior corneal stromal opacification, a lamellar rather than a penetrating keratoplasty is the treatment of choice.

Refractive Surgery

Refractive corneal surgery involves changing the refractive power of the eye by surgically modifying the shape of the cornea. There are a variety of procedures employed, only the most common of which will be discussed.

Radial keratotomy, the most common refractive surgery performed, is used to correct myopia. Partial-thickness radial cuts are made in the cornea, sparing the visual axis (Figs. 3.11 and 3.12). This pattern of incisions tends to flatten the central cornea, thereby reducing the myopic refractive error. The procedure generally is performed under topical anesthesia. The amount of correction can be modified by varying the size of the spared central optical zone, the number of radial incisions, and the depth of the incisions. The predictability of radial keratotomy depends upon the degree of myopia being treated. Patients with low to moderate myopia have an 80 to 90% chance of obtaining 20/40 or better uncorrected visual acuity. Chances of obtaining better visual acuity decrease with increasing myopia.

Surgical complications are rare, though many patients note glare and fluctuating visual acuity in the early postoperative period that tends to resolve with time. Repeat procedures are sometimes required, and if the result still does not offer adequate uncorrected visual acuity, the patient has to return to spectacle or contact lens wear. Questions have been raised about the stability of radial keratotomy: some patients demonstrate gradual increased effect of the surgery over a period of several years. There is also concern that deep radial incisions may weaken the structural integrity of the cornea, rendering it more susceptible to traumatic rupture.

Other refractive procedures include corneal relaxing incisions, compression sutures, wedge resection, epikeratophakia (application of a donor cornea), and keratomileusis (grinding a new curvature on the cor-

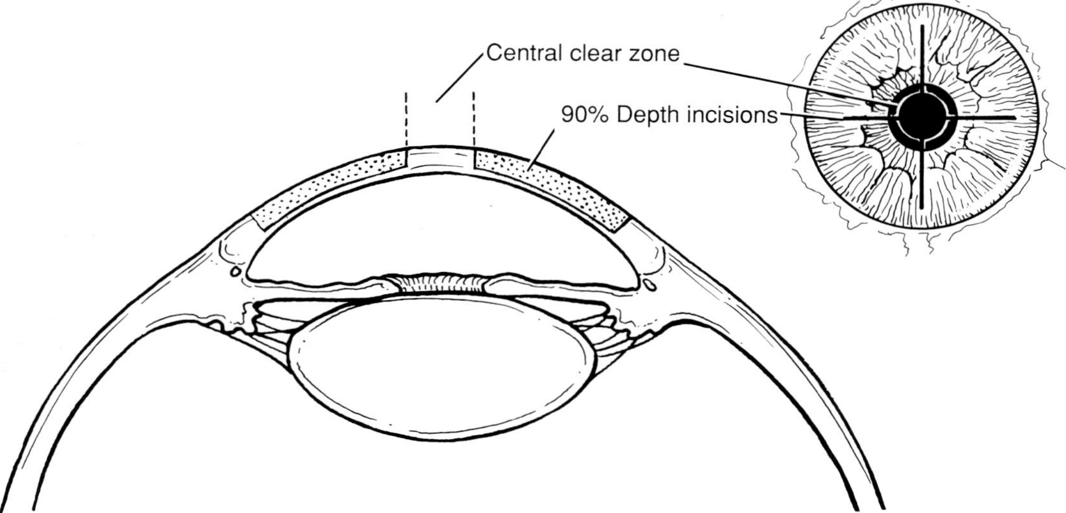

Figure 3.11. Radial keratotomy.

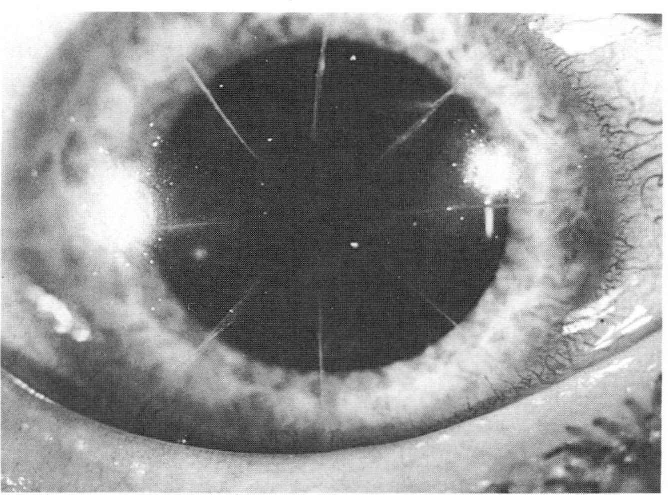

Figure 3.12. Eight-incision radial keratotomy.

nea). Patients with congenital astigmatism or residual postoperative astigmatism usually can be managed with glasses or contact lenses. If astigmatism is excessive, surgical alternatives include relaxing incisions, compression sutures, and wedge resection. Relaxing incisions centered on the steep axis of the corneal astigmatism cause flattening of the cornea in that meridian, thereby reducing the amount of astigmatism. Corneal compression sutures and wedge resections are used to steepen a flat corneal meridian. Visual rehabilitation following wedge resection is much longer than with relaxing incisions. Corneal compression sutures have a variable effect and may not be permanent. The predictability of astigmatic surgery is less than ideal, but in patients with excessive postoperative astigmatism there is nothing else to offer for visual rehabilitation.

Epikeratophakia and keratomileusis are examples of refractive procedures using lamellar keratoplasty. Epikeratophakia is used primarily to correct aphakia in patients who are contact lens intolerant and are not good candidates for a secondary intraocular lens. The procedure involves suturing a commercially prepared lenticule of corneal tissue on top of the recipient cornea after the corneal epithelium has been removed. Recovery is fast and the procedure easily repeatable if necessary. Keratomileusis involves shaving off a thin anterior section of the patient's own cornea, freezing it, lathing it to the desired power and shape, thawing it, and resuturing it into its original site. This procedure is reserved for highly myopic patients who cannot be corrected otherwise and who do not want glasses or contact lenses. The procedure requires expensive equipment, the use of which can be difficult to master. Major drawbacks of the procedure include poor predictability, irreversibility, and the potential for surgically induced irregular corneal astigmatism.

One of the most exciting developments in corneal surgery has been the introduction of the Excimer laser, which is capable of vaporizing tissue with high precision. Clinical trials are underway to evaluate the potential for laser sculpting of the anterior cornea to produce refractive change. If the encouraging preliminary results hold up over the long term, this laser could revolutionize the practice of ophthalmology.

Pterygium

A pterygium is a plaque-like extension of fibrovascular tissue onto the superficial cornea. Pterygia characteristically originate nasally from pinguecula (accumulation of connective tissue that thickens the conjunctiva) and grow onto the adjacent corneal surface. The cause of pterygia is unknown, but the incidence seems to correlate with exposure to ultraviolet light.

Pterygia commonly remain restricted to the peripheral cornea, where they do not interfere with visual acuity. Some cause localized irritation that can be controlled with topical lubricants and vasoconstrictors. However, some pterygia extend toward the visual axis

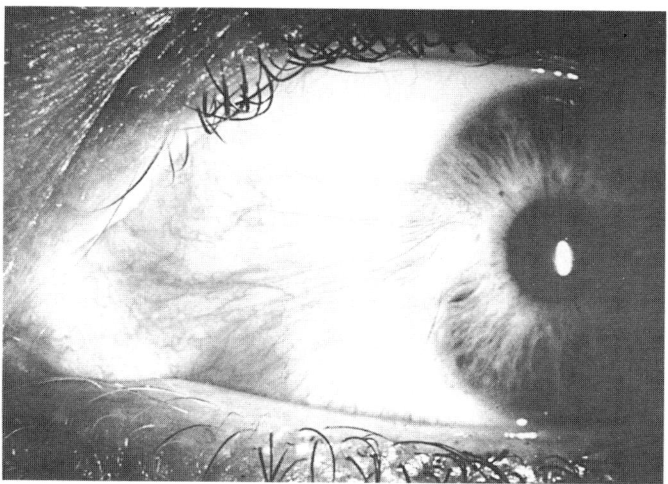

Figure 3.13. Recurrent pterygium.

with resultant induced corneal astigmatism and visual distortion. If a pterygium grows into the visual axis, it may interfere with visual acuity by causing opacification and obscuration of the central cornea. Surgical excision is recommended when vision begins to be distorted before the pterygium encroaches on the visual axis.

Surgery usually is done under local anesthesia. The pterygium is dissected off the corneal surface with a fine lathe. Small cautery burns to the conjunctiva outlining the proposed graft site are helpful in delineating the proposed donor conjunctival site, because once the initial incision into conjunctiva is made, retraction of the tissue makes these measurements difficult. The graft is carefully sewn into place over the pterygium excision site taking care not to turn the donor tissue inside out.

Recurrence rates after primary pterygium removal vary between 10 to 50%, but tend to be lower in northern latitudes where there is less ultraviolet light exposure. The recurrence rate may be diminished by the use of a conjunctival transposition to cover the exposed bed of the excised pterygium. To decrease the chance of recurrence, beta irradiation and/or topical antimetabolites (mitomycin, thiotepa) have been advocated.

A recurrent pterygium may become more extensive than the original one. Excessive scarring and cicatrization ensue with involvement of underlying extraocular muscles, which can restrict ocular motility and cause double vision. Thus, pterygium surgery is best avoided unless it is absolutely necessary because of visual restriction, recurrent irritation, or cosmetic disfigurement. Before proceeding with surgery, the patient must be made well aware of the potential for recurrence (Fig. 3.13).

Surface Disorders

Ocular surface disorders include dry eye syndrome, exposure keratopathy, and neurotrophic keratitis. Dry eye syndrome (keratitis sicca) most commonly occurs as an isolated finding in menopausal women but can also occur as part of Sjogren's syndrome, ocular pemphigoid, or Stevens-Johnson syndrome. Exposure keratopathy results from inability of the lids to cover the entire corneal surface on blinking or during sleep. It occurs in Bell's palsy and in ocular trauma, where localized scarring of the lids prevents full corneal coverage. Neurotrophic keratitis is caused by dysfunction of the sensory nerve supply to the cornea as occurs in neurologic diseases affecting the first division of the trigeminal nerve.

The result of all ocular surface disorders is desiccation of the corneal epithelium and conjunctival squamous metaplasia and keratinizations. Patients commonly complain of ocular irritation and foreign body sensation. Supplemental liquid tear substitutes and bland ointment may be all that are necessary to promote ocular comfort and maintain the integrity of the corneal epithelium. Occluding the puncta (shown in Fig. 3.37) with silicone plugs, cautery, or hyfrecation can also enhance ocular surface lubrication. In cases of severe dry eyes, however, permanent punctal occlusion may be necessary.

Patients with severe dry eye syndrome, exposure keratopathy, or neurotrophic keratopathy can be helped by tarsorrhaphy. The procedure involves sewing the edges of the superior and inferior lid margins together, usually preceded by splitting the lid margin or excising a thin superficial layer of lid margin to create two opposing raw surfaces that remain permanently adjoined once the sutures are removed. Because a tarsorrhaphy is cosmetically disfiguring, it is reserved for patients with severe ocular surface disease and a potential for corneal ulceration and melting. Once the cornea has completely healed, the tarsorrhaphy can be separated by a simple excision. The potential for recurrent epithelial breakdown remains, however.

A conjunctival flap is an alternative but is resorted to only when the patient refuses a tarsorrhaphy or when the visual potential of the involved eye is poor.

Oculoplastic surgery is a third alternative to correct other eyelid deformities that result in corneal exposure. Conjunctival cicatrizing disorders such as ocular pemphigoid and Stevens-Johnson syndrome are often resistant to all surgical and medical attempts to improve the ocular surface environment. In such cases the only alternative is a keratoprosthesis in which a small telescope is sewn through the cornea into the eye and then brought out through a small opening in the eyelids that are otherwise sewn closed. Although excellent results can be obtained for a few months to years, the long-term prognosis is poor.

Diseases of the Anterior Chamber

Glaucoma is a disease characterized by an increased level of ocular pressure that interferes with the normal functioning of the optic nerve head, leading to atrophy of the optic nerve with progressive loss of the visual field. If untreated, glaucoma can lead to total, irreversible blindness. Prevention of lost vision depends on

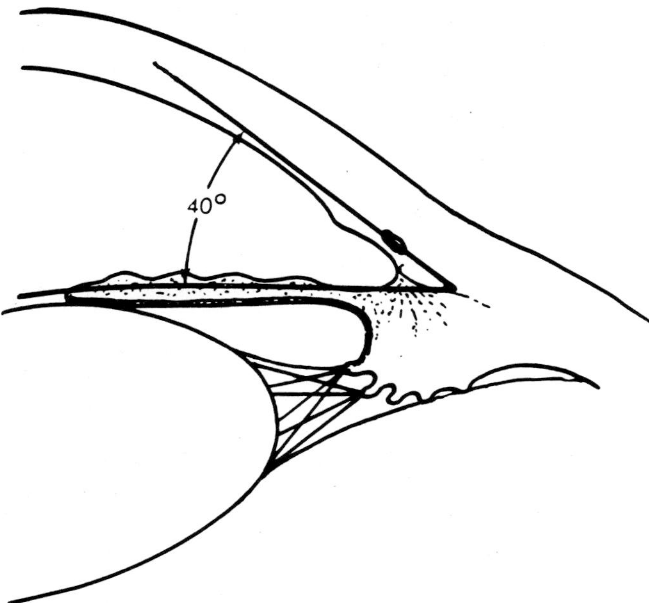

Figure 3.14. Typical configuration in open-angle glaucoma. The angle of the anterior chamber (indicated by arrows) is formed by the cornea and iris.

early detection and proper treatment of glaucoma, either by medication or surgery. Intraocular pressure depends on the relationship among aqueous production, aqueous outflow, and episcleral venous pressure. Normal intraocular pressure is 16 mm Hg (normal pressure ranges between 10 and 22 mm Hg). Some patients, however, have optic nerves that can withstand pressures greater than 22 mm Hg. These patients, even though they do not show optic nerve damage or visual field changes, are considered ocular hypertensives or glaucoma suspects. Glaucoma is commonly categorized according to the cause of the altered resistance to aqueous outflow, as well as to the clinical appearance of the anterior chamber angle. Glaucoma can be primary, secondary, or congenital.

Primary Glaucoma

Primary glaucoma is classified as chronic open-angle, narrow-angle (also called angle-closure), or mixed.

Chronic Open-Angle Glaucoma. Chronic open-angle glaucoma is the most common form of glaucoma: 2% of the general population over the age of 65 is at risk (Fig. 3.14). In chronic open-angle glaucoma, the trabecular meshwork appears anatomically normal but its ability to remove aqueous from the anterior chamber is diminished. This type of glaucoma is treated topically with such medications as timolol maleate, levobunolol, betaxolol, or pilocarpine, as well as systemically with carbonic anhydrase inhibitors. If these medications fail to reduce intraocular pressure to a safe level (i.e., if further loss of vision is occurring at the present pressure) or if the patient is unable to tolerate the medications, then a laser trabeculoplasty may be attempted. Like laser iridotomy, laser trabeculoplasty is performed under topical anesthesia and involves the use of a special gonioscopic mirror to allow angle visualization. Using a laser, approximately 75 spots are placed into the anterior trabecular meshwork in an area of 180°. Usually, a 50-micron, spot-sized, blue-green argon laser is used with wattage varying from 800 to 1200 mw. The mechanism by which a laser trabeculoplasty effects change is not well understood, but the procedure reduces intraocular pressure by about 25% in approximately 65–75% of patients. Although the procedure may relieve pressure for only months to a few years, it has few side effects and is sometimes used even before systemic medications.

If a patient is still losing vision, a surgical procedure may be required. In the United States, the most common surgical procedure is a trabeculectomy, a filtering procedure effective in 75–90% of cases (Fig. 3.15). A trabeculectomy usually is performed under local anesthetic on an outpatient basis. After adequate anesthesia and prep using an iodine/Proviodine solution, a lid speculum is inserted beneath the lids. The eye is rotated inferiorly, the superior rectus muscle is grasped with a forceps, and a 4-0 suture is passed under the muscle for traction. A peritomy is performed with blunt scissors and can be either fornix-based (the conjunctiva and Tenon's capsule are opened at the limbus) or limbus-based (the conjunctiva and Tenon's capsule are opened approximately 8–10 mm behind the limbus). Cautery is used to obtain hemostasis, and the sclera is cleaned by scraping with a fine blade. Using a very fine diamond knife, a half-scleral-thickness incision is made perpendicular to the limbus and extended approximately 3–4 mm behind it. Another, parallel incision is made approximately 4 mm away and is joined to the first one with an incision parallel to the limbus and 3–4 mm behind it. This area is then dissected forward with a blunt blade. The flap is carried into clear cornea. The shape of the half-scleral-thickness flap may be triangular, rectangular, or even rhomboid; studies have shown there is little difference in outcome resulting from the shape of the flap. A full-thickness piece of trabecular meshwork, approximately 1.5–2 mm, is removed. A small iridectomy is performed to prevent closure of the opening by iris. The flap is resutured, using 10-0 sutures at the posterior edge of the incision. Conjunctiva and Tenon's capsule are resutured in place. Even after a trabeculectomy, patients may require additional medication to control the pressure.

Narrow-Angle Glaucoma. Narrow-angle (angle-closure) glaucoma is caused by a mechanical blockage of the angle by the iris (Fig. 3.16). Symptoms of acute angle closure are halos around lights, headaches, nausea, and ocular pain. Signs are a steamy cornea, a partly dilated nonreactive pupil, a gonioscopically closed angle with high intraocular pressure, and red, injected eyes.

The blockade usually is easily broken by producing a laser iridotomy (with either a yttrium-argon-garnet (YAG) or an argon laser), which creates a conduit for aqueous humor to flow from the posterior to the anterior chamber. This procedure deepens the anterior chamber and opens the angle by allowing the iris to fall back to its original position. After topical anesthesia a specially designed lens is used to focus the laser onto the iris surface. A YAG laser is then used to photodisrupt (or an argon laser to burn) the iris, producing a hole that breaks the pupillary block.

Occasionally, when the cornea is hazy and a laser cannot be used, a surgical iridectomy is performed (Fig. 3.17). After adequate anesthesia a small 3–4 mm peritomy is performed, usually superiorly, which releases the conjunctiva from its limbal attachments. The surgical limbus is identified and the anterior chamber is entered with a knife. A forceps is used to grasp and retract the iris, and a small piece of iris is removed with scissors. The limbal incision is closed with a small 9-0 or 10-0 suture and the peritomy closed over that.

Mixed Chronic Open- and Narrow-Angle Glaucoma. In nearly 95–100% of patients with acute narrow-angle glaucoma and with most nonchronic forms of glaucoma, either the laser or surgical iridectomy is effective in preventing further attacks. Because a chronic, low-grade, narrow-angle attack may lead to damage of the trabecular meshwork, however, a patient may develop a mixed chronic open- and narrow-angle glaucoma requiring medication even after the iridectomy or iridotomy has been performed.

Secondary Glaucoma

Secondary glaucoma is characterized by associated ocular or systemic abnormalities that appear to account for the diminished resistance to aqueous outflow. Such glaucomas may be associated with intraocular tumors or hemorrhage; corneal endothelium, pigmentary, lens, or retinal disorders; ocular inflammation, trauma, or surgery; steroid ingestion; or elevated episcleral venous pressure.

Neovascular glaucoma is a secondary glaucoma in which new blood vessels form in the angle of the eye and on the iris. Histologically, connective tissue is also present with these vessels. The neovascularization often starts at the pupillary margin. Eventually, vessels can cover the iris and then progress into the angle. The fibrovascular membrane that is formed is contracted, leading to ectropion uvea (the posterior pigment layer of the iris is pulled into the pupil and then onto the anterior surface) and also to anterior synechiae (the iris is pulled into the angle).

The cause of neovascular glaucoma is not fully understood. A common property of the many causes of rubeosis iridis appears to be hypoxia, either anteriorly or, more commonly, posteriorly. Many think there is an angiogenesis factor released that leads to the new vessels forming. Some of the more common causes of rubeosis iridis include diabetes mellitus, retinal vein occlusion, retinal artery occlusion, carotid artery disease, and intraocular surgery.

In general, the treatment for rubeosis is panretinal photocoagulation to reduce the stimulus for angiogenesis factor(s). Later stages may need surgery, including setons (plastic one-way valves that drain externally). If these are unsuccessful cyclocryotherapy, laser therapy, or alcohol injections may be necessary.

Congenital Glaucoma

Congenital glaucoma is a rare, usually bilateral disease that affects approximately 1 in 20,000 live births. The exact mechanism that triggers this disease is not known, but the angle acts as if there were a membrane over the trabecular meshwork. The signs and symptoms of congenital glaucoma are photophobia, buphthalmos (large eye), large corneas, tearing, and corneal edema. Medications do not work well in affected infants and surgery is required.

The two primary procedures for correcting congenital glaucoma are goniotomy and trabeculotomy. In goniotomy, favored by most surgeons, a fine knife is passed across the anterior chamber to incise the trabecular meshwork (and usually Schlemm's canal) for approximately 120° (Fig. 3.18). The angle of the anterior chamber is viewed through a gonioscope, which breaks the total internal reflection and allows the angle to be viewed. In trabeculotomy, the incision is made at the limbus, dissecting both conjunctiva and Tenon's capsule. The surgical limbus is identified using a very sharp knife, such as a diamond knife. Schlemm's canal is identified from the outside often by visualizing aqueous reflux and then threading a fine-wire gauge (trabeculotome) into the canal to tear into the anterior chamber. Both procedures accomplish the same end and both have advantages and disadvantages. For example, in a goniotomy a cloudy cornea can limit anterior chamber visibility, and in a trabeculotomy the canal of Schlemm cannot always be identified. Either procedure may have to be performed two or three times, but intraocular pressure can be controlled in approximately 80–90% of patients. For those in whom it cannot, a standard trabeculectomy (as described above for chronic open-angle glaucoma) is performed.

Diseases of the Lens

Cataract Formation

The lens of the eye is an avascular structure that grows throughout an individual's life. It is composed of a dense nucleus surrounded by softer cortex and is sequestered in a capsule. The lens epithelium produces new lens material analogous to the layers of an onion. A cataract is any clouding of the lens of the eye, and may occur anywhere within the lens (Fig. 3.19). The most common opacities occur within the nucleus, which naturally yellows and hardens with age. Opacities can occur in the anterior and posterior cortical areas as well as in the posterior subcapsular area.

Etiology. Many factors can be involved in the etiology of cataracts. Family history, general health, age, trauma, diabetes, steroid use, intraocular inflammation, or exposure to radiation may all play a role. The lens is not only vulnerable to trauma, but because it is an avas-

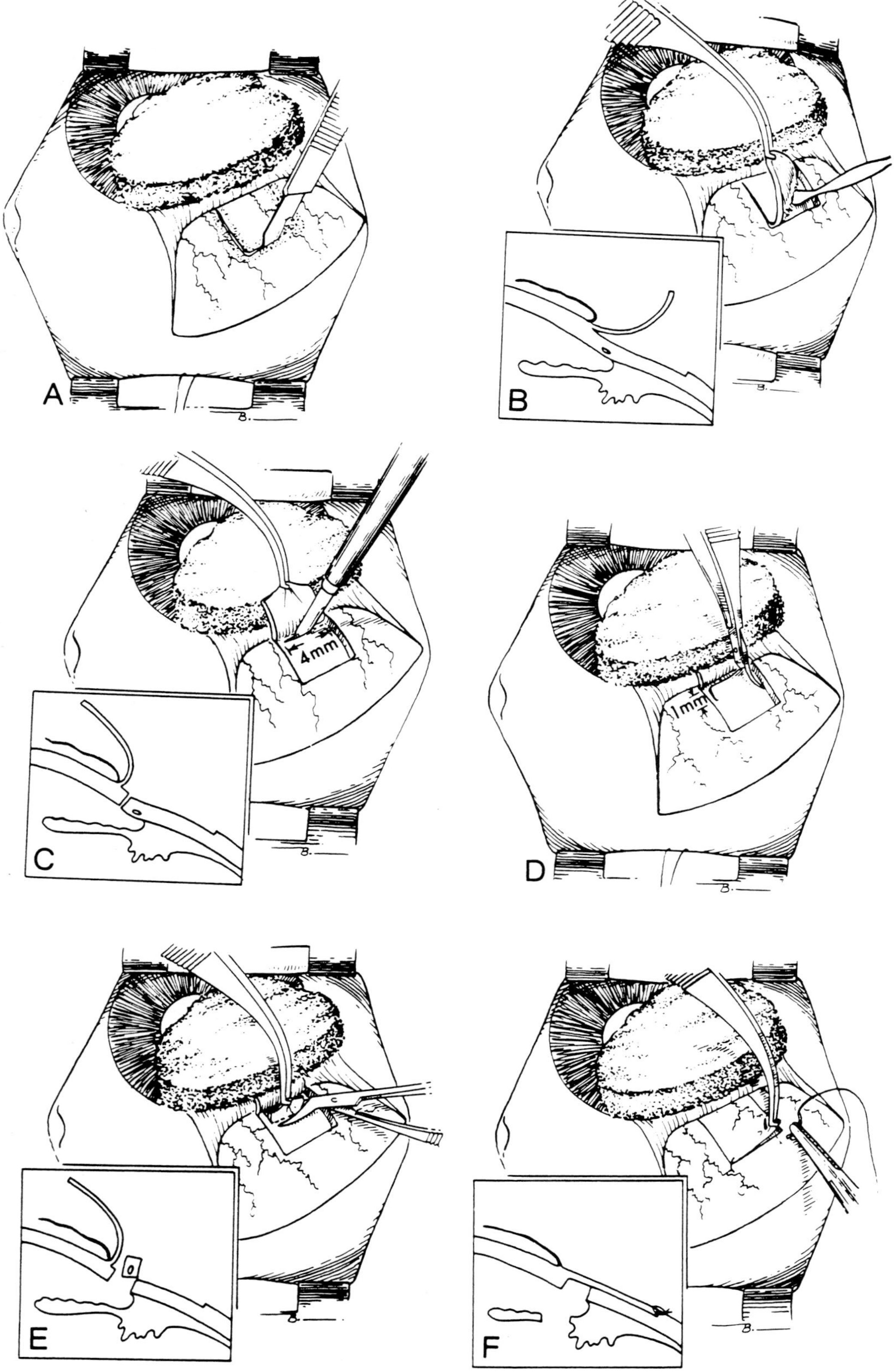

Figure 3.15.—*continued*

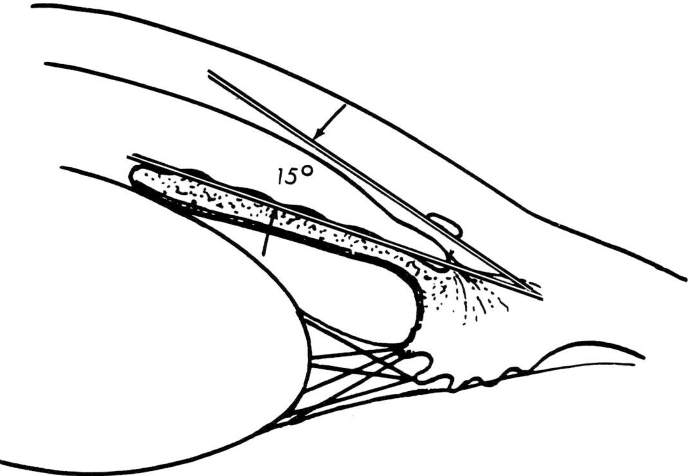

Figure 3.16. Narrow angle that typically precedes most forms of angle-closure glaucoma. (From Shields, MB. A study guide for glaucoma. Baltimore: Williams & Wilkins, 1982:137.)

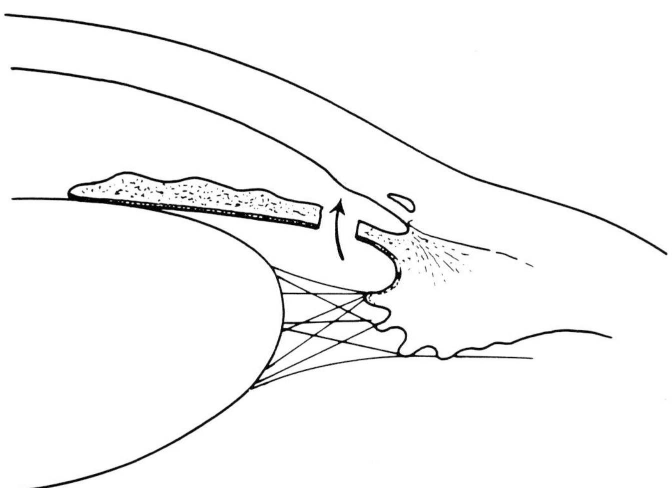

Figure 3.17. Mechanism of iridectomy. Communication between anterior and posterior chambers (**arrow**) bypasses the pupillary block, which relieves the relatively higher pressure in the posterior chamber, allowing peripheral iris to fall away from the trabecular meshwork. (From Shields MB. A study guide for glaucoma. Baltimore: Williams & Wilkins, 1982:478.)

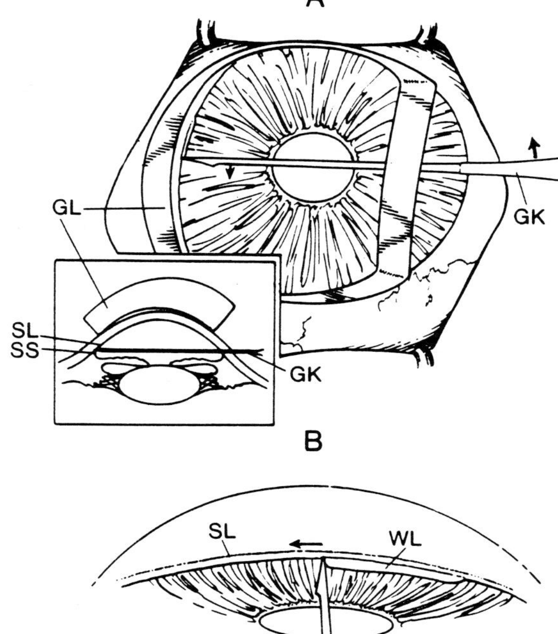

Figure 3.18. Goniotomy. **A**, With a surgical goniolens (**GL**) positioned on the cornea, a goniotomt knife (**GK**) is inserted through peripheral cornea and passed across the anterior chamber to the angle in the opposite quadrant. **B**, Under direct gonioscopic visualization, angle tissue is excised between Schwalbe's line (**SL**) and scleral spur (**SS**) for approximately one-third of the chamber angle circumference. This creates a white line (**WL**) as the cut edge of tissue retracts from the incision. **Arrows** indicate the direction of knife movement during incision of angle tissue. (From Shields MB. A study guide for glaucoma. Baltimore: Williams & Wilkins, 1982:489.)

cular structure it cannot rid itself easily of any metabolic insult.

A senile or age-related cataract is seen as a yellowing of the lens, the result of natural by-products of the aging process. Density and coloration of the lens are extremely variable. In some early aging syndromes the lens may yellow at 30–35 years of age. While almost all patients over 65 have some form of hardening or yellowing of the nucleus, some patients in their 80s and 90s have little lenticular change.

Blunt trauma, even without ocular perforation, may cause cataract formation, typically seen as a petal-form anterior cortical opacification in the central region of the lens (Fig. 3.19). It appears quite commonly in boxers who receive repeated blows to the head, but may be seen after a single blow. Another common cause for this type of cataract is racquet sports, particularly racquetball and squash, in patients who do not wear protective eye gear.

Systemic and long-term topical steroid use can produce a posterior subcapsular cataract. Many feel this to be a dose-dependent phenomenon, although the mechanism is not known. Another cause of such cataracts is intraocular inflammation, as seen in anterior and posterior uveitis syndromes such as sarcoidosis, Reiter's syndrome, and other human leukocyte antigen B27 (HLA-B27) subgroups. Swelling of the lens caused by high glucose levels in diabetics can initiate a classic

Figure 3.15. Trabeculectomy, basic technique. **A**, Margins of scleral flap are outlined by partial-thickness incisions. **B**, Dissection of scleral flap. **C**, Anterior chamber is entered with a knife just behind the hinge of the scleral flap. **D**, Completion of anterior and lateral margins of deep limbal incision with scissors. **E**, Flap of deep limbal tissue is excised by cutting along scleral spur. **F**, Approximation of scleral flap. (From Shields MB. A study guide for glaucoma. Baltimore: Williams & Wilkins, 1982:464. Portions reprinted with permission from *Ophthal Surg* 1980;11:498.)

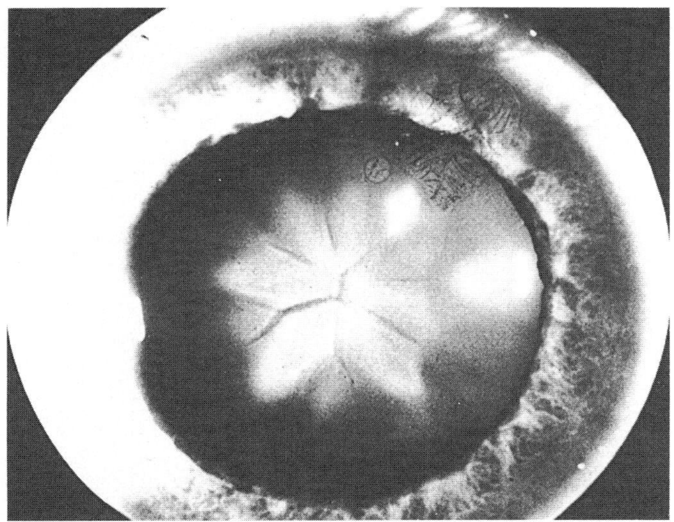

Figure 3.19. Petal-leaf formation in a traumatic cataract.

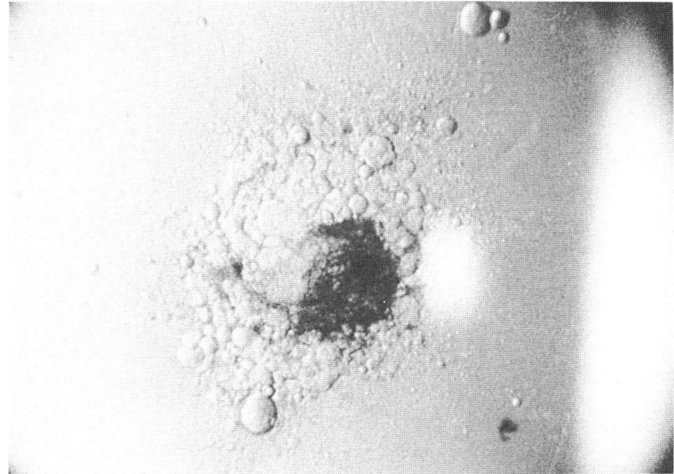

Figure 3.20. Light scattering from a posterior subcapsular cataract.

water cleft type of cataract. In uncontrolled diabetics, glucose enters the lens structure where aldose reductase transforms it into sorbitol, which cannot leave the lens. This process causes an osmotic gradient, resulting in a swelling of the lens. While the condition may be reversible, repeated offenses may lead to permanent lens changes.

Radiation exposure, usually in excess of 400 rads, may also cause cataract formation. Radiation treatment for cancer around the head and neck is of particular concern. Some epidemiologic studies suggest that exposure to ultraviolet light over long periods of time, as seen in farmers and fishermen, may also induce more rapid cataract formation.

Indications for Surgery. Indications for surgery vary with every patient. Visual function is reduced by cataract, but its subjective effect on the patient is the most important consideration. A senile cataract induces a myopic shift in refraction by increasing the refractive index of the lens, thus causing light to focus in front of the retina. This shift can result in the patient's ability to read without glasses, a phenomenon called "second sight." The cataract also decreases night vision, increases glare at night, and because it absorbs blue light leads to a dulling of colors (or "browning effect"). Until well developed, however, the cataract does not usually affect reading and other close activities. In patients with poor distance vision (20/60 or less) who are nevertheless happy, surgery is not indicated.

In contrast to a nuclear cataract which usually affects the elderly, a posterior subcapsular cataract often occurs in young patients, especially those taking steroids. Such a cataract diffracts light and, depending on its location (central or peripheral), can cause severe disability in reading (Fig. 3.20). It can also cause extreme sensitivity to light and to glare from oncoming headlights. A patient may have 20/25, 20/30, or even better distance vision but may be unable to read a newspaper. Individuals with excellent distance vision but with occupations

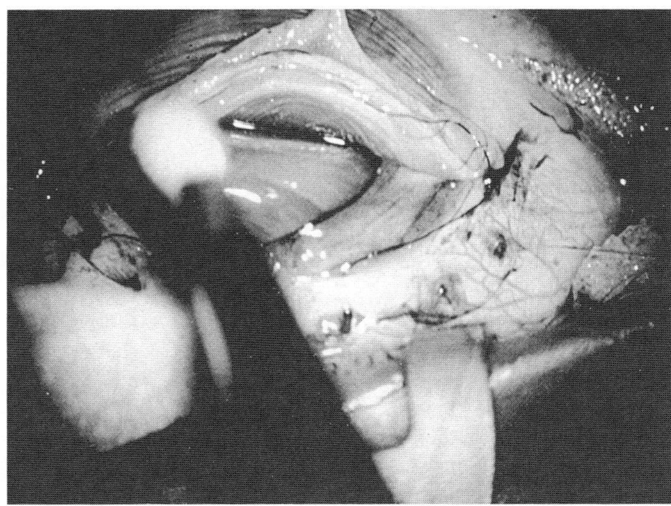

Figure 3.21. Freezing probe removing cataract including the capsule (intracapsular cataract extraction).

requiring good close vision may thus require surgical intervention quite early.

Since a cataract does not harm the eye, indications for its removal are quite variable, requiring knowledge of the patient's capabilities, lifestyle, and desires. Although cataract extraction has a success rate approaching 99%, a detailed discussion of its potential risks and benefits must be undertaken in advance of surgery. Except in rare circumstances, potential for good vision does not decrease by delaying cataract surgery.

Cataract Extraction

Technique. Before the late 1970s most cataract extractions were done by removing the entire lens, usually by cryosurgery. A probe reaching approximately −20°C was attached to the lens capsule, allowing a complete removal of the lens and its capsule as a unit (intracapsular cataract extraction, Fig. 3.21). This tech-

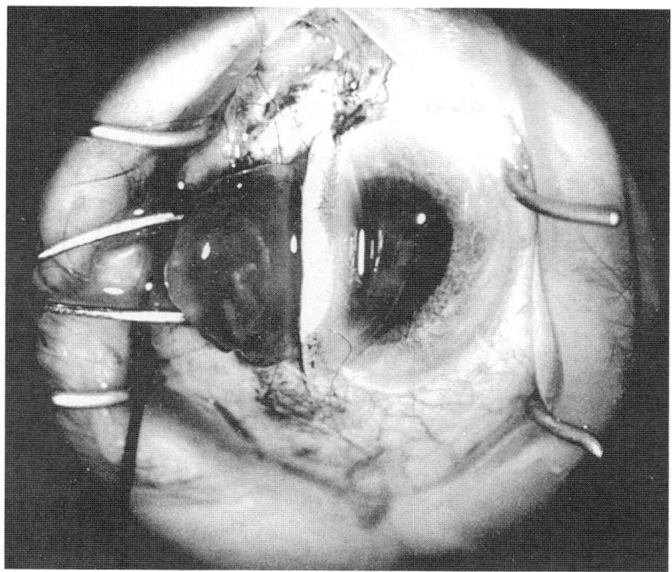

Figure 3.22. Nucleus removed by extracapsular cataract extraction by a lens loop.

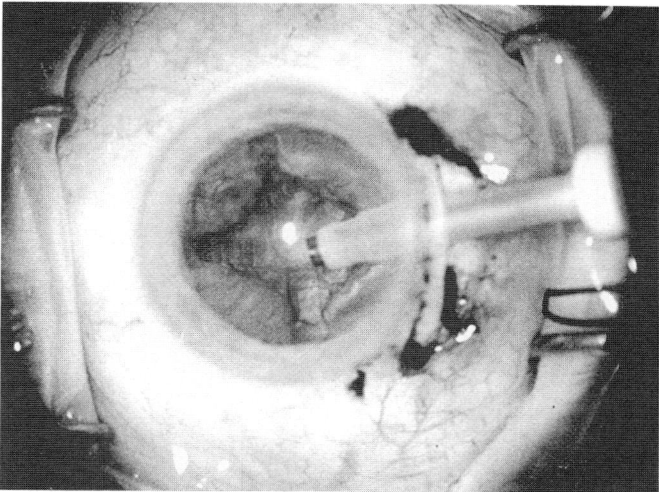

Figure 3.23. Phacoemulsification of the nucleus of a cataract.

nique had several drawbacks. It required a large incision that resulted in a slow healing process. Also, the removal of the lens capsule structure and possible rupture of the anterior vitreous face led to a relatively high incidence of postoperative problems, such as retinal detachment and cystoid macular edema. In the late 1960s the invention of the phacoemulsification technique by Charles Kelman, M.D., renewed interest in extracapsular cataract extraction. This technique, in which a cataract is emulsified and aspirated with a low-frequency ultrasonic needle, leaves the posterior capsule intact for support. This support, good for the integrity of the eye itself, becomes support for an implanted posterior chamber intraocular lens.

The two techniques for extracapsular cataract extraction are manual extraction and phacoemulsification. In the manual technique the nucleus of the lens is removed whole. After conjunctiva and Tenon's capsule are dissected away from the surgical limbus, a 10.5–11 mm incision is made at the surgical limbus. The anterior capsule is opened (capsulotomy), and a central disk of this capsule is removed. The nucleus is freed from its cortical attachments, usually by hydrodissection or by movement of the nucleus with an intraocular instrument. The nucleus is then moved into the anterior chamber and removed by means of a lens loop (Fig. 3.22). Cortical material remaining within the capsule is removed by a unit with an irrigation and aspiration port. In most cases, an IOL is implanted between the posterior and remaining peripheral anterior capsule, and the corneal wound is closed with 9-0, 10-0, or 11-0 suture material (usually nylon, although Mersilene is also being used).

In the phacoemulsification technique, ultrasound vibrates a titanium-tipped needle 27,000–54,000 cycles/sec to emulsify the nucleus, which is then aspirated through the tip of the needle (Fig. 3.23). The advantage of this technique is that it can be performed through a 2.7–3.2 mm incision. The incision is then enlarged to accommodate an intraocular lens—anywhere from 3.5 mm for a foldable silicone or hydrogel lens to 7.0 mm for a large optic lens. The smaller incision improves the patient's recovery time and minimizes postoperative astigmatic changes occurring with larger incisions. There are also disadvantages to this technique. Because it requires skills different than those for the manual technique, it can be difficult to learn, especially if there is no experienced surgeon available for instruction and assistance. Also, this technique requires expensive equipment (up to $60,000 per instrument), tying one to the instrumentation much more than does the manual technique. Nevertheless, there has been a distinct trend toward this procedure: while in 1984 only 15% of cataract surgeons used phacoemulsification, today nearly 50% use it.

Complications. There are several serious complications of cataract surgery. First, a choroidal hemorrhage may occur during the surgery. This complication occurs in approximately 1 of every 10,000 procedures, usually in elderly patients with arteriolar sclerosis. Choroidal hemorrhages usually lead to severe if not total loss of vision. The risk of choroidal hemorrhage approaches zero with the technique of phacoemulsification.

Endophthalmitis is also an unusual but devastating event, often occurring 3 days to 2 weeks after surgery. Classically, a patient presents with severe ocular pain, eyelid swelling, and white blood cells layering in the anterior chamber (hypopyon). The patient's outcome depends on the microbe involved and how quickly the condition is managed. Commonly seen microbes are *Staphylococcus aureus*, *Streptococcus epidermides*, and *Propionibacterium acnes* in late onset endophthalmitis. Management must include early diagnosis and treatment with appropriate antibiotics. A culture and Gram's stain from around the eye is taken, as well as an anterior chamber aspirate and often a vitreous aspirate. Intraoc-

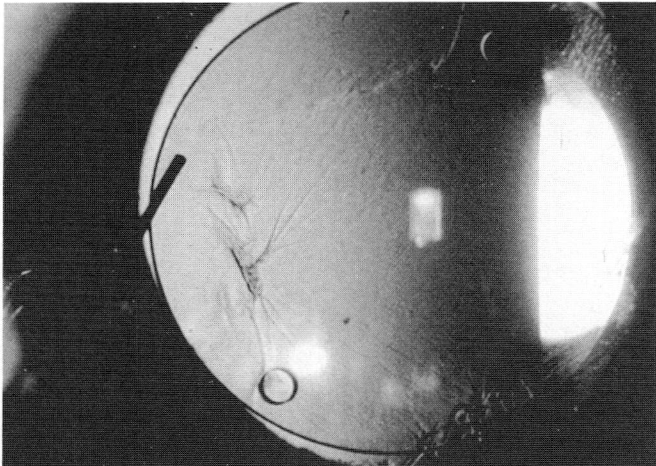

Figure 3.24. Intraocular lens.

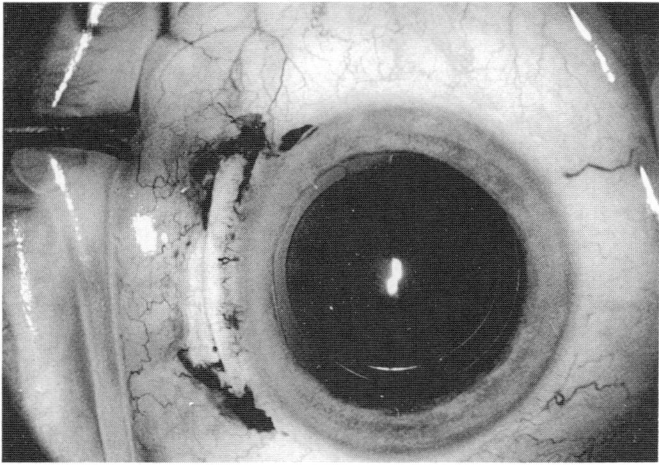

Figure 3.25. Well-positioned posterior chamber ("in-the-bag") intraocular lens.

ular broad-spectrum antibiotics are injected while awaiting culture results. A retinal detachment may also occur after cataract extraction. While the incidence of retinal detachment is approximately 5% in patients who have undergone intracapsular cataract extraction, the incidence in uncomplicated extracapsular cataract surgery now approaches the spontaneous rate for that age group, which is below 1%.

Any surgical procedure causes release of prostaglandins into the eye, which may lead to swelling at the foveal region in the posterior segment. Studies have shown that this swelling, known as cystoid macular edema (CME), occurs temporarily in nearly all patients who have undergone cataract extraction. Once the blood-aqueous barrier has been stabilized, the macular edema clears spontaneously. In 0.1–1% of patients, however, this edema may be a persistent and annoying problem, since it causes distortion of central vision. Treatment of CME may include posterior injection of steroids or systemic treatment with nonsteroidal anti-inflammatory agents.

Optical Correction after Surgery

Removal of the lens requires an optical correction with either glasses, contact lenses, or an intraocular lens implantation. Glasses can provide good optical correction but only at large magnification compared to contact lenses: 25% rather than 7%. The brain is unable to fuse images seen by one eye as 25% disparate in size from those seen by the other eye, and barely able to fuse images seen with a 7% disparity. Peripheral vision is better with contact lenses, but some patients have problems inserting and removing them. An IOL implantation resolves problems of both glasses and contact lenses (Fig. 3.24). Improvements in IOL design and quality control since Harold Ridley launched the era of IOL implantation in 1947 in England have made IOLs the standard of care. There are two major types. Anterior chamber lenses are placed on top of the iris with footplates (called haptics) resting in the anterior chamber angle. Posterior chamber lenses, on the other hand, are placed within the remaining capsule, thus isolating the lens from the very sensitive tissues in the eye. The posterior (or "in-the-bag") implantation is preferred (Fig. 3.25). After a few weeks the lens becomes quite stable in the capsule and dislocations are rare. However, because the capsule still contains live epithelial cells, 10–25% of patients may experience a clouding of the posterior lens capsule following cataract surgery. This clouding, termed a secondary cataract because its symptoms resemble those of the primary cataract, can be treated with a YAG laser, which opens the capsule causing the immediate return of vision. In pediatric patients, where the eye has not attained adult structure, contact lenses remain the treatment of choice.

Diseases of the Retina and the Vitreous

Retinal Breaks and Detachment

Full-thickness retinal defects are known as retinal breaks. These may be small, atrophic holes or tears due to vitreoretinal traction. Most retinal tears occur following a spontaneous or traumatic posterior vitreous detachment (PVD), in which the posterior attachments of the vitreous separate from the retina and the vitreous body collapses anteriorly. The vitreous remains firmly attached over the vitreous base (a circumferential zone straddling the ora serrata peripherally). Other areas of relatively firm vitreoretinal adhesions include: retinal scars, areas of vitreoretinal degeneration (i.e., lattice degeneration), and major retinal blood vessels. The vitreoretinal traction induced by a PVD may cause tearing of the retina along any of these regions.

Most PVDs are spontaneous; their prevalence increases with age (affecting 63% of persons over age 70) and following cataract surgery. A PVD may also be induced following blunt or penetrating eye trauma. The symptoms of a PVD and possible retinal tear are those

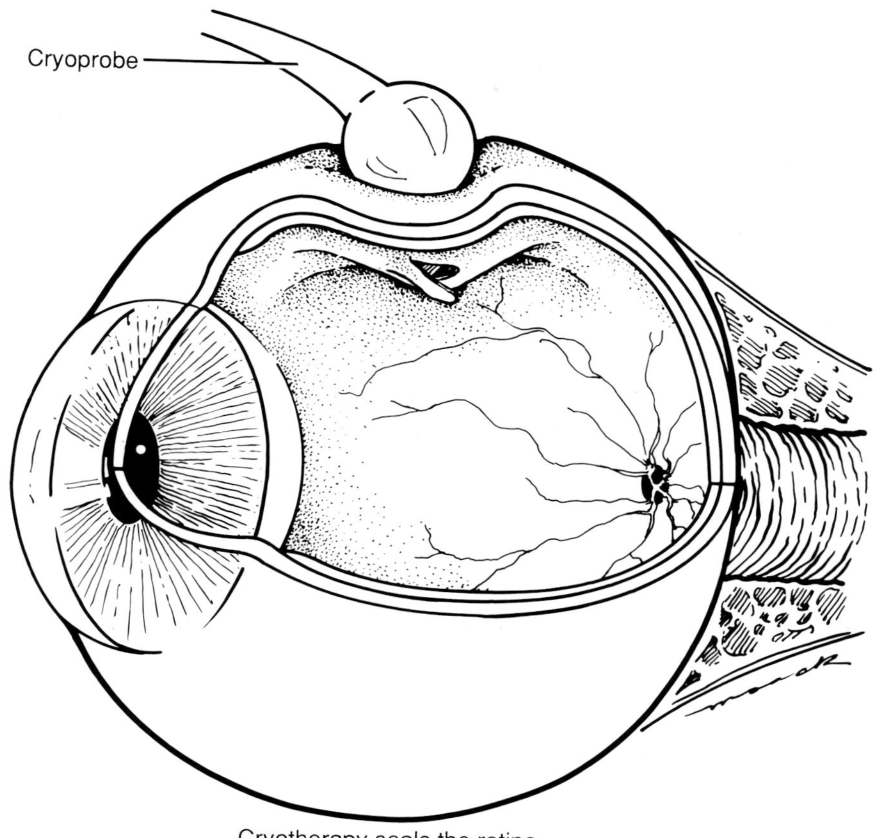

Figure 3.26. Cryotherapy treatment. Cryotherapy seals the retina.

of floating spots and/or flashing lights in the field of vision of one eye. The floaters are the result of shadows cast upon the retina by vitreous opacities such as condensed collagen fibers, glial tissue from the previous attachment of the posterior vitreous to the optic nerve (Vogt's ring), or hemorrhage. Flashing lights are caused by physical stimulation of the retina by vitreous traction. Any patient who presents with a new onset of flashing lights and floaters should have an immediate full dilated funduscopic examination to look for evidence of any retinal tears or detachment. Of all patients who present with a new onset PVD, approximately 10% will be found to have a retinal tear. The presence of vitreous hemorrhage is an ominous sign: as many as 70% of these patients will be found to have a retinal tear, whereas less than 4% of patients without vitreous hemorrhage are found to have a tear.

Retinal Breaks. Retinal breaks can be either asymptomatic or acute. Asymptomatic retinal holes are seen in approximately 6% of the population. Of this group, only 1 person in 10,000 each year develops retinal detachment. Acute symptomatic retinal tears (especially those associated with persistent vitreoretinal traction), however, are dangerous and carry a much higher risk of retinal detachment. Patients who have had previous cataract surgery, are highly myopic, have a family history of retinal detachment, or have had a retinal detachment in their other eye are particularly at risk. Prophylactic treatment of these retinal breaks is thus indicated.

The goal in prophylactic treatment of a retinal break is to prevent a retinal detachment by creating a firm chorioretinal scar that keeps liquid vitreous from leaking through the break into the subretinal space. The two most common methods of achieving this scarring are cryotherapy and laser photocoagulation. Both methods are effective; the decision on which method to use is dictated by the location of the tear, the presence of any subretinal fluid, and the surgeon's personal preference. In both methods, the goal is to surround the break with confluent treatment so as to prevent subretinal fluid accumulation and retinal detachment. Cryotherapy is normally performed transconjunctivally, allowing the freeze to penetrate the sclera, choroid, and retina. Visualization is performed using the indirect ophthalmoscope. The "iceball" effect is then allowed to thaw, the cryoprobe is moved slightly, and the process repeated until the break is completely surrounded (Fig. 3.26). Laser photocoagulation treatment is normally performed in conjunction with a fundus contact lens and either a slitlamp or indirect ophthalmoscopic delivery system. Multiple 300–500 micron spots are placed until there are 2–3 rows of confluent surrounding treatment (Fig. 3.27). All patients are reexamined within 1 week to assess the adequacy of the treatment. (Laser

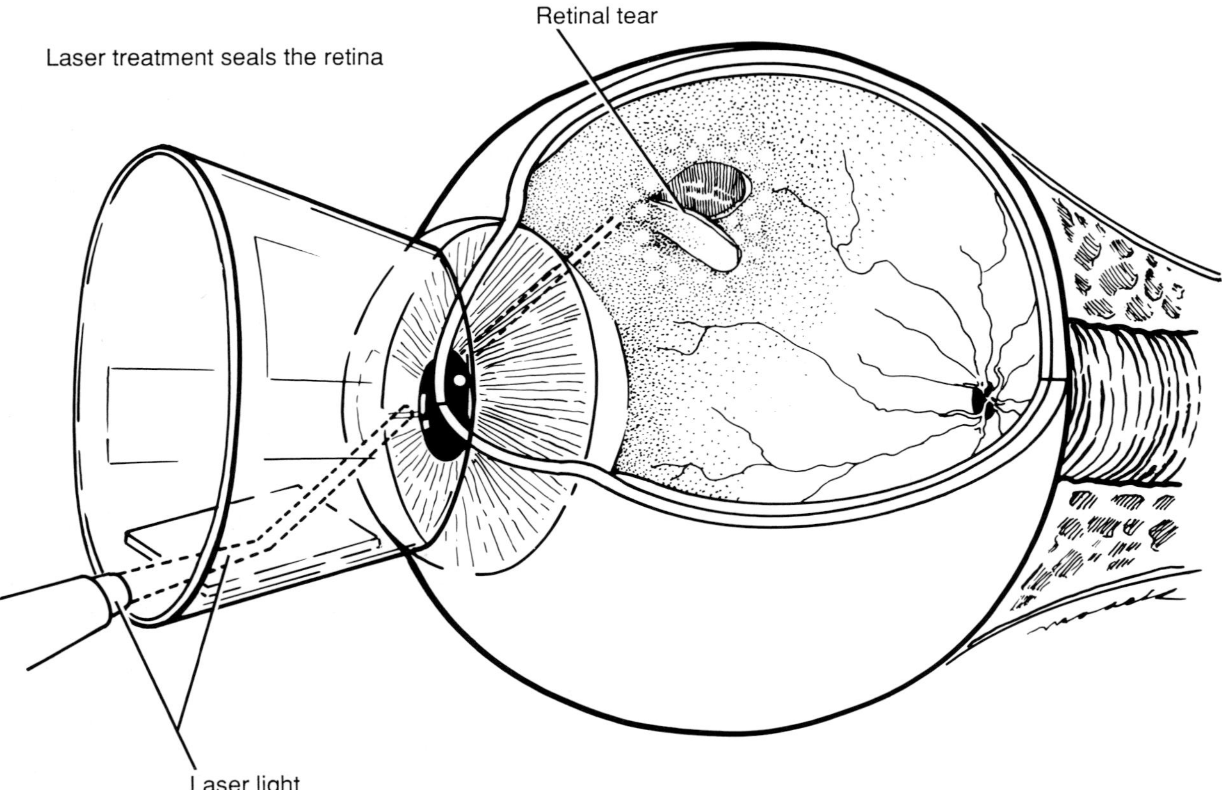

Figure 3.27. Laser treatment.

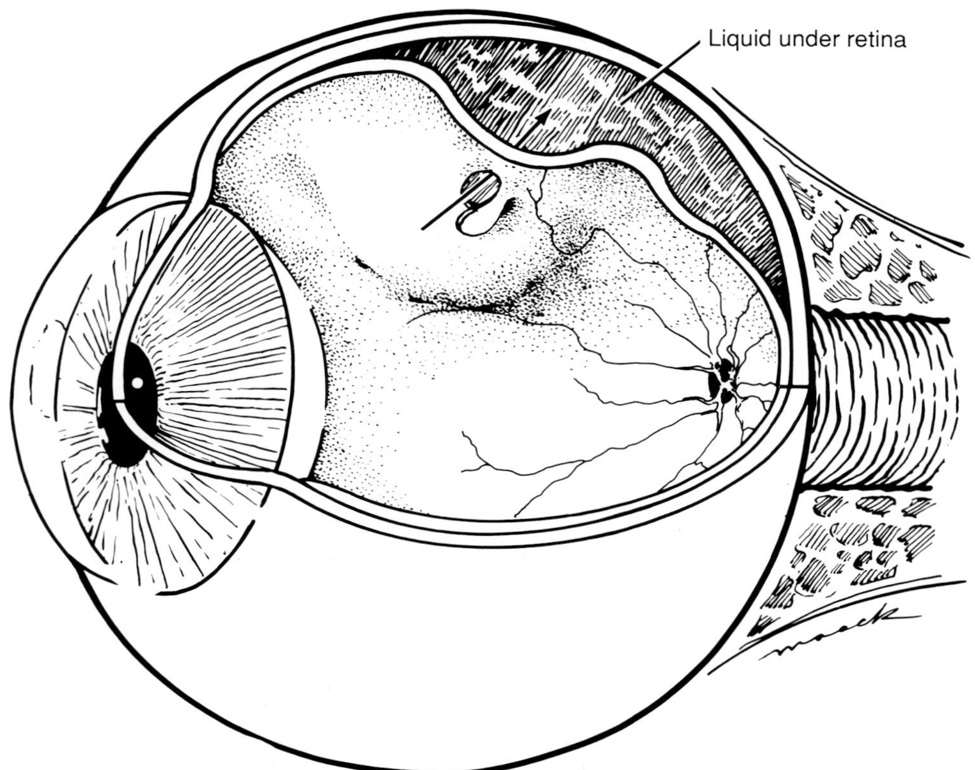

Figure 3.28. Large retinal detachment.

photocoagulation treatment is discussed in greater detail at the end of this chapter.)

Retinal Detachment. Retinal detachments are most commonly the result of a retinal break, that is, they are rhegmatogenous (from the Greek rhegma, to break). They may also be tractional, as in severe proliferative diabetic retinopathy, or exudative, as in some intraocular tumors or cases of severe uveitis. This section will discuss the surgical management of rhegmatogenous retinal detachments.

When subretinal fluid accumulates from an open retinal break, a retinal detachment exists (Fig. 3.28). Patients often present with the same symptoms as in PVD (floaters and flashing lights), but may also have a "dark curtain" obscuring a part or all of their vision. Upon examination the detached retina is typically found to have a corrugated appearance and often undulates with eye movement. To manage retinal detachment a thorough preoperative examination to locate all retinal breaks is imperative. Regardless of which surgical technique is used, the principles of retinal detachment surgery are: (*a*) locate all retinal breaks, and (*b*) close all retinal breaks. Following these principles, 90–95% of all retinal detachments can be anatomically reattached. The major reasons for failure are the physician's not locating and closing all retinal breaks (early failure) or the patient's developing proliferative vitreoretinopathy (PVR). PVR is a fibrocellular response that causes membrane formation, contracture, and the reopening of retinal breaks or tractional retinal detachment.

The success of restoring good vision in retinal detachment repair depends on whether and for how long the macula was detached before surgery. If the retina is reattached before macular detachment, then the probability of the patient's retaining good central vision is excellent. If the macula has been detached for more than one week, only half of affected patients will regain better than 20/70 vision.

The most widely accepted technique for retinal detachment repair is the scleral buckle procedure. Surgery is usually performed under a general anesthetic but may also be performed with local retrobulbar anesthesia. After retinal breaks are located, they are treated with cryotherapy as previously described. The breaks are then closed by suturing either a solid silicone or a silicone sponge to the sclera of the eye overlying the retinal breaks (Fig. 3.29). A buckling effect is created, which serves both to reoppose the break against the retinal pigment epithelium and to negate persistent vitreous traction. Once the breaks are closed, the subretinal fluid is reabsorbed spontaneously, usually within 24 hours. Occasionally, the retinal breaks cannot be closed with the buckle alone. In such cases the subretinal fluid is drained into the subretinal space by means of a small sclerotomy and micropuncture, allowing the retina to settle against the buckle and the breaks to close. The conjunctiva is then carefully closed over the sclera and buckling elements. The patient is normally hospitalized 1–3 days and is kept at minimal physical activity for at least 1 week.

The complications from scleral buckling surgery include subretinal or vitreous hemorrhage, intraocular infection, strabismus with associated double vision, glaucoma, cataract formation, and retinal re-detachment. The silicone buckling elements are left permanently in place unless signs of infection or extrusion occur.

Alternative techniques for retinal detachment repair include: a temporary scleral buckle and pneumatic retinopexy. In a temporary scleral buckle, an inflatable balloon is placed subconjunctivally over the retinal break, which is then treated as previously mentioned with either laser photocoagulation or retinal cryopexy. The balloon is deflated and removed once an adequate chorioretinal scar has formed (usually 1 week). This technique is particularly useful in small anteriorly located tears with little vitreous traction. In pneumatic retinopexy sterile filtered air or expansile gas (C_3F_8, SF_6) is injected into the vitreous through the pars plana. The patient is then positioned so that the bubble either creates an internal tamponade of the open break or breaks, allowing spontaneous resorption of the subretinal fluid. The breaks are treated with either cryotherapy or laser photocoagulation. The overall success of the pneumatic retinopexy is somewhat less than that of scleral buckling surgery. However, because pneumatic retinopexy can be performed on an outpatient basis, thus avoiding the need for hospitalization and general anesthesia, it is an increasingly popular technique. The major complications include recurrent retinal detachment, cataract, glaucoma, and intraocular infection.

Vitreous Surgery

As indicated, most retinal breaks and resultant retinal detachments are the result of a posterior vitreous detachment. Indeed, most severe retinal problems requiring surgery are directly related to the vitreous. This section will discuss the principles behind vitreous surgery, the indications for it, and some of the specialized techniques involved.

Principles of Vitreous Surgery. Vitreous surgery is performed in the hospital using the operating microscope, with the patient usually under general anesthesia. A multiport system is used with the entry sclerotomies to the vitreous cavity performed through the pars plana (3–4 mm posterior to the corneal limbus). One port is used to provide a constant infusion of a balanced salt solution to maintain normal intraocular pressure. The other two ports are "working" ports through which various instruments are passed: a fiberoptic light, vitreous cutter, intraocular forceps, microscissors, or endolaser photocoagulation probes (Fig. 3.30).

The goals in vitreous surgery depend upon specific indications, but include:

1. Removing opaque vitreous (for example, vitreous hemorrhage).
2. Releasing vitreoretinal traction.
3. Releasing or removing epiretinal membranes.
4. Closing retinal breaks.
5. Treating ischemic retina (i.e., endolaser photocoagulation).

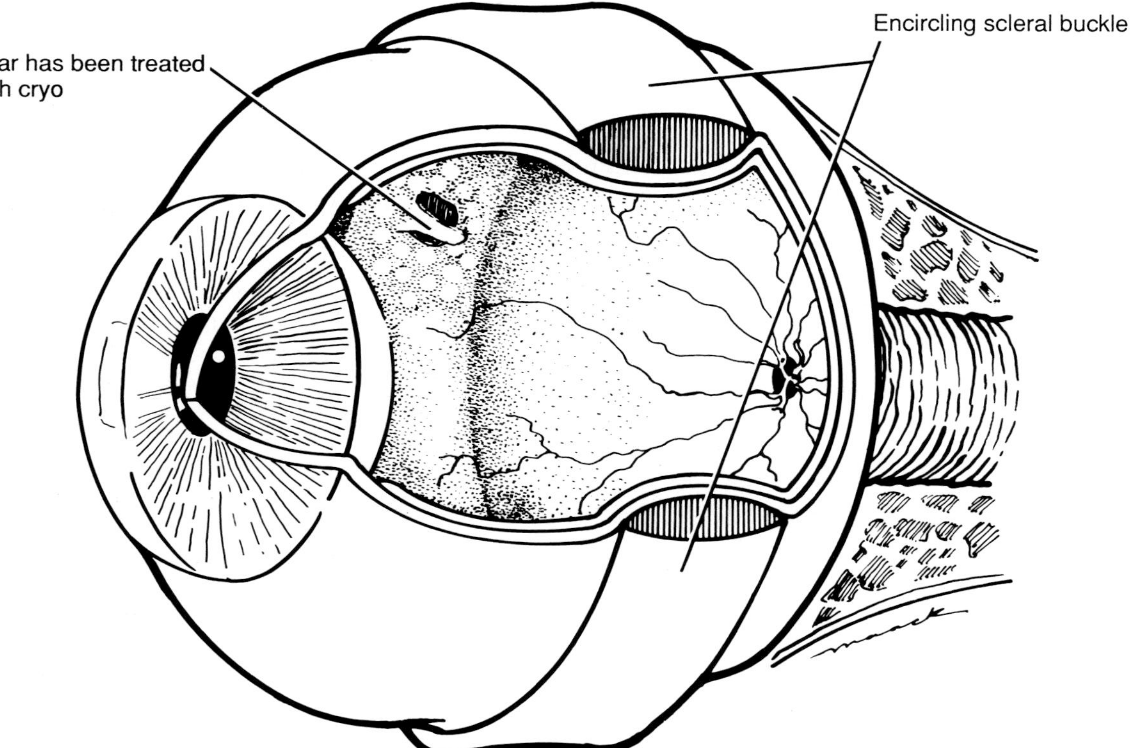

Figure 3.29. Scleral buckling surgery for retinal detachment.

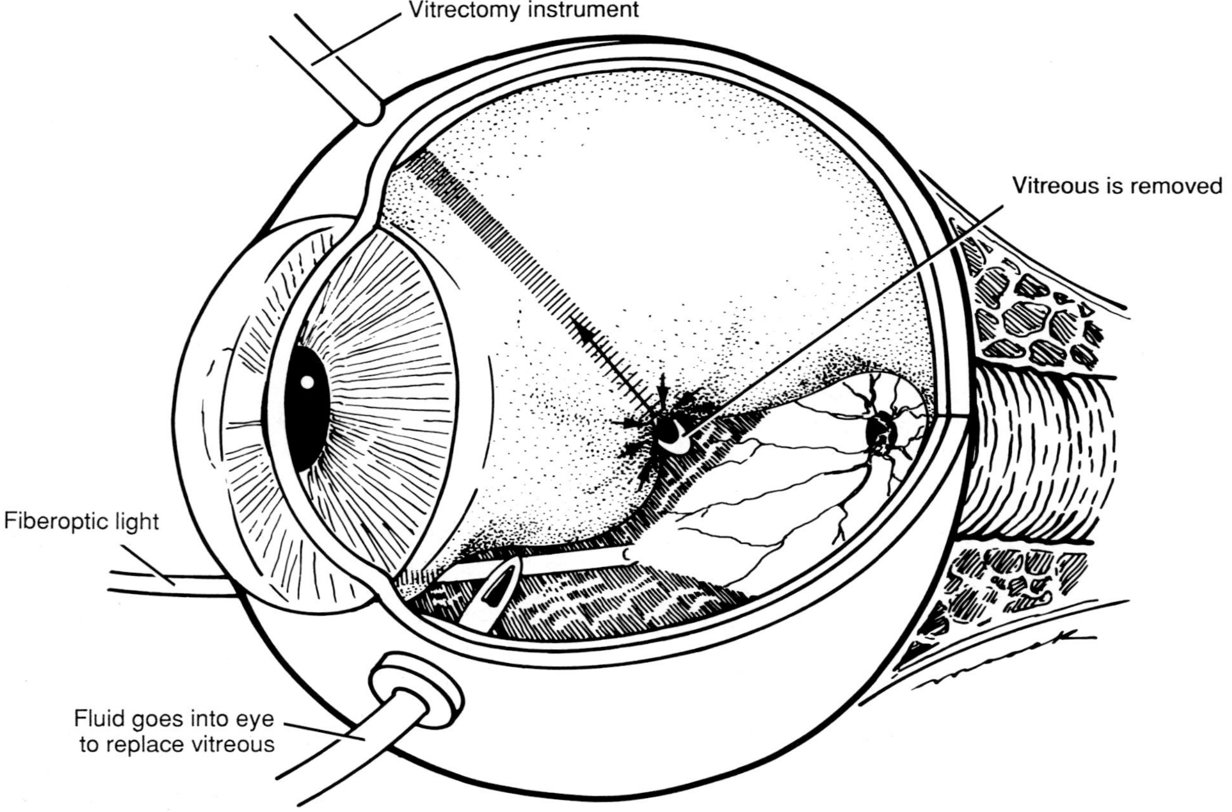

Figure 3.30. Vitrectomy.

6. Obtaining material for culture or cytologic examination.

Indications

Complex Retinal Detachments. As mentioned, some retinal detachments cannot be repaired by scleral buckling techniques alone. These include eyes with advanced proliferative vitreoretinopathy, retinal detachments with opaque media (such as vitreous hemorrhage), or eyes with large, complicated, retinal tears. Vitreous surgery in these eyes allows for improved visualization, release and/or removal of tractional membranes, and replacement of the vitreous with long-acting gas for prolonged internal tamponade. Even with these advanced techniques, however, the prognosis is poor.

Proliferative Diabetic Retinopathy. Vitreous surgery in proliferative diabetic retinopathy (PDR) produces visual improvement in approximately 75% of eyes with vitreous hemorrhage alone and approximately 60% of eyes with retinal detachments involving the macula. Patients with diabetes mellitus who have developed proliferative retinopathy are at risk for vitreous hemorrhage. In the absence of associated retinal detachment, it is usually recommended that vitreous surgery be deferred for several months to allow for possible spontaneous clearing. Approximately 25% of vitreous hemorrhages, however, fail to clear and vitrectomy surgery is indicated for visual rehabilitation. Of patients so treated, 75% will have visual improvement. In other diabetic patients, continued fibrovascular proliferation and contracture may result in either tractional or combined traction/rhegmatogenous retinal detachment requiring vitreous surgery. Of patients with retinal detachments involving the macula who are treated with surgery, 60% have visual improvement.

Trauma and Intraocular Foreign Bodies. The initial approach to any eye suspected of having a possible rupture, penetration, laceration, or retained intraocular foreign body (IOFB) is to protect the integrity of the globe by covering it with a protective shield and obtaining immediate ophthalmologic consultation. Any significant trauma to the eye can lead to severe retinal problems, possibly necessitating vitreous surgery. In managing an eye with suspected trauma, the goal is to restore the integrity of the eye by achieving a watertight closure. Further surgery depends upon specific indications, such as intraocular infection (endophthalmitis), ruptured lens with admixture of lens and vitreous, vitreous prolapse through the wound, retinal detachment, and the kind of IOFB. A retained IOFB should be suspected in an eye suffering a projectile injury (such as from an explosion or from hammering metal on metal). The eye should be examined carefully and evaluated radiologically. Most retained IOFBs should be removed as soon as possible once they have been properly localized, especially those toxic to the eye (such as copper and iron). On rare occasion, small inert IOFBs may be left in the eye if they are not a threat to vision.

Penetrating eye injuries frequently develop late complications related to intraocular cellular proliferation, membrane formation, and possible retinal detachment. Vitrectomy surgery is thus indicated to remove the scaffolding upon which these membranes proliferate. The timing of vitreous surgery following penetrating eye trauma is controversial. Some vitreoretinal surgeons advocate early intervention within the first 1–3 days, while others prefer to defer for 7–10 days. The advantages of deferring are (*a*) decreasing the chances of significant intraoperative hemorrhage and (*b*) allowing the vitreous to detach from the retina spontaneously, thus facilitating complete vitreous removal.

Blunt injuries to the globe can also cause a scleral rupture. Signs of a potential rupture include conjunctival chemosis and hemorrhage, a deep anterior chamber, low intraocular pressure, and severe vitreous hemorrhage. Such signs indicate the need for immediate exploration and repair under general anesthesia.

Miscellaneous Indications for Vitreous Surgery. Other less common indications for vitreous surgery are to manage endophthalmitis, to remove epiretinal membranes (macular pucker), to aid in the diagnosis of intraocular malignancies (large cell lymphoma), and to remove other causes of vitreous opacities such as amyloidosis or inflammatory debris from chronic uveitis. Potential complications in vitreous surgery include retinal tears and detachment, hemorrhage, cataract, and glaucoma. Diabetic eyes are particularly susceptible to the development of iris neovascularization (rubeosis iridis), especially when vitreous surgery is combined with lens removal. Iris neovascularization may lead to neovascular glaucoma and possible loss of the eye.

Laser Photocoagulation Surgery

Laser photocoagulation treatment has become widely used over the past 20 years for a variety of ocular diseases. Most laser photocoagulation treatments are performed in an outpatient setting under topical or occasionally local retrobulbar anesthesia. The specific wave length or type of laser used depends on surgeon preference, the specific entity being treated, and availability. In ophthalmology, the argon blue-green, argon green, krypton red, and YAG are the most commonly used lasers. Most treatments are performed using a fundus contact lens with the patient seated comfortably at a slitlamp delivery system. (For further detail on the physical properties of the laser and the pathophysiologic effects of laser photocoagulation treatment, refer to the suggested reading section.)

Laser photocoagulation is used to (*a*) treat retinal breaks, (*b*) treat retinal ischemia, (*c*) ablate choroidal or retinal neovascularization, (*d*) create a chorioretinal adhesion or scar, (*e*) stimulate resorption of retinal or subretinal fluid. In the anterior segment of the eye laser photocoagulation surgery is used to treat glaucoma and posterior lens capsule opacification after cataract surgery. In the posterior segment of the eye the most common disease for which laser photocoagulation is used is proliferative diabetic retinopathy, the leading cause of blindness in the developed world. Untreated, many eyes progress to vitreous hemorrhage and fibrovascular proliferation with retinal detachment. Diabetic retinopathy studies show the risk of severe visual loss can be reduced with photocoagulation treatment. The exact means by which this treatment causes regression of PDR is unknown. One theory is that by treating or ablating the ischemic retina, there is a decrease in production of a "vasoproliferative factor" with subsequent regression of neovascularization. A similar response occurs when laser photocoagulation is used in other ophthalmic diseases that produce retinal ischemia and neovascularization, such as branch and central retinal vein occlusion and sickle cell retinopathy.

Laser photocoagulation is also used to treat macular edema in patients with diabetic retinopathy. Macular edema is the most common cause of visual loss in diabetics. Leakage from macular capillary or microaneurysms may result in either focal or diffuse areas of retinal thickening and edema. Lipid exudation may also be present. Studies have shown that by treating the areas of macular edema with either a focal or "grid" pattern it is possible to reduce or eliminate the edema in a majority of cases. The benefits of this treatment are stabilization and often improvement in central vision. This form of treatment has also been found to be beneficial for other retinal vascular disorders that result in macular edema (such as branch retinal vein occlusion).

Another use for laser photocoagulation is in the destruction of choroidal neovascularization, which may develop in a number of ocular disorders, including age-related macular degeneration (ARMD), presumed ocular histoplasmosis syndrome (POHS), or virtually any condition that disrupts the integrity of Bruch's membrane, which separates the retina from the underlying choroid. Macular choroidal neovascularization may cause hemorrhaging in the subretinal, retinal, or vitreous spaces. A fibrous "disciform" scar may form, resulting in permanent loss of central vision. The purpose in laser photocoagulation treatment is to destroy the choroidal neovascularization before it involves the central macula (fovea). Since the laser treatment scar itself produces a permanent scotoma, choroidal neovascularization involving the fovea is not generally treated.

The side effects and potential complications of laser photocoagulation, frequent but rarely severe, include loss of peripheral vision; decrease in night vision and dark adaptation; transient (and sometimes permanent) loss of central visual acuity; retinal holes; subretinal, retinal, or vitreous hemorrhage; recurrence of choroidal neovascularization; and accidental treatment of the fovea. In spite of the potential hazards, however, laser photocoagulation treatment is an invaluable tool in the treatment of many eye diseases. It has clearly lowered the risk of severe visual loss in both diabetic retinopathy and age-related macular degeneration, the two most common causes of blindness in our country.

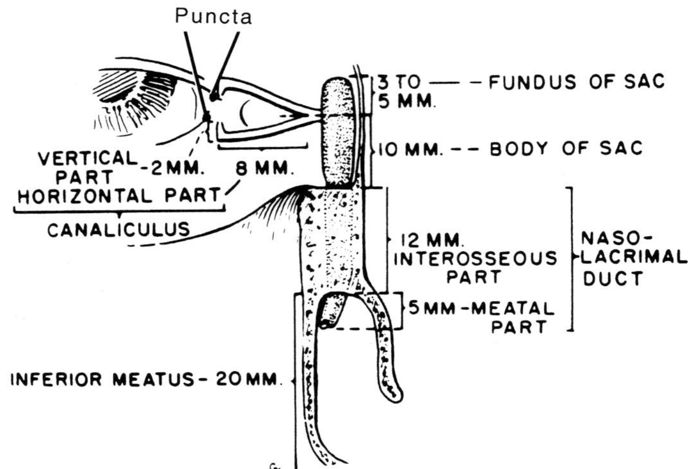

Figure 3.31. Lacrimal excretory system.

Diseases of the Nasolacrimal System, Eyelids, and Orbit

Oculoplastic surgery is the interface between the specialties of ophthalmology and plastic surgery. The oculoplastic surgeon is concerned with those conditions of the periocular bones and soft tissues that directly affect the health and functioning of the eyes: the nasolacrimal system, the eyelids, and the orbit. The oculoplastic surgeon is also concerned with removing the eye should it become necessary.

Nasolacrimal System

The nasolacrimal system is the conduit for drainage of tears from the conjunctival sac to the inferior meatus of the nose (Fig. 3.31). The system is made up of paired upper and lower eyelid puncta and canaliculi that run just below the mucocutaneous junction of the eyelids, beginning approximately 5 mm temporal to the angle of the medial canthus. The system converges into a short common canalicular segment that empties into the nasolacrimal sac. At this point the flow of tears progresses down the nasolacrimal sac into the nasolacrimal duct, which subsequently opens into the inferior meatus. Located along this route are a series of valves that help to maintain unidirectional flow. Additionally, the medial canthal region attachments of the orbicularis muscle are situated so as to create a negative pressure within the lumen of the nasolacrimal sac with each blink. This "pumping" action actively draws tears into the system and thus insures rapid turnover of the tear film.

A block at any point in the nasolacrimal system results in epiphora or the symptomatic complaint of tearing. Of more concern, blockage leads to the creation of a blind pouch in which infection and even abscess formation is frequent. The various forms of blockage are quite variable, but in general are distinguished as being either congenital or acquired obstructions.

Congenital Obstruction. In approximately 40% of normal infants, the opening of the nasolacrimal duct into the inferior meatus is occluded by a vestigial membrane at the time of birth. By 3 months of age this membrane has become patent in approximately 95% of infants. Conservative measures such as massaging the area overlying the nasolacrimal sac are useful in attempting to open the remaining 5%. If after 6 months of age the child is noted still to have epiphora, the nasolacrimal system needs to be probed and the membrane physically opened. With the child placed under either mask or general anesthesia, a small metallic Bowman probe is introduced through either the upper or lower lid puncta. Once inside, the probe is gently passed through the canalicular system into the lumen of the nasolacrimal sac. After contacting the medial wall of the nasolacrimal sac, the probe is rotated inferiorly 90° and passed into the nasolacrimal duct, where it is gently advanced and the membrane ruptured. For the majority of infants this is all that is required. In the event that epiphora or infection recur, however, the procedure may be repeated using a soft silicone stent simultaneously to intubate the full length of the system. The stent is left in position and secured within the nose to remain for approximately 6 weeks. After the stent is removed, the nasolacrimal duct remains patent in the majority of children.

Acquired Obstruction. Acquired lacrimal system obstructions, most frequently seen in adults, usually occur at the level of the nasolacrimal duct. Obstruction can result from trauma, infection, or tumor, but more often is the result of an idiopathic fibrosis related to chronic inflammation. The second most frequent site of obstruction is at the level of the canalicular system. Trauma, topical eye medications, viral infections, and tumors are most commonly responsible for obstructions at this level.

The management of acquired obstructions is almost entirely surgical. The adult drainage system is much more rigid than the child's and does not respond to probing or dilating maneuvers. In fact, these manipulations often result in more scarring and stenosis. The two procedures performed most often have in common the creation of an osteotomy through the lacrimal and maxillary bones. Through this site vertical incisions are made in both the nasolacrimal sac and the nasal mucosa. The mucosal surfaces of each are united, creating a mucosa-lined tract through which tears are conducted. If the nasolacrimal duct was the original site of obstruction, this new tract bypasses the blockade. This procedure, known as a dacryocystorhinostomy, is completed with the passage of a soft silicone stent through the intact canalicular system, which is then brought out through the newly created mucosa-lined osteotomy site. The stent is secured inside the ala of the nose to ensure patency of the newly created tract during the postoperative healing process. The stent is removed after 3–6 months.

With a canalicular obstruction, after creation of a nasal osteotomy the entire canalicular system must be bypassed. This is done by inserting a Jones tube (a hollow glass tube measuring anywhere from 6–25 mm in length and 3–4 mm in diameter) through an incision in the caruncle and the underlying soft tissues into the osteotomy site. The conjunctival portion of the tube is fluted in order to facilitate the entry of tears into the lumen and to help position it properly deep within the medial canthus. The Jones tube then remains in place, to be removed only for a yearly cleaning.

The Eyelids

Protection of the cornea and anterior segment of the eye depends on the correct position and functioning of the eyelids. Malposition of the eyelids can lead to a multitude of problems with the ocular surface, all of which can quickly lead to decreased vision or blindness. The importance of proper lid function cannot be overstressed.

In the hospitalized patient, the most common eyelid malposition is lagophthalmos, an inability to close the eyelids completely resulting in corneal exposure. Causes of lagophthalmos include eyelid retraction, proptosis, and seventh nerve palsies. However, it is most frequently encountered in an intensive care setting where typically the patient is comatose or obtunded. The resultant decrease in orbicularis tone allows the eyelids to open partially and the cornea to be exposed. Topical ointment applied to the ocular surface at intervals varying from once a day to as often as every hour is the mainstay of therapy. Should this prove insufficient, it may be necessary to perform a tarsorrhaphy, which is the surgical creation of permanent or temporary adhesions between the upper and lower eyelids. The entire lid margin or only a portion of it may be apposed. If there is full neurologic recovery, the entire tarsorrhaphy may be taken down. On the other hand, in the presence of a residual neurologic deficit such as Bell's palsy, a partial tarsorrhaphy may be left permanently to ensure adequate protection of the cornea.

Ptosis is the condition in which the upper eyelid margin droops, resulting in a narrowing of the palpebral fissure. It may be congenital or acquired and may be either unilateral or bilateral: congenital ptosis is most frequently the result of a poorly developed or nonfunctional levator muscle, while acquired ptosis results typically from a disinsertion of the levator aponeurosis from its attachment to the rigid tarsus, the major supporting structure of the lid (Fig. 3.32). Acquired ptosis occurs most frequently with aging but can occur following intraocular surgery, trauma, or protracted inflammatory conditions. Several other conditions can lead to acquired ptosis and must be considered when evaluating a patient: myasthenia gravis, myotonic dystrophy, and third nerve palsies. The fact that each of these conditions may be life threatening underscores the importance of recognizing ptosis during a general physical exam.

Surgical correction of ptosis largely depends on the amount of levator muscle function present. In most

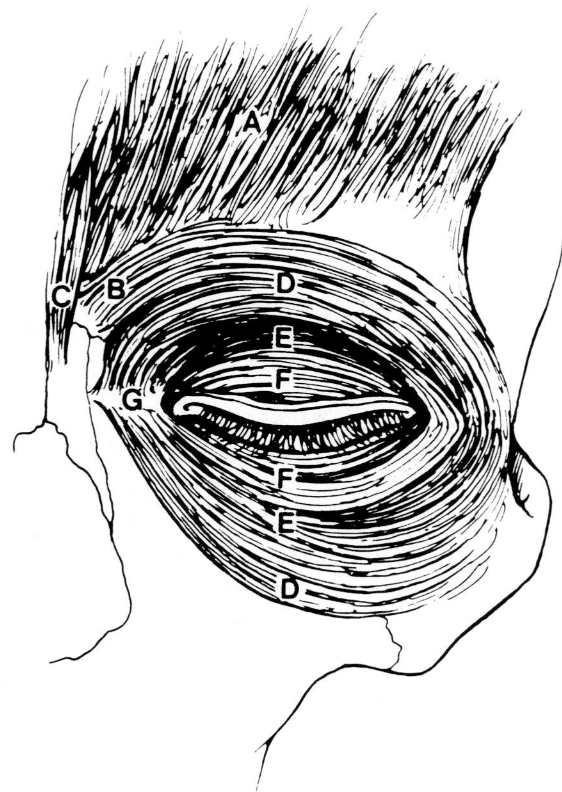

Figure 3.32. Musculature of the brow and eyelids. **A**, Frontalis muscle. **B**, Corrugator superciliaris muscle. **C**, Procerus muscle. **D**, Orbital orbicularis muscle. **E**, Preseptal orbicularis muscle. **F**, Pretarsal orbicularis muscle. **G**, Medial canthal tendon.

cases the preferred approach is to make a skin incision along the lid crease of the eyelid through which the levator aponeurosis is isolated. The aponeurosis is first resected an appropriate amount to correct the ptosis and then reattached to the tarsus. If levator function is very poor, the upper eyelid is connected to the overlying frontalis muscle by a sling made of alloplastic material or fascia lata harvested from the thigh.

Ectropion and entropion are terms that relate to a turning outward or inward, respectively, of the eyelid margin. Each condition is related to an imbalance of forces between the outer surface of the eyelid (made up of the skin and orbicularis muscle) and the inner surface (made up of the eyelid retractors and the conjunctival surface). Age-related involutional changes and cicatrizing inflammatory conditions are the most frequent causes of these conditions, which can produce serious corneal exposure or marked corneal irritation from inward turning eyelashes. These malpositions are corrected surgically by tightening the lax structures and lysing adhesions. Frequently, skin grafts or mucous membrane spacer grafts are required.

Eyelid tumors may be responsible for the development of almost any form of eyelid malposition. The most frequent tumors of the eyelids derive from skin. In order of relative frequency, these include basal cell carcinomas, squamous cell carcinomas, sebaceous gland carcinomas, and malignant melanomas. While basal cell carcinoma is capable only of local spread, the other three have metastatic potential. Surgical management of these lesions requires resection of the tumor under frozen section monitoring to insure complete excision. Frequently, the major portion of the eyelid must be removed, followed by immediate eyelid reconstruction to insure the safety of the eye. This process is complex and requires the combined use of myocutaneous tissue flaps, composite tissue grafts, and other plastic surgical techniques.

Orbital Disease

Because the orbit is one of the most complex areas of the body, the pathologic processes involving the orbit are numerous and varied. The most common physical findings produced by orbital disease are proptosis and weakness of a particular cranial nerve or extraocular muscle. As in many areas in oculoplastics, the causes of orbital disease can be differentiated between those found in children and those found in adults.

The most common cause of proptosis in children is periocular infection, usually in the form of preseptal cellulitis or orbital cellulitis. It is important to differentiate between these two as true orbital cellulitis is a medical emergency. Preseptal cellulitis is distinguished by the presence of eyelid swelling and erythema in the presence of a white and quiet eye with normal vision and ocular motility. The inflammatory process is limited to the periocular soft tissues and does not penetrate posterior to the orbital septum. It is most frequently caused by bacterial infection of an insect bite or a traumatic laceration.

In contrast, orbital cellulitis, in addition to periocular swelling and erythema, is associated with an inflamed ocular surface and the presence of either or both decreased vision and extraocular motility disturbance (Fig. 3.33). In this process the infection is located posterior to the orbital septum and thus can spread to involve the eye, cranial nerves, and orbital vessels. Of graver concern is that the infection can penetrate to the middle cranial fossa through the superior orbital fissure, which can result in meningitis and brain abscess. Most frequently the process is an extension of paranasal sinusitis that extends through the thin lamina papyracea of the medial wall of the orbit. Proper management requires hospitalization for intravenous antibiotics, and, if vision is compromised, immediate surgical decompression and evacuation of the abscess.

Other causes of proptosis in children include orbital pseudotumor, hemangiomas, lymphangiomas, dermoid cysts, neurofibroma, and various tumors including optic nerve glioma, neuroblastoma, and rhabdomyosarcoma. The rapid development of unilateral proptosis in a child in the absence of inflammatory signs should be regarded as indicative of rhabdomyosarcoma until proven otherwise. Such development is an indication for an emergent biopsy to prove or disprove the diagnosis, as the tumor is capable of doubling

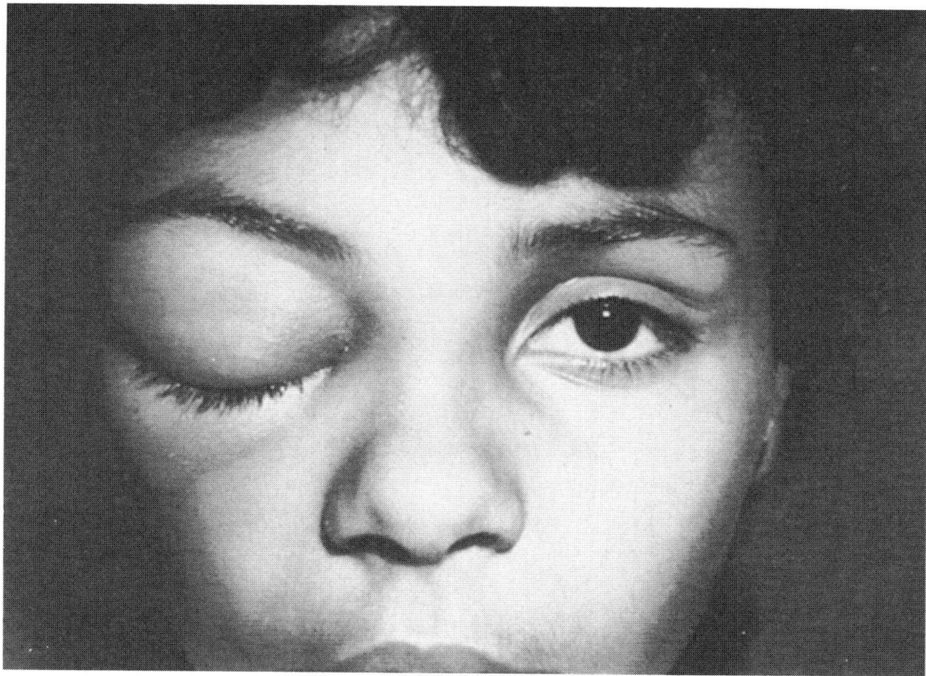

Figure 3.33. Clinical appearance of a patient with orbital cellulitis and subperiorbital abscess.

in size in a 24-hour period. When limited to the orbit, rhabdomyosarcoma is curable with a combination of chemotherapy and radiation therapy in up to 90% of cases.

The most common cause of either unilateral or bilateral proptosis in adults is Graves' ophthalmopathy (Fig. 3.34), followed by orbital pseudotumor, cavernous hemangioma, lymphangioma, and lymphoma (Fig. 3.35). Metastatic carcinoma, sphenoid meningioma, and lacrimal gland tumors are much less common.

While neuroimaging studies such as computed tomography and magnetic resonance imaging have aided immensely in the evaluation of orbital disease, in many cases a correct diagnosis can be reached only with tissue biopsy. Surgical approaches to the orbit are based on the location of the lesion—whether they are intraconal or extraconal (inside or outside the space bounded by the extraocular muscle cone). Intraconal lesions most frequently are approached by way of either a transcranial superior orbitotomy, which involves the removal of the roof of the orbit, or by way of a lateral orbitotomy, which requires the removal of a portion of the zygomatic bone and the greater wing of the sphenoid. While both approaches provide excellent visualization of the intraconal structures, the lateral approach is preferred as it avoids the morbidity associated with a craniotomy. The orbital apex is the only location within the orbit which needs a superior approach. A third approach for lesions located on the medial side of the optic nerve involves the disinsertion of the medial rectus muscle followed by retraction of the globe laterally in order to visualize the intraconal space. This technique is somewhat limited in terms of exposure and visualization.

Many techniques exist for approaching lesions located outside the muscle cone. For the most part, these lesions can be reached through well-camouflaged incisions placed within the lid crease or directly through the conjunctiva.

Removal of an Eye

The following are indications for removal of an eye.

1. A blind eye that is causing intractable pain and is unresponsive to conservative treatment.
2. An irreparably traumatized eye that is at risk of inciting sympathetic ophthalmia, an autoimmune condition that can result in blindness in the patient's remaining eye.
3. The presence of a untreatable intraocular malignancy.
4. A blind eye that is cosmetically disfiguring and not satisfactorily corrected by a cosmetic scleral prosthesis.
5. Removal of a blind eye for diagnostic purposes if vision in the remaining eye is threatened.

The two procedures used to remove an eye are enucleation and evisceration. Each has its own indications and limitations with which the oculoplastic surgeon must become familiar. Further information concerning the merits of each procedure can be found in the references listed under Suggested Readings.

An enucleation involves the removal of the eye in its entirety. The rectus muscles are transected at their in-

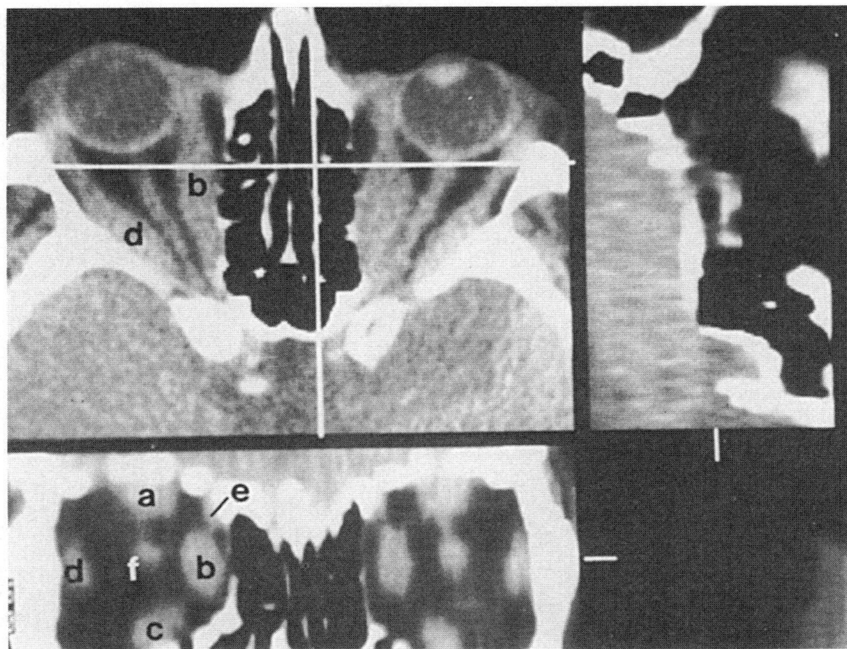

Figure 3.34. Orbital examination by computerized tomography of a patient with thyroid ophthalmopathy showing greatly enlarged extraocular muscles and posterior compression of the optic nerve. The direct scan was made in the axial plane at a midorbital level. Computer reconstructed coronal (*below*) and sagittal (*right*) sections provide multiplanar views of orbital structures. (Notations: **a**, superior rectus muscle; **b**, medial rectus muscle; **c**, inferior rectus muscle; **d**, lateral rectus muscle; **e**, superior oblique muscle; **f**, optic nerve.)

sertions and the optic nerve is severed. The space previously occupied by the globe is taken up by an alloplastic implant such as a sphere. The extraocular muscles are attached to the implant, giving it motility that parallels the natural movement of the contralateral eye. The procedure is completed by closing the conjunctiva and related periocular soft tissues over the face of the implant.

Evisceration of an eye involves removing the entire contents of the eye through an incision in the scleral coat, leaving the extraocular muscles and the optic nerve attached to the sclera. An alloplastic implant is inserted into the scleral shell and the wound closed. Frequently, the cornea is excised as well, as it has little inherent strength and is at risk of rupturing and causing extrusion of the implant. Six to eight weeks after undergoing an enucleation or evisceration, the patient is fitted with an ocular prosthesis hand-painted to resemble the remaining normal eye.

Diseases of the Extraocular Muscles

Anatomy

Structure and function are closely related in extraocular muscle activity. The four recti muscles insert on the globe either horizontally or vertically; their primary action is as adductors or abductors (medial and lateral recti, respectively) or as elevators and depressors (superior and inferior recti, respectively) (Fig. 3.36). The orbit is pear shaped with its stem oriented posteriorly and medially. The superior and inferior recti therefore insert onto the globe in a slightly outward angle, affording these recti a secondary function of adduction. The inferior and superior oblique muscles insert obliquely on the globe; their primary action is to extort and intort the eye, respectively (Figs. 3.37 and 3.38).

Because the superior division of the ocular motor nerve enervates the levator and superior rectus muscles, lid elevation is intimately associated with up-gaze. The inferior division enervates the medial rectus, inferior rectus, and inferior oblique muscles. It also carries the parasympathetic fibers responsible for pupillary constriction. The trochlear nerve enervates the superior oblique muscle, and the abducens nerve enervates the lateral rectus muscle. All of the extraocular muscles have a basal level of tone. This is manifest by esotropia caused by an unopposed medial rectus in sixth nerve palsy.

The blood supply to the extraocular muscles also supplies most of the anterior segment of the eye. Two anterior ciliary arteries course through every recti except the lateral rectus, which has only one artery. Operating on more than two recti muscles at a time is not indicated, as doing so could lead to anterior segment ischemia.

Pathology

Strabismus, a misalignment of the eyes, is categorized as follows:

1. Esotropia: an inward turning;
2. Exotropia: an outward turning;

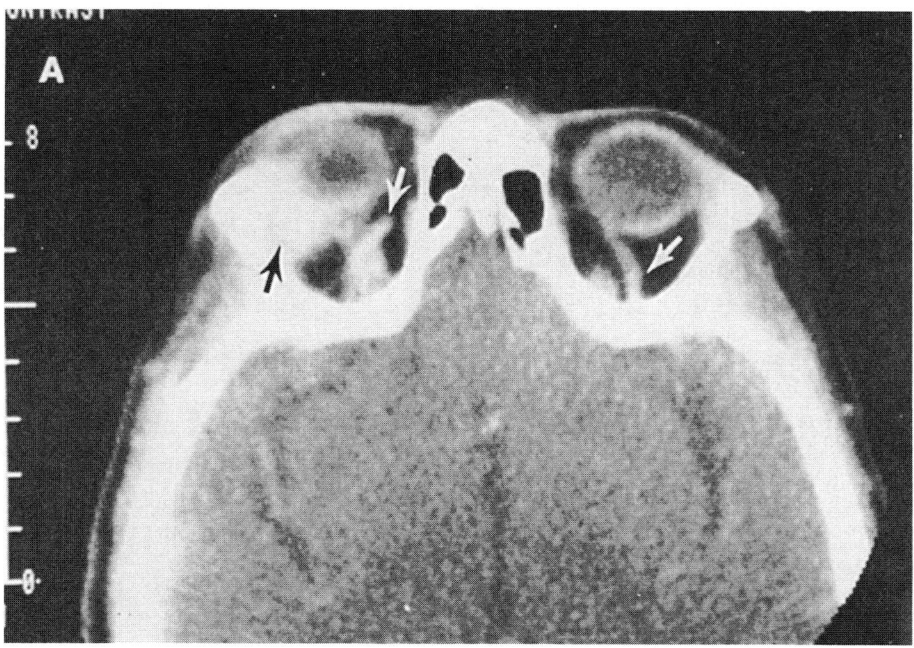

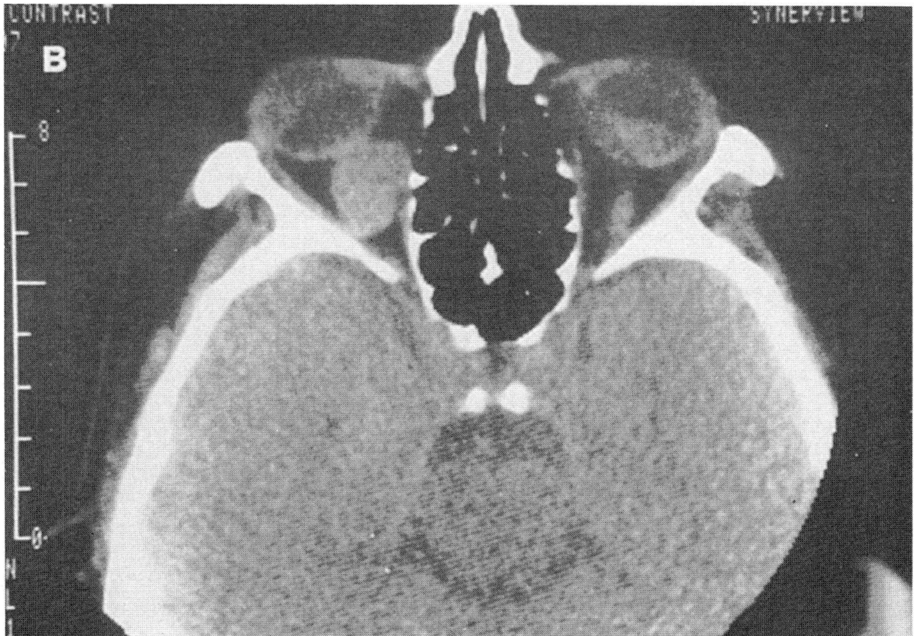

Figure 3.35. **A**, Axial CT scan of a patient with lymphoma in the superolateral portion of the right orbit (**small black arrow**). Note the superior ophthalmic veins crossing the orbit from lateral to medial on both sides (**white arrows**), **B**, CT scan of a patient with a well-circumscribed cavernous hemangioma within the muscle cone of the right orbit.

3. Hypertropia: an upward deviation;
4. Hypotropia: a downward deviation.

Pseudostrabismus refers to changes in the tissues surrounding the eye which simulate strabismus.

Congenital esotropia, usually apparent shortly after a child's birth, is a leading indicator for strabismus surgery. Ideally, surgery is done at 6 months of age; delay in correcting the condition denies the patient the prospect of using both eyes together. If the surgery is delayed past 10 months of age, there is a reduced chance of obtaining some element of single binocular vision. Perceiving one image in the brain from the visual input of two eyes is the most rudimentary form of single binocular vision. Actual depth perception (stereopsis) is a higher order of binocular vision and is rarely

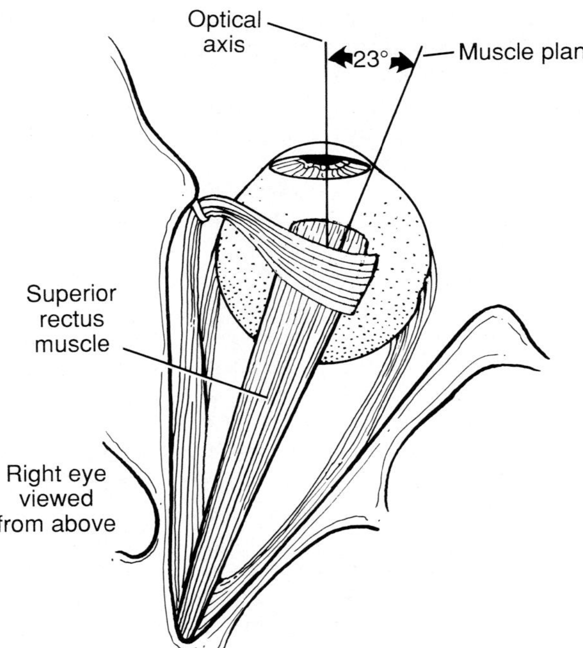

Figure 3.36. Muscle attachments and action.

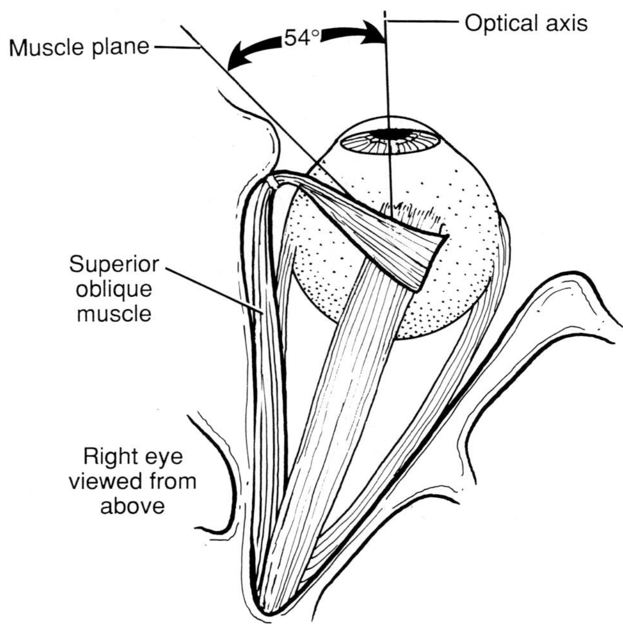

Figure 3.38. Primary action of superior oblique muscle.

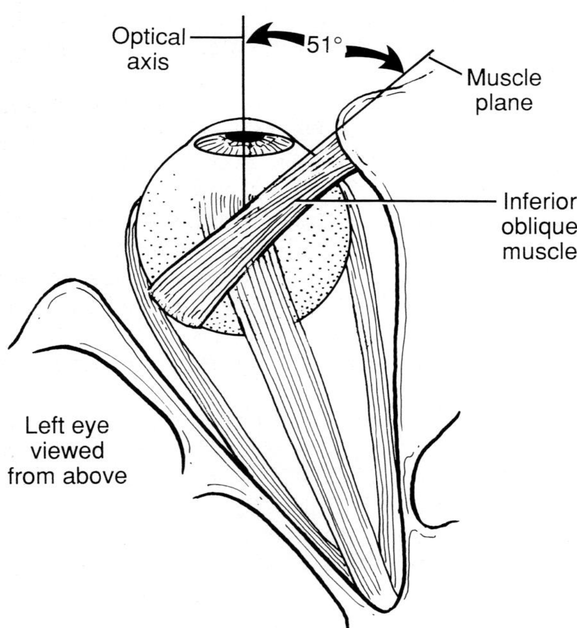

Figure 3.37. Muscle attachment and orbit orientation.

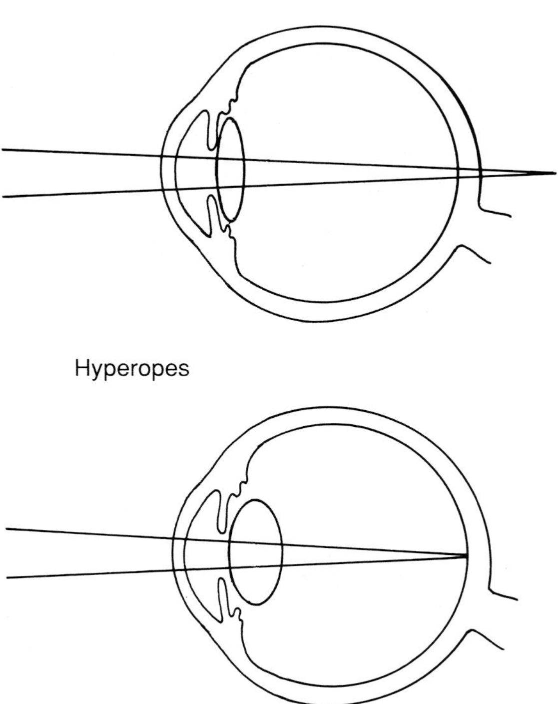

Figure 3.39. Hyperopia: lens requires focusing even at infinity.

attained with surgical correction of the congenital esotropia. It is imperative that the general physician realize that treatment is surgical; the eyes do not have a tendency to realign spontaneously. There are other situations, such as Duane's syndrome and congenital sixth nerve palsy, that may simulate congenital esotropia, but these are beyond the scope of this discussion.

Esotropia can also be caused by excessive convergence. Because children tend to be hyperopic (light focuses behind the eye), the lens of their eye accommodates or changes shape to focus light on the retina (Fig. 3.39). Because accommodation is tied to convergence, hyperopic children need to accommodate for clear distance vision. If this effort passes a critical level, it may lead to esotropia.

Exotropia, the tendency of the eye to deviate outward, increases with age. Often there is exotropia in the

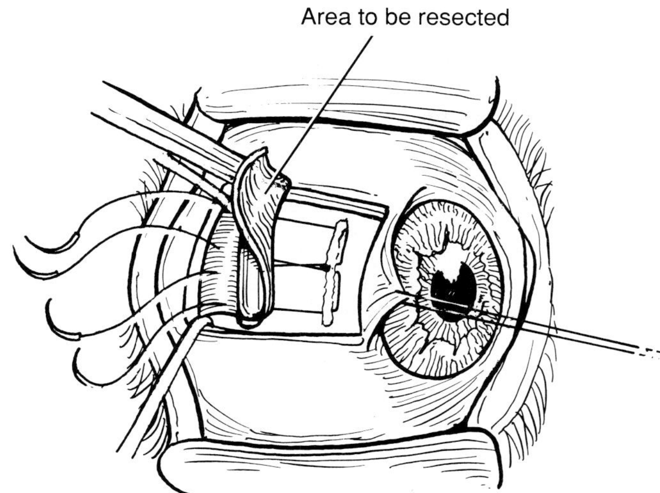

Figure 3.40. Resection of lateral rectus muscle.

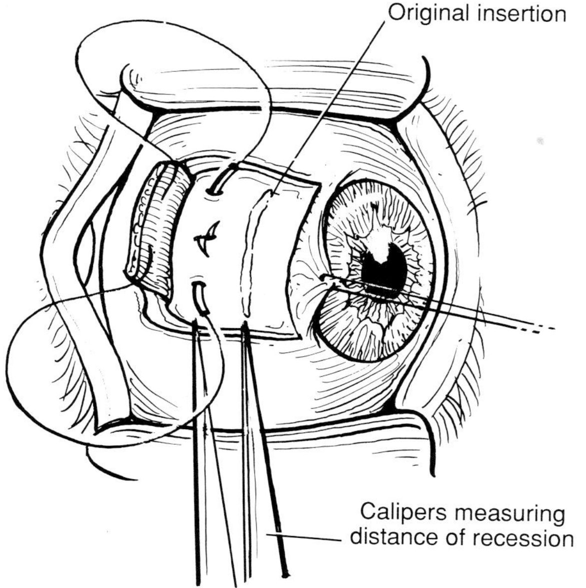

Figure 3.41. Recession of medial rectus muscle.

blind eye of elderly patients whose ability to fuse images previously kept the eyes aligned, preventing diplopia. In the case of one blind eye, obviously there can be no diplopia; therefore, there is no incentive for spontaneous realignment (fusional convergence).

Hypertropic and hypotropic deviations are less commonly encountered as isolated entities, but may often be seen as a part of the congenital esotropic complex.

Surgery

During the preoperative evaluation of the strabismus patient, it is imperative to perform a full ophthalmological examination including a dilated fundus exam. Objective measurement of ametropia (myopia or hyperopia) and degree of eye turn is always indicated to rule out the possibility of an accommodative component to strabismus. If amblyopia is present, occlusion of the better-seeing eye is done prior to surgery to force the amblyopic eye to be used. The earlier occlusion therapy is initiated, the greater the probability that the amblyopic eye will see better.

Surgical correction of strabismus involves tightening or relaxing the extraocular muscles. In esotropia, the lateral rectus may be tightened or resected (Fig. 3.40) and the medial rectus relaxed or recessed (Fig. 3.41). This procedure results in more effective pulling by the lateral rectus and less effective pulling by the medial rectus, causing an outward turning of the esotropic eye. Alternately, both medial recti can be recessed. There are circumstances in which the surgeon would choose this technique, understanding that it involves surgery on both eyes whereas recess/resect surgery involves surgery on only one eye. In exotropia, surgical correction could involve resection of the medial rectus and recession of the lateral rectus in one eye; medial rectus resection in both eyes; or lateral rectus recession in both eyes. The approach depends on what is thought to be the underlying problem: for example, a patient with poor ability to converge (convergence insufficiency) might require bimedial resection. Superior and inferior rectus surgery is similar to horizontal rectus surgery, except that a small amount of muscle or tendon is resected or recessed to yield a greater effective change in alignment.

In performing muscle surgery, the conjunctiva is opened to gain access to the extraocular muscles. A peritomy is often performed at the limbus, although some surgeons prefer to open the conjunctiva more posteriorly or directly over the muscle insertions. A 6.0 Vicryl traction suture may be used at the limbus to help pull the muscle being operated on into the surgeon's view. Once the muscle is visualized, it is isolated by slipping a muscle hook beneath it. Blunt dissection further isolates the muscle and frees it from intermuscular attachments.

In resection surgery, blunt dissection must be more extensive than in recession surgery in order to expose the area of muscle to be resected. A caliper is used to measure the distance between the muscle insertion and the anticipated resection site where the muscle clamp is to be placed. Scissors are used to disinsert the muscle from the globe, leaving a small (<1 mm) stump. Two double 5.0 Vicryl sutures are placed, often in a mattress technique, to suture the remaining stump to the area of the muscle posterior to the clamp (Fig. 3.40). The excess muscle is excised and the muscle clamp removed.

In recession surgery, the muscle is isolated and hooked as in resection surgery. A 6.0 Vicryl suture is placed just posterior to the muscle insertion, and the muscle is disinserted from the globe with scissors. Because the muscle is to be placed more posteriorly on the globe, it is important to cut the muscle insertion flush with the globe, leaving as small a stump as possible. Calipers are used to mark the intended distance posterior to the original insertion, and a partial-thickness

Vicryl suture is placed in the sclera, suturing the muscle in place (Fig. 3.41).

Results and Complications

The goal of strabismus surgery in congenital esotropia is the attainment of some degree of single binocular vision. This goal requires that the eyes be aligned to within 10 prism diopters or 5° of orthophoria (being straight). Of 106 cases of congenital esotropia, all of those that had surgical alignment by 6 months of age attained some degree of binocular vision, but only 40% of those aligned after 24 months attained any degree of single binocular vision. Statistics concerning surgical treatment of exotropia vary widely. In new onset exotropia, especially in an adult, surgical alignment is accomplished with the expectation of treating diplopia. If exotropia is long-standing, the patient may develop suppression to alleviate his or her diplopia. In this case, success may be defined as adequate cosmesis.

The greatest risk of complication in strabismus surgery is secondary to general anesthesia. In adult strabismus surgery, local anesthesia is almost always preferred. In the pediatric patient, malignant hyperthermia is rare but potentially fatal if it occurs. Early signs include tachycardia or tachypnea with trismus or other muscular rigidity. Later signs include rapid increase in body temperature, metabolic acidosis, and cyanosis, followed by myocardial ischemia, hyperkalemia, and renal failure. If there is a family history of this condition, the patient should have a preoperative evaluation of serum creatine phosphokinase (CPK) and pharmacological testing of a muscle biopsy.

Poor alignment is the most common complication of strabismus surgery. Excessive relaxing of the muscle in recession surgery leads to overcorrection, while too little relaxing leads to undercorrection. The same logic applies to muscle tightening in resection surgery. The level of alignment noted in the immediate postoperative condition is often transient, and its instability may ultimately lead to a more or a less aligned permanent outcome. The use of adjustable sutures in the adult strabismic patient has decreased the incidence of this complication. Another complication is loss of muscle arising from retraction of the muscle into the orbit after disinsertion. It can be avoided by always locking the muscle clamp and releasing it only after sutures have been placed. Yet another complication is postoperative slippage of the sutured muscle. It may be avoided by placing sutures deep into the muscle tendon and not into the outer muscular capsule.

To prevent changes in the size of the palpebral fissure in inferior rectus surgery, it is important to dissect attachments free carefully. The inferior rectus is closely attached to the inferior oblique muscle and indirectly attached to the retractors of the lower lid. If the inferior rectus is recessed without separating its attachments to the eyelid retractors and orbital septum, the lid margins may be pulled inferiorly, thereby opening the palpebral fissure and leading to fissure asymmetry.

Perforation of the globe can lead to another complication in recession surgery. If the globe is perforated as the muscle is disinserted and resutured more posteriorly to the sclera, the result is usually a benign chorioretinal scar. However, in some instances perforation has led to endophthalmitis—infection of the globe. Presenting signs are pain, lid swelling, conjunctival injection, white blood cells layering in the anterior chamber (hypopyon), and fever. Endophthalmitis usually occurs within 2–5 days after surgery.

Finally, foreign body granulomas may appear at the incision site, as may conjunctival inclusion cysts. These and other sequelae that lead to elevated conjunctiva near the limbus may interfere with tears reaching the corneal surface, causing subsequent focal corneal dehydration and thinning referred to as dellen. Excessive scarring or an excessive muscle resection may also lead to restriction in ocular motility.

Ocular Disorders

The Red Eye

An acute red eye may be caused by a number of conditions, including conjunctivitis, corneal abrasion or ulceration, lid disorders, angle-closure glaucoma, or trauma. The most common cause is conjunctivitis. Conditions threatening loss of sight and therefore requiring immediate referral include corneal ulcer, acute iritis, angle-closure glaucoma, hyphema, and lacerated globe. The causes of red eye, diagnostic clues, and recommended therapy are listed in Table 3.2.

Visual Field Defects

Visual field testing is an important part of the ophthalmic examination. The visual field is defined as that portion of space visible to the fixating eye. The defects found on visual field testing are useful in localizing the site of pathology. Confrontation visual fields are easy to perform and can yield a great amount of information. More formal forms of visual field testing include use of a tangent screen or computerized automated perimetry. These means are useful in following the progress of a disease and in assessing the effect of treatment on it. Examples of visual field defects are shown in Figure 3.42.

Papillary Disorders

Any swelling of the optic nerve with an accumulation of abnormal fluid is known as disc edema. Swelling that is associated with raised intracranial pressure is known as papilledema, while swelling associated with inflammation is known as papillitis.

Papilledema is marked by loss of central cup, indistinct disc margins, loss of spontaneous venous pulsations, and hyperemia of the disc tissue. There may be disc hemorrhages, dilated veins, and exudates. Patients usually do not have any symptoms, although some may experience transient blurring of vision. Papillitis, on the other hand, is marked by loss of vision, particularly central vision, and by an afferent pupillary defect. Visual field examinations are useful in distinguishing

Table 3.2.
Red Eye: Causes, Diagnostic Clues, and Recommended Therapies

Area	Condition	Diagnostic Clues	Therapy
Lid (vision fine)	Ectropion	Lid not against globe.	Refer for surgery.
	Entropion	Lashes against globe.	Refer for surgery.
	Chalazion	Not hot, minimal pain, slow evolution, lump in lid.	Hot compresses; if no resolution, may excise.
	Hordeolum externa	Acute onset, abscess on lid margin.	Hot compresses followed by I&D (incise and drain). Topical antibiotics (gentamycin 0.3 mg/mL q.i.d.).
	Lid cellulitis (hordeolum interna)	Swollen, red, warm lid of acute onset. Often follows a stye.	Oral antibiotics (cephalexin 500 mg p.o. q.i.d. or similar). Follow closely! If getting worse refer promptly!
	Blepharitis	Red lid margin with scales and debris on lashes.	Clean lid margins b.i.d. Intermittent topical antibiotic ung. (Garamycin or erythromycin b.i.d.). Chronic condition so refer for severe irritation or corneal complications only.
	Trachoma	Tarsal plate scarring. Superior corneal pannus.	Tetracycline or erythromycin p.o. or topical. Typical Rx: tetracycline ung. b.i.d. × 4 weeks then first 5 days of each month × 3 months.
Conjunctiva (vision fine if discharge removed)	Allergic conjunctivitis	Redness and swelling of conjunctiva with clear discharge. Itching. Chronic. Seasonal.	Topical astringents (Naphcon or Naphcon-A q.i.d.). Opticrom q.i.d. more severe cases. Steroids on referral only!
	Bacterial conjunctivitis	Conjunctival redness and swelling with a purulent discharge. Acute onset.	Topical antibiotics (sulfacetamide or Garamycin q.i.d.). Acute and severe consider gonococcus. If Gram's stain suggestive, penicillin G 100,000 U/mL one drop q.1 h. around the clock and get immediate ophthalmological coverage!
	Vernal conjunctivitis	Children with large bumps on upper tarsal plate. Atopic children. Photophobic.	Opticrom q.i.d. If unsuccessful refer to ophthalmologist for steroid treatment.
	Viral conjunctivitis	Conjunctival redness and swelling with a serous or seromucoid discharge. Acute onset.	Scrupulous hygiene (do not pass this around). Topical antibiotics as for bacterial conjunctivitis if not sure. Refer for any corneal complications!
Cornea (vision often decreased)	Abrasion	Fluorescein stain shows epithelial defect. No corneal infiltrate. Vision OK. Marked pain.	Antibiotic (e.g., Garamycin ung.) and tight pressure patch. Monitor epithelial healing daily. Refer for nonhealing or evidence of any infitrate. Make sure there is no foreign body on upper tarsal plate!
	Corneal foreign body	Visible. Irregularity in fluorescein staining. Use magnifier. Painful.	Remove foreign body with bevel of 25-gauge needle. Remove all rust easily removable. Patch and follow as corneal abrasion.
	Corneal ulcer	Epithelial defect with infiltrate! Marked pain and photophobia.	Emergency! Prompt referral! If any delay start Garamycin solution q.30min. around the clock.
	Corneal herpes	Irregular (dendritic) epithelial defect. Not much pain.	Zovirax ung. q.4h. while awake and refer.
	Pterygium	Advancing fleshy growth on cornea. Usually nasal.	Sunglasses. Artificial tears (Liquifilm tears q.i.d.). Astringents (Naphcon q.i.d.). If advancing on cornea refer for surgery.
Iris	Iritis	Photophobia. Redness perilimbal. Vision may be decreased. Pain variable but usually more severe than casual exam would predict. Irregular iris and deposits on back surface of cornea.	Refer for appropriate workup and treatment
	Angle-closure glaucoma	Acute onset pain, photophobia and blurred vision. Nausea common. Cornea has "ground glass" appearance.	Emergency! Prompt referral critical. May start pilocarpine 2% drops q.10min. × 3 and Diamox 250 mg p.o. if any delay likely.

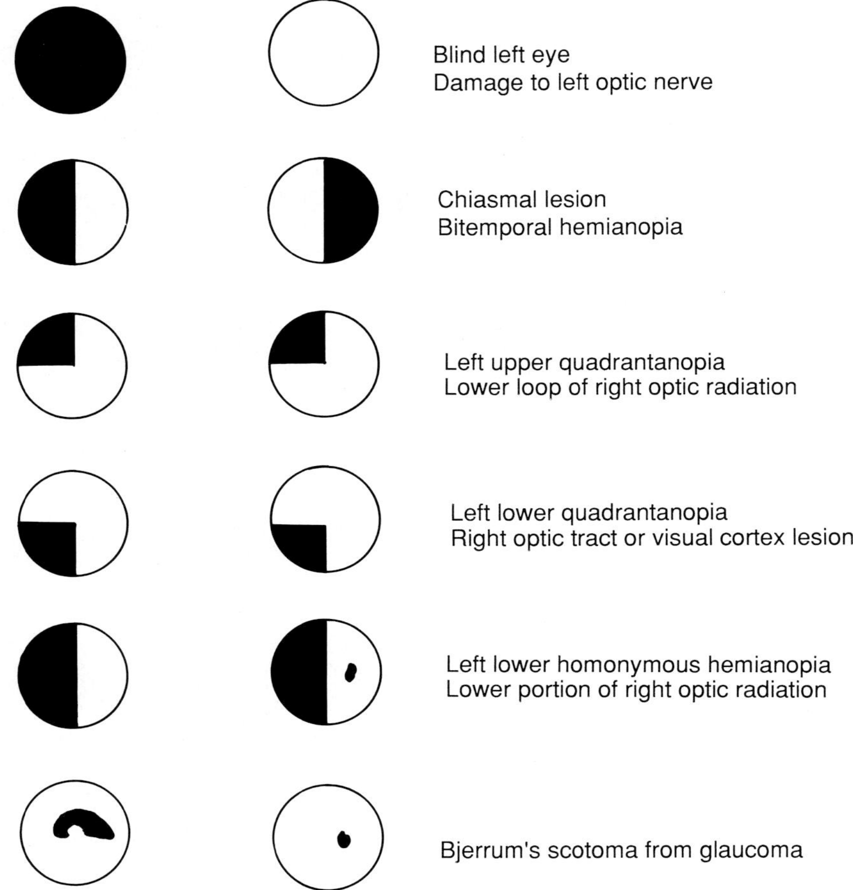

Figure 3.42. Example of visual field defects.

between the two. In papilledema there is an enlarged blind spot and constriction of the peripheral isopters, while in papillitis there is a central scotoma.

A special form of disc edema is associated with cranial arteritis (giant cell), and is known as ischemic optic neuropathy. It classically presents as sudden visual loss (usually an altitudinal field defect) with pale disc swelling and few hemorrhages. Systemic symptoms include weight loss, loss of appetite, pain on mastication, headache, and tenderness on the forehead over the temporal artery. Most patients have an elevated sedimentation rate. Because those affected respond dramatically to steroids, it is important to make the correct diagnosis. Ischemic optic neuropathy can also be caused by atherosclerosis.

Hypertensive Retinopathy

Hypertension can cause vascular changes in the eye which are of value both in diagnosing the hypertension and in gauging its severity. In the early stages, there may be focal narrowing of the arterioles (Fig. 3.43), beginning after the diastolic blood pressure is over 120 mm Hg. Disc hemorrhages may occur early as well. Long-standing hypertension produces a more generalized effect on the vessels. As the arterial wall thickens

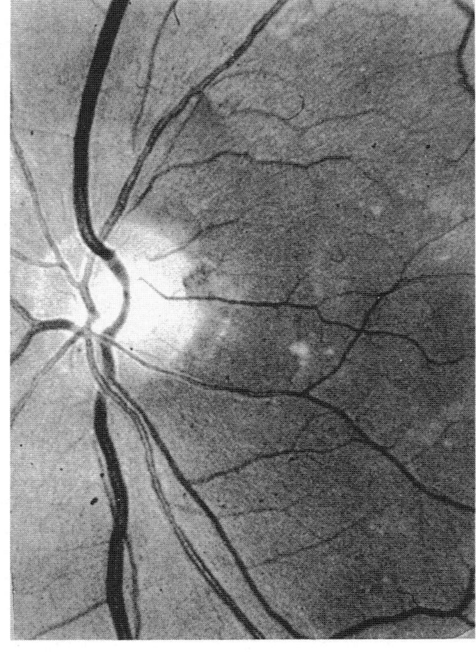

Figure 3.43. Arterial spasm—hypertension.

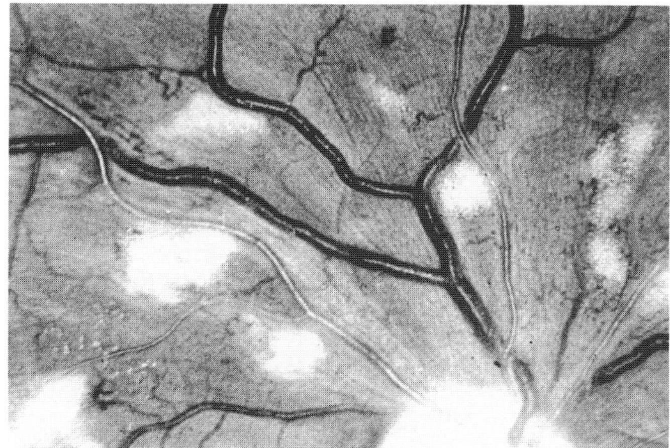

Figure 3.44. Copper wiring appearance in hypertensive retinopathy.

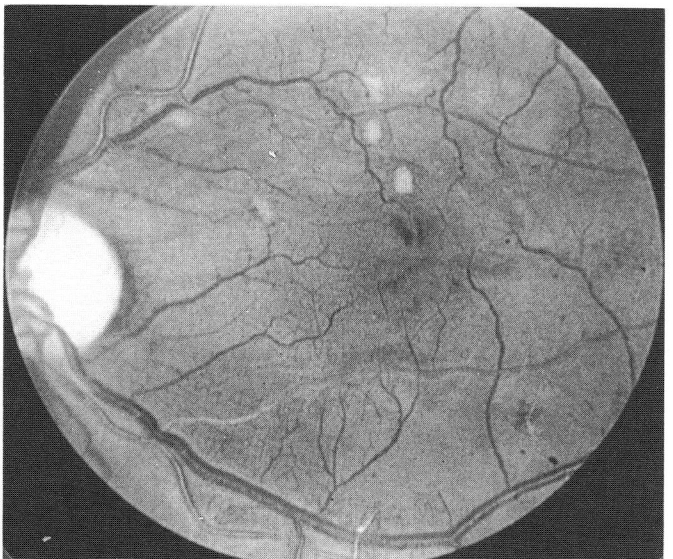

Figure 3.45. Silver wiring appearance in hypertensive retinopathy.

the light reflex is altered. This condition may progress to give a copper wiring appearance to the eye (Fig. 3.44) and eventually to a silver wiring appearance (Fig. 3.45), signifying low blood flow and retinal ischemia. Arteriolar venous crossing changes also signify hypertensive changes. These occur because the arteriole and the vein share a common adventitial sheath.

Retinal Vein Occlusion

Central retinal vein occlusion is a common problem, especially in the elderly. Vein occlusions are either nonischemic or ischemic. Ischemic vein occlusions have a worse visual prognosis and are often associated with neovascular glaucoma and retinal neovascularization, both of which may lead to blindness. The most common ocular cause of vein occlusion is glaucoma. An increased incidence of vein occlusion is also associated

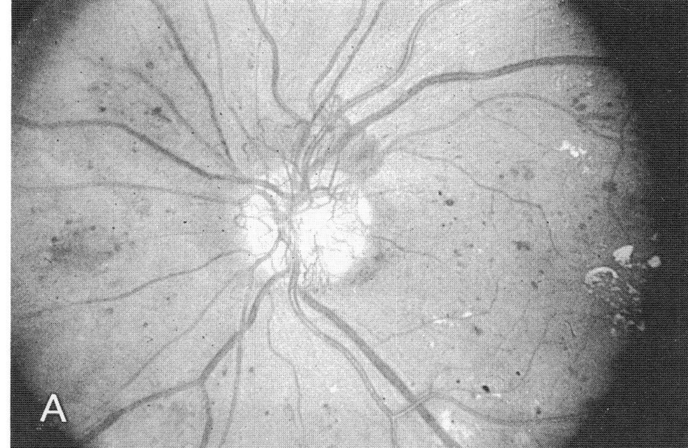

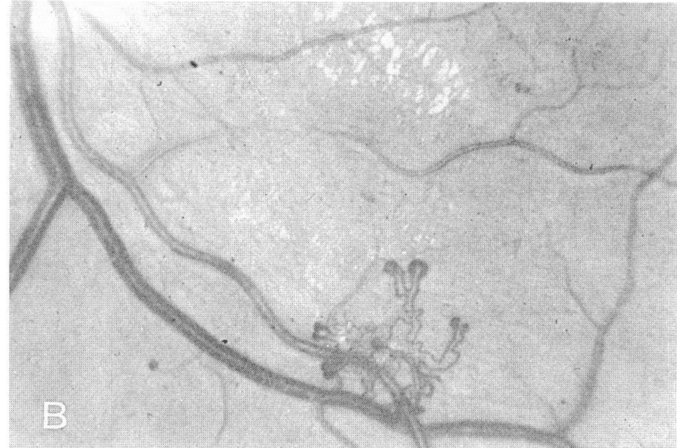

Figure 3.46. Diabetic neovascularization. **A**, Disc. **B**, Elsewhere.

with certain systemic diseases, including hypertension, diabetes mellitus (Fig. 3.46**A**, **B**), hyperviscosity syndromes, and collagen vascular diseases (especially systemic lupus erythematosus).

Amaurosis Fugax

Amaurosis fugax is a temporary loss of vision. It is confined to one eye and may last 5–10 minutes. Retinal emboli are the cause of these transient ischemic attacks. There are three main types. A fibrin platelet embolus (Fisher plug) arises from the carotid bifurcation, other great vessel, or heart and represents platelet aggregates (Fig. 3.47). A calcific embolus arises from cardiac valves and appears as solid plaque (Fig. 3.48). A cholesterol embolus (Hollenhorst's plaque) is formed from shed atheromatous plaque, usually from the carotid artery, and are composed of fibrin and cholesterol. Calcific plaques are dull, white, and "chalky," while cholesterol plaques are bright orange or yellow and tend to "glisten."

Third Nerve Palsy

The third nerve innervates the pupil, the medial rectus, superior rectus, inferior rectus, the levator of the

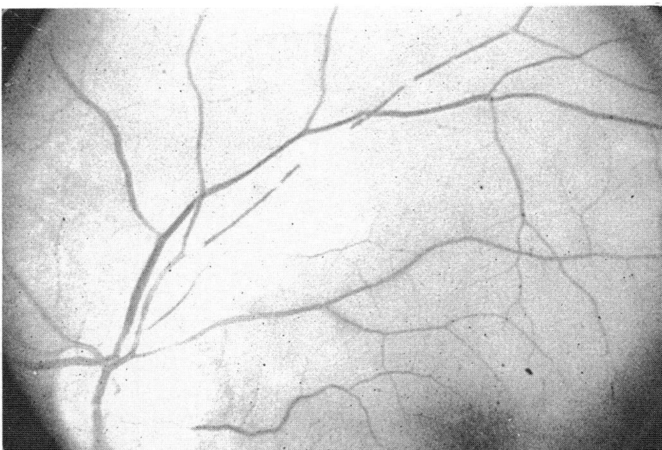

Figure 3.47. Fibrin embolus.

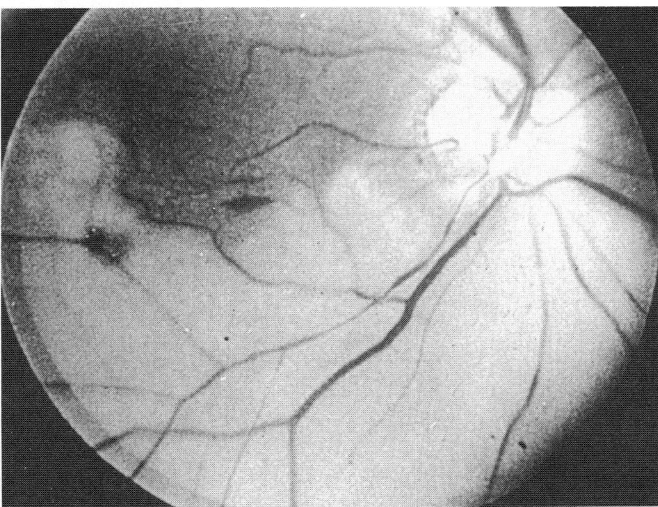

Figure 3.48. Calcific embolus.

lid, and the inferior oblique. With total palsy there is ptosis, the eye is deviated down and out, the pupil has no reaction, and accommodation is down. In an adult, a third nerve palsy with pain usually is due to compression from an aneurysm or from ischemic disease such as diabetes. Trauma may also cause third nerve damage.

Sixth Nerve Palsy

The sixth cranial nerve has a long intracranial course, which makes it susceptible to injury. It may be damaged by lesions in the orbit, cavernous sinus, or pontine lesions. Isolated sixth nerve palsies in adults may be induced by trauma but are most often due to vascular problems. Affected patients present with a horizontal diplopia.

Diplopia

Diplopia means double vision. A patient with true double vision should return to single vision if either eye is occluded. "Monocular" diplopia can occur as a result of ocular causes, such as corneal disease or cataract formation, and should not be classified as diplopia. True diplopia requires that both eyes see (and have developed together since birth). If diplopia exists, it becomes necessary to differentiate between horizontal diplopia and vertical diplopia, because the muscles involved and the nerve pathways are different. Each eye is examined separately and the individual muscles evaluated. For example, when evaluating the right lateral rectus muscle (innervated by the sixth cranial nerve), the patient is asked to move the eye to the right (laterally) in a horizontal plane. In this manner, the muscle involved can be isolated.

SUGGESTED READINGS

Ocular Disorders

Amaurosis Fugax Study Group: Amaurosis fugax (transient monocular blindness), a consensus statement. In: Bernstein EF, ed. Amaurosis Fugax. 1988:Heidelberg, Springer-Verlag.

Arruga J, Sanders M. Ophthalmologic findings in 70 patients with evidence of retinal embolism. Ophthal 1982;89:1336.

Hayuh SS. Hypertensive retinopathy, introduction. Ophthalmologic 1989;198:173.

Keith NM, Wagner HP, Barker NW. Some different types of essential hypertension, their course and prognosis. Am J Med Sci 1989;197: 332.

Michels RG, Gass JDM. Natural course of retinal vein obstruction. Trans Am Acad Ophthalmol Otolaryngol 1974;78:166.

Diseases of the Cornea

Brightbill F, ed. Corneal surgery. St. Louis Missouri: CV Mosby, 1986.

Bruner WE, Stark WJ, Maumenee AE, eds. Manual of corneal surgery. New York: Churchill Livingstone, 1986.

Kaufman HE, McDonald MB, Barron BA, Waltman SR, eds. The cornea. New York: Churchill Livingstone, 1988.

Leibowitz H, ed. Corneal disorders: clinical diagnosis and management. Philadelphia: WB Saunders, 1984.

Smolin G, Thoft R, eds. The cornea: scientific foundations and clinical practice. Boston: Little, Brown, 1987.

Diseases of the Anterior Chamber

Epstein DL. Trabeculectomy. In: Chandler PA, Grant WM, eds. Glaucoma. 3rd ed. Philadelphia: Lea & Febiger, 1986:204–218.

Kolker AE, Hetherington J Jr eds. Becker-Shaffer's diagnoses and therapy of the glaucomas. 5th ed. St. Louis, Missouri: CV Mosby, 1983.

Ritch R, Shield MB, Krups T, eds. The glaucomas. St. Louis, Missouri: CV Mosby, 1989.

Diseases of the Lens

Clayman H. Intraocular lenses. In: Tasman W, Jaeger E, eds. Duane's clinical ophthalmology. Vol 5. Philadelphia: JB Lippincott, 1989:1–29.

Kelman C. Phacoemulsification and aspiration: the Kelman technique of cataract removal. In: Tasman W, Jaeger E, eds. Duane's clinical ophthalmology. Vol 5. Philadelphia: JB Lippincott, 1989:1–13.

Kratz RP, Olson P, Johnsen S, Farley M. Phacoemulsification associated with intraocular lens. In: Waltman S et al, eds. Surgery of the eye. New York: Churchill Livingstone, 1988:181–140.

McIntyre D. Manual catacract extraction. In: Waltman S et al, eds. Surgery of the eye. New York: Churchill Livingstone, 1988:119–130.

Weinstein G. Cataract surgery. In: Tasman W, Jaeger E, eds. Duane's clinical ophthalmology. Vol 5. Philadelphia: JB Lippincott, 1989:1–52.

Diseases of the Retina and Vitreous

Kini MM. Retina and vitreous. In: Pavan-Langston, D ed. Manual of ocular diagnosis and therapy. Boston: Little, Brown, 1980:133–155.

Kini MM. Vitreous. In: Vaughan D, Asbury T, eds. General ophthalmology. 9th ed. Los Altos, California: Lange Medical, 1980:135–143.

Kini MM. Retina. In: Vaughan D, Asbury T, eds. General ophthalmology. 9th ed. Los Altos, California: Lange Medical, 1980:144–166.

Parker AJ, ed. Manual of retinal surgery. New York: Churchill Livingstone, 1989.

Michels R. Vitreous surgery. In: Rice TA et al eds. Ophthalmic surgery. 4th ed. Boston: Butterworth, 1984:209–254.

Diseases of the Nasolacrimal System, Eyelids, and Orbit

Smith BC, Della Rocca RC, Nesi FA, Lisman RD, eds. Ophthalmic plastic and reconstructive surgery. St. Louis, Missouri: CV Mosby, 1987.

Stewart WB et al, eds. Ophthalmic plastic and reconstructive surgery. American Academy of Ophthalmology, 1984.

Diseases of the Extraocular Muscles

Greenwald MJ. Amblyopia. In: Tasman W, ed. Duane's clinical ophthalmology. Vol 1. Philadelphia, JB Lippincott, 1989.

Greenwald MJ, Marshall MP: Treatment of amblyopia. In: Ophthalmology. Vol 1. Philadelphia: JB Lippincott, 1989.

Hoyt CS, ed. Surgery of the eye. New York: Churchill Livingstone, 1988:761–826.

Parks MM. Sensorial adaptations in strabismus. In: Tasman W, ed. Duane's clinical ophthalmology. Vol 1. Philadelphia: JB Lippincott, 1989.

Parks MM. Sensory tests and treatment of sensorial adaptations. In: Tasman W, ed. Duane's clinical ophthalmology. Philadelphia: JB Lippincott, 1989.

Parks MM, Wheeler MB. Concomitat esodeviations. In: Tasman W, ed. Duane's clinical ophthalmology. Philadelphia: JB Lippincott, 1989.

Reinecke RD. Muscle surgery. In: Tasman W, ed. Duane's clinical ophthalmology. Philadelphia: JB Lippincott, 1989.

Von Noorden GK. Atlas of strabismus. 4th ed. St. Louis Missouri: CV Mosby, 1983.

Skills

1. Dilate the pupil. Place one drop of tropicamide 1% in each of the patient's eyes. Place one drop of phenylephrine 2.5% in each of the patient's eyes. This combination will usually work but may be repeated twice.
2. Identify a corneal abrasion by means of fluoresein staining. Fluorescein comes in sterile strips that can be placed in the cul-de-sac of the patient's eye or in 2% drops that can be placed in the eye.
3. Identify a cataract through use of an ophthalmoscope. Place the ophthalmoscope on +6 or +8 magnification and observe the eye from a distance of approximately 6 inches. If a cataract is present, it can be seen with a red reflex in the background.
4. Perform a confrontation visual field (perimetry) test by comparing the patient's visual field with your own. Position yourself about 1 meter from the patient. Have the patient cover one eye and then fixate on your eye. By moving your fingers or red balls, you can check the extent of the patient's central and peripheral field vision.

Study Questions

DISEASES OF THE CORNEA

1. A patient presents with a yearlong complaint of decreasing vision in her left eye. She has corneal edema OS (left eye) with legal blindness and a healthy right eye. She has a history of cataract and intraocular lens implant surgery in the left eye. Discuss your diagnosis and treatment plan, including risks, as you would with the patient. How would your treatment plan change if this woman also had a history of herpes simplex keratitis in that eye?
2. A patient with a recent corneal transplant, currently taking a small amount of topical steroid, is on the telephone complaining of increased redness and irritation in the operated eye. Discuss how you would approach this problem over the telephone, specifically addressing medications and patient instructions with attention to the patient's inquiry, "Doctor, I don't want to see you if I don't have to. Can't I just increase my steroid medicine a bit?"
3. You are asked to consult on a patient who recently had an acoustic neuroma removed from the right side successfully. The patient has no specific eye complaints, although you notice immediately that the eye is quite red and the eyelids function poorly. Explain your evaluation, treatment plan, and justification for either medical or surgical treatment.
4. A 30-year-old moderately myopic electrical engineer presents complaining "I would like to get rid of my glasses. I hate contact lenses and I've been to many ophthalmologists who have always had a hard time refracting me just right. The image just never seems as sharp as I like." Discuss your evaluation, differential diagnosis, and appropriate treatment strategy.
5. A visiting professor from India presents with a complaint of a pterygium that is growing over the left eye. He has a history of successful pterygium removal in the right eye years ago. On examination you note a small pterygium 2 mm onto the left cornea, visual acuity of 20/25, and an irregular photokeratoscope picture. Explain your treatment plan. What if this pterygium had been removed about 2 months ago when the patient was in India?

DISEASES OF THE ANTERIOR CHAMBER

1. What are the symptoms of chronic open-angle glaucoma?
2. What are the signs and symptoms of narrow-angle glaucoma?

3. Describe a goniotomy.
4. What is the use of laser surgery for open-angle glaucoma?

DISEASES OF THE LENS

1. What are the different types of cataracts?
2. Name a cause for posterior subcapsular cataract formation.
3. Describe the signs and symptoms of postoperative endophthalmitis.
4. What is the difference in the size of incisions between extracapsular cataract extraction and phacoemulsification?
5. Describe intraocular lenses.

DISEASES OF THE RETINA AND VITREOUS

1. A patient complains of recent onset of flashing lights and new floaters. What is your differential diagnosis and what do you need to do to examine the patient?
2. A young patient presents with a 12-year history of diabetes mellitus. What are you looking for and what advice do you give the patient?
3. Describe the principles of retinal detachment surgery.
4. On what principle does retinal laser surgery work?

DISEASES OF THE NASOLACRIMAL SYSTEM, EYELIDS, AND ORBIT

1. What is the most frequent cause of proptosis in children?
2. A 65-year-old man presents to the ophthalmologist's office after noting the sudden onset of "drooping" of his right upper eyelid shortly after awakening this morning. What specific, additional physical findings should be looked for in order to evaluate properly this patient's ptosis?
3. The production of a cicatricial ectropion of the lower eyelid typically results from shortening of which layers of the eyelid?

DISEASES OF THE EXTRAOCULAR MUSCLES

1. Give the actions of the six extraocular muscles.
2. What is the principle behind glasses for esotropia?
3. Why do patients develop amblyopia and at what ages does it occur?

4 Plastic Surgery: Diseases of the Skin and Soft Tissue, Face, and Hand

David B. Reath, M.D. and
Brent V. Stromberg, M.D.

ASSUMPTIONS

The student has a basic knowledge of wound healing.

The student is familiar with the anatomy and physiology of the skin, subcutaneous tissue, facial skeleton, and upper extremity.

OBJECTIVES

1. Discuss the different types of wounds and their management.
2. Understand the different types of skin grafts and flaps used in the reconstruction of soft tissue defects, and their appropriate applications.
3. Describe the clinical presentation and indications for treatment of benign skin lesions, including nevi, keratoses, hemangiomas, cysts, and lipomas.
4. Differentiate hypertrophic scar and keloid formation from normal wound healing.
5. Describe the initial assessment of a patient with facial trauma, and the repair of soft tissue injuries.
6. Describe the evaluation, diagnosis, and treatment of facial fractures.
7. Discuss the examination of the hand, diagnosis of acute hand injuries, and their initial treatment.
8. Describe the clinical features and indications for treatment of paronychia, felon, tenosynovitis, and human bites of the hand.
9. Understand the evaluation and treatment of common tumors of the hand.
10. Understand the development of prepalatal and palatal structures and their relationship to cleft lips and cleft palates.
11. Understand the objectives and different types of postmastectomy breast reconstruction.
12. Describe the different types of aesthetic operations, the goals, and their appropriate uses.

The field of plastic and reconstructive surgery is concerned with the reconstruction or improvement of both the form and function of many areas of the body. Rarely can either form or function be sacrificed one for the other, but frequently one may be of greater concern. The majority of this chapter will be concerned with reconstructive surgery, which is required because of abnormalities of the skin and soft tissues resulting from trauma, malignancies, congenital deformities, or other diseases. Reconstructive surgery is differentiated from aesthetic surgery, which is directed at the cosmetic improvement of *normal* structures.

As the field of plastic surgery almost always involves surgery of the skin, this chapter will begin with an understanding of the structure, healing, and reconstruction of the skin. (A more complete discussion of wound healing is covered in EGS2, Chapter 11.)

Skin Structure

The skin or integument is the largest organ of the body and completely envelops its surface. The skin functions both as our primary defense against the environment and as our principal means of communicating with it. The skin also serves important functions in terms of homeostasis and thermoregulation. The integument is, in fact, an indispensable organ: total destruction of the skin is incompatible with life.

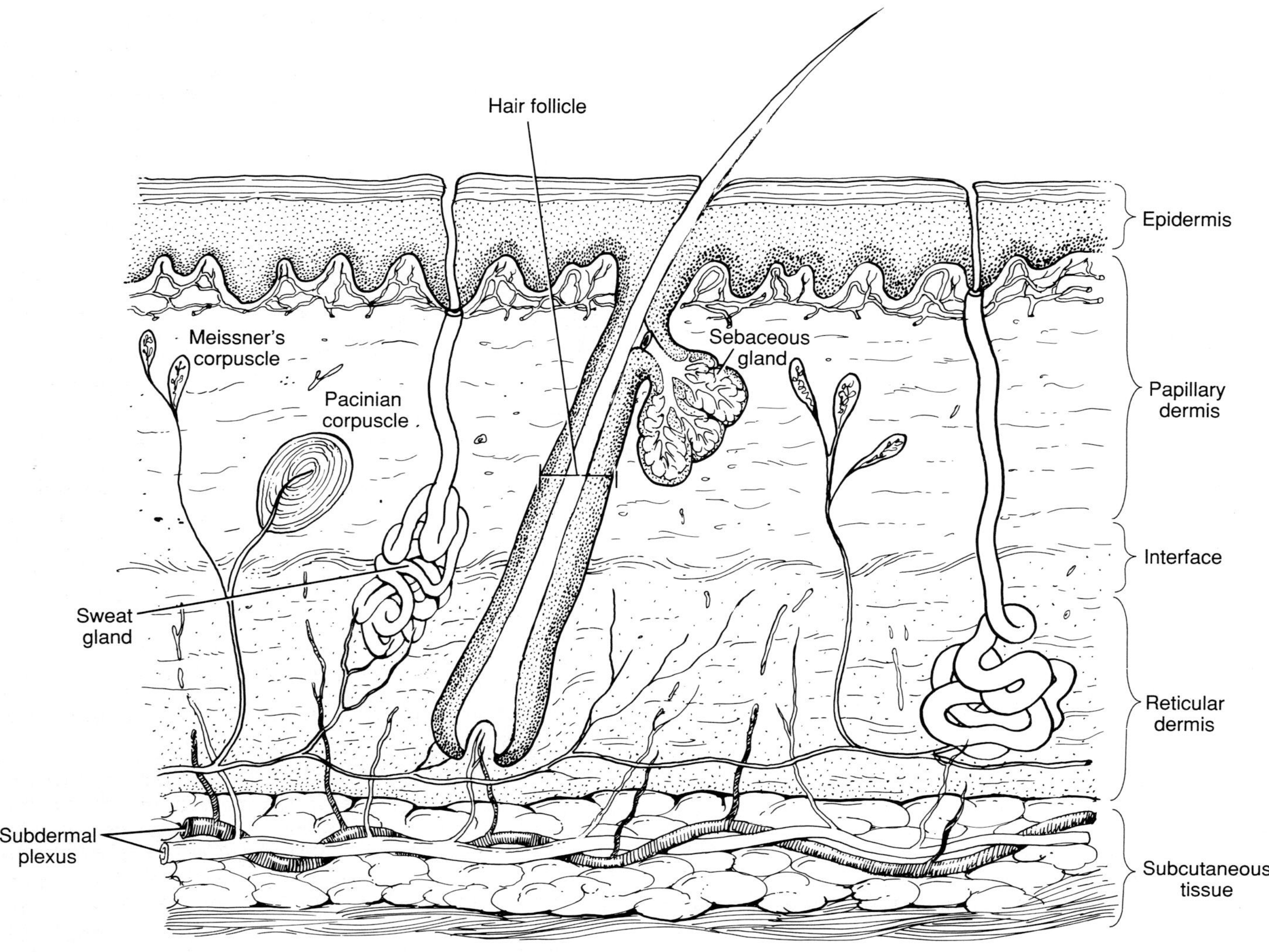

Figure 4.1. Cross-section anatomy of the skin.

The skin is divided into two embryologically distinct layers: the epidermis and the underlying dermis (Fig. 4.1). The epidermis consists of five distinct strata, the cells of which all derive from the innermost of these strata, the stratum germinativum or basal layer. Mitosis of this layer, with transformation of these cells as they migrate outward, forms the other strata of the epidermis. Located within the basal layer are the pigment-containing melanocytes. The epidermis is devoid of vasculature and receives its nourishment from the underlying dermis. Epidermal projections known as rete pegs extend down into the underlying dermis.

The dermis, which is 15 to 40 times thicker than the epidermis, is divided into the thin papillary dermis, located beneath the epidermal rete pegs, and the thicker subjacent reticular dermis. The papillary dermis contains reticular and elastic fibers intermingled with a rich capillary network. The reticular dermis contains dense bundles of collagen parallel to the skin's surface. This layer is responsible for much of the tensile strength of the skin. Also contained within the dermis are pilosebaceous apparata, eccrine and apocrine units, and important nerve end organs such as pacinian and Meissner's corpuscles.

Wound Healing

Wound healing consists of three phases. The initial or inflammatory phase is characterized by inflammation around the edges of the wound, a nonspecific reaction to injury of any sort. Leukocytes function to remove debris and bacteria. Toward the end of this relatively brief phase, the activated macrophages appear and direct the next phase. While the inflammatory phase lasts approximately 4 days in wounds with little contamination, it may be significantly prolonged in contaminated wounds. The second or proliferative phase is characterized by collagen production by fibroblasts. Tissue fibroblasts synthesize collagen at an increased rate for about 6 weeks in a normal wound. This synthesis causes a rapid gain in wound tensile strength that peaks at the end of this phase (Fig. 4.2). The third or maturation phase consists of the remodeling of collagen by the formation of intermolecular cross-links. The third phase,

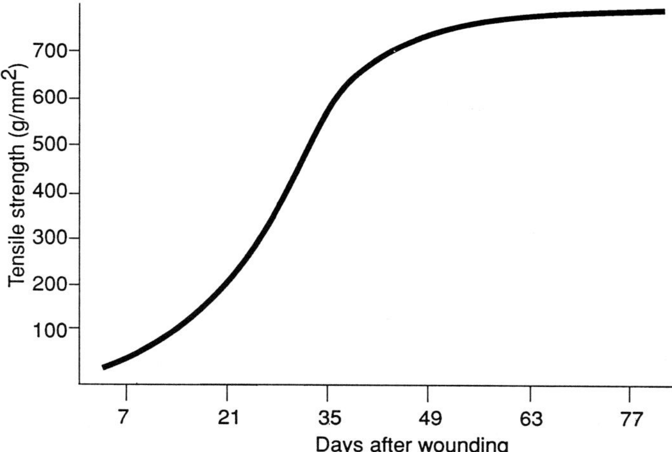

Figure 4.2. Wound tensile strength as a function of days.

which lasts from 6 to 18 months, leads to a flatter, paler scar, with little increase in tensile strength. This phase is characterized by a dynamic balance of collagenolysis and collagen synthesis.

Wound healing is classified as healing by primary, secondary, or tertiary (delayed primary) intention. Healing by primary intention involves recent, clean wounds that are managed by simple repair. These wounds are first gently irrigated and debrided to minimize the inflammatory process. Debridement consists of removing foreign material and devitalized tissue. After debridement the tissue planes should be approximated accurately to provide optimal healing. At the peak of collagen synthesis the scar itself looks mildly inflamed; it is raised, red, and often pruritic. Over the course of time, the scar flattens, thins, and becomes much lighter in color. The process takes at least 9 to 12 months in an adult and somewhat longer in a child. The final appearance of a scar depends on the initial injury, the amount of contamination and ischemia, and the method and accuracy with which the wound was closed. Wound healing may be delayed by impaired circulation, immunosuppression, infection, or inadequate nutrition. Generally, absorbable sutures are used below the skin surface, and nonabsorbable sutures are used for the outer closure since they are less reactive (Fig. 4.3).

Wounds left open to heal without surgical intervention are said to heal by secondary intention. This secondary closure is characterized by a prolonged inflammatory phase that persists until the wound is covered with epithelium. Wounds treated in this manner will eventually heal, unless such factors as infection and foreign bodies are present. Epithelialization from the wound margins proceeds at a rate of approximately 1 mm/day in a concentric pattern. The wound contraction greatly reduces the size of the wound, although it never approaches the final appearance of a primarily closed wound. Healing by secondary intention is indicated in infected or severely contaminated wounds, since an open wound will not develop an abscess or wound infection.

Delayed primary closure, or healing by tertiary intention, involves the subsequent repair of a wound that was initially left open or not repaired. This method is indicated for wounds with a high bacterial content (e.g., a human bite), a long time lapse since initial injury, or a severe crush component with significant tissue devitalization. Successful closure depends on the cleanliness of the wound, preparedness of the wound edges, and absence of significant bacterial colonization (less than 10^5 bacteria per gram of tissue).

Abnormal healing may take the form of *hypertrophic scars* or keloids. Hypertrophic scars are raised, widened, red, may be pruritic, with tissue remaining within the boundaries of the scar (Fig. 4.4**A**). *Keloids*, on the other hand, have an abnormal growth of tissue that usually mushrooms over the edges of the wound, extending outside the boundaries of the scar (Fig. 4.4**B**). Keloids are more common in blacks and Asians. Differentiating between the two scars is important since their treatment differs. A hypertrophic scar will often improve with time or may be improved by a surgical revision. A keloid, however, may actually be made worse by revision and is instead treated with topical steroids or anti-inflammatory medication.

Types of Wounds and their Treatment

Different wounds have specific etiologies and treatment guidelines.

Lacerations. Lacerations consist of cut or torn tissue. Care includes gentle handling of tissue and cleansing the wound of clots, foreign material, or necrotic tissue. Mild irrigants, such as normal saline, rather than strong antiseptics should be used to cleanse the wound. Administering a local anesthetic before the final cleansing is helpful. Once cleansed, lacerations should be closed with an atraumatic technique. Careful closure of wound margins gives the best chance for ideal healing with minimal scarring (Fig. 4.5). Dressings should consist of sterile material that will protect the wound as well as allow some absorption of wound drainage. Immobilization may be helpful in complex extremity wounds.

Abrasions. Abrasions are injuries in which the superficial skin layer has been removed. They may be of variable depth. Abrasions should be gently cleansed of any foreign material. Occasionally, more vigorous rubbing with a scrub brush is appropriate. Again, a local anesthetic can help facilitate cleansing. Dirt and gravel must be removed to prevent permanent discoloration, known as traumatic tattooing. It is important that the wound be cleansed within the first day of injury. Subsequent to this cleansing, an abrasion can be cared for by any method that keeps it clean and moist. Use of topical antibiotic ointment and/or gentle protective dressings or bandages is appropriate.

Contusions. A contusion is an injury that results from a forceful blow to the skin and soft tissues. In contusions the entire outer layer of skin is intact, although it is injured. Contusions require minimal early care.

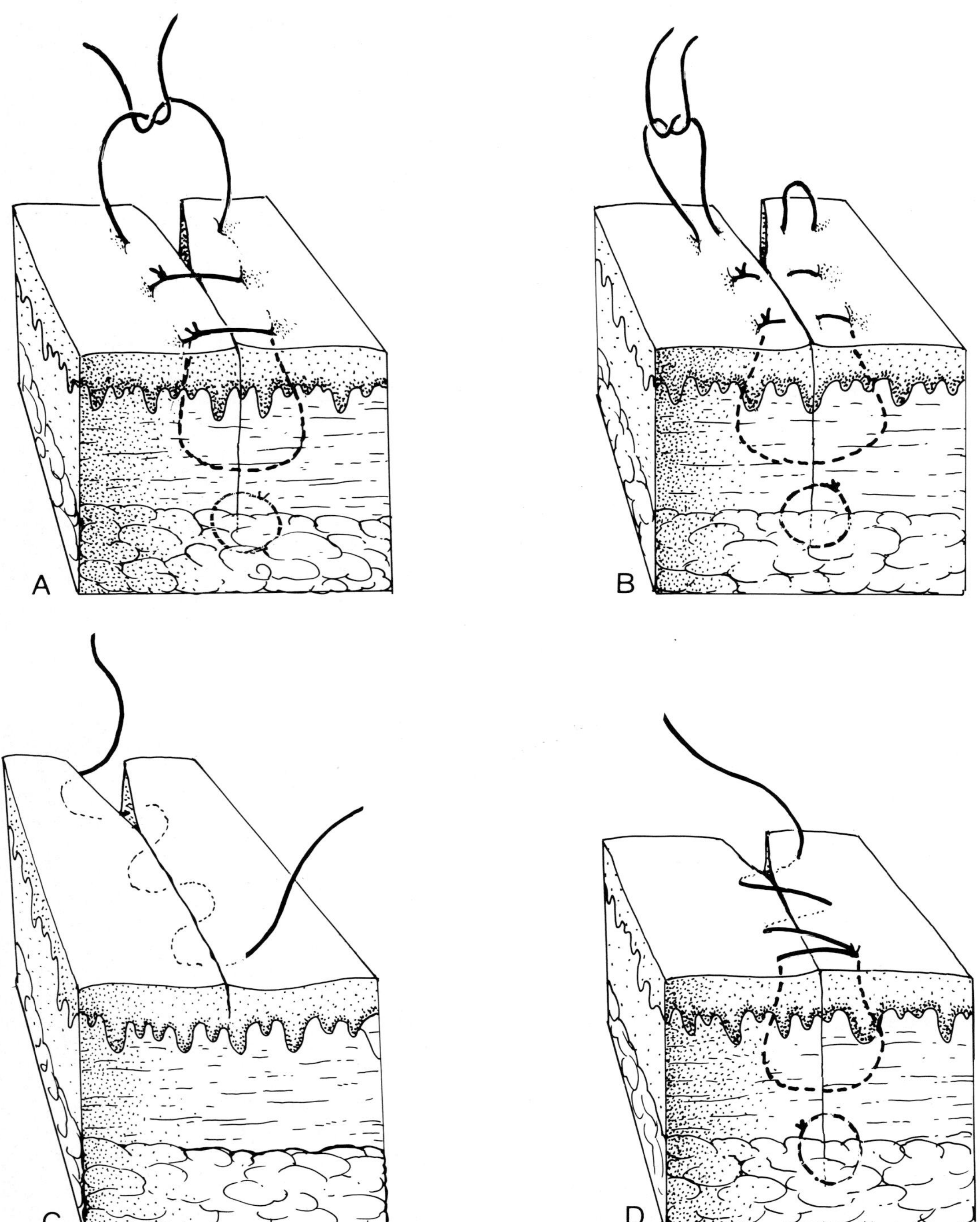

Figure 4.3. Techniques of skin closure. **A**, Simple interrupted sutures. **B**, Vertical mattress sutures. **C**, Running subcuticular sutures. **D**, Continuous simple sutures.

They should be evaluated early, however, to diagnose a possible deep hematoma or tissue injury. To minimize edema and limit expansion of a hematoma, a contusion can be cooled for the first 24 hours. After that, warmth may speed the absorption of the blood and edema.

Avulsions. In avulsions tissue has been torn off, either partially or totally. In partial avulsions the tissue is elevated but still attached to the body. If this raised portion of tissue is adequately vascularized and appears viable, showing good capillary refill and normal skin color (i.e., not cyanotic), the tissue should be gently cleansed, irrigated, and simply sutured into its anatomic location. If the tissue is not viable, although still attached, it is usually best to excise it and use an alternative method of closure, such as a skin graft or local flap (discussed later). Completely avulsed tissue usu-

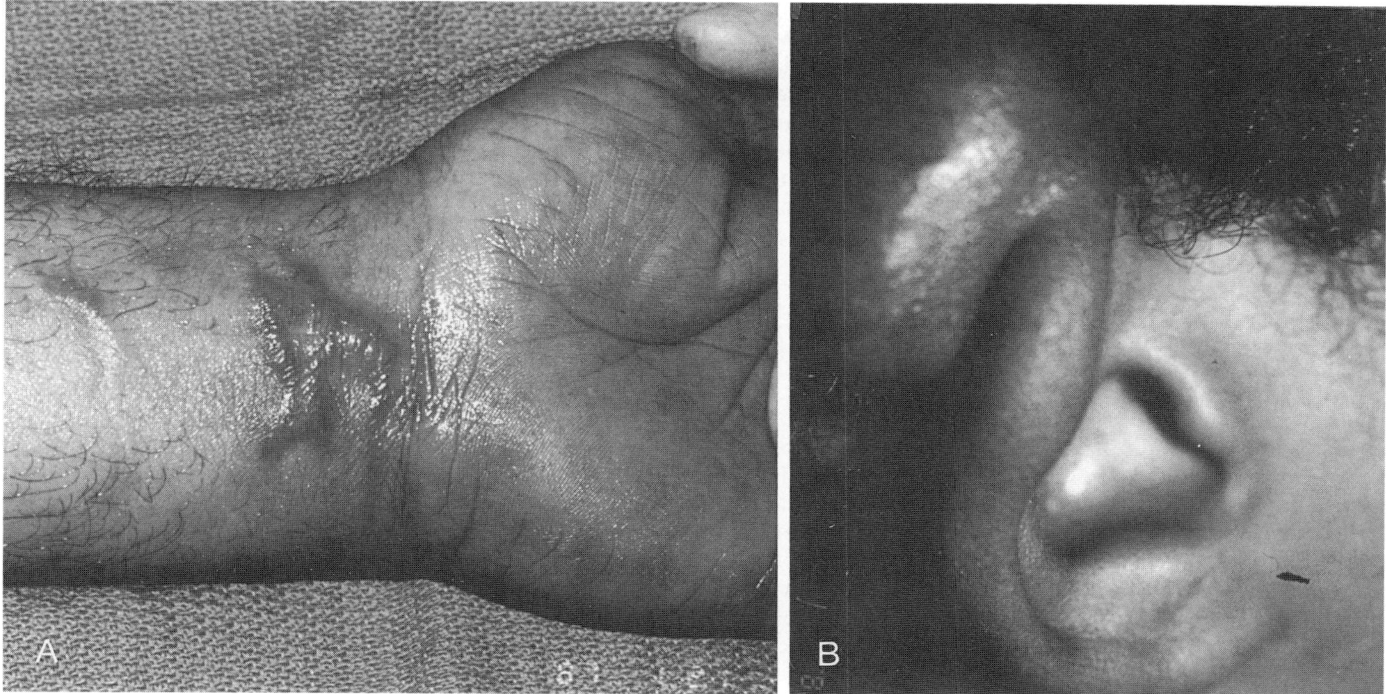

Figure 4.4. **A**, Hypertrophy of a scar on the volar wrist. Note that the scar does not extend beyond the boundaries of the original scar. **B**, Keloid of scar of the helical rim. The scar tissue mushrooms out beyond the boundaries of the original scar.

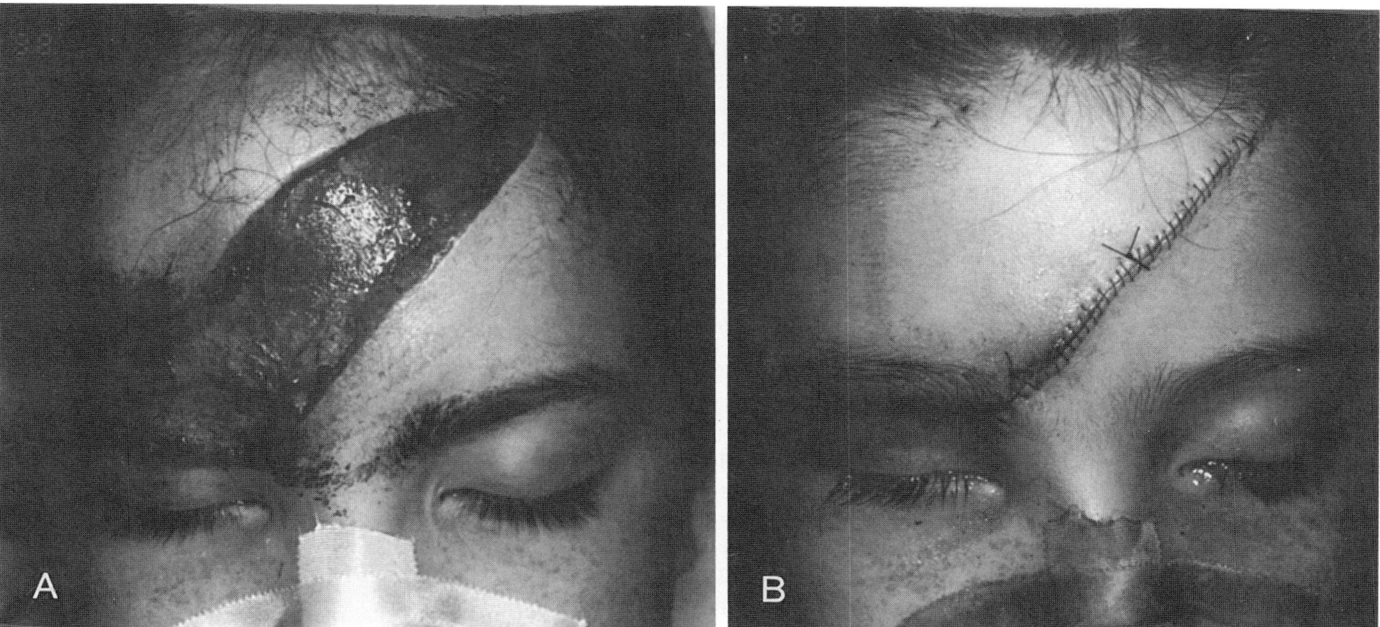

Figure 4.5. Complex laceration of the forehead and eyelid, **A**, before and **B**, after debridement and closure.

ally cannot be replaced, because it would act as a graft. Such a graft would be too thick to insure reliable take. However, if the tissue has been preserved and is gently handled, it may be possible to use only the avulsed skin as a graft, after debulking and defatting it. Since there are some exceptions to replacing avulsed tissue in infants, specialty consultation should be obtained.

Major avulsions, such as amputation of extremities, fingers, ears, nose, scalp, and eyelids, need specialty evaluation and care. Since replacement of avulsed tissue is possible if it is appropriately handled, the patient should be rapidly referred and transported to the specialty team. For appropriate techniques, see the discussion below on amputation of the upper extremity.

Bites. Bites from animals and humans are a major problem because they are heavily contaminated by bacteria. Most animal bites can be irrigated, debrided, and often closed with the expectation of uneventful healing. Although dog bites may be appropriately left open for wound care, most of these bites, if handled appropriately and closed, will heal without infection. Human bites, because of their much heavier bacterial contamination, should be irrigated, debrided, and left open. Broad-spectrum antibiotics should be administered following a human bite. Human bites to the hand are a special topic and will be discussed later. Immobilization and elevation of extremity wounds will be helpful in the healing of these heavily contaminated wounds.

Contaminated Wounds. A contaminated wound is one that has been exposed to bacteria from the body or local environment. The management of acute, significantly contaminated wounds consists of debridement, irrigation, consideration of antibiotics, and often secondary or delayed primary closure. Use of antibiotics is reserved for specific indications, such as severely contaminated wounds in immunocompromised patients and contaminated wounds involving deeper structures (such as joints and fractures) or when obvious infection is present. Choice of antibiotic depends on the most likely encountered organisms given the etiology of the injury. Coverage of *Staphylococcus aureus* is recommended in cutaneous wounds requiring antibiotics; an antibiotic resistant to penicillinase or a first-generation cephalosporin is commonly used. Contaminated wounds should be closed cautiously, depending on the degree of contamination and location of the wound. Deep sutures, if required, should be kept to a minimum and should be monofilament. Patients with contaminated wounds should be reevaluated within 24 to 48 hours. If there are any signs of deep infection on reevaluation, at least a portion of the wound should be opened by removing the sutures.

Contaminated Chronic Wounds. Lacerations and old open injuries of greater than 24 hours require debridement and irrigation. With few exceptions, systemic antibiotics are usually not helpful in controlling bacterial colonization within a chronic, contaminated wound. Antibiotic penetration into a chronic wound, with its granulating fibrous bed, is poor and unpredictable. Topical antibiotic creams such as silver sulfadiazine (Silvadene), bacitracin, and Neosporin may be helpful. Some of these topical agents inhibit epithelialization and initial aspects of wound healing, however. Highly toxic solutions such as alcohol or hydrogen peroxide may have an adverse affect on wound healing. Contaminated wounds should be closed only after bacterial contamination has been controlled. Chronic wounds that show no evidence of epithelialization or contraction, or that are any color but the beefy red of a granulating bed, usually contain significant bacterial contamination and may be clinically infected. Although the type of organism is important, the principal determinant of wound sepsis seems to be total bacterial load per gram of tissue.

Wound Management

The initial care of the wound is a major determinant in its healing. The cardinal principle is the gentle, careful handling of all injured tissue. The methodical assessment of the injury, followed by meticulous closure technique, will minimize deformity and maximize functional result. Evaluation should include an assessment of tissue injury, amount of tissue lost, and degree of injury to deeper structures. Treatment of a wound begins after the patient is evaluated and stabilized. After careful debridement and hemostasis, the injury pattern and tissue deficit are defined before the appropriate reconstructive technique is selected. Early care of the soft tissue injury involves controlling bleeding: direct pressure is usually adequate. It is an unusual wound that requires hemostats or vessel ligatures. Should direct pressure fail to control bleeding, proximal pressure may be applied directly with compression over the feeding vascular supply. Proximal pressure will cause less tissue damage than inappropriate clamping deep in a pool of blood. Tourniquets can increase venous bleeding or cause limb ischemia. Once bleeding has been controlled, the wound should be gently irrigated with a physiologic solution such as normal saline.

After the wound is cleaned, the viability of the wound margins is assessed. Clean lacerations have minimal surrounding tissue injury. Contused, contaminated wounds, on the other hand, have a crush component or surrounding ischemic tissue. In general, recent, clean wounds without tissue loss can be gently irrigated and closed. Crushed, contaminated wounds, however, have areas of tissue injury and devitalization that may require debridement and closure, delayed closure, or even the use of skin grafts or flaps to resurface injured areas that have inadequate overlying tissue. Specialized tissues, such as eyebrows, eyelids, ears, and lips—and other tissues that are difficult to replace precisely—should be debrided only by a physician experienced in complicated wound care. Some areas of the body, such as the face, have a rich vascular supply and tend to heal well, although initially the viability of portions of these wounds may be in question. As a rule, any questionable tissue should be gently irrigated and left for a reexamination 24 to 48 hours later. While contused, crushing injuries predictably have a less favorable outcome, precise reconstruction of these defects can optimize the results.

All penetrating injuries and many nonpenetrating injuries, such as abrasions and burns, require consideration of tetanus immunization status. Appropriate guidelines for wounds that may be tetanus prone should be followed (Table 4.1).

Reconstruction of Large Wounds and Tissue Defects

Wounds that cannot be repaired by simple approximation of the wound margins will frequently require an alternative method of reconstruction, such as a graft or flap. When choosing the appropriate method of recon-

Table 4.1.
Immunization Recommendations

History of Immunization	Tetanus Prone		Nontetanus Prone	
	Tetanus Toxoid	Tetanus Immune Globulin	Tetanus Toxoid	Tetanus Immune Globulin
Unknown or incomplete	0.5 mL[a]	250 units	0.5 mL[a]	No
Complete, last booster <5 yr ago	0.5 mL	No	No[b]	No
Complete, last booster <5 yr ago	No	No	No	No

[a]In unimmunized children, DT (diphtheria, tetanus) or DPT (diphtheria, pertussis, tetanus) is used. Completion of immunizations is necessary.
[b]Yes, if booster >10 years ago.

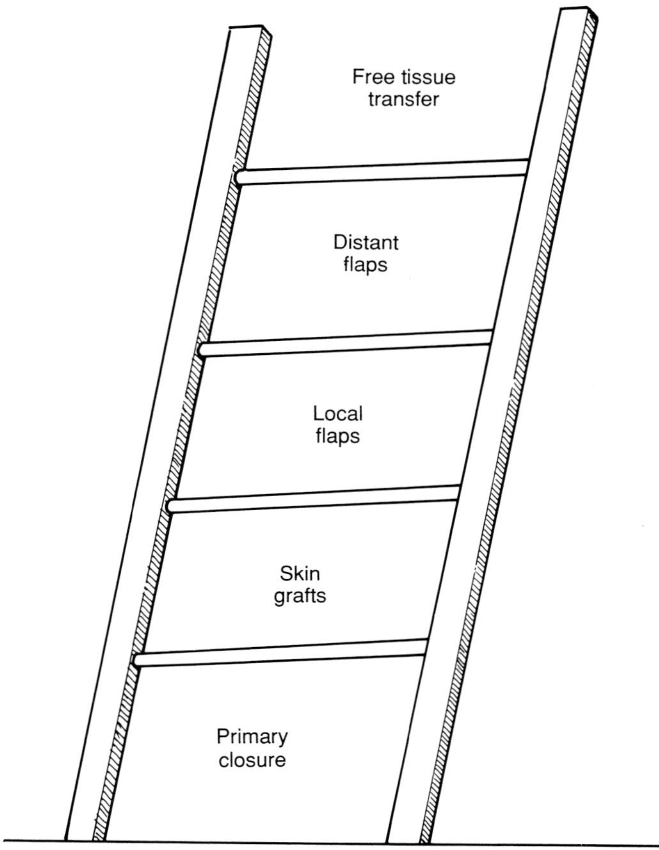

Figure 4.6. Reconstructive ladder.

struction, the concept of a "reconstructive ladder" must be borne in mind (Fig. 4.6). This reconstructive ladder is a classification of the methods of wound reconstruction according to increasing complexity of design. While simpler methods may often be the best, they will not always suffice. The different "rungs" of the ladder are discussed in this section.

Skin Grafts

A skin graft is defined as a portion of the skin consisting of the epidermis and a variable amount of dermis that is completely removed from its original location (donor site) and transferred to another area of the body (recipient site). No underlying tissue is included. Because of its separation, a skin graft must derive all of its nutritional supply from its recipient bed. It carries along no vasculature nor any lymphatic or nerve structures. Skin grafts are categorized according to species and thickness.

Species Classification. An autograft is a graft taken from one place on an individual and transplanted to another place on the same individual. Thus, immunologic compatibility is assured and the graft is considered permanent. An allograft (homograft) is a graft taken from one individual (usually a cadaver) and transplanted to another individual of the same species. In general, these grafts are useful for resurfacing defects for brief periods of time. Rejection eventually occurs, except in cases of transplantation among identical twins or, potentially, in permanently immunosuppressed individuals. The third type of species graft, the xenograft (heterograft), is a graft from a donor of one species to a recipient of a different species. A xenograft, commonly used in clinical practice, entails the use of porcine skin to cover large skin and soft tissue defects on a temporary basis. Both allografts and xenografts should be viewed as temporary methods of wound closure, or as biological dressings.

Thickness Classification. A split-thickness skin graft includes the epidermis and a portion of the dermis (Fig. 4.7). The graft includes a variable amount of dermal appendages, depending on the thickness of the dermis taken with the graft. The success of the skin graft increases with the thinner grafts, since they require less early diffusion to maintain their viability. Thinner grafts can also be expanded to a greater degree than thicker grafts. They are used in areas of large skin loss (Fig. 4.8), over areas of granulating tissue, and in areas of marginal vascularity of potential contamination. They are usually obtained using an air- or electric-powered dermatome, or a specialized free-hand knife. The donor site, representing a partial-thickness loss, heals by reepithelialization from wound edges and from residual deeper skin dermal appendages scattered throughout the wound base. The donor site itself requires ongoing care to prevent secondary infection, which, if present, can convert it to a full-thickness loss. This care consists of keeping the wound moist while minimizing contamination, pressure, and desiccation. The donor site should be treated as a clean abrasion. Split-thickness skin grafts are generally taken from the buttock or high thigh area because of the large amount of surface area available and the relatively inconspicuous location of the donor site.

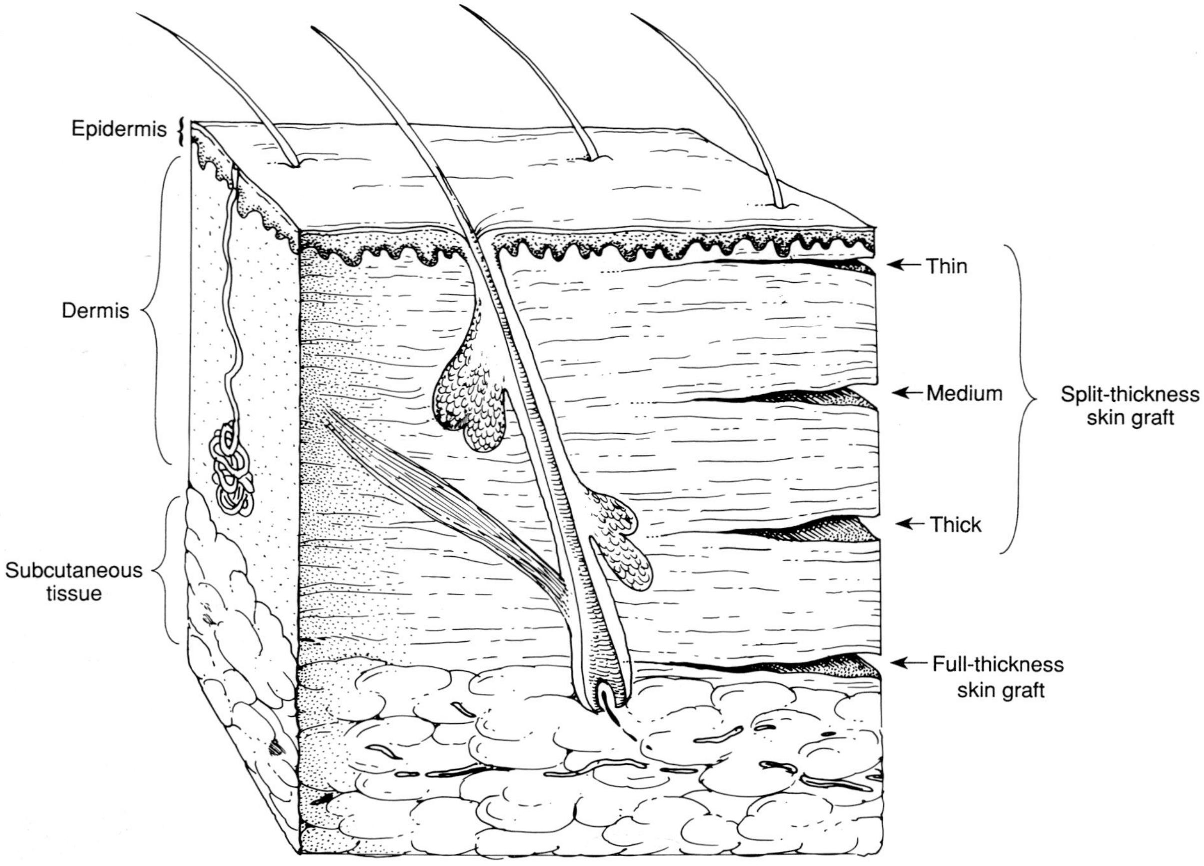

Figure 4.7. Different levels of thickness of skin grafts.

A full-thickness skin graft consists of the epidermal layer and the entire thickness of the dermis (Fig. 4.7). In contrast to a split-thickness graft, it provides a more durable cover, its appearance is more normal, and it carries an increased number of dermal appendages. However, because of its greater thickness and slower revascularization, it may be less likely to succeed than the split-thickness skin graft. The absolute thickness may vary according to the thickness of the dermis at the donor site. A thin full-thickness skin graft may be obtained from the eyelid or postauricular areas. Thicker full-thickness skin grafts can be obtained from the cervical and groin areas. Full-thickness grafts are usually used on the face because of their better color match, on the fingers to avoid joint contractures, and on any place that a thicker skin and smaller secondary contraction is desired. Because the donor site is a full-thickness defect, it must be managed by either primary closure or split-thickness skin grafting. This factor limits the size of full-thickness skin grafts. These grafts are usually taken from the groin, postauricular, upper eyelid, supraclavicular, or scalp areas. The last four locations are useful for reconstruction in the head and neck because of proper color match, but have a limited amount of skin available (Fig. 4.9).

When a graft is harvested, it immediately contracts after it is freed from the surrounding tissue. This phenomenon, primary skin graft contraction, is related to the number of elastin fibers in the graft. Thus, the thicker the graft—because it contains more elastin fibers—the greater the primary contraction. Secondary contraction occurs during the healing phase (Fig. 4.9). As healing occurs, the graft contracts to leave a smaller surface area. The thicker the graft, the less that secondary contraction occurs. This phenomenon is related more to the percentage of dermis in the graft than the actual thickness. Thus, a graft taking 50% of the dermis would be predicted to contract less than a graft containing 30%. Secondary contraction is mediated by myofibroblasts, which are specialized fibroblast-like cells containing smooth muscle contractile elements, within the wound itself. The dermis of the skin has been shown to suppress the myofibroblast population. Greater suppression is seen with greater thickness of the dermis.

Contraction must be taken into account when planning reconstruction. Thus, reconstruction of defects or scar contractures may need more graft placed than initially predicted. Secondary graft contraction, on the other hand, may be used to an advantage. A large defect can be surfaced with a thin split-thickness skin graft in expectation that the total surface area will shrink with the skin graft contraction. A secondary procedure can then be performed to excise a portion of the defect and leave a much smaller defect.

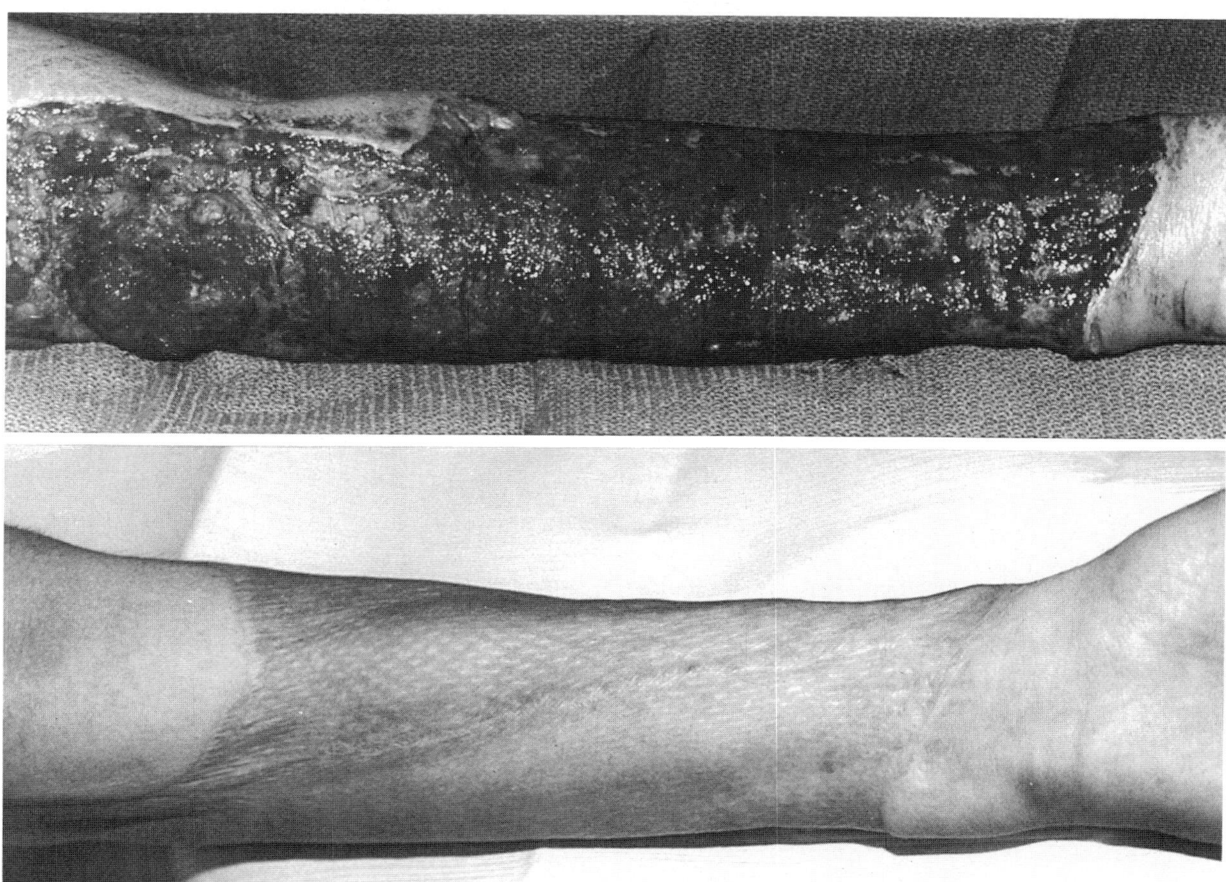

Figure 4.8. Open wound of the forearm **A**, prior to split-thickness skin grafting and **B**, after successful healing of a meshed graft.

Split thickness	Full thickness
Easier take (more reliable)	Difficult take
Less 1° contraction	Greater 1° contraction
Greater 2° contraction	Less 2° contraction
Donor site heals by re-epithelialization	Donor site must be closed
May be used in most wounds	Used in specialized situations

Figure 4.9. Comparison of split-thickness and full-thickness skin grafts.

Skin Graft Healing. As the skin graft is completely isolated from its original nutrient source, it must survive initially by recipient bed diffusion into the graft itself. The diffusion of nutritional elements and fluid from the recipient site and the subsequent diffusion back to the host bed of metabolic waste products is called plasma imbibition. This process allows skin graft survival for the first 48–72 hours after graft placement. Vascular ingrowth begins shortly after placement of the skin graft on the host bed. However, adequate nutritional exchange to maintain tissue viability does not occur until 48–72 hours after graft placement. The new ingrowth of capillary tissue into the graft (neovascularization) is called inosculation.

The recipient bed should be prepared by minimizing bacterial concentration and preparing for good vascularization. Wounds may need to be debrided at the time of grafting or even several days before grafting. Adequate vascular supply must be assured, particularly in the compromised extremity. While physical examination is usually sufficient, Doppler examinations or arteriography may be necessary. Should local blood flow be thought inadequate, a vascular bypass or other procedure may be necessary. The well-vascularized recipient site, if kept clean, will show signs of local capillary proliferation. The mixture of capillary buds and connective tissue, called granulation tissue, is usually a beefy red color and bleeds easily to the touch. In most cases it forms a good recipient bed for skin grafting, but because it represents a chronic open wound, it also supports bacterial growth.

The graft should be immobilized on the recipient site to prevent shear forces from dislodging the tenuous ingrowth of new capillaries. Separation of the graft from its bed will prevent both the diffusion of nutrients and the ingrowth of new vascular tissue, resulting in loss of the skin graft. Because skin grafts require a well-vascularized recipient bed, they do not take on relatively

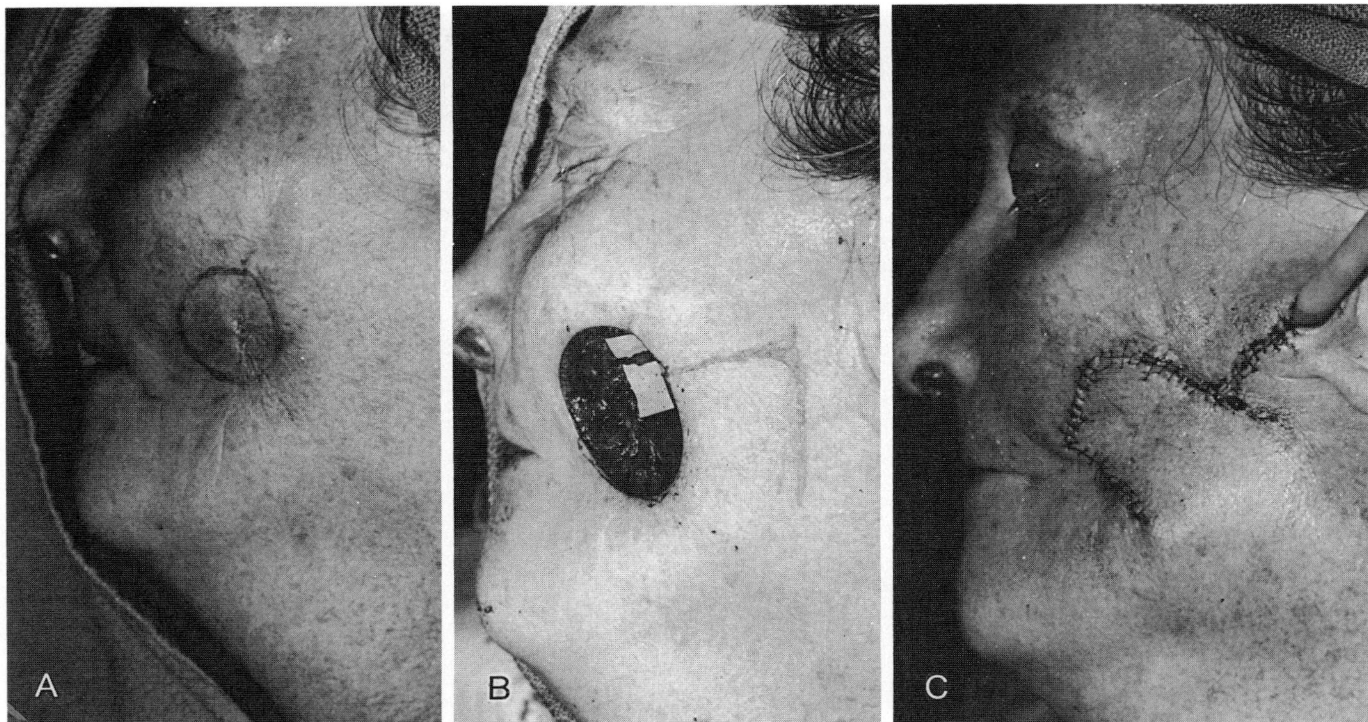

Figure 4.10. **A**, This recurrent basal cell carcinoma of the cheek required, **B**, resection, and **C**, coverage with a random pattern skin flap of adjacent cheek skin. The length-to-width ratio of the flap is about 1 to 1.

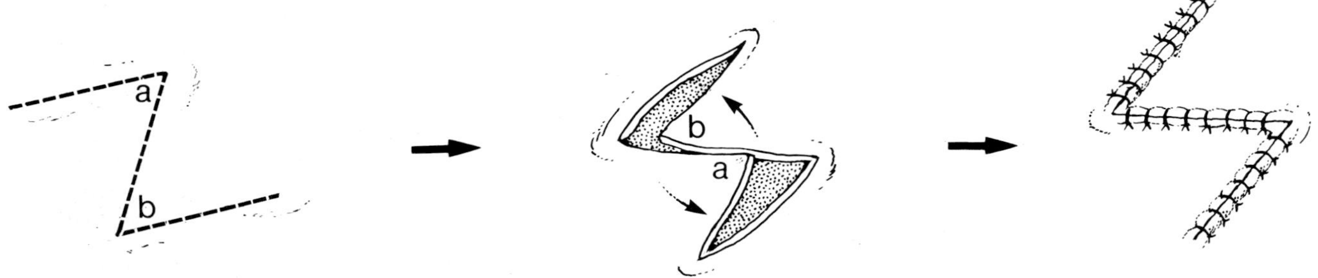

Figure 4.11. Z-plasty: a Z-plasty is used to reorient a scar and lengthen the scar (distance A to B) at the expense of width.

avascular structures such as bone, tendon, heavily irradiated areas, and infected wounds. On the other hand, skin grafts take well on periosteum, paratenon, and perichondrium.

Graft failure is usually a result of mechanical blockage of diffusion, such as hematoma or seroma under the graft, presence of shearing forces dislodging the graft from its recipient bed, or inadequate recipient site (either because of contamination or poor blood supply). Systemic factors, such as malnutrition, sepsis, and medications, may also play a role in the success of the skin graft. Systemic steroids, antineoplastic agents, and vasoconstrictors (nicotine) may adversely affect skin graft survival, as well as wound healing in general.

Flaps

Tissues transferred from one location to another that are supported by an intact blood supply are commonly known as flaps. They are generally used to replace tissue lost to trauma or surgical excision. They may be used to provide temporary or permanent skin coverage in critical areas that require a good soft tissue bulk for underlying structures (such as tendons and joints). They also may provide increased padding over bony prominences (such as in pressure sore reconstruction). They bring in a better blood supply to relatively poorly vascularized areas and, on occasion, may be used to improve sensation to an area by bringing in an accompanying nerve supply. In addition, they can be used to carry specialized reconstructive

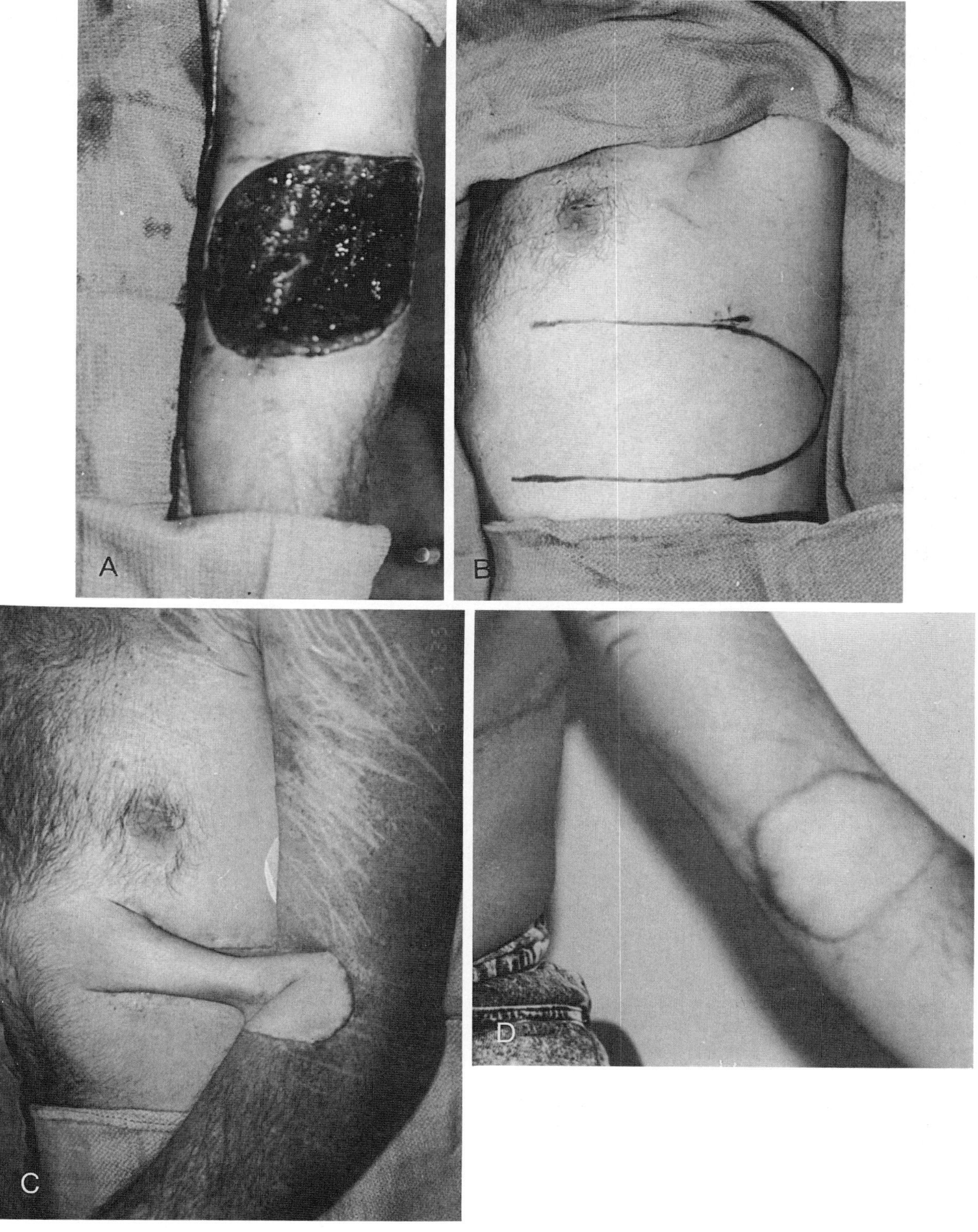

Figure 4.12. **A**, Open wound of the antecubital fossa. **B**, A thoracoepigastric axial pattern skin flap is designed. Note that its length greatly exceeds its width. **C**, The flap is attached as a pedicled flap and is left for several weeks prior to division of the pedicle. **D**, The pedicle has now been divided, inset, and has healed.

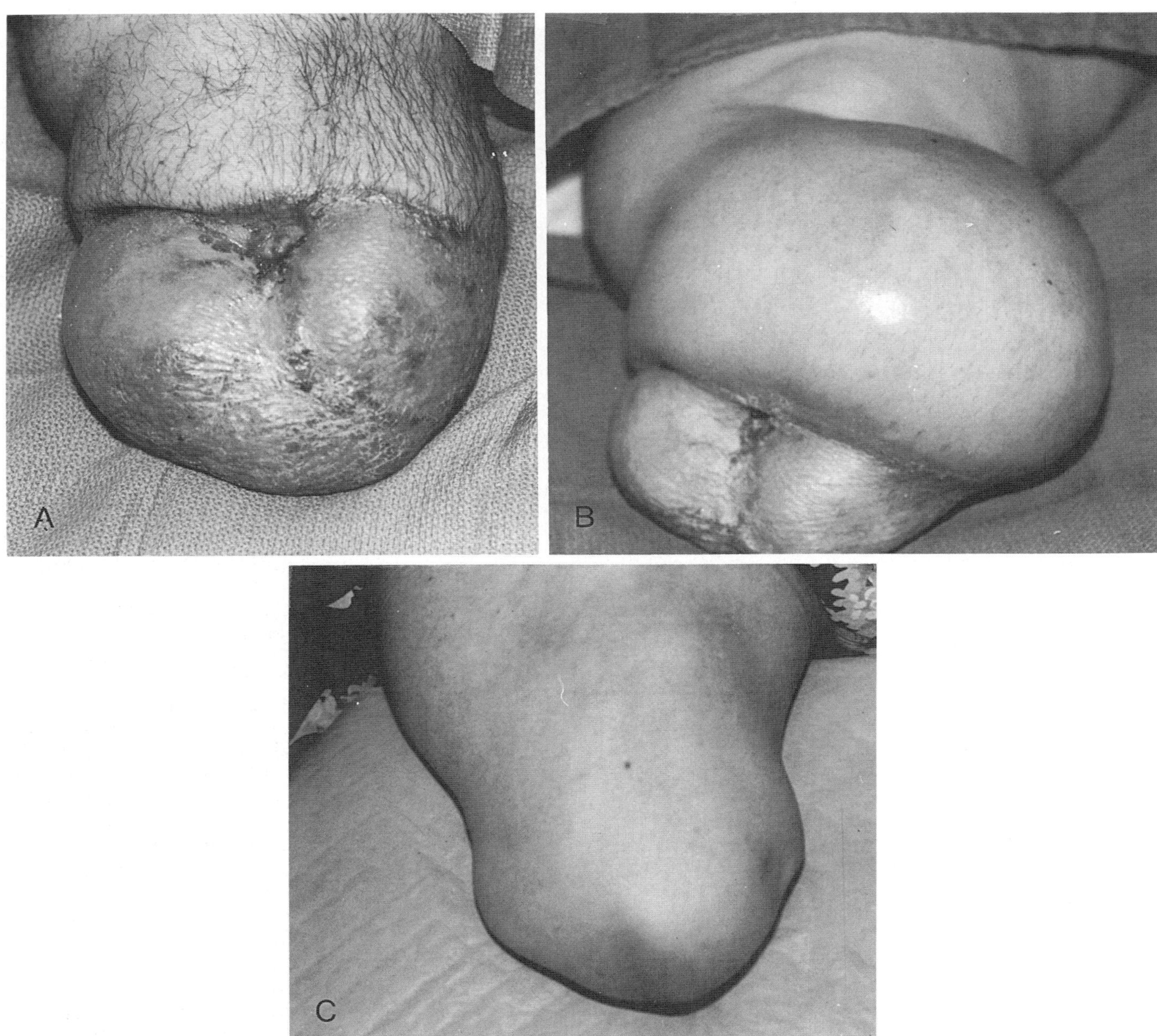

Figure 4.13. **A**, This patient presents with inadequate skin graft coverage of a below-knee amputation stump. **B**, A tissue expander is placed anteriorly and has now been fully inflated. **C**, The skin graft has been removed and the expanded skin used to cover the distal stump.

tissue such as bone or cartilage. They may consist of skin, subcutaneous tissue, muscle, bone, cartilage, and such specialized tissues as jejunum, bowel, omentum, or fascia. Skin flaps may be classified according to their vascular anatomy as random or axial and according to their anatomic location as local, regional, or distant.

A random skin flap consists of an area of skin and subdermal tissue without a specifically defined vascular distribution (Fig. 4.10). For viability, the flap depends mostly upon the random dermal and subdermal plexus of vascular structures. It has a limited length-to-width ratio (usually 1:1) to assure that enough blood vessels will be included to provide nutrition throughout its length. Random flaps may be raised in any location, assuming normal vascularity of the skin. Random flaps on the face may be raised with a slightly greater ratio (1.5:1 or 2:1), because of the excellent vascularity of the face.

Z-plasties represent specific use of random pattern skin flaps. These involve the raising of two random flaps in the shape of a Z, which are then interdigitated with one another (Fig. 4.11). In so doing, two things are accomplished. Most importantly, the scar is lengthened at the expense of width. Also, the direction of the scar is reoriented. Z-plasties are frequently employed when scar contractures have developed.

Axial pattern or arterialized flaps are similar to random pattern flaps with the exception that the tissue includes a named blood supply (Fig. 4.12). It is important that the underlying vasculature be well mapped and that the flap outline be designed to maximize the vascular supply; it must include a direct artery and accompanying vein(s). Specific axial pattern skin flaps have been described in different anatomic locations taking advantage of known cutaneous arteries. Because of this known arterial supply, generally a greater length-to-width ratio (up to 5 or 6 to 1) is possible than with the random flap. Certain axial flaps may be used as free flaps (see below).

Tissue expansion is a comparatively new technique that uses the ability of skin to relax and expand as a result of tension applied to it. When local tissue directly adjacent to the wound is the best option for reconstruction, the two-staged process of tissue expansion is used. An inflatable prosthesis is placed beneath the skin or other tissue to be expanded. Then, after initial healing, the expander is serially inflated through a valve or injection port, usually on a weekly basis. Once full expansion is achieved, the expander is removed at a second operation and the expanded tissue is used as a local flap to reconstruct the wound (Fig. 4.13).

Myocutaneous flaps are the next most complex form of flaps used for reconstruction (Fig. 4.14). The skin overlying many muscles of the body is supported by vessels that course directly from the muscle to the skin, known as musculocutaneous perforators. Thus, large amounts of skin left attached to the underlying muscle can be transferred from one location to another as long as the blood supply to the underlying muscle is preserved. Knowledge of the blood supply to these muscles has allowed the rotation or transposition of the tissue from the donor site to the reconstructed wound using the location of the dominant vasculature as the pivot point for the arc of rotation. In certain circumstances a muscle alone is transferred and subsequently skin grafted.

If local skin flaps or regional myocutaneous flaps are not available for wound reconstruction, free flaps raised from a distant site may be used. These flaps are transplanted from one site of the body to another by isolating the dominant artery and vein(s) to a flap and performing a microscopic anastomosis between these and vessels in the recipient wound. While muscle and skin are most commonly used, bone, nerves, tendons, jejunum, and omentum may also be transferred. These flaps are predominantly used in lower extremity, breast, and head and neck reconstructions, although they may be applied to almost any reconstruction situation (Fig. 4.15).

Management of Benign Skin Lesions

Types of Lesions

Skin lesions are either benign or malignant, and differentiation is important in providing appropriate care. Common benign lesions include nevus, keratosis, verruca, fibroma, and hemangioma. Common malignant lesions include basal cell carcinoma, squamous cell carcinoma, and melanoma. (Malignant lesions are discussed in EGS2, Chapter 28.)

The *nevus* is the most common lesion in the adult. It is usually brown, slightly raised, and it may have hair (Fig. 4.16). Nevi are subclassified according to appearance and depth of active proliferating cells. Some nevi, dysplastic nevi, have a potential for malignant transformation; they are typically smooth with irregular borders and display various shades of brown. While it is impractical to excise all nevi, suspicious pigmented lesions having a recent change in size, elevation, color (brown to black or gray), or irregular borders (notching) should be excised. Other lesions that should be excised are those with a surface discharge, a tingling sensation, bleeding, itching, or those that are constantly irritated, as those under a belt line or bra. All significant nevi should be carefully observed.

The second most common type of benign lesion is the *keratosis*. It is subclassified into seborrheic, senile or actinic, and keratoacanthoma. The seborrheic keratosis is elevated, brown, and has a greasy feeling. It can be treated by freezing, scraping, cauterizing, or excision. If the diagnosis is uncertain, it should be excised. The senile or actinic keratosis is a rough, irregularly shaped, brownish patch, most commonly seen in the elderly. Because it may be premalignant, it should be removed.

The *verruca* (wart) usually has a viral etiology. It is characteristically self-limiting and spontaneous disappearance is the rule. Surgical excision is occasionally indicated, especially if the lesion occurs on pressure points and is symptomatic (soles of feet and palms of hands).

The *keratoacanthoma* is a rapidly growing, elevated lesion. It may have a central crater or ulceration (Fig. 4.17). It usually resolves spontaneously in 4 to 6 months. Concern over its growth and appearance, however, justifies excision for diagnosis.

Fibromas present as solid lesions just below the skin surface and may involve skin structures. They are subclassified into fibromas, neurofibromas, and dermatofibromas. All three types should be excised. If the neurofibromas occur as a neurofibromatosis syndrome (von Recklinghausen's disease), they may be too numerous to excise. Symptomatic and enlarging lesions should be removed.

The *hemangioma* is the most common benign tumor of infancy. It consists of an abnormal collection of blood vessels. Several classifications exist based on the likelihood of proliferation or regression. Treatment is observation unless these tumors become physiologically or functionally important—producing visual or airway obstruction, bleeding, or ulceration.

Techniques for Excision

The goal in excising small skin lesions or other subcutaneous lesions (such as cysts or lipomas) is to completely remove the lesion while leaving as inconspicuous a scar as possible. Some factors contributing to the achievement

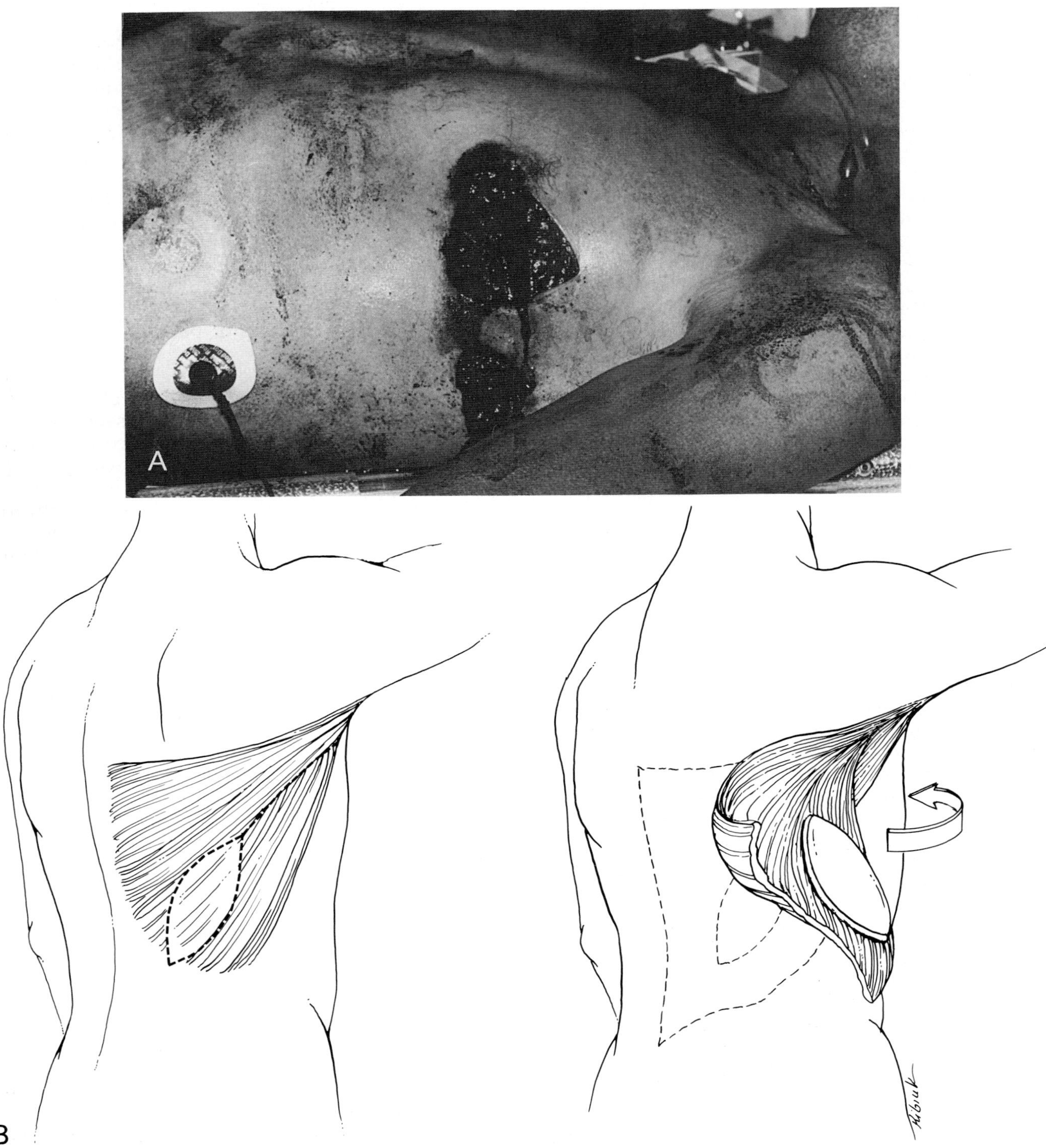

Figure 4.14. **A**, This patient has sustained a point-blank shotgun blast to the chest. **B**, The defect will be closed with a latissimus dorsi myocutaneous flap. **C**, Once the flap is elevated, it is tunneled into the defect on the chest. **D**, The patient following successful reconstruction.

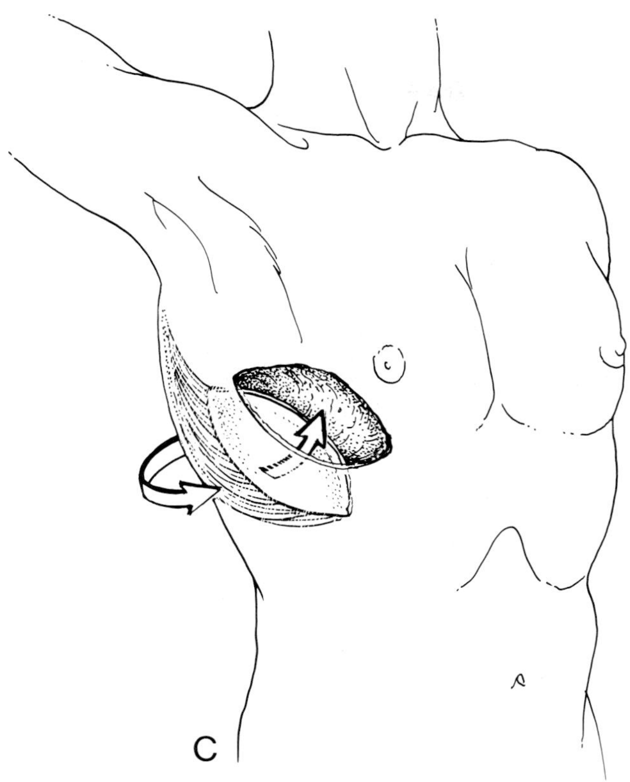

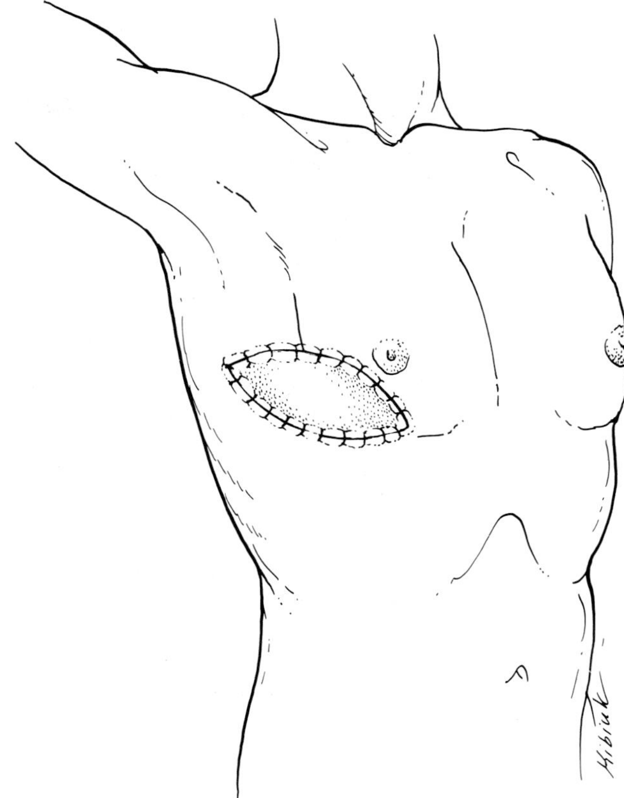

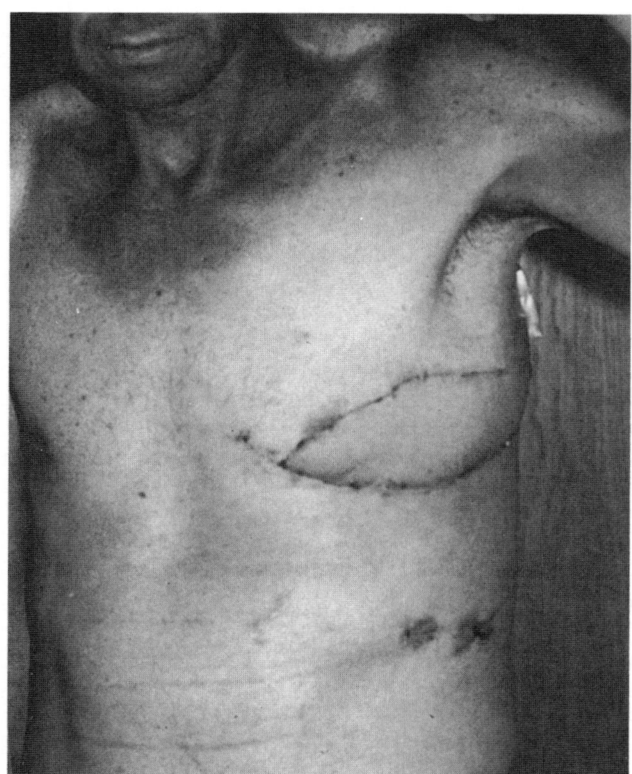

Figure 4.14. *(continued)*

of this goal are not under the control of the surgeon: location, size, and orientation of the lesion, and overall health and age of the patient. Operative technique, however, is controllable. A spindle-shaped or lenticular incision is made, with the total length of the spindle being about twice the diameter of the lesion. The long axis of the incision should parallel lines of relaxed skin tension, so that the ultimate scar is as inconspicuous as possible. The incision should be distinctly into the subcutaneous tissue but not penetrate into fascia or deeper structures. Gentle undermining can help decrease tension on the closure. A careful, layered closure will provide the best result. The specimen should always be sent to the pathologist, even when it appears to be benign.

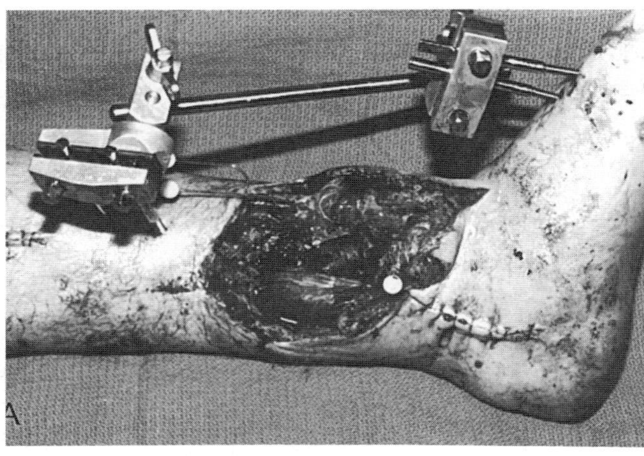

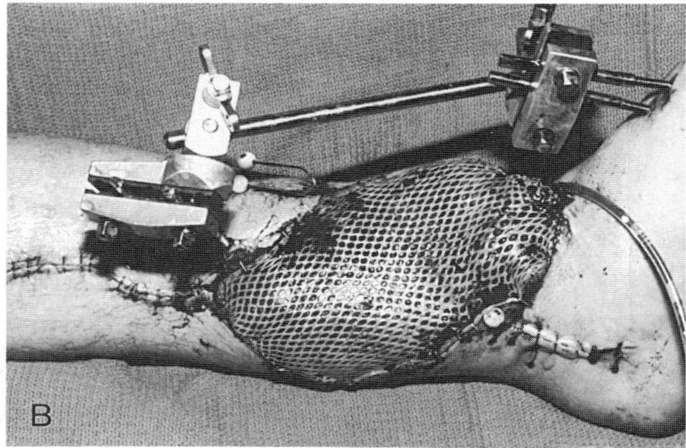

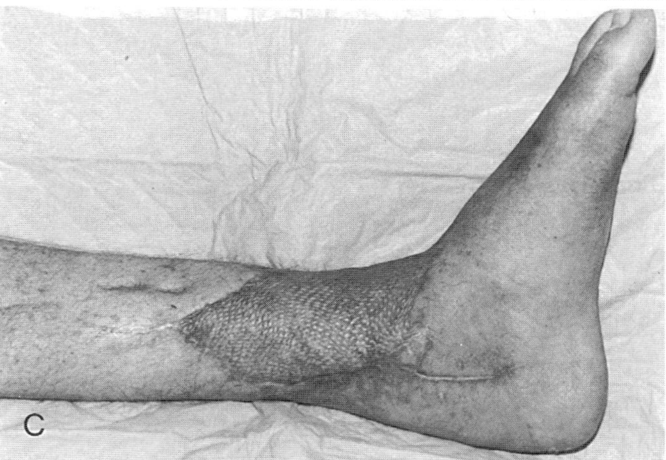

Figure 4.15. A close-range shotgun blast to the ankle has required external fixation of the ankle, and vascular reconstruction. **B**, The ankle is seen immediately following reconstruction with a free muscle flap and skin graft. **C**, Long-term result showing satisfactory reconstruction of the ankle.

Facial Trauma

The care of the patient with facial injuries requires early wound care; precise diagnosis by history, physical examination, radiographic studies; and appropriate wound repair and fracture stabilization. Facial fractures should be reduced and stabilized within the first 7 to 10 days. If the patient's general condition allows and evaluation of the facial injuries is complete, early repair is preferable. If, on the other hand, the patient has other significant injuries (such as closed head, intrathoracic, or intra-abdominal injuries), medical attention to these injuries takes priority over repair of the facial fractures. Secondary revision of facial injuries may be required but should be delayed until scars have matured and fractures healed (6–12 months). Skin grafts and flaps are occasionally required for large soft tissue defects.

Emergency Care

Initial care of the facially injured patient focuses on managing the airway and controlling bleeding. Foreign material and blood should be removed from the airway either by hand or by suction. Tracheostomy is seldom indicated when the injury involves only the facial soft tissues. However, with difficult problems involving facial fractures, bleeding, and potential cervical spine injuries, early tracheostomy or cricothyroidotomy may be appropriate. After the airway is clear, bleeding should be controlled. Direct pressure usually is adequate. Dressings wrapped around the face rarely ensure prolonged control of bleeding. Vessels should not be clamped until the injury can be adequately visualized, since blind clamping risks injury to important facial structures, such as the facial nerve. Circulating blood volume should be restored as hemorrhage is controlled.

After the extent of injury is assessed, the wound is meticulously cleansed. As previously noted, irrigation and debridement are important. All foreign material should be carefully removed. Gentle, manual palpation of the wound may demonstrate retained foreign material that is not otherwise evident. All wounds should also be palpated or gently explored for the possibility of underlying injury to bony structures. Manual physical examination is the most sensitive means of evaluating the presence of facial fractures. After initial wound care and hemostasis, the underlying structures can be repaired.

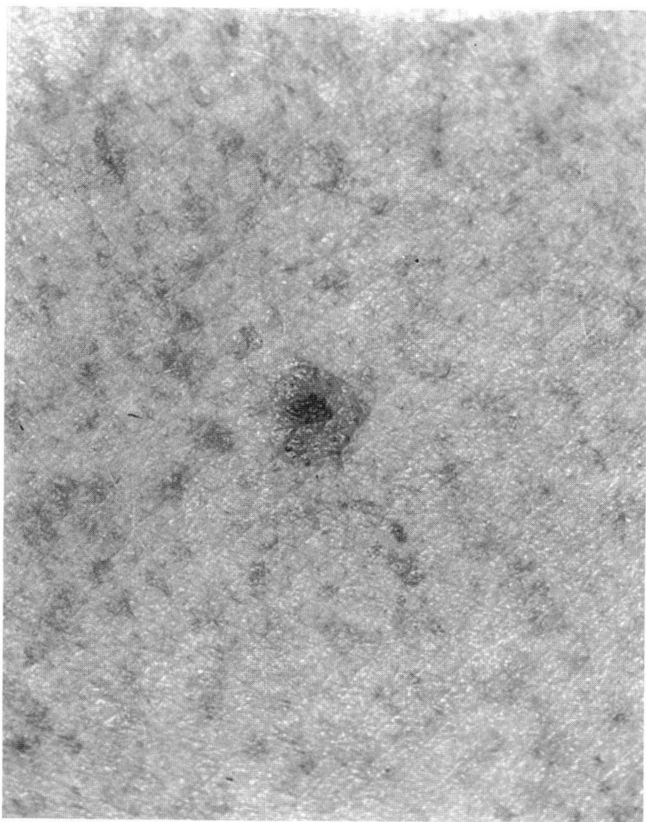

Figure 4.16. Benign nevus.

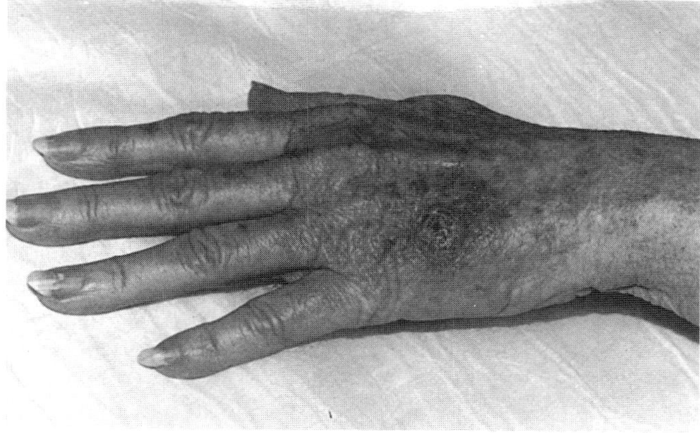

Figure 4.17. Keratoacanthoma of the hand; note the central crater or ulcer.

Soft Tissue Defects

As soon as the patient's general condition allows, soft tissue injuries are treated. Ideally, treatment would follow within the first several hours after injury. If the patient's general condition is not good, primary wound closure may be delayed. Because of the excellent vascular supply of the face, facial wounds can be closed up to 24 hours after injury if necessary.

Soft tissue repair of the face requires gentle cleansing, minimal debridement, and restoration of all available parts. Most injuries result in little or no tissue loss once they are evaluated. The illusion of skin loss is the result of skin elasticity and retraction. Although nonviable tissue should be removed, questionable areas of skin should be put back in place gently.Most promptly repaired facial wounds do not require antibiotics. Tetanus prophylaxis, however, should always be considered.

Early skillful repair of soft tissue injuries provides the best result. Local anesthetics containing epinephrine should be used to allow adequate wound cleansing and assist with hemostasis. After the wound is irrigated and debrided, it should be carefully closed. The possibility of injury to deeper structures such as the facial nerve, lacrimal apparatus, or parotid duct should be considered next (Fig. 4.18). Although rapid assessment of facial nerve function is possible in the awake, cooperative patient, it can be extremely difficult in the multiply injured or comatose patient. Ideally, facial nerve injuries should be identified on initial physical examination so that repair may be planned. Parotid duct injuries should be suspected when a cheek laceration crosses a line from the tragus of the ear to the base of the nose.

Injuries about the eyelids should also be carefully evaluated because of the precision of repair required and the possibility of injury to the lacrimal apparatus. Debridement must be conservative in such specialized areas as the eyebrows, eyelids, nose, ears, and lips. Because these areas are extremely difficult to reconstruct, it is better to repair questionably ischemic areas, even if a minor revision is required later, than to sacrifice large portions of tissue. However, obviously nonviable tissue must always be debrided.

Treatment of specific injuries, such as abrasions and lacerations, is similar to that in other parts of the body. Lacerations about the lip and other such areas require independent reconstruction of the muscle layers. For most injuries, topical antibiotic ointments are adequate to keep the wound clean and moist (their antimicrobial component has minimal effect). Systemic antibiotics are not routinely required in facial injuries unless there has been massive and gross contamination or open injuries to deeper structures such as cartilage or bone. Sutures should be left in place for 5–6 days. In significantly contused and crushed tissue, sutures may be left a few days longer. Although an individual's initial injury and genetic makeup are the main determinants in healing outcome, appropriate initial handling of the wound is also an important factor.

Simple lacerations are appropriately repaired by a generalist using careful technique. Extra care should be taken in reapproximating the vermilion border of the lips and repairing eyelids; eyebrows should not be shaved. More complex injuries involving stellate lacerations, crush injuries, or devitalized or avulsed tissue should be referred to a specialist. Likewise, significant injuries to the eyelids and injuries involving deeper structures (nerve injury, parotid duct injury, fractures) require prompt referral.

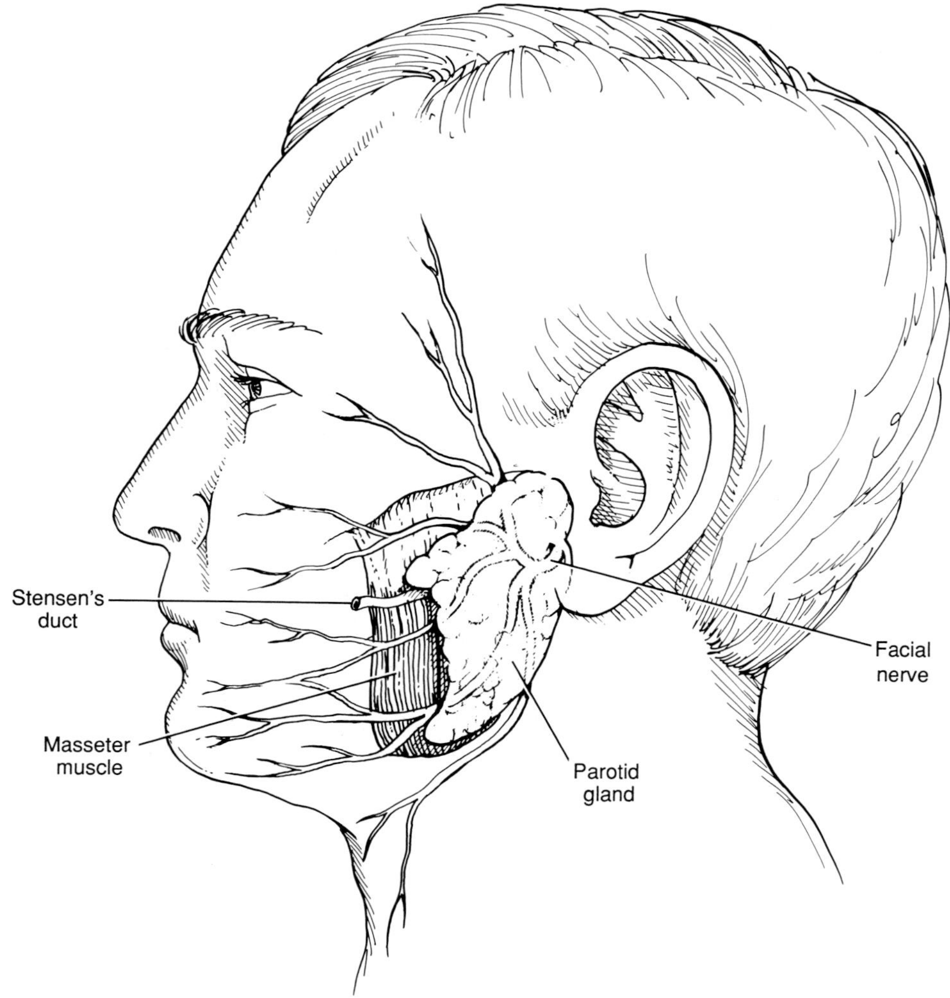

Figure 4.18. Anatomy of the parotid gland showing Stensen's duct and the relationship of the facial nerve to the parotid gland and the face.

Facial Fractures

General Principles. Facial fractures are relatively common in the traumatized patient. The usual etiology is a motor vehicle accident or an altercation. Other causes include sports injuries and penetrating trauma. These fractures may be open or closed injuries. However, overlying tissue may be significantly injured or contused in closed injuries. A history of the injury will often indicate the facial area involved. The nasal bone and zygomatic-malar area are the most commonly injured areas, followed by the mandibular area. Maxillary fractures, although less common, also are seen frequently. A high percentage of patients have multiple facial fractures.

Most facial fractures can be diagnosed on the basis of physical examination, which should include gentle examination and palpation of the facial bones. A fracture is to be suspected if there is any mobility of facial bones, asymmetry, palpable bony step-offs, extraocular muscle irregularities, sensory loss, localized pain or tenderness, or malocclusion of the teeth. This examination should be followed by a radiographic evaluation, first ensuring that the cervical spine is uninjured. Of patients with significant facial injuries, 15–25% have concomitant cervical spine injuries. The possibility of skull fractures and intracranial injuries should also be evaluated.

X-ray evaluation consists of a complete facial bone series, which includes the Water's, anterior-posterior, and lateral views. The Water's view demonstrates most clearly the entire facial complex and is most helpful. Currently, however, computed tomography (CT) scans in both axial and coronal planes are the most accurate method of visualizing complex fractures. Mandibular x-ray evaluation is best obtained with the panorex (panoramic x-ray) view. This specialized x-ray is superior to plain films of the mandible. Its disadvantage, however, is that in most facilities the patient must be in an upright position, a difficult position for the patient with multiple injuries.

After facial fractures have been identified, the urgency of their treatment should be assessed. Urgency depends on the likelihood of continued bleeding, cerebral spinal fluid leak, or loss of airway because of shift-

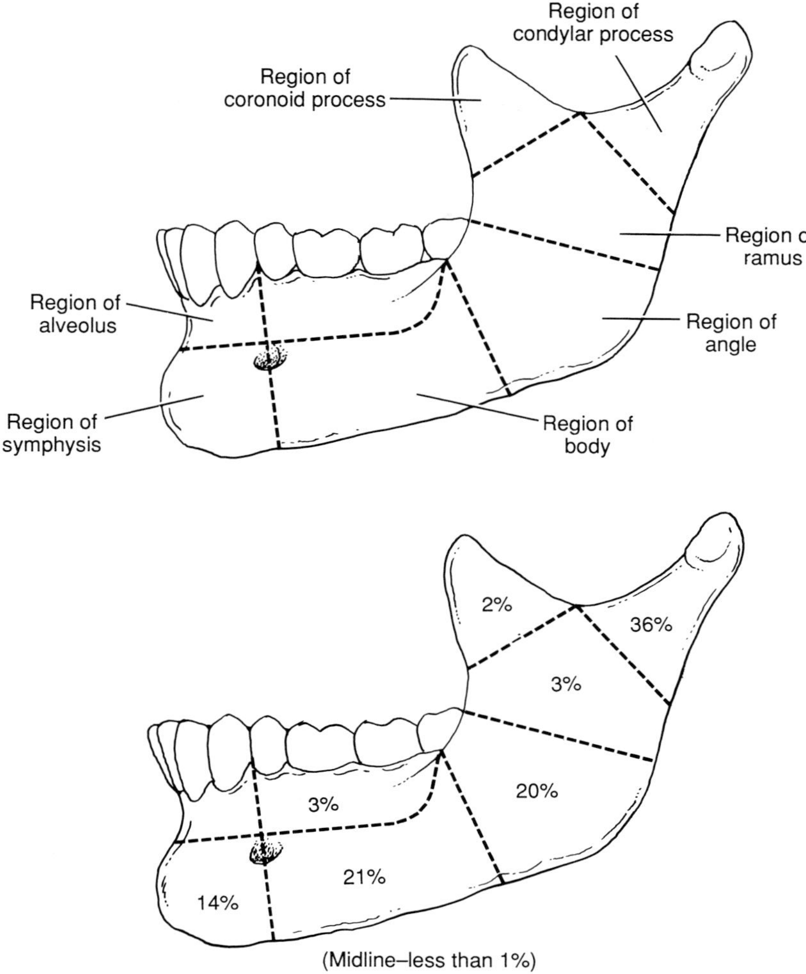

Figure 4.19. **A**, Anatomy of mandibular regions. **B**, Frequency of fractures by mandibular regions.

ing oropharyngeal structures. Early consultation with all services treating facial fractures should be made. If the patient is stable and treatment not urgent, repair of the facial fractures may be appropriately delayed for up to a week without adverse effects. This interval gives adequate time for evaluation and treatment of other injuries and for reduction of facial edema.

The principal goal of facial fracture reconstruction is the restoration of normal (premorbid) function and appearance. This goal is achieved by precise, anatomic reconstruction of all fractured bone segments, usually by open reduction and internal fixation. While closed reduction may be adequate for simple fractures, internal fixation with interosseous wires or with plates or screws is most commonly performed. Currently, the replacement of unusable fragments of bone with immediate bone grafts is favored.

Mandibular Fractures. Mandibular fractures occur frequently in facial trauma and are rarely isolated to one location. In patients with mandibular fractures, 94% have associated fractures in a second area of the mandible because of its ring structure: when force is applied at one point sufficient to produce a fracture, a second fracture site is likely as the force is transmitted to the entire ring. Some regions are more frequently associated with multiple fractures (Fig. 4.19). Fractures of the mandibular condyle are often associated with fractures of the symphysis and the corresponding condyle on the contralateral side. Mandibular body fractures are associated with fractures of the contralateral mandibular angle.

The classification of mandibular fractures is similar to that of long bone fractures. Simple fractures show no break in the overlying skin. Greenstick fractures, unusual in the mandible, exhibit bending of the bone with an incomplete fracture involving the cortex. These fractures are more likely to occur in children. Compound or open fractures, extremely common in the mandible, involve an external or internal (intraoral) wound associated with a break in the bone. Although the overlying skin may not be broken, fractures into the tooth-bearing area are essentially open and should be treated as such. Alveolar fractures involve only the alveolar process and not other portions of the main body of the bone. These are more common in the maxillary than in the mandibular area. Multiple fractures, as previously mentioned, are common. Anatomically, most mandibular fractures occur in the condylar area. The mandibular body in the molar region accounts for the next most common location, followed by the angle.

Dislocation of the mandibular condyle, which is occasionally seen, may be unilateral or bilateral. Signs are inability to close the jaw, malocclusion, and pain. The dislocation is reduced by pressing downward on the mandible and sliding it posteriorly into position. Because the muscles of mastication (primarily the masseter and temporalis) quickly go into spasm, reduction may require sedation and occasionally general anesthesia. Recurrence is relatively common.

Evaluation. The first priority in evaluating the patient with a mandibular fracture is assessment of the airway. Manual displacement of the mandible forward will usually relieve obstruction by the tongue. In certain cases emergent definitive airway management may be needed. Routine complaints include alteration of normal dental occlusion, abnormal position of the teeth, and abnormal mobility of the mandible. Manual palpation shows disjointed movement of the mandible and some separation between mandibular fragments. Patients almost uniformly complain of pain. The presence of crepitus is unusual in mandibular fractures but when present is virtually pathognomonic of a fracture. Patients may also demonstrate lacerated gingiva or mucosal ecchymosis. Occasionally, patients will complain of anesthesia in the lower teeth, a condition secondary to an injury or contusion to the inferior alveolar nerve.

Fractured mandibles are usually displaced. Appreciation of the normal pull of the muscle of mastication can be used to predict motion of the mandibular fragments. By evaluating the location of the mandible fracture and taking into account the location of muscle insertion and vector of pull, one can accurately predict the direction of displacement and give an estimate of ultimate stability of the fracture. If the normal muscle pull tends to reduce the mandibular fracture, the fracture is termed a *favorable* fracture. If the normal muscle pull tends to distract the bony fragments, the fracture is termed *unfavorable*. This distinction can be helpful in determining whether a closed reduction is adequate or whether an open reduction will be required.

Treatment. Treatment methods include closed reduction, open reduction and internal fixation, or external fixation. A minimally displaced fracture can be treated by *closed reduction* (wiring the teeth together into normal occlusion). Good dentition with a reliable and stable occlusion is necessary for this type of treatment. This method involves the placement of maxillary and mandibular arch bars that are wired or banded together in what is known as intermaxillary fixation. From 4 to 6 weeks of fixation are necessary in adults, and 2 to 4 weeks in children. *Open reduction*, with direct visualization of the fractures and wiring or plating in some configuration, is frequently necessary. The advantage of this method is better approximation of the fracture site. In addition, internal fixation prevents displacement and movement of the fracture, which provides more precise restoration of occlusion. Open reduction can be accomplished both extraorally (through a neck incision) or intraorally. Intermaxillary fixation is almost always used with internal fixation methods to help with fracture alignment. The open technique carries a higher incidence of infection (4–5%) than the closed technique. *External fixation* with an external appliance may be used in complicated fractures, or fractures with significant bone loss.

Complications. Mandibular fractures may have multiple complications. Delayed healing occurs in the presence of inadequate or loosened fixation, infection, or a fault in the reduction and fixation technique. Loosened fixation is associated with either initially poor technique, poor patient compliance, or secondary infection. Malunion is due to lack of adequate treatment or lack of patient compliance regarding proper oral hygiene and wound care. Malunion essentially allows healing to take place in a nonanatomic position, resulting in a significant amount of functional difficulty due to the resultant malocclusion. Malunion may require further surgery. Nonunion is the result of delayed healing, which is frequently secondary to inadequate fixation or infection. Treatment of nonunion consists of debriding the area and inserting a bone graft.

Special Cases. Mandibular condyle fractures deserve separate consideration. Patients routinely complain of tenderness and pain in the preauricular area. The mandible may deviate toward the fractured side upon opening because of pterygoid muscle function. Mandibular movement is limited and there may be malocclusion and preauricular swelling. On examination, there is pain on palpation of the anterior wall of the external auditory canal. Occasionally, hemotympanum or external auditory canal laceration is noted. Radiographically, a panorex view is the best diagnostic tool. Only rarely is a CT scan helpful in evaluating a difficult mandibular fracture.

Treatment of mandibular condyle fractures is usually by closed reduction, which is accomplished by intermaxillary fixation with the patient in correct occlusion. When adequate occlusion cannot be obtained by closed reduction, open reduction of the condylar fracture is indicated. Complications of mandibular condyle fractures include ankylosis, temporomandibular joint dysfunction, limited postoperative motion, malocclusion, occasional sequestration of a dislocated fragment, and chorda tympani nerve damage (especially with dislocation). In children, aseptic necrosis with disruption of mandibular growth may occur with condylar fractures. Rarely, seventh nerve paralysis occurs in association with open reduction of the condylar fracture.

Edentulous patients with mandibular fractures are a therapeutic problem. Signs and symptoms are basically the same as for patients with dentition. However, bilateral body fractures are more common because of the atrophy of the mandibular segment in that area. Edentulous patients also have a much higher incidence of nonunion because of poorer bony stock and decreased strength of the small atrophic mandible.

During the period of intermaxillary fixation, attention to oral hygiene is necessary. Although it is difficult

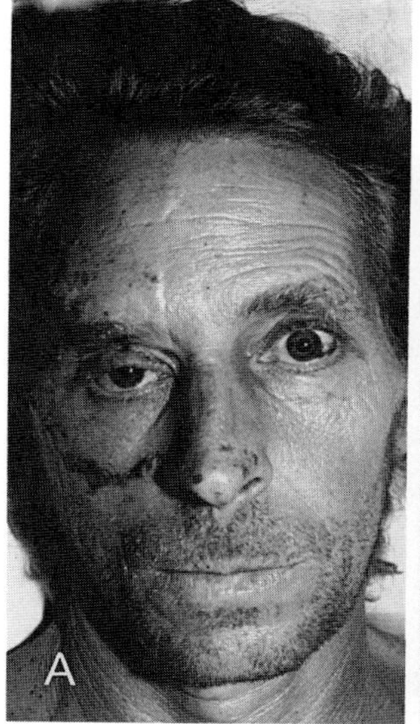

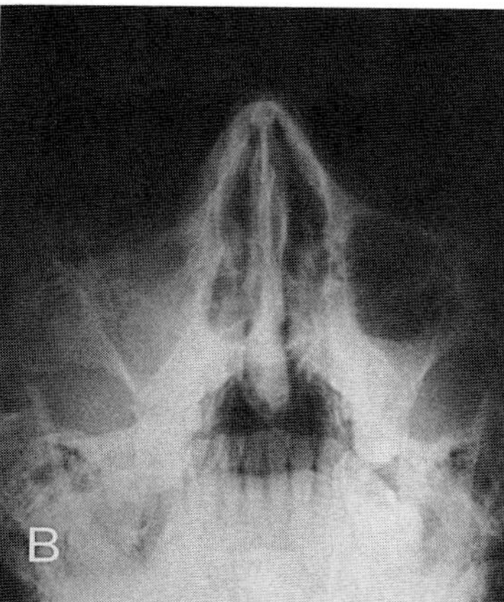

Figure 4.20. **A**, Grossly displaced right zygomatic maxillary complex fracture can be seen. **B**, X-ray shows the fracture lines, as well as clouding of the right maxillary sinus.

to brush the teeth normally, frequent cleansing with one of the pulsatile water hygiene devices or with a mouthwash can be very helpful.

Zygomatic Maxillary Complex Fractures. The anatomy of the zygomatic and orbital regions has several important features. The orbit is composed of the maxilla, lacrimal, frontal, sphenoid, palatine, zygoma, and ethmoid bones. The orbital rims are composed of a confluence of bones that is relatively strong. By comparison, the floor and walls of the orbit are composed of bone that is quite thin and easily fractured. The eyelids are attached by ligaments at the medial and lateral canthi. The lateral canthal ligament is attached to the zygoma, while the medial canthal ligament is attached to the lacrimal bone. Each canthus may be displaced by certain fractures. The orbit also contains (and protects) many important structures. Cushioned within a layer of periorbital fat are the globe, optic nerve, ophthalmic artery, extraocular muscles, and their accompanying nerves. Injury to the structures in specific fractures is not uncommon.

Evaluation. Periorbital injuries and fractures are extremely common (Fig. 4.20). Patients routinely present with chemosis (subconjunctival hematoma), which results in a ballooning effect of the conjunctiva, and with swelling over the cheek area. Palpation, however, reveals a flatness of the bones on that side. The injury may be missed if the examiner is unaware that overlying edema tends to mask the depression. Patients may have limited mandibular opening because the depressed zygomatic arch impinges on the temporalis muscle as it inserts on the choronoid process of the mandible. They may exhibit anesthesia in the distribution of the infraorbital nerve, which traverses the floor

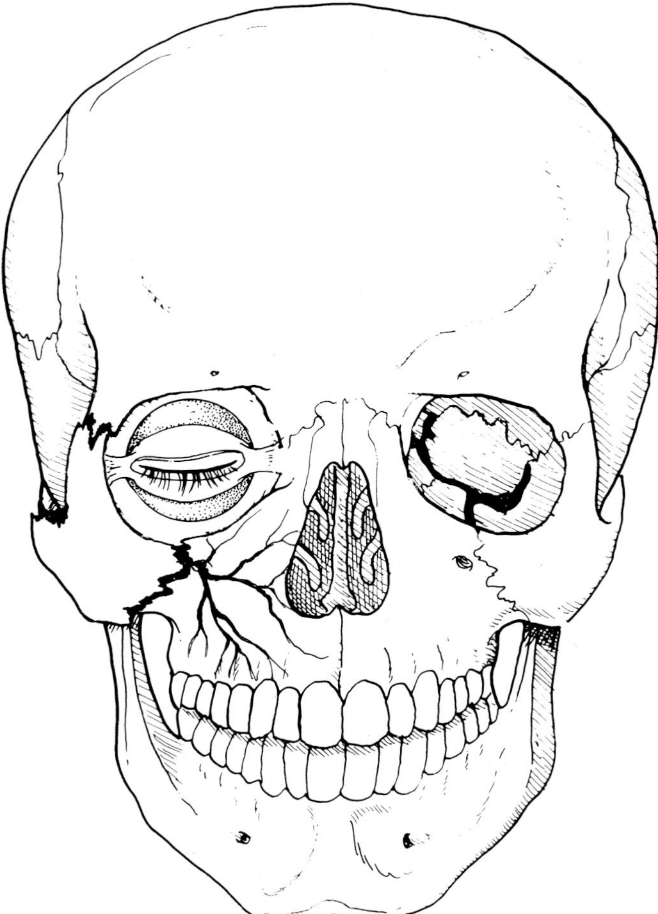

Figure 4.21. Zygomaticomaxillary complex fracture. Note that the fracture through the infraorbital rim extends through the infraorbital foramen, where it can injure this sensory nerve.

of the orbit. An oblique canting of the eye may be caused by depression of the lateral palpebral fissure caused by displacement of the lateral canthus (Fig. 4.21). Periorbital edema and ecchymosis are also present. Careful evaluation may reveal enophthalmos, diplopia (secondary to entrapment of periorbita), and step-offs at the inferior and lateral rims. The patient should be examined for intraoral buccal ecchymosis. A limitation of gaze in multiple planes is associated with corresponding entrapment of orbital contents. Loss of suspensory ligaments or herniation of fat into the maxillary antrum may result in a downward displacement of the globe.

Radiographically, the patient should be evaluated by routine facial x-rays. X-rays often reveal separation of suture lines, fracture fragments, rim discrepancies, and opacification of a maxillary sinus. Unilateral opacification of a maxillary sinus is considered a presumptive sign of a facial fracture until proven otherwise. A submental vertex view is important because it may show depression of the zygomatic arch. CT scans in the axial and coronal planes will most clearly define the location

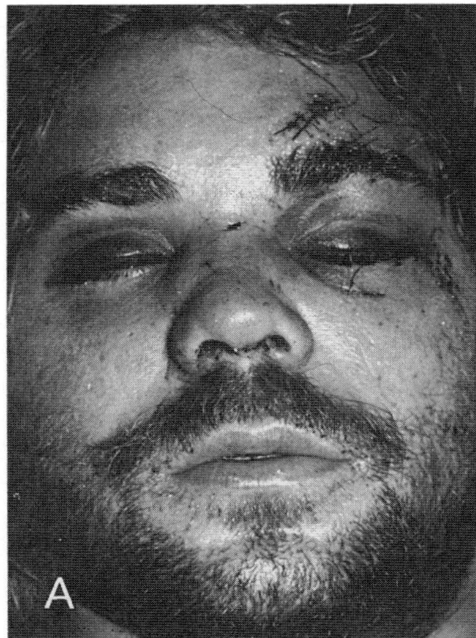

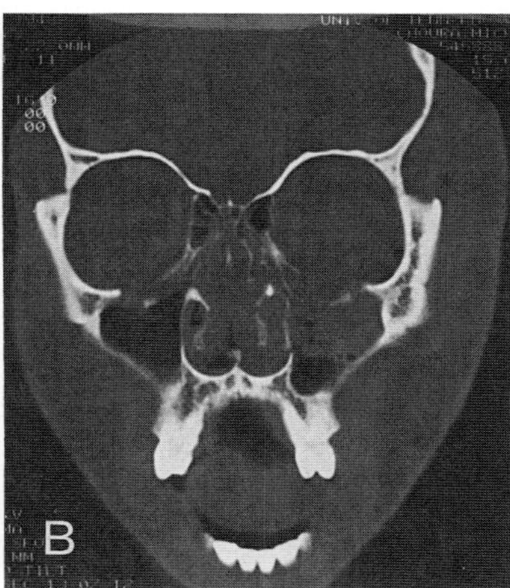

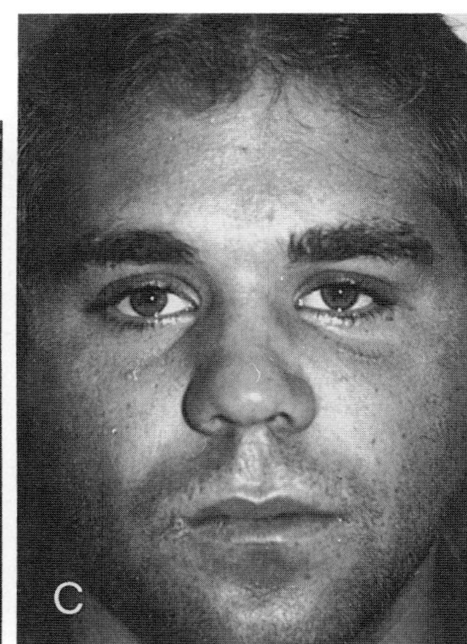

Figure 4.22. **A**, Patient following an assault in which he was beaten about the face. **B**, Coronal CT scans show bilateral orbital floor (blow-out) fractures. **C**, Only the left orbital floor fracture was symptomatic and required reconstruction.

of fractures. Three-dimensional CT scans, where available, may also be of help.

Treatment. Treatment of zygomaticomaxillary complex fractures usually requires open reduction with internal fixation of the fracture segments at several locations. Orbital floor exploration may be necessary to rule out floor fracture. The infraorbital nerve is commonly contused, resulting in some anesthesia to the area of its distribution. Return of sensation may take several weeks or months. It is rare, however, for this nerve to be lacerated.

Complications. Because of the possibility of ocular injury in any significant facial injury, an ophthalmologic evaluation and consultation should be sought. Retrobulbar hematoma, usually diagnosed by proptosis of the globe, may occasionally occur and should be treated immediately. In addition, the optic nerve may be involved and loss of vision may occur. The presence of any of these symptoms requires immediate ophthalmologic consultation. Residual entrapment of the orbital contents may occur after treatment. If there is residual entrapment, reexploration is required. Late enophthalmos can occur and is thought to be secondary to atrophy of periorbital fat with retrusion of the intraorbital structures. Surgical correction of this condition depends upon the patient's symptoms.

Orbital Blow-out Fractures. Blow-out fractures of the orbit ("racquetball" fractures) are a relatively common fracture complex. A blow-out fracture is an isolated fracture of the orbital floor in which a segment of the orbital floor and a portion of the periorbital contents are displaced downward into the maxillary sinus with or without extraocular muscle entrapment. In a pure blow-out fracture there is no infraorbital rim fracture. However, a blow to the globe may transmit a force to the orbital floor, causing the thin bone to break. Alternatively, a blow to the orbital rim may cause a momentary deformation in the rim that causes the floor to buckle and break without causing an associated rim fracture. Either mechanism causes the floor to fracture into the maxillary antrum, creating a "blow-out" of the orbital region.

Evaluation. The patient presents with decreased extraocular muscle function and some diplopia. Evaluation may be difficult because of surrounding swelling, edema, and ecchymosis. There may be some evidence of enophthalmos. In addition, there may be paresthesia of the infraorbital nerve and some inequality in pupil height. Because all of these findings are relatively mild in most cases, confirmation with radiographic studies is usually indicated. Plain radiographs rarely demonstrate any findings other than clouding of the maxillary scar. CT scans, however, will more accurately display any fractures (Fig. 4.22).

Treatment. Operative treatment of orbital floor fractures depends on the associated symptoms. Patients who are asymptomatic or complain of transient diplopia require no treatment. However, persistent diplopia, enophthalmos, displacement of the globe into the maxillary sinus, or a large fracture seen on CT scan are indications for operative repair. This repair involves the exploration of the orbital floor, reduction of periorbital contents back into the orbit, and reconstruction of the orbital floor with bone grafts or prosthetic materials. Long-term complications are generally those of posttraumatic enophthalmos or diplopia (especially if the fracture has been inadequately treated).

Nasal and Nasoethmoidal Fractures. The nasal bone is the most commonly fractured bone of the face because of its relative weakness and prominent position. The thin nasal bones fuse laterally with the frontal process of the maxilla and superiorly with the frontal bone. Internally, the perpendicular plate of the ethmoid articulates posteriorly with the sphenoid and the vomer. In addition, there is a cartilaginous skeletal anatomy consisting of upper lateral, lower lateral, septal, and accessory cartilages.

Evaluation. The mechanism of injury will affect the nature of the fracture. Anterior blows usually produce a comminuted fracture with flattening of the bridge or telescoping (shortening) of the nose, while lateral blows depress the affected side and cause a convex deformity on the other side. Patients always present with significant swelling, which may make precise examination of nasal deformities difficult. Epistaxis, facial asymmetry, nasal airway obstruction and periorbital ecchymosis are usually signs. However, crepitus over the nasal bones and septal hematomas are not uncommon. Nasoethmoidal fractures present with all of the above symptoms as well as telecanthus (an increase in the inner canthal distance), severe depression of the nasal bridge—generally with telescoping of the nasal bones and fractures of the inferior orbital rims. CSF rhinorrhea, pneumocephalus or anosmia may also be present. Simple nasal fractures are best evaluated by physical examination alone, whereas nasoethmoidal fractures require visualization on CT scans. Comparison of the patient's appearance to previous photographs is helpful in determining the extent of deformity.

Treatment. Treatment of nasal fractures can rarely be achieved early due to the amount of edema that rapidly develops. Once the edema has resolved (usually in 3–4 days), operative repositioning of the nasal bones, or closed reduction, may be achieved. Delays of greater than 10 days make this quite difficult. Septal hematomas, if present, should be drained immediately. Repositioning of the nasal septum may be required. Generally, the nasal bones are stabilized with external splints and internal packs. Patients who present with obvious nasal deformities and minimal or no acute swelling may have old nasal fractures that cannot be treated with closed reduction.

Nasoethmoidal fractures will usually require open reduction and internal fixation. Although a number of approaches are available, the best is through a bicornal incision that allows exposure of the glabellar, medial canthal, and superior orbital regions. Significant lacerations may also be used as an approach to the fractures. The goal of fixation is to reestablish or repair the nasal pyramid, medial canthal region, and medial orbits. Interosseous wiring, plate and screw fixation, transnasal wiring of the medial canthal ligaments, and immediate bone grafting may be used.

Complications. Postoperatively, nasal and nasoethmoidal fractures may be complicated by residual nasal and septal deformities with resultant nasal airway obstruction. Deformities of the medial canthi are common. They usually result from inadequate treatment and produce telecanthus, which requires secondary correction. CSF rhinorrhea may complicate more significant fractures. Damage to the lacrimal apparatus is very common and is repaired secondarily.

Maxillary Fractures. Maxillary fractures may be subdivided according to the LeFort classification. While not all fractures fit this classification, it remains a useful one.

LeFort I Fractures. The LeFort fracture is defined as a transverse fracture extending through the maxilla and pterygoid plates above the floor of the maxillary sinus (Fig. 4.23**A**). Etiology is usually traumatic and most commonly from a central midline blow. The patient presents with consistent findings of malocclusion and mobility of the maxilla. On examination, patients will have ecchymosis in the buccal vestibule, some crepitus in the maxillary area, and false motion of the lower maxilla with stability of the upper nose and orbits. Patients occasionally present with airway obstruction, noticeable lengthening of the face, nasal septal deformities, and paresthesia in the distribution of the infraorbital nerve. The patient should be evaluated by routine facial x-rays and CT scans if appropriate.

Treatment of LeFort I facial fractures involves establishing the mandible as a foundation on which to base other repairs. Mandibular injuries are thus usually repaired before maxillary injuries. In most instances, intermaxillary fixation gives sufficient reduction and stabilization. Bone grafts may also be needed if severe comminution is present. Complications of LeFort I facial fractures commonly include malocclusion, paresthesia, nasal septal deformities, or facial asymmetry.

LeFort II Fractures. LeFort II fractures consist of a zygomatic midfacial fracture with a floating fragment shaped like a pyramid (Fig. 4.23**B**), from which the term "pyramidal fracture" is derived. The central portion of the face is free-floating, while the lateral orbits and cranium are stable. The patient presents with a flattening of the nasoorbital region and mobility across the nasal bridge. Epistaxis is common. The examiner finds that the maxilla is mobile and moves with the nasal bridge and the medial component of the inferior rim, while the lateral orbital rim and forehead remain stable. Open bite deformities and malocclusion are also common. Palpation along the orbital rims and nasofrontal areas usually demonstrates step deformities. CSF leaks are also relatively common. The patient may also have some lengthening of the midface and paresthesia of the infraorbital nerve. Diplopia and decreased intraocular muscle function may occur when there is significant disruption of the orbital floor. Although most fractures can be diagnosed on physical examination, CT scans are usually indicated.

Treatment of the LeFort II facial fracture involves restoration of anatomic configuration and structure. Intermaxillary fixation is first performed (after stabilization of mandibular fractures, if present). Direct fixation in the areas of the lateral maxilla, infraorbital rim, and nasofrontal angle is then achieved with plate and screw

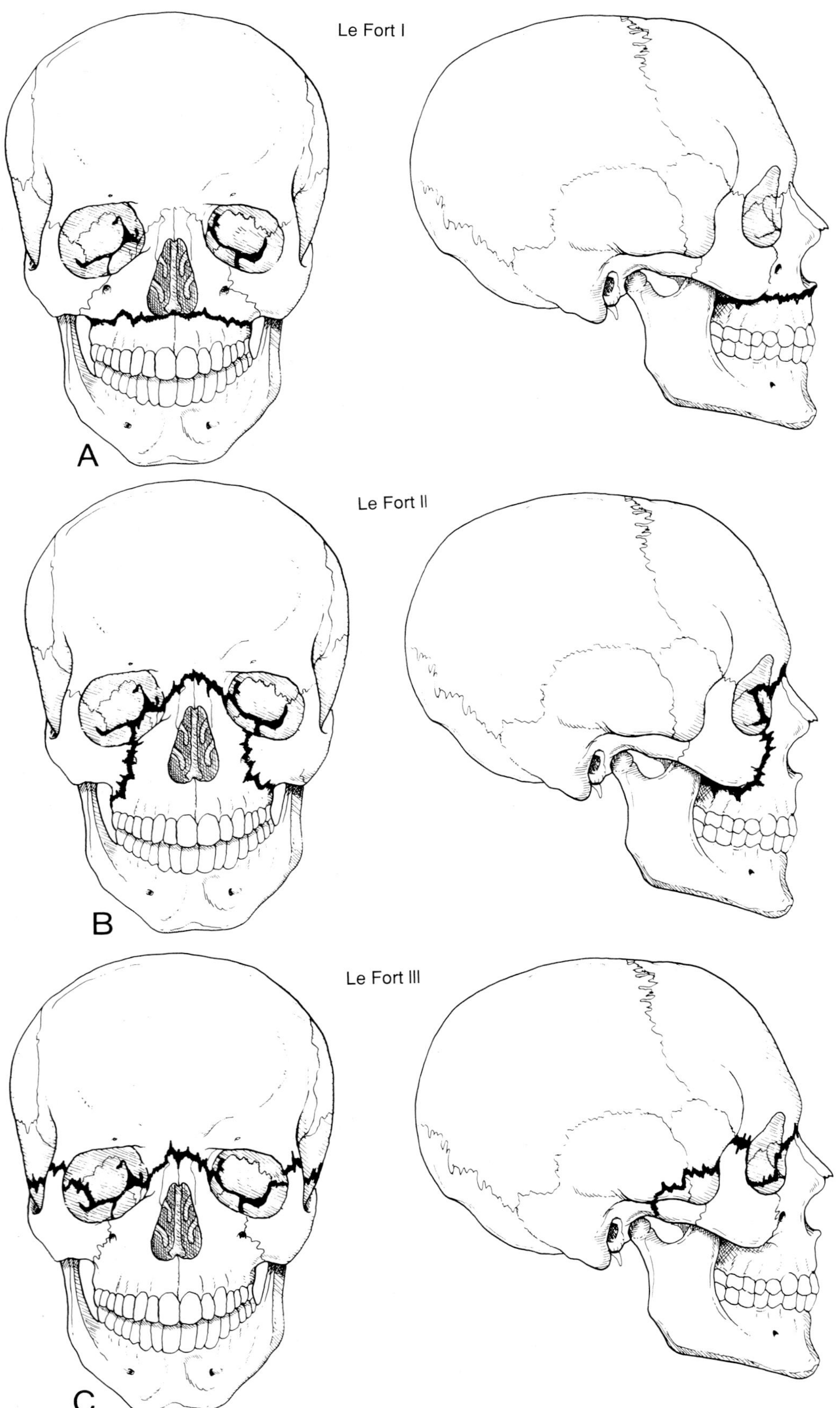

Figure 4.23. LeFort classifications of maxillary fracture: **A**, LeFort I fracture; **B**, LeFort II fracture; **C**, LeFort III fracture.

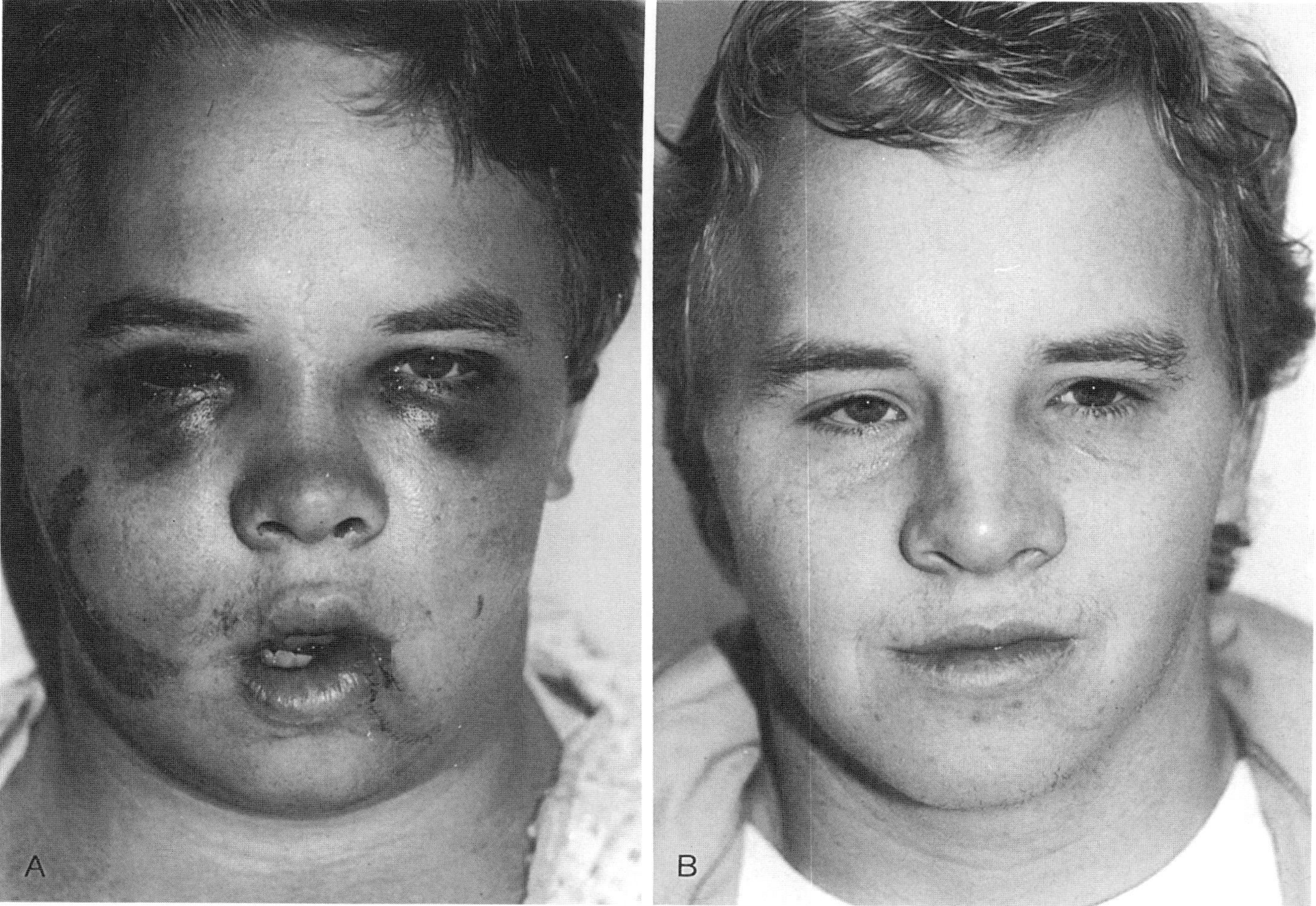

Figure 4.24. **A**, Patient with multiple facial fractures including a LeFort III fracture. Note the "racoon eyes." **B**, Following fracture fixation and facial reconstruction.

fixation, which will allow early motion and release of intermaxillary fixation. Again, bone grafts are used if necessary in cases of severe comminution or bone loss.

Basic complications of the LeFort II facial fracture are the same as those of the LeFort I fracture. If the fracture is incorrectly or inadequately corrected, the midface might be lengthened. There is a higher incidence of orbital injuries, CSF leaks, nasal deformities, and midface abnormalities involving the lacrimal system.

LeFort III Fractures. LeFort III fractures are severe fractures that completely separate the midface from the upper face, a separation known as "craniofacial disjunction" (Fig. 4.23**C**). Signs and symptoms of the LeFort III facial fracture are similar to those of the LeFort II fracture, with additional signs associated with basilar skull fractures. Depressed zygomatic arches are often found with the inferior rims intact. Relatively common findings are Battle's sign (ecchymosis in the mastoid region), bilateral orbital ecchymosis (raccoon's eyes) (Fig. 4.24), CSF otorrhea, and hemotympanum.

Diagnosis revolves around the facial examination. Upon manipulation of the maxilla, movement will be felt at the frontonasal angle and frontozygomatic sutures. However, the entire midface remains intact. Zygomatic arch fractures are also palpated. Radiographic diagnosis is usually made by CT scans, which will also evaluate cranial vault fractures and intracranial injuries.

As in other facial fractures, the goal is anatomic restoration of the fracture complex. The general treatment protocol is the same as that for the LeFort II fractures, with the exception that the inferior orbital rims are no longer available for superior stabilization. Stabilization must thus be achieved at the frontozygomatic sutures and zygomatic arches. Complications of the LeFort III facial fractures are basically the same as those of the LeFort II facial fractures, with the possible addition of injuries to the cranial base with neurologic damage.

Pan Facial Fractures. Patients who have sustained facial trauma as a result of high levels of kinetic energy, such as high speed motor vehicle crashes, frequently have multiple different fracture complexes (Fig. 4.25). When these involve all areas of the face, they are referred to as pan facial fractures. The same principles of

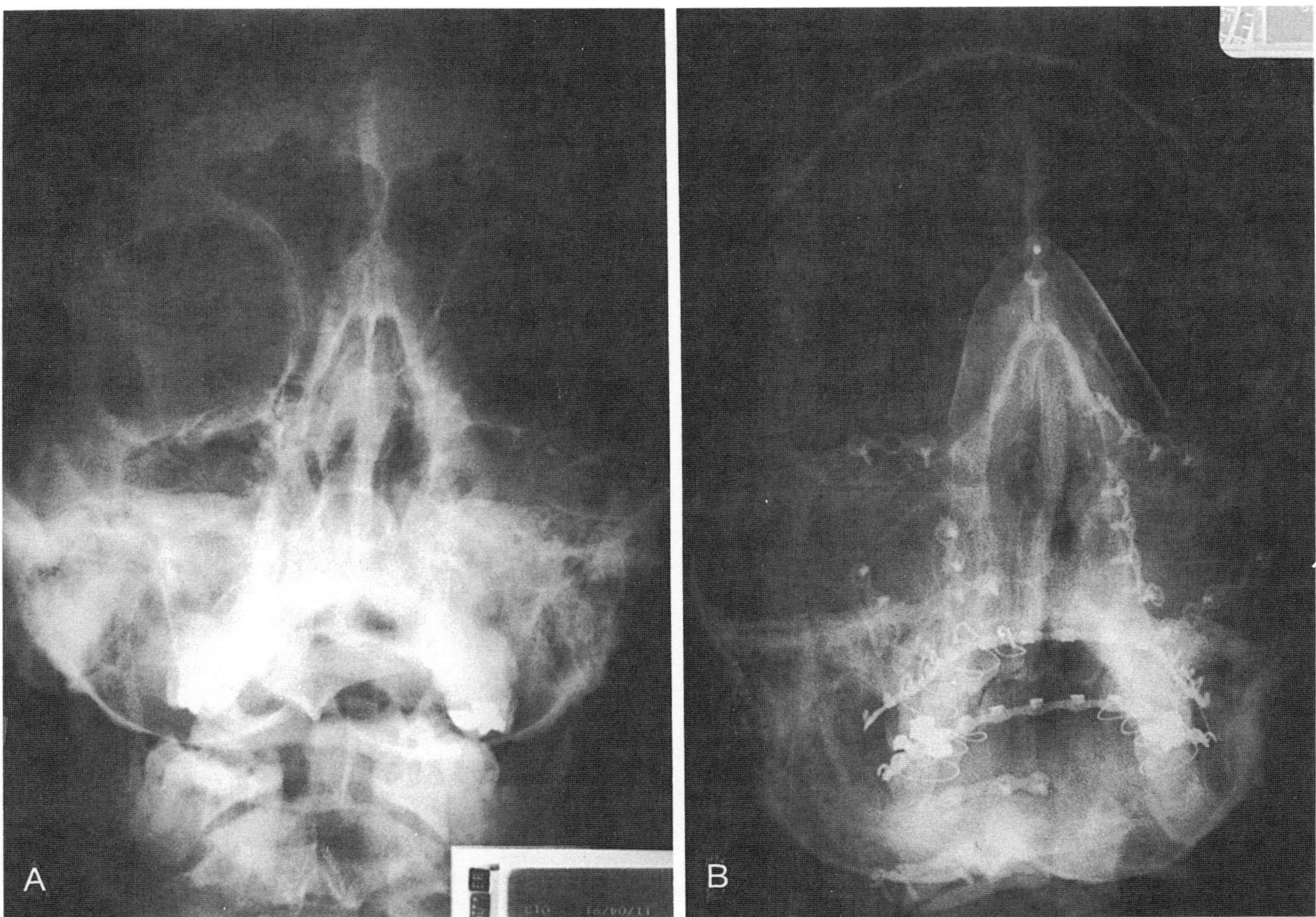

Figure 4.25. X-rays of a patient with pan facial fractures **A**, before and **B**, after fixation using both intermaxillary fixation and rigid internal fixation.

diagnosis and treatment that are used in isolated fracture complexes are applied to these complex injuries. To avoid serious soft tissue contraction of the overlying facial skin, early fixation of these fractures is generally indicated.

CSF Rhinorrhea. CSF rhinorrhea may occur in as many as 25% of high-level midface injuries that involve the paranasal sinuses. The majority of these will be manifest by symptoms of leakage within the first 48 hours after injury. Less commonly, rhinorrhea may be demonstrated 5 to 7 days later. Clinically, midfacial fractures are associated with fracture of the cribiform plate and a dural tear. Subsequent to this injury, the clear, watery CSF fluid begins to leak out slowly. The patient may notice a salty taste in the mouth or throat. If the patient remains in a dorsal supine position, fluid will drain down the posterior pharynx and the patient may not be aware of any leakage. CSF rhinorrhea will occasionally be confused with nasal mucous secretions.

CSF rhinorrhea is usually diagnosed by clinical suspicion. A "double-ring" test may be used, in which the nasal discharges are collected on filter paper and allowed to dry. If the leakage is cerebrospinal fluid, a homogeneous ring will form about the drop of dried fluid. If the leakage is serum or mucus, several rings will form about the drop. If a CSF leak is diagnosed, the patient should generally remain supine and avoid head-down positioning. Nasal packing should be avoided, and any attempt at passing a nasogastric or nasoendotracheal tube is contraindicated. In addition, extreme care should be taken if mask positive pressure ventilation is required.

Early reduction of facial fractures will usually stop CSF leakage within a few days. Prophylactic antibiotics should probably only be used perioperatively. The diagnosis of a CSF leak should prompt a neurosurgical consultation. If the leak has not decreased after several days, direct dural repair should be considered. The most significant complication associated with CSF leakage is the upward migration of bacteria to cause meningitis and subsequent brain abscess. In such cases specific antibiotic coverage should be instituted.

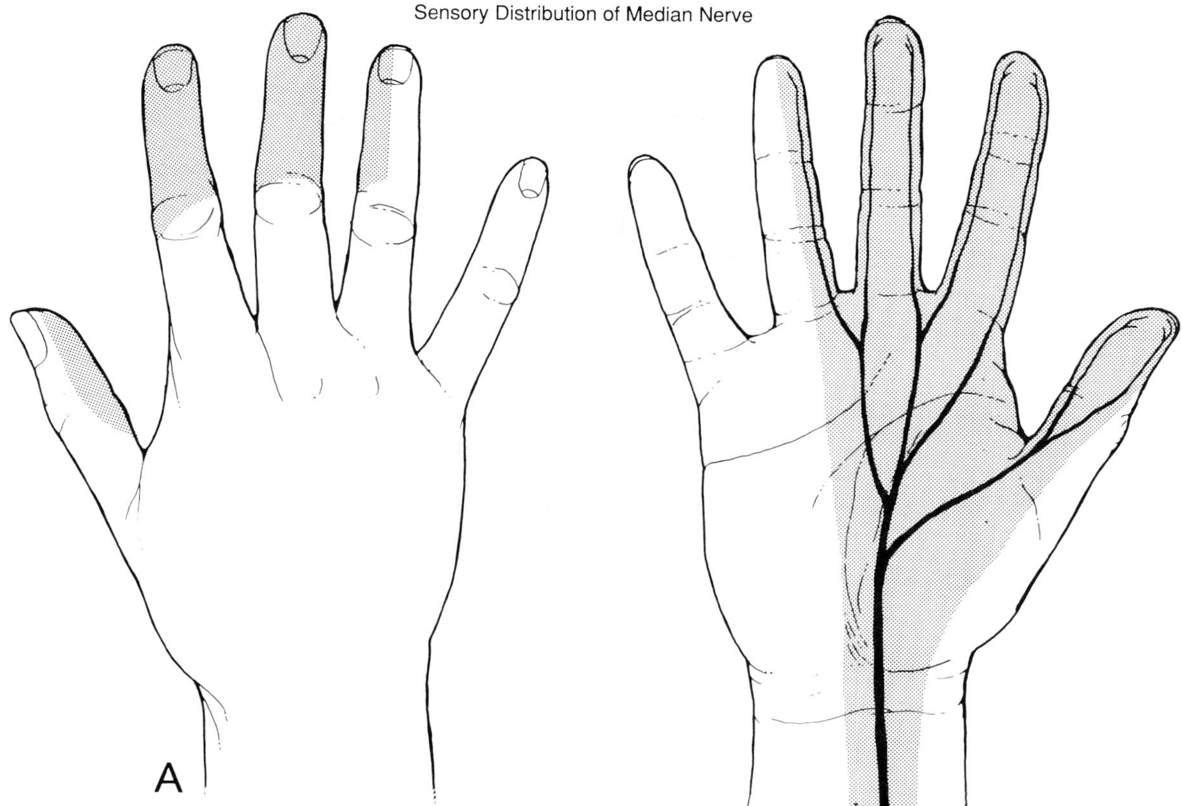

Figure 4.26. Sensory innervation of the hand: **A**, median nerve; **B**, ulnar nerve; **C**, radial nerve.

Hand Surgery

The hand and upper extremity are a unique functional organ system enabling a complex interaction between an individual and the environment. The hand is able both to manipulate the external environment and to receive sensations from it. Because hand injuries are seen often in clinical practice, all physicians should have a basic knowledge of hand anatomy and injuries in order to assess the need not only for primary treatment but for referral. As definitive treatment of the hand is usually performed by a specialist, emphasis will be given to diagnosis and early treatment of the injured or diseased hand. Second only to back injuries, injuries to the hand and upper extremity are the most common reason for loss of workdays in the United States.

Functional Anatomy and Examination

The hand is composed of multiple, finely balanced functional units. Disturbances of these units, of their interaction with one another, or of their innervation will result in dysfunction and ultimate disability of the patient. To properly treat diseases and injuries of the hand, an understanding of hand anatomy is required. We will discuss the nervous anatomy, the motor anatomy, the bony anatomy, and, lastly, the vascular anatomy.

Nervous Anatomy and Evaluation. Three principal nerves supply sensory innervation to the hand: the median, ulnar, and radial nerves. The *median nerve* (Fig. 4.26**A**) enters the hand at the wrist through the carpal tunnel. The motor median nerve branch to the thenar musculature arises within the carpal tunnel or just distal to it. The median nerve then divides into sensory branches that serve the volar aspect of the thumb, index, and long finger, and radial half of the ring finger. The *ulnar nerve* (Fig. 4.26**B**) also enters the hand at the wrist through a less well-defined tunnel and then branches to provide sensation to the volar and dorsal aspects of the ulnar half of the ring finger and to the entire small finger. Within the hand, motor branches to the intrinsic muscles arise from the ulnar nerve. The *radial nerve* (Fig. 4.26**C**), which lies dorsally, provides sensation to the dorsal aspects of the thumb, index, and long fingers, and half of the ring finger. It is important to understand that significant overlap in these nerves may be present. Sensory innervation of the digits, especially on their volar surfaces, is critical to their proper functioning. The major sensory nerves first divide into proper digital nerves within the hand, subsequently giving rise to digital nerves that run along the ulnar and radial aspect of the digits.

When examining the hand, tests of the normal functions of the nerves can be performed. Sensory functions are generally tested by light touch from a wisp of cotton or fine filament, and by two-point discrimination. The

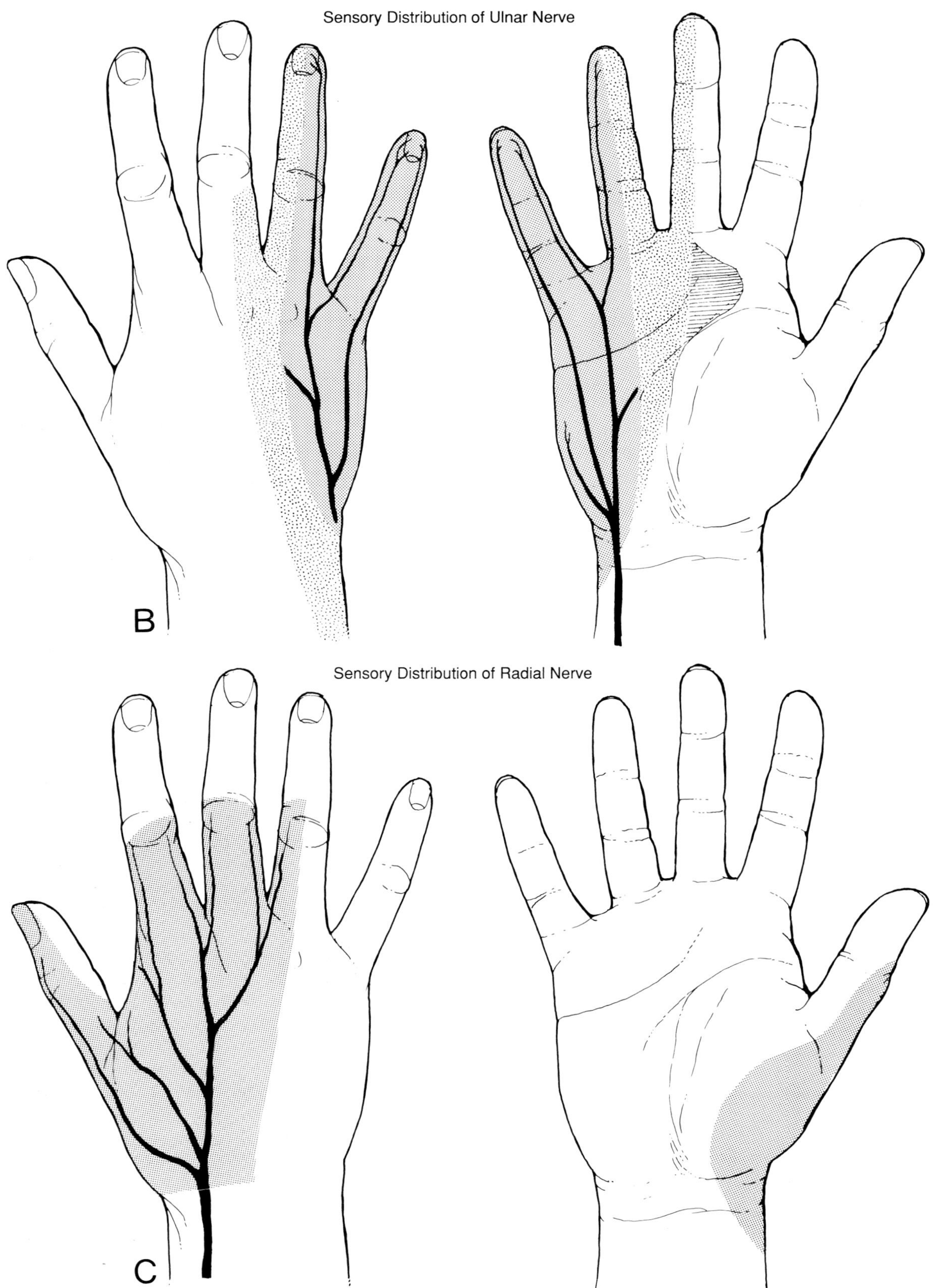

Figure 4.26. *(continued)*

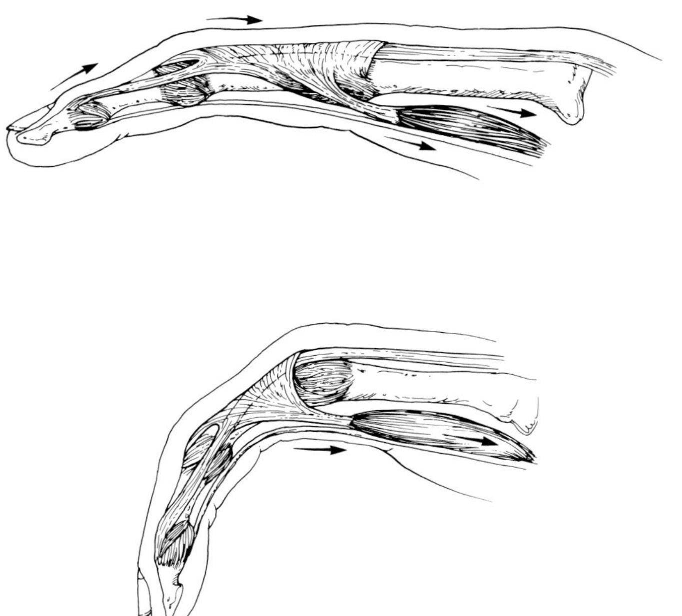

Figure 4.27. Lumbrical muscle anatomy and function. **A**, The insertion of the lumbrical muscle onto the extensor apparatus allows the extension of the DIP and PIP joints on contraction of the lumbrical muscle. **B**, Because the lumbrical tendon passes on the volar surface of the MP joint, flexion of the MP joint is achieved on contraction of the lumbrical muscle.

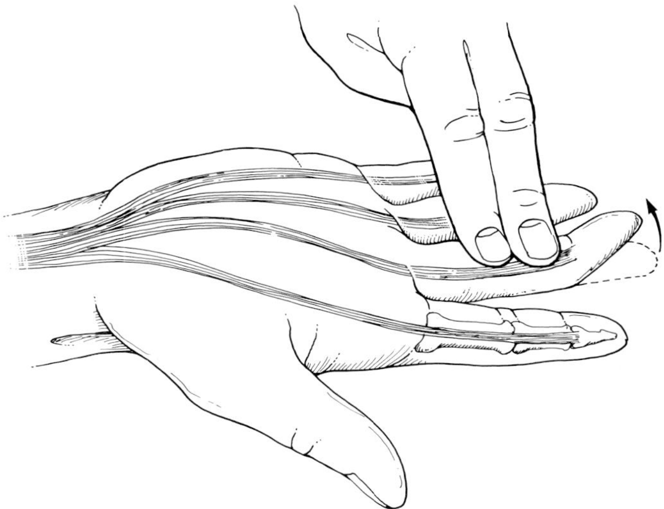

Figure 4.28. Examination of the flexor digitorum profundus. Integrity of the flexor digitorum profundus musculotendinous unit is examined by blocking flexion at the PIP joint and observing flexion at the DIP joint of the finger in question.

patient should be told to look away from the hand during the exam. If it is not clear whether there has been sensory loss, the exam should be repeated at a later time. Motor functions are tested to assess the peripheral nerves. The patient is assessed for the ability to extend the wrist against resistance in a test of the proximal radial nerve, which innervates the major wrist extensors. In a test of the integrity of the proximal median nerve, which innervates the major finger flexors in the forearm, the patient is asked to grasp an object (such as the examiner's finger). Since the thenar muscles are median controlled, asking the patient to touch the thumb to the small finger tests the distal motor function of the median nerve. The interosseous muscles, which abduct and adduct the fingers, are mostly controlled by the ulnar nerve distally. The function of this nerve is tested by asking the patient to spread the fingers against resistance or to hold a piece of paper between opposing surfaces of adjacent fingers while the examiner attempts to withdraw it.

Motor Unit Anatomy. The motor functions of the hand can be divided into three important functions: *finger flexion*, *finger extension*, and *thumb opposition* or prehension. While the motor functions of the wrist and forearm have an important effect, they will be discussed only briefly. Certain muscles, the intrinsic muscles, reside totally within the hands, while others, the extrinsic muscles, are in the forearm and reach the hand by tendons that travel through the wrist.

Flexor Anatomy and Examination. Flexion of the metacarpal phalangeal (MP), proximal interphalangeal (PIP), and distal interphalangeal joints (DIP) are each served by separate musculotendinous units. The lumbricales, which are intrinsic muscles, arise within the hand and insert into the proximal phalanges, crossing the MP joint (Fig. 4.27). These, along with the interossei, are responsible for MP flexion (and also for DIP and PIP joint extension). The extrinsic flexors, the flexor digitorum superficialis and the flexor digitorum profundus, are responsible for flexion at the PIP and DIP joints, respectively.

The *flexor digitorum profundus* (FDP) muscle originates in the forearm and gives rise to four tendons that run through the wrist within the carpal tunnel to insert at the base of the distal phalanges of the fingers. Its function is tested by blocking flexion at the PIP of the involved finger and observing flexion at the DIP (Fig. 4.28). Since a single muscle gives rise to all four deep flexion tendons, the flexor digitorum profundus acts as a unit, and independent DIP flexion is not observed. PIP flexion is achieved through the action of the *flexor digitorum superficialis* (FDS), which is also located in the forearm and sends four flexor tendons through the carpal tunnel to ultimately insert on the base of the middle phalanges of the fingers. Separate muscle fibers give rise to each of the tendons, allowing independent flexion. To test the function of the flexor digitorum superficialis, passive extension of adjacent fingers is maintained (to block the deep flexor unit), while flexion of the PIP joint of the affected finger is observed (Fig. 4.29).

Extensor Anatomy and Examination. Finger extension is achieved through the action of both intrinsic and extrinsic muscles that insert into a complex tendinous system on the dorsum of the fingers, known as the extension apparatus. The *extensor digitorum* is a common extrinsic extensor muscle that inserts onto the extension

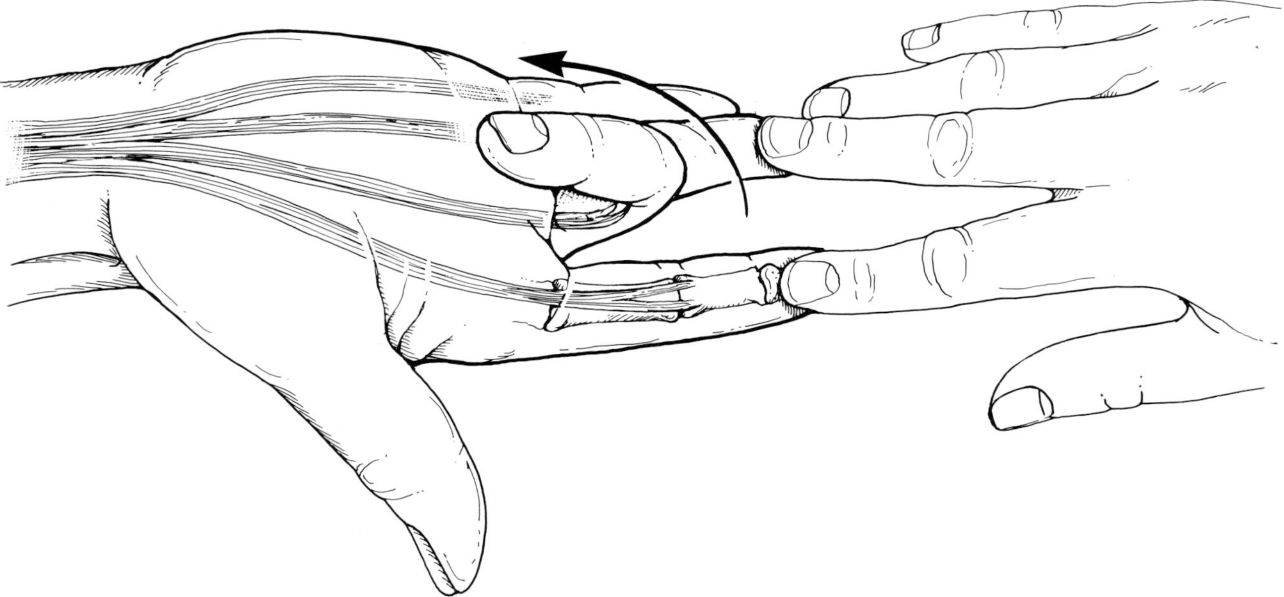

Figure 4.29. Examination of the flexor digitorum superficialis. Because the flexor digitorum profundus tendons have a common muscular origin, the action of this musculotendinous unit can be blocked by maintaining adjacent fingers in extension. Flexion of the finger in question then will be a function of only the flexor digitorum superficialis function.

apparatus (Fig. 4.30) and provides MP extension, as a unit, of the index, large, ring, and small finger. Independent extension of the index and small fingers is provided by two independent extensors, the extensor pollicis and the extensor digiti minimi, respectively. PIP and DIP joint extension is achieved through an interplay of both the common extensors and the intrinsic muscles of the hand (the lumbricales and interossei). These intrinsic muscles, which also provide MP flexion, travel volar to the axis of rotation of the MP joint to insert into the lateral bands of the extensor apparatus (Fig. 4.27). This unique position, along with the movement of the MP joint acting as a "cam" joint, allows the intrinsic muscles to act as both flexors (at the MP joint), by crossing the volar aspect of the MP joint, and as extensors, by inserting into the lateral bands of the extensor apparatus.

Examination of the extensor function of the hand involves observation of extension, with or without resistance, of each of these elements. As independent extension of the index and small fingers is provided, these digits must be evaluated both separately and as a unit with the long and ring finger.

Thumb extension is also provided by intrinsic and extrinsic muscles. The extensor pollicis longus muscle located within the forearm gives rise to a tendon that inserts on the base of the distal phalanx and allows IP joint extension. The intrinsic extensor, the extensor pollicis, inserts onto the base of the proximal phalanx and allows MP joint extension. Thumb extension is also assisted by abduction of the thumb by the abductor pollicis longus, which crosses the wrist to insert on the thumb metacarpal. The area between the tendons of the flexor pollicis longus and the abductor pollicis longus on the dorsum of the wrist is known as the "anatomic snuff box."

Thumb Opposition. Opposition of the thumb, allowing pinch function, is a unique ability of our hands. It is provided by the muscles of the thenar eminence, the opponens pollicis, the flexor pollicis brevis, and the abductor pollicis. The pinch function is assisted by the flexion of the thumb IP joint, which is provided by the flexor pollicis longus, an extrinsic flexor whose tendon travels through the carpal tunnel and inserts on the base of the distal phalanx.

Bony Anatomy. The bony anatomy of the hand can be divided into three segments: the phalanges, the metacarpals, and the carpal bones (Fig. 4.31). While the fingers each have three phalanges, the thumb has only two. The five proximal phalanges all articulate with their respective metacarpals. The metacarpals in turn articulate with the carpal bones, which as a unit form the wrist joint, articulating with the radial head. Because of its frequency of injury and subsequent complications, the scaphoid deserves special note. As a portion of the carpus, the scaphoid articulates with the base of the thumb metacarpal and the radial head. Injury to this area will give tenderness on palpation of the anatomical snuff box.

Vascular Anatomy. Both the radial and ulnar artery contribute to the blood supply of the hand (Fig. 4.32). Usually, the ulnar artery is dominant. Together they form two arches or arcades within the hand, from which the digital arteries arise. The separate digital vessels travel along the radial and ulnar sides of the digits with their respective digital nerves forming neurovascular bundles. While the integrity of these vessels may

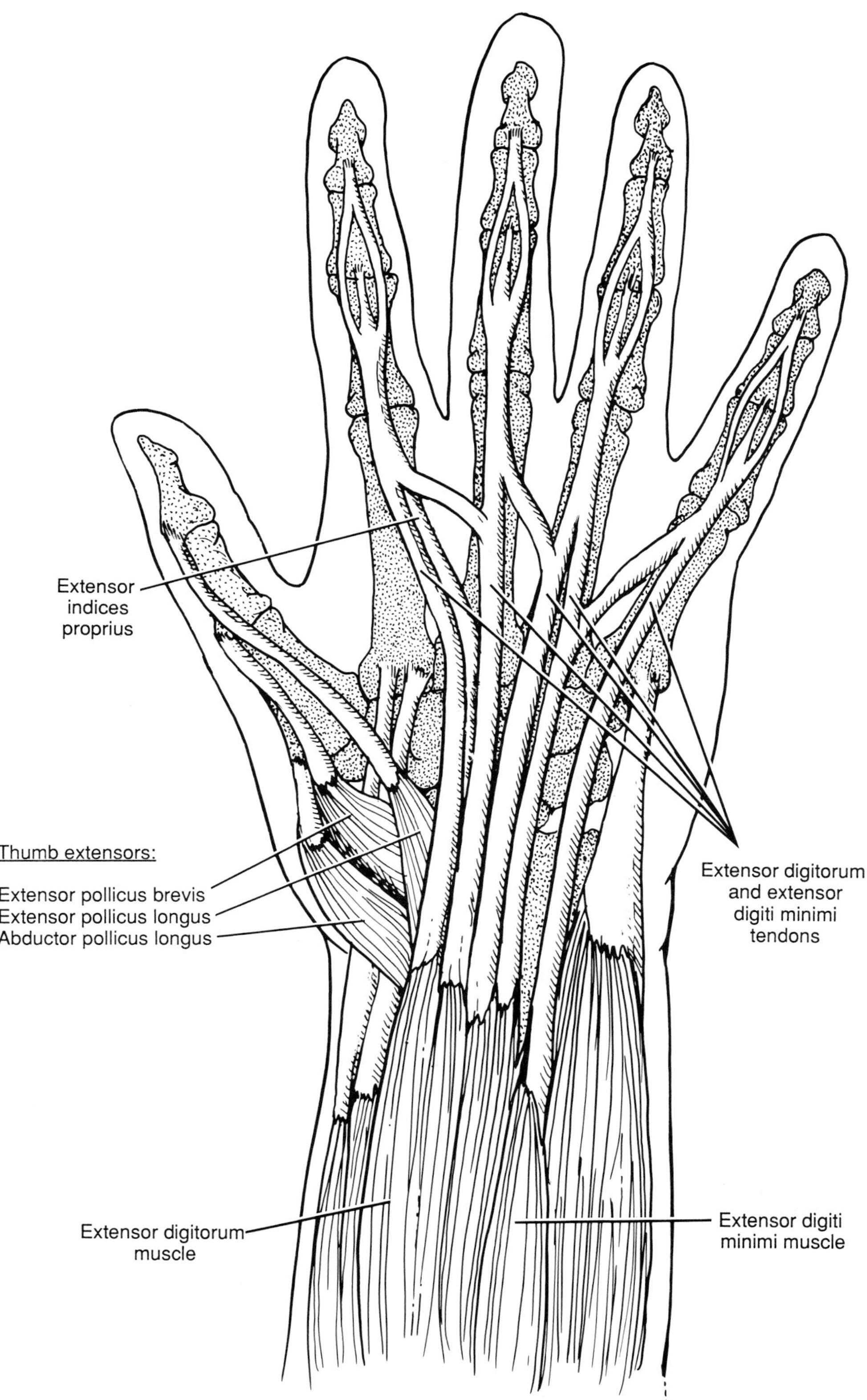

Figure 4.30. Anatomy of the extensor tendons to the hand.

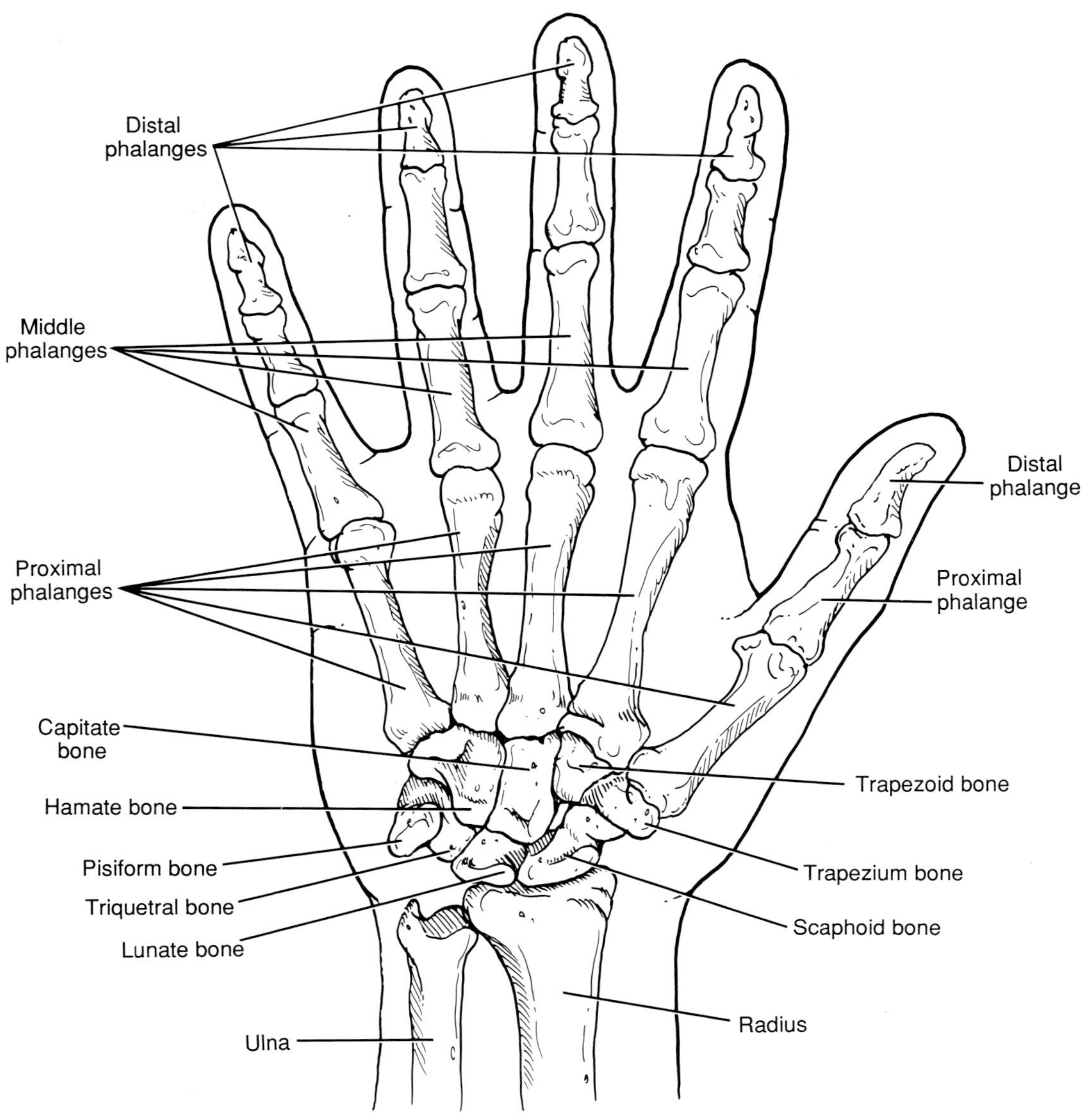

Figure 4.31. Skeletal anatomy of the hand.

be checked by observing capillary refill, the radial and ulnar arteries themselves may be examined using the Allen's test. To test the radial artery, the patient is asked to make a tight fist. The ulnar artery is compressed and the hand opened. If the radial artery is intact, the hand will be pink when the fist is opened. If the radial artery is not intact, the hand will be pale or blanched when the fist is opened but will "pink up" when compression of the ulnar artery is released. The ulnar artery may be similarly tested by compressing the radial artery after the patient makes a fist. If vascular integrity is still uncertain, Doppler examination may be helpful.

Diagnosis of Hand Injuries

Due to the complexity of the hand's anatomy and function, and the potentially severe consequences of hand injuries, most significant injuries should be treated by a hand specialist. However, the nonspecialist may be the first person to evaluate these injuries and thus must be able to evaluate, initially treat, and, if appropriate, subsequently refer these patients for specialty consultation.

As always, the evaluation of the hand begins with a proper history. The time and mechanism of the injury along with the environment within which the injury occurred are of paramount importance (particularly in cases of injuries with open wounds). The patient's overall medical condition, allergies, medications, tetanus immunization status, and previous injuries are next documented. The patient's hand dominance, occupation, and avocations play an important role in therapeutic decision-making and should be noted and communicated to the hand specialist.

Before the hand is examined in detail, its vascular integrity should be evaluated so that if it is in need of revascularization the patient can be immediately re-

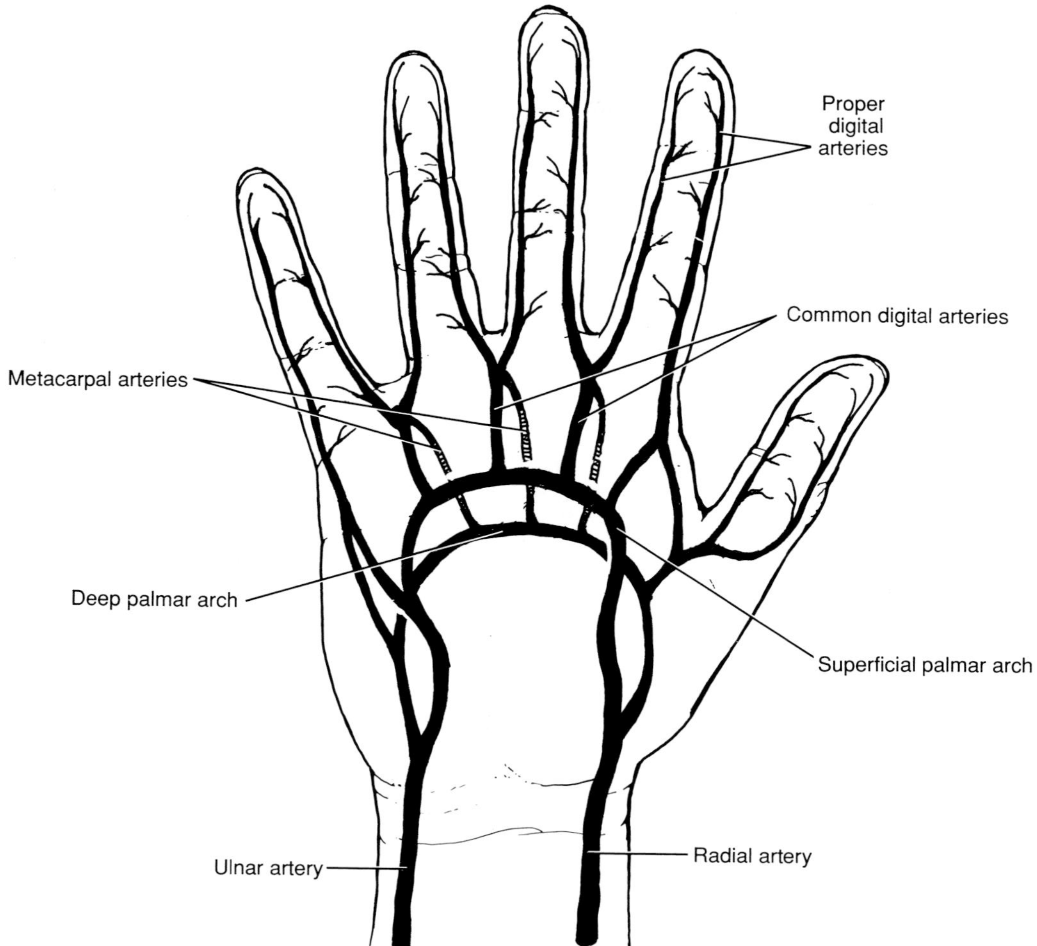

Figure 4.32. Vascular anatomy of the hand.

ferred. Bleeding should be controlled with direct pressure alone. Bleeding vessels should not be clamped because of the risk of damaging accompanying nerves or of further damaging reparable vessels. A pneumatic tourniquet should be used only in extreme cases. The nail bed of each digit should be examined for capillary refill, and the wrist and forearm should be checked for pulse. Doppler examination can be used to confirm patency of the ulnar and radial arteries, palmar arch, and digital arteries. If major portions of the hand appear ischemic, plans should be set in motion to evacuate the patient to a replantation center with microvascular capabilities (or to the operating room).

A careful examination of all motor and sensory units should next be performed. The distribution of each of the major sensory nerves and digital nerves should be tested and recorded. Each flexor and extensor tendon should be individually examined as previously outlined. When fractures are suspected, appropriate radiographs should be obtained. Complex injuries involving multiple tendons and nerves can be simply and well delineated with a thorough exam. As always, careful documentation of these injuries is required.

During the initial evaluation of the hand, fractures should be suspected and diagnosed. Inspection of the hand often is diagnostic, when localized swelling, angulation, or rotational deformity of the hand is seen. Tenderness to palpation over the fracture site is generally the rule; there may be limitation of motion of the involved finger. A survey x-ray of the entire hand should be obtained, followed by anterior-posterior and lateral x-rays of the affected part, taken at 90° of one another. If suspected fractures are not well visualized with these, oblique views may be obtained.

Treatment of Hand Injuries

Soft Tissue Injuries. Open wounds of the hand should be copiously irrigated with a physiologic solution. Multiple liters of saline irrigation may be required for highly contaminated wounds. If no sensory or motor injuries have been sustained, these wounds can be simply closed in a sterile manner. Antibiotics are recommended for contaminated wounds or for open wounds with underlying bone, joint, or tendon injuries. Tetanus immunization status must always be ascertained.

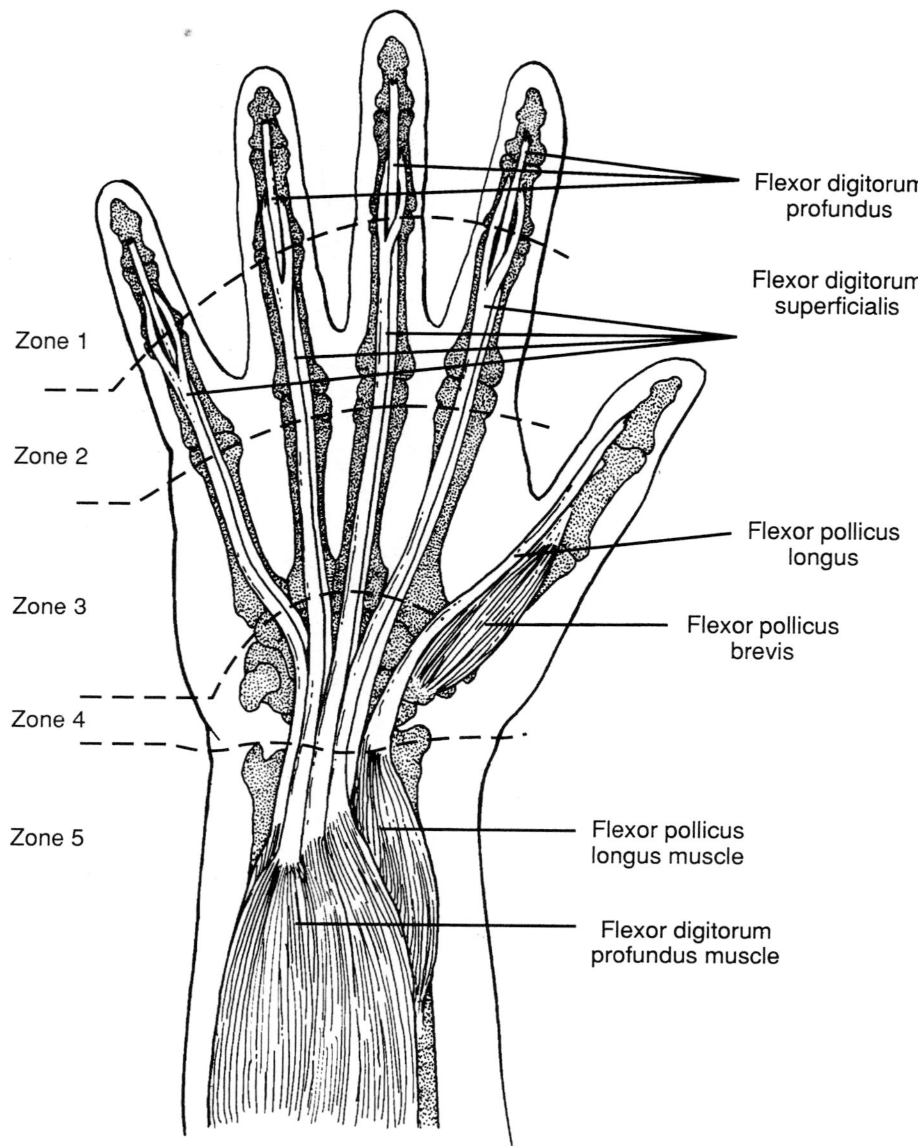

Figure 4.33. Zones of flexor tendon injuries.

If a nerve has been lacerated, it will require microscopic repair in the operating room. Such an injury does not need to be repaired immediately if it is not convenient; repair can be delayed for several days.

Flexor tendon injuries must also be repaired in the operating room. These injuries can be classified according to different zones (Fig. 4.33). Injuries within Zone II ("no-man's-land") can be the most difficult to manage. The deep and superficial flexor tendons run within the flexor sheath in this location. Once they are repaired, adhesions may form that can restrict normal motion. A flexor tendon laceration can be repaired immediately or within several days. Simple skin closure and referral for repair within a few days is acceptable management of these injuries.

Many extensor tendon injuries can be repaired in the emergency room at the discretion of the hand surgeon. Laceration of the extensor tendon in the hand will disallow extension of the entire finger (Fig. 4.34**C**). Injuries to the central portion of the extensor mechanism at the PIP joint will produce a "boutonnière deformity" (Fig. 4.34**B**). Injuries to the extensor tendon overlying the DIP joint will produce a "mallet finger" (Fig. 4.34**A**).

Fractures of the Hand. Fractures of the hand are a common component of the injured hand. The treatment goal is proper reduction of the fracture and maintenance of the reduction by means of splinting, casting, or internal fixation, in order to achieve as near normal function as possible. In certain fractures, minor discrepancy in final bone alignment can be tolerated, whereas in other fractures anatomic reduction is required. Due to the complexity of the hand and its fractures, nearly all fractures will require the consultation of a hand surgeon.

Closed fractures are generally treated electively as the localized swelling will allow. Proper splinting until

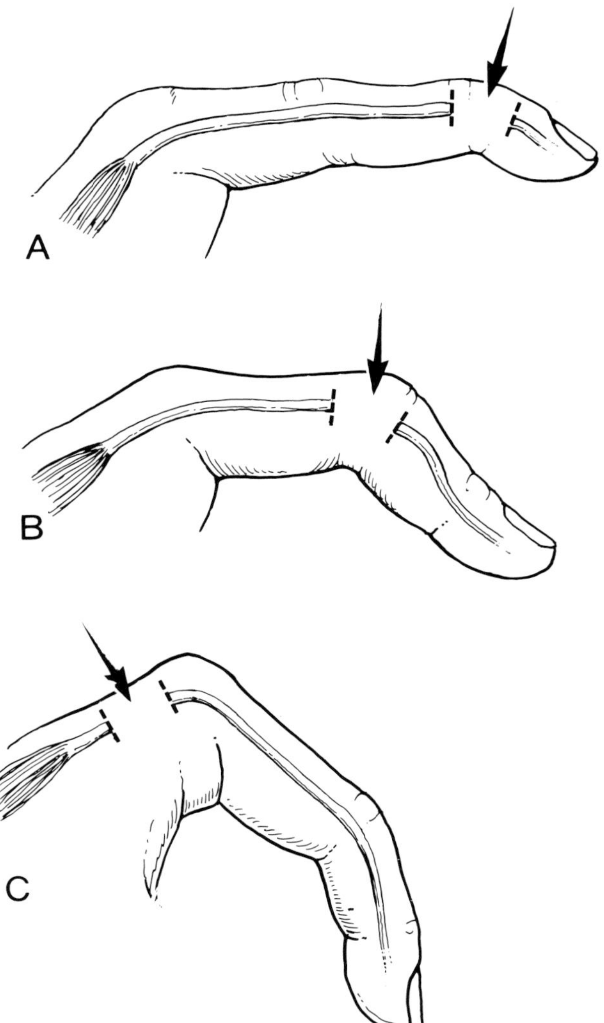

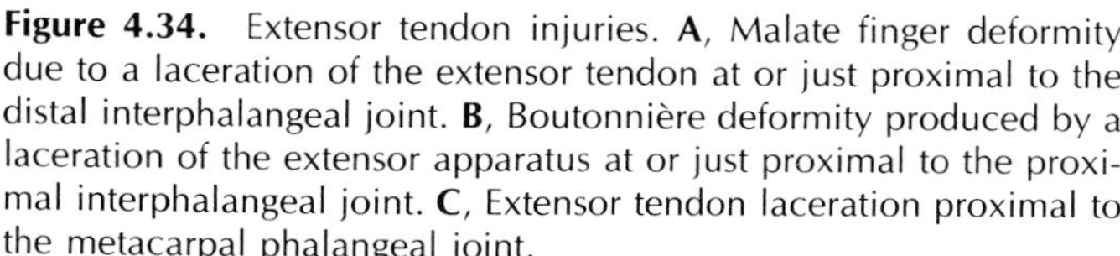
Figure 4.34. Extensor tendon injuries. **A**, Malate finger deformity due to a laceration of the extensor tendon at or just proximal to the distal interphalangeal joint. **B**, Boutonnière deformity produced by a laceration of the extensor apparatus at or just proximal to the proximal interphalangeal joint. **C**, Extensor tendon laceration proximal to the metacarpal phalangeal joint.

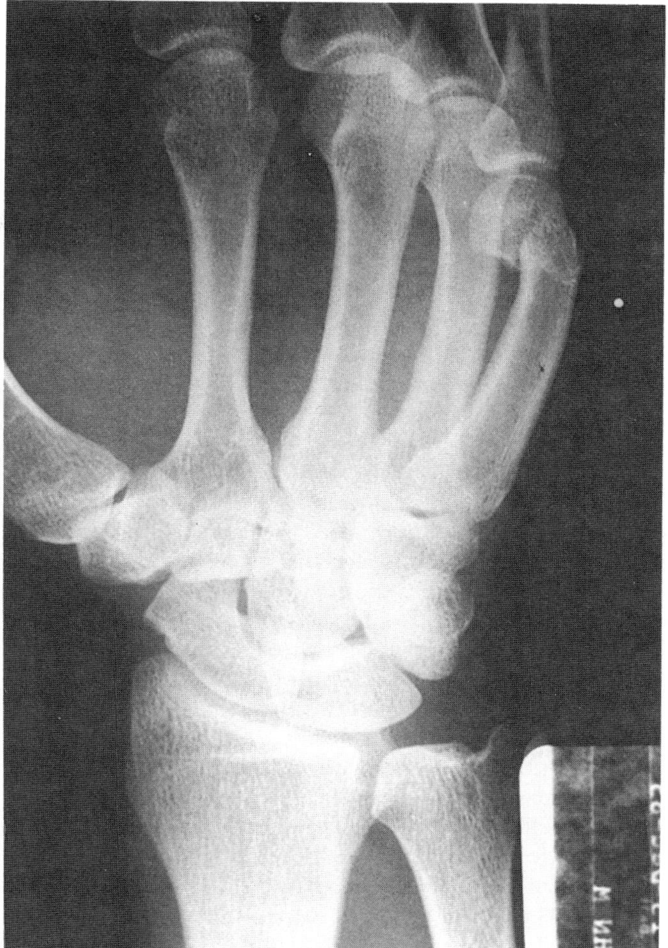
Figure 4.35. Boxer's fracture.

fixation will decrease patient discomfort and the amount of swelling. All open fractures should be treated acutely as the patient's overall condition will allow. With the exception of very minor fractures, or of those treated with casting alone, all definitive reduction and fixation should be done in the operating room. Although in-depth discussion of specific hand fractures is beyond the scope of this chapter, a few will be mentioned.

Probably the most commonly seen fracture is that of the end of the distal phalanx or distal tuft. Because the fracture occurs distal to the insertion of the extensor and flexor tendons, precise anatomic reduction is not required. These fractures can be easily treated with splints for 2 to 3 weeks, generally without complications. Seriously crushed tips may require some molding during splinting to achieve the best result. If the fracture involves the DIP joint space or any tendinous insertion, referral should be sought. Fractures of the middle and proximal phalanges are also common. Stable fractures are treatable with splints and casts. However, unstable, comminuted, or spiral fractures, as well as those involving the joint space, may require internal fixation.

Fractures through the shaft of the metacarpals frequently result from altercations. A "boxer's fracture" is one through the fourth or fifth metacarpals, usually the result of a blow to another object (such as an opponent's chin) (Fig. 4.35). Angulation or rotational deformity will frequently be seen. Whereas up to 20–30° of volar angulation of the fourth and fifth metacarpals may be acceptable, little or no angulation of the other metacarpals is acceptable. Likewise, rotational deformity is unacceptable because of its interference with normal motion. Whereas boxer fractures and other stable, nondisplaced metacarpal fractures may be treated with casting alone, most others will require additional methods of fixation.

Fractures of the scaphoid usually occur following a fall on the outstretched hand. This history and tenderness over the anatomical snuff box are key to making the diagnosis. Initial radiographs may not show a frac-

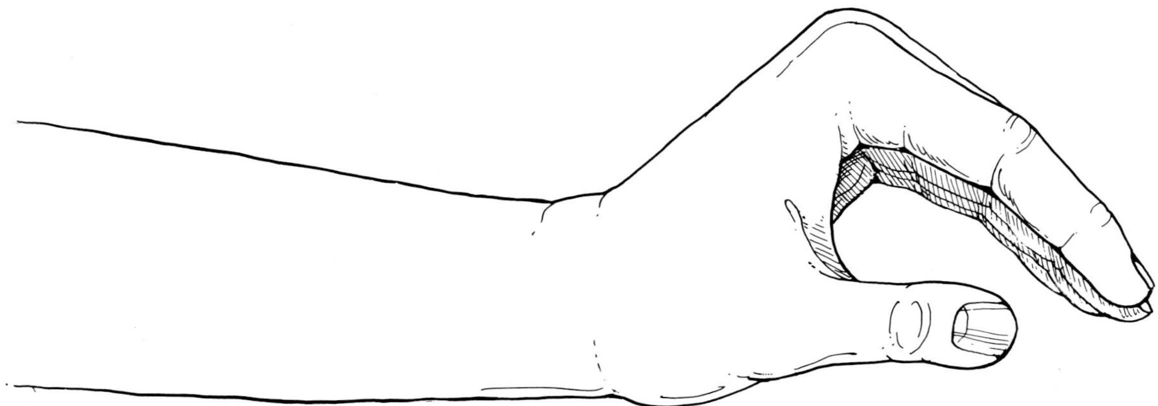

Figure 4.36. "Safe position" for immobilization of the hand.

ture, whereas repeat films in 1–3 weeks may. Because of the problems with nonunion in improperly treated scaphoid fractures, those suspected of having sustained such injuries but in whom initial x-rays are negative should be cast and treated as though they do in fact have this fracture. Aseptic necrosis is a common complication of this fractured scaphoid.

Splinting of the injured hand is quite important and deserves special note. Prolonged splinting in an inappropriate position may result in joint stiffness, shortening of musculotendinous units, and ultimate loss of some function. While certain specific fractures or tendon injuries may require splinting in different positions, most injured hands should be splinted in the "safe" position to preserve function (Fig. 4.36). In this position, the wrist should be in 20–30° of extension, the MPs are flexed at 80–90°, and the IP joints are straight or nearly so. The thumb is held in opposition. Generally, splints to maintain this position are placed on the volar surface of the hand, wrist, and forearm.

Special Injuries

Fingertip Injuries. Although fingertip injuries can be quite common, their care can be very complex due to the structure and function of the fingertip. The goals of treatment are to maintain adequate length and normal sensibility. Whereas very simple distal skin losses can be treated with dressings alone and allowed to heal by contraction, injuries involving the distal phalanx or nail bed require complex repairs. If the distal amputated part is available, it should be gently handled and properly attended to (see below).

Amputations. Particular care must be given to amputated parts. Frequently, the injuries in which digits or significant portions of digits have been amputated occur as industrial accidents in untidy settings. The amputated part should be rinsed with saline to remove debris and gross contamination. The part should next be wrapped in moist gauze and placed in a sealed watertight plastic bag, which is then inserted into a container filled with iced saline. The amputated part should not be allowed to become waterlogged by being placed directly in saline. X-rays of the part should be obtained before it is transferred.

Although not all amputated parts can or should be replanted, the ultimate decision regarding replantation should be made by the replantation surgeon. Those patients who have sustained thumb amputations, amputations distal to the PIP joint, multiple digit amputations, bilateral amputations, hand or hemi-hand amputation, or who are pediatric patients are considered for replantation. Replantation of severely crushed or avulsed parts is generally not indicated, nor is that of parts having undergone warm ischemia for a period greater than 6–12 hours. The ultimate decision regarding replantation should be made by the team that will be performing such an operation.

Thermal Injuries. The thermally injured hand offers a challenge to the initial treating physician: correct early treatment significantly improves patient outcome. The hand should be cleansed gently with physiologic solution and, if necessary, a mild soap. All foreign material such as burned clothing should be removed. Blisters should be left intact; they are a sign of a second-degree burn and offer protection to the underlying tissue. When these blisters eventually break on their own, they should be gently debrided. The capillary refill of all burned digits should be checked, since circumferential burns can interfere with distal circulation. This interference may take several hours to develop; if it does, escharotomies may be required.

Once the hand is cleaned, an antibiotic ointment such as Silvadene is applied and the hand is placed in a bulky dressing and splinted in the safe position. Therapy consists of daily whirlpool baths, dressing changes, and aggressive range-of-motion exercises to prevent joint contracture. Individuals sustaining significant partial-thickness burns or full-thickness burns that will require skin grafting should be referred.

Hand Infections The complex structure of the hand offers multiple sites for infection. While superficial cellulitis and subcutaneous abscesses can occur in the hand as in other locations, some infections are peculiar to the hand. Such infections can occur within the lateral nail bed (paronychia), at the finger pulp (felons),

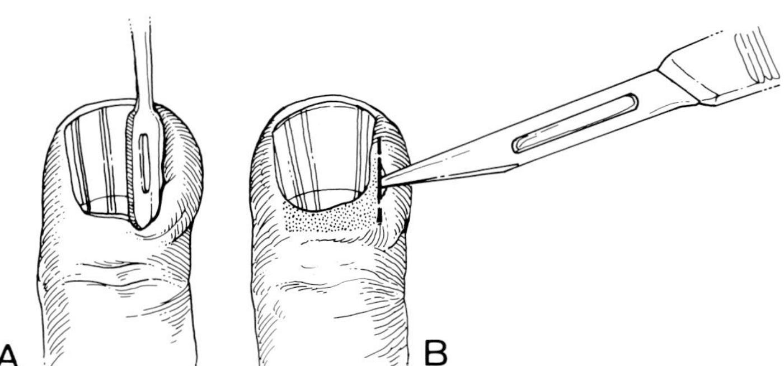

Figure 4.37. Treatment of paronychia. **A**, Elevation of the nail fold. **B**, Placement of an incision.

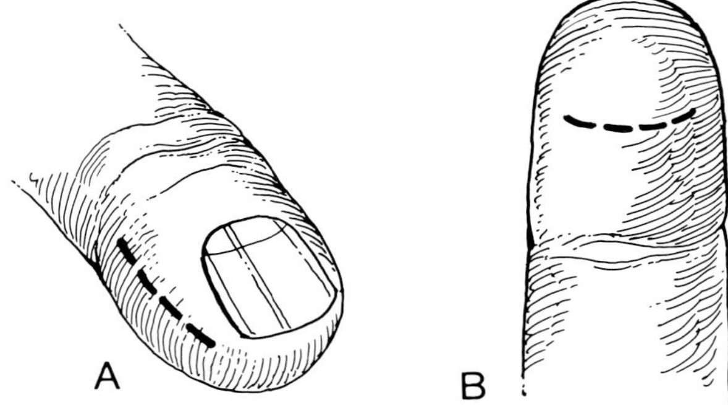

Figure 4.38. Drainage approaches for a felon. **A**, Incision on the lateral aspect of the finger. **B**, Transverse incision across the pulp of the finger.

in the tendon sheaths (tenosynovitis), and in the deeper structures of the hand (deep space infections). Human bites to the hand are also a common infectious problem. Successful management of hand infections depends on a knowledge of both hand anatomy and the specific treatment of each infection.

In the hand, progression of infection usually is rapid. Without prompt diagnosis and treatment the infection can spread quickly along fascial planes, causing damage to adjacent structures. In addition, this rapid spread can lead to massive tissue necrosis, which may require amputation of the extremity, or, at a minimum, result in a stiff, nonfunctional extremity. Treatment of suppurative infections of the hand is based upon adequate surgical drainage. Although systemic symptoms may be present, symptoms and signs are generally localized to the hand. Serious infections of the hand usually are treated in the operating room under regional or general anesthesia, with tourniquet control. Appropriate aerobic and anaerobic cultures are taken. After adequate surgical drainage, the hand is immobilized in the protective, splinted position and elevated. Antibiotics are routinely administered, generally a first-generation cephalosporin or an antibiotic resistant to penicillinase. After surgical drainage, the hand should be reevaluated frequently. Further extension of the infection is possible, and adequate drainage should be verified by progressive resolution of pain and swelling.

Paronychia. Paronychia, an infection of the lateral nail fold, usually presents as a small collection of purulent material at the side of the nail. If seen early, it is properly treated by elevating the skin over the nail or excising a small lateral, longitudinal portion of the nail in order to drain the purulent material (Fig. 4.37). More advanced infection may require incision within the nail fold for drainage. This procedure is followed by soaking the finger in warm water several times a day. Chronic paronychia usually implies secondary colonization with more complex organisms. Antibiotic treatment for chronic paronychia should await results of cultures. Fungal nail infections or herpetic infection ('herpetic whitlow') may be confused with chronic paronychia. Proper diagnosis is vital because operating on a fungal or herpetic infection may worsen the condition and result in delayed wound healing.

Felon. A *felon*, a purulent infection of the pad of the finger, is usually extremely painful. Fibrous septae within the tip of the finger allow a significant amount of pressure with only a minimal amount of purulent material present. This condition also increases local tissue pressure to the point of interrupting capillary flow, which can produce ischemia and necrosis. The felon can be drained by various methods (Fig. 4.38). If skin necrosis is present, the incision can be made over it, or the incision can be made at a point of maximum tenderness. Alternatively, it can be drained through a small stab incision laterally on the digit pad. In draining a felon it is important to adequately disrupt the fibrous septae to provide enough drainage.

Tenosynovitis. Tenosynovitis is a painful inflammation of the tendon sheath. Suppurative tenosynovitis usually results from a puncture wound over the volar aspect of the hand, although it can develop from extension of a felon (Fig. 4.39). Diagnosis is usually made by observing (Kanavel's) four signs: (*a*) finger held in slight flexion, (*b*) fusiform swelling of the finger, (*c*) tenderness over the tendon sheath, and (*d*) pain on passive extension. Usually the fourth sign is the key to proper diagnosis.

Prompt and appropriate treatment of this infection is required to prevent complications. Although some very early infections can be treated with intravenous antibiotics, elevation, and immobilization, more advanced infections require surgical drainage of the tendon sheath. Such drainage must be carried out in the operating room by a hand surgeon.

Deep Space Infections. Infection of the deep spaces of the hand or thenar eminence can also occur. The presenting symptom is usually pain and swelling. Although the primary problem may be in a volar location, there will almost always be more dorsal swelling. Treatment is surgical drainage of the affected spaces. The complexity of the anatomy of the deep spaces of the hand complicates their drainage and thus usually requires referral to a hand surgeon.

Human Bites. Human bites to the hand can produce devastating complications due to the degree of wound contamination from human saliva. Frequently,

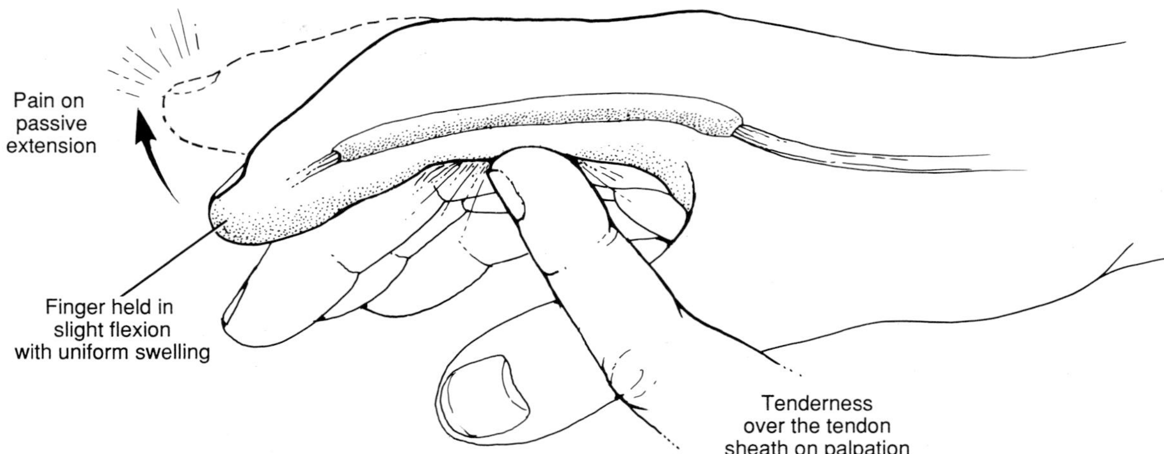

Figure 4.39. Flexor tenosynovitis. The diagnosis is made by Kanavel's four signs: finger held in slight flexion, fusiform swelling of the finger, tenderness over the tendon sheath, and pain on passive extension.

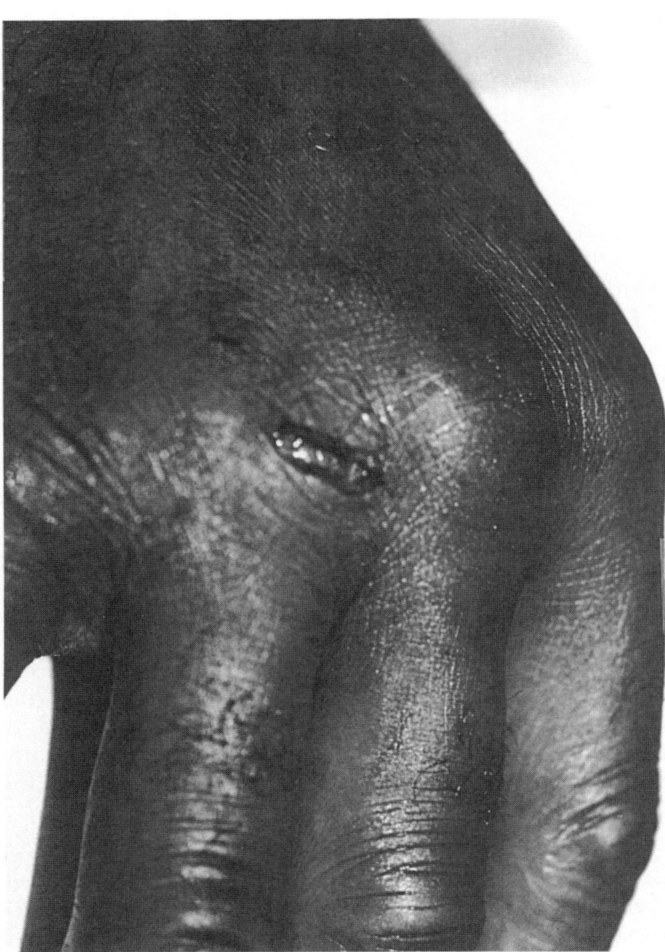

Figure 4.40. Human bite to the MP joint. This is the typical appearance of a "fight bite."

the diagnosis is complicated by an inaccurate or misleading history given by the patient. Lacerations overlying the dorsal MP joint (knuckle) should always be suspected of being a "fight-bite" (Fig. 4.40). Lacerations from human bites should never be closed but be left open to drain. Patients should be admitted for 24–48 hours of intravenous antibiotics, with the hand elevated and immobilized. Bites not treated within 24 hours will require longer hospitalization and more complex treatment, whereas those properly treated within 24 hours will virtually always have a favorable outcome.

Tumors of the Hand

Benign Tumors

Ganglion Cyst. By far the most common soft tissue mass of the hand is a ganglion cyst, which can occur in several anatomic locations. The ganglion represents an outpouching of the synovium, usually of a joint or tendinous structure. The most common location is on the dorsal radial aspect of the wrist where it originates from the ligament joining the scaphoid and lunate bones. It may also occur on the volar radial area of the wrist or along the palmar surface of the hand or finger overlying the flexor tendon sheath. Symptomatic ganglion cysts are surgically removed. Untreated, they tend to increase in size slowly but progressively. Other methods of treatment, such as bursting, aspiration, and injection with either steroids or sclerosing materials, are generally ineffective.

Mucous Cyst. A mucous cyst is not a true cyst at all, but a ganglion arising from the dorsum of the finger overlying the distal interphalangeal joint. Surgical resection is complicated by the need to excise the cyst usually with some overlying skin, and underlying periosteum. Small skin grafts or skin flaps may be required for closure.

Giant Cell Tumor. Another soft tissue tumor that occurs in the wrist or finger is the giant cell tumor (xanthoma). This slowly growing, yellow/brown tumor invades surrounding structures. It has a high recurrence rate after resection. Surgical excision should be carefully performed under low power magnification.

Malignant Tumors. Squamous and basal cell carcinomas of the skin are relatively common in the hands and are usually a result of aging and sun exposure. Treatment is as in other parts of the body: wide local excision, followed by proper soft tissue reconstruction.

Miscellaneous

Arthritis. Some of the more common problems with the hands involve the presence of either degenerative or rheumatoid arthritis. These conditions are extremely debilitating and may cause permanent disability. The primary treatment of both diseases is medical. Surgical treatment is reserved for maintaining or restoring functional ability of the patient. Many patients can be improved by early surgical intervention for joint reconstruction, muscle and tendon rebalancing, and synovectomies.

Dupuytren's Disease. Dupuytren's disease is a progressive fibrosis of the palmar fascia of the hand. The etiology of the disease is unclear but it has a definite hereditary pattern. It usually presents after the age of 40, is more common in males by a 7:1 ratio, and occurs bilaterally in over 50% of cases. It is manifested by increasing contraction of the fibrous palmar fascia that presents as nodules and bands in the hand. The natural course of the disease is progressive contracture of the hand and inability to fully extend the digits. There is no known medical treatment for this disorder. Indications for surgery include limited finger extension, rapid progression of the disease, and the presence of painful nodules. The best results of Dupuytren's contracture surgery occur when the patient is evaluated early and the surgical resection done before the formation of joint abnormalities or fixed joints. At the time of surgery, the involved palmar fascia is removed, and the skin is repaired to alleviate scar contractures. Care must be taken, since the neurovascular bundles may be encased in the diseased tissue.

Compression Neuropathies. Although compression neuropathies can occur in many locations of the upper extremity, the most common location is the carpal tunnel. The median nerve is compressed as it passes through the wrist within the carpal tunnel, which is bounded dorsally by the carpal bones and volarly by a tough ligament, the volar carpal ligament. Nine flexor tendons accompany the median nerve through the carpal tunnel, the four tendons of the FDS, the four of FDP, and the tendon of the flexor pollicis longus. Patients usually present with numbness and tingling, felt particularly at night, within the median nerve sensory distribution of the hand. They may also complain of a difficulty grasping objects. Frequently these patients have occupations which require a large amount of manual work. Usually symptoms of pain and tingling can be reproduced by percussing the median nerve within the carpal tunnel (Tinel's sign). In advanced cases, atrophy of the thenar musculature can occur. Nerve conduction studies usually demonstrate delays.

Treatment is directed at relieving the amount of compression and resultant inflammation of the median nerve. In early cases, splinting or alteration of work habits may be helpful. However, these measures are usually only of transient help. Definitive operative treatment involves the division of the volar carpal ligament, and occasionally an internal neurolysis of the median nerve. Surgery should not be delayed until thenar atrophy develops, since this condition can be permanent.

Congenital Defects

Congenital Defects of the Hand

Congenital defects of the hand can occur alone or in association with multiple other medical syndromes. Early diagnosis allows planned treatment. Common defects include webbed fingers (syndactyly) (Fig. 4.41) and extra digits (polydactyly). Syndactylies are routinely repaired before the infant is 6 to 12 months of age. Repair should not be delayed past 12 months of age unless there are other associated medical problems. If the two digits fused together are of unequal length (such as the ring/small digit or thumb/index digit), a progressive contracture and bony angulation will occur as the child grows. Another reason to proceed early with separation is the presence of complex syndactyly

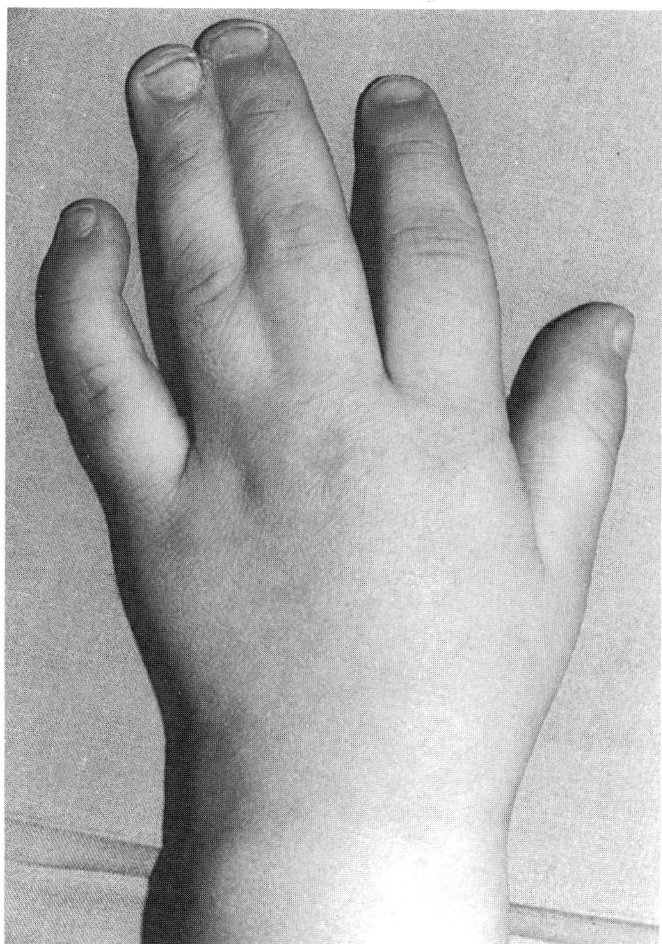

Figure 4.41. Case of simple syndactyly.

in which fusion of adjacent phalanges occurs. This fusion causes significant growth abnormalities if the phalanges are not divided early.

Surgical care of polydactyly usually involves amputation of the extra digits. However, amputation should be done only after complete evaluation has been made of the functional status and potential of all the digits. Such an evaluation may require waiting for several months or even over a year until it is evident which digit will be the most functional. Occasionally, combining some elements of one digit with those of the other during the amputation is indicated.

Two congenital hand problems require early treatment. One is a constriction ring deformity in which a band of tissue forms a tourniquet around the digit. It may also form a tourniquet around other parts of the body, such as the wrist, leg, or toes. The constriction must be at least partially relieved early as it tends to limit circulation. A second defect that benefits from early treatment is the significantly deviated hand, such as a radial clubhand. Very early splinting of this defect prevents increasing angulation and deformity.

Cleft Lip and Palate

The most common developmental anomalies of the face are the cleft lip and cleft palate. The incidence of clefts is between 1:600 and 1:1000 live births. A cleft of the left lip and palate occurs more frequently in males and has a hereditary component; a cleft palate alone is seen more often in females and does not have a hereditary component. The etiology of clefts is not completely understood, but because heredity is known to play a significant role, many patients are concerned about the risk of clefts in their offspring. If one parent has had a cleft, a child has a 7% chance of having a cleft; this figure increases to 14% if there is already a sibling with a cleft. When two normal parents already have a child with a cleft, a second child has a 4.5% chance of being born with a cleft.

The lip and palate structures can be divided anatomically into prepalatal (primary palate), and palatal (secondary palate). The incisive foramen located in the midline on the hard palate just behind the alveolus divides the prepalatal and palatal clefts, as their embryology is different. The prepalatal structures form during the 4th to 7th week of fetal life and arise from three mesenchymal islands, one central and two lateral. Incomplete migration and fusion of these elements can lead to the clefts seen. Prepalatal clefts involve the lip, alveolus, nose and nasal cartilages. Cleft lips can be unilateral or bilateral, and complete or incomplete. The palatal structures at 7 weeks are composed of two palatal shelves that are vertically oriented along the sides of the tongue. As the neck of the fetus straightens, the tongue drops and the palatal shelves rotate upward to become horizontal by the 12th week. Palatal clefts can involve the hard palate, soft palate, and uvula. Various combinations of clefts of the prepalatal and palatal structures can be seen.

Treatment of the cleft lip is directed at returning the different lip elements to their normal position to improve appearance and correct such minor functional problems as lisping (Fig. 4.42). The timing of cleft lip repairs remains controversial. Generally, repairs are begun when the infant is aged 6–12 weeks and completed by age 6–9 months. Treatment of the nasal deformity is much more difficult because of the underdevelopment and malposition of the nasal cartilages. The cleft lip nasal deformity may require many revisions extending into the teenage years, although primary treatment of the nose at the time of lip repair is gaining wider acceptance because of recent promising results.

Whereas the cleft lip is repaired primarily for the sake of appearance, the cleft palate is repaired to ensure function, specifically the function of speech. The competent palate is able to elevate and come into contact with the posterior pharyngeal wall (creating velopharyngeal closure) during speech and swallowing. The inability to do this produces abnormal speech, which can range from hypernasal speech to nearly unintelligible speech. The various cleft palate repairs are designed at reorienting the musculature of the palate, closing the cleft, and lengthening the palate. As with the lip, the timing of cleft palate repair varies. While some surgeons complete the repair by the time the infant is 3 months of age, other surgeons will not attempt repair until 18 months. Many surgeons now prefer earlier closure to allow for more normal speech development.

Because of the abnormal orientation of the palatal musculature around the pharyngeal opening of the eustachian tube, middle ear infections are very common in these patients. Almost all of these children will require myringotomy tubes if long-term hearing problems are to be avoided. Another relatively uncommon cleft disorder is the Pierre Robin syndrome, in which the palatal cleft is associated with a small or retropositioned mandible and a posteriorly displaced tongue. Emergency treatment may be required to maintain the airway.

The child with a cleft palate may have numerous developmental problems; treatment should thus be conducted by a team of specialists under the direction of the plastic surgeon.

Other Congenital Head and Neck Anomalies

Branchial Cleft Cysts. Multiple other anomalies are possible within the head and neck area. The most common are variations of the branchial cleft cyst or sinus. This anomaly involves an epithelial tract along the lateral neck, which is seen along the anterior border of the sternocleidomastoid muscle. The cyst or sinus tract can range from a small blind pouch to a tract extending completely into the oral cavity. Treatment consists of surgical resection, the timing of which may be varied according to the patient's symptomatology.

Thyroglossal Duct Cyst. A thyroglossal duct cyst or sinus presents as an opening or defect in the absolute midline of the neck around the hyoid bone. The defect may present as either a small blind pouch or a sinus tract extending into the base of the tongue at the

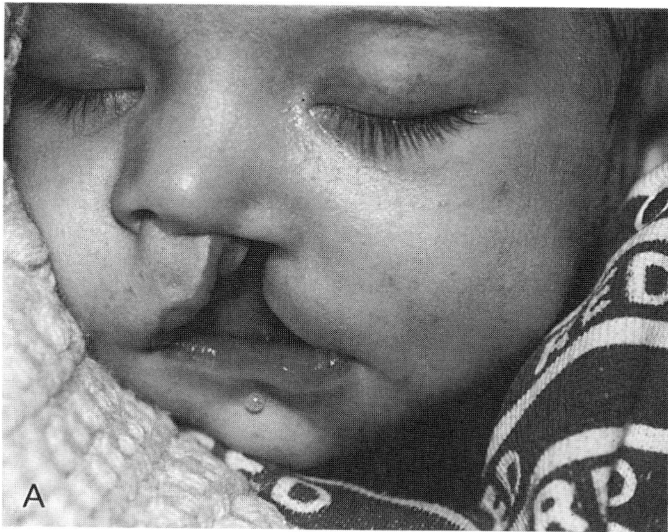

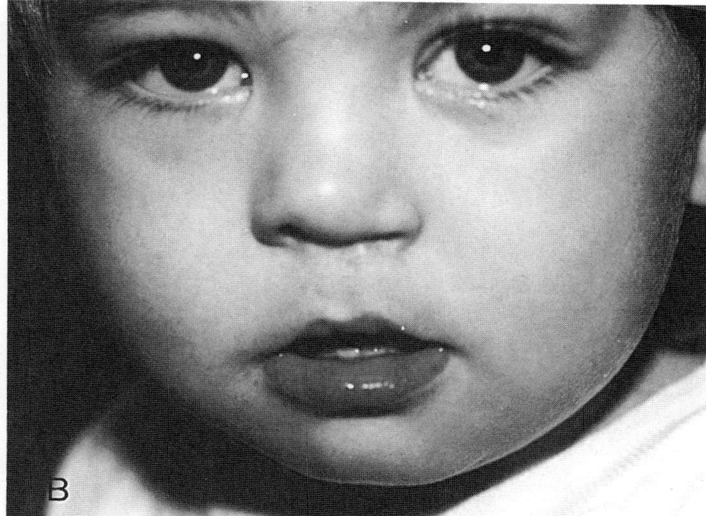

Figure 4.42. **A**, Four-week-old child seen with a complete cleft of the left lip. **B**, Same child at 2 years of age following lip repair using a rotation advancement method.

foramen cecum. Occasionally, as in the branchial cleft cyst, infection may occur and a brief course of antibiotics may be required. However, the definitive treatment for the sinus itself is surgical excision. Because a thyroglossal duct cyst routinely goes through the middle of the hyoid bone, adequate resection requires removing the central portion of the hyoid bone as well as the complete sinus, usually all the way to the base of the tongue.

Congenital Ear Deformities. Another type of congenital deformity is an ear deformity. Although complete absence of the ear (anotia) is rare, abnormally forming cartilage (protruding ears) and deficient cartilage (microtia) are relatively common. Anotia or microtia require the reconstruction of the cartilaginous framework of the ear. A large piece of cartilage is harvested, usually from the patient's rib, and carved to resemble the scaffolding of the ear. It is implanted and covered with adequate skin. Although the technique is difficult and demanding, expert hands can produce excellent results. The amount of reconstruction depends upon the severity of the defect. Routinely, three to four surgical procedures are required. Microtia repairs can be performed when a child is 6 years old, since the ear is almost adult size and adequate rib cartilage is available.

Congenital protruding ears are repaired by removing some of the conchal cartilage and plicating the remains to the mastoid fascia. Acquired ear deformities, as in partial amputation, can be repaired using techniques similar to those used for the reconstruction of congenital defects.

Acquired Deformities

Treatment of acquired soft tissue deformities frequently requires reconstructive surgery. Several factors are important to a successful reconstruction, beginning with a careful consideration of the etiology of the deformity and the natural history of the disease producing the deformity. Next, the deformity itself should be considered. Both the amount and type of tissue missing and the function of this tissue are important. Through such an evaluation, the patient's reconstructive needs can be understood. Finally, the reconstructive surgeon must choose the most appropriate method of reconstruction, keeping in mind the reconstructive ladder.

In many cases, several reconstructive options may be appropriate, or at least possible. A careful and comprehensive discussion of these options with the patient is important, since the patient is an important part of the decision-making process. Furthermore, since each patient's needs, desires, and expectations are different, it is very difficult to follow a "cookbook" approach that always treats certain wounds with specific operations. Each patient must be considered individually in order to appreciate his or her unique differences and needs.

Postmastectomy Breast Reconstruction

During the last 25 years, major advances have taken place in postmastectomy breast reconstruction. Technical advances include the development of tissue expanders, improvement in breast prostheses, and new methods of flap reconstruction. Psychological considerations have also come to be appreciated. The patient's psychological well-being and recovery may be significantly affected by proper breast reconstruction. As general surgeons have come to understand the methods of breast reconstruction, better collaboration with the reconstructive surgeon has resulted. Surgeons now understand that breast reconstruction can often be begun or completed at the time of mastectomy, and that the method chosen must take into account the patient's body habitus, life-style, healing capabilities, and desires. All options must be discussed with the patient and the patient's preference elicited. In fact, in cases where two

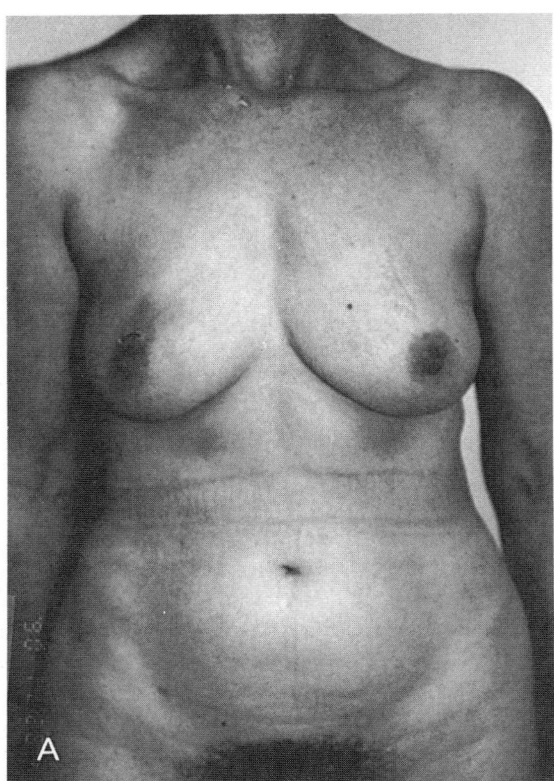

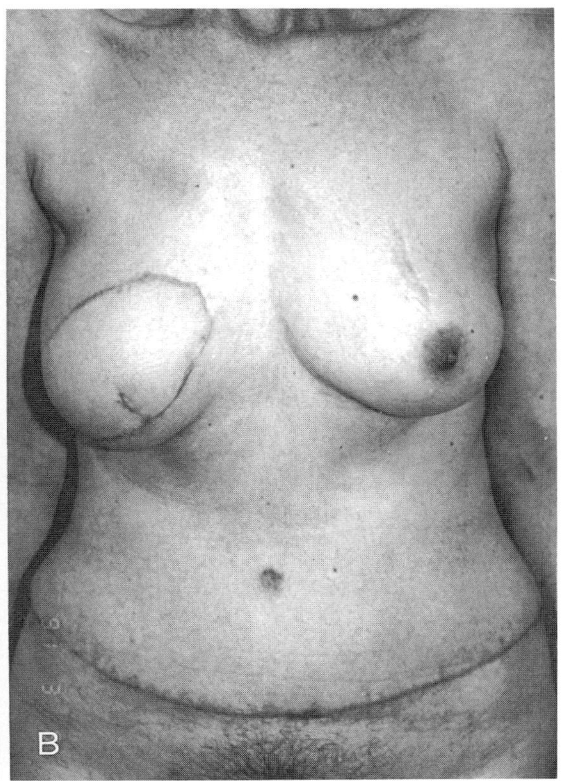

Figure 4.43. **A**, A 44-year-old woman with biopsy-proven carcinoma of the right breast prior to mastectomy. **B**, Status of patient after right modified mastectomy and immediate breast reconstruction with a TRAM flap.

options are equally appropriate—or nearly so—the patient herself may choose the operation she prefers.

Before undertaking breast reconstruction, the surgeon must determine whether the procedure should be performed, what the timing should be, and what method should be followed. While some form of reconstruction is possible for most patients, others (because of advanced disease, associated illness, or unrealistic expectations) should be counseled instead about external prostheses. The timing of reconstruction can be immediate, starting with mastectomy, or delayed, beginning after the mastectomy wound has healed. While a number of considerations come into play at this juncture, frequently the patient's desires are the most important. Finally, the appropriate technique should be considered.

Reconstruction of the breast can be divided into reconstruction of the breast mound and of the nipple-areola complex. For the breast mound, local or distant tissue may be used in conjunction with an implant. A small or moderate-sized implant placed beneath the chest wall skin and the muscles of the chest wall (pectoralis major and serratus anterior) often gives an acceptable breast mound. If local tissue is not available in sufficient quantity to cover the implant size chosen, a tissue expander may first be placed in these patients to be followed by the permanent implant at a second operation.

When local tissue is either not available or not preferred, distant tissue can be used. The most common source of such is the lower soft tissue of the abdominal wall or transverse rectus abdominis myocutaneous (TRAM) flap (Fig. 4.43). A transverse paddle of skin and fat from just above the umbilicus down to the pubic hairline can be elevated and supported by the deep superior epigastric vessels that lie within the rectus abdominis muscle. By maintaining the attachment to one or both rectus abdominis muscles, the tissue can be transferred to the chest to create the breast mound. This procedure not only provides the best breast reconstruction aesthetically but also improves the donor site by providing an abdominal lipectomy. Back skin and fat transferred with the underlying latissimus dorsi supported by the thoracodorsal vessels may also be used. This flap is exceedingly reliable and can be used when other options are unavailable or not preferred. A small breast implant can be placed beneath these flaps to provide the necessary breast mound projection. Free flaps have also been used. The TRAM flap can be based on the deep inferior epigastric vessels and transferred as a free flap with only a small amount of underlying muscle. Other potential donor sites are the buttock and lateral thigh.

Reconstruction of the nipple and areola, which completes breast reconstruction, is chosen by many patients. The nipple is created by a flap of local tissue folded upon itself to give adequate projection or by a free graft from the contralateral nipple, if it is quite large. The areola can then be mimicked by intradermal tattooing to match the color of the normal areola or by a full-thickness skin graft from the upper inner thigh (skin that is darker).

Since many options for breast reconstruction are available, adequate time must be spent with the patient to determine how to suit her needs. The patient should also be counseled about what to expect regarding her operation, her recovery, and the ultimate aesthetic results. Frequently, the reconstructed breast can look as good or better than the contralateral breast. At other times, the reconstruction may appear only adequate (especially when the patient is fully clothed) but is superior to an external prosthesis.

Lower Extremity Reconstruction

The soft tissues of the leg frequently require reconstruction of defects caused by trauma, vascular disease, or diabetes. Trauma is the most common cause for reconstruction, and high energy blunt trauma (such as that sustained in motor vehicle accidents, crush injuries, or falls) is the most complex to repair. Wounds can involve the skin, bone, and vasculature of the leg. Loss of soft tissue will cause the exposure of fracture sites, orthopedic hardware, or vascular reconstruction, allowing infection, which in turn will cause loss of fixation, disruption of vascular anastomoses, or osteomyelitis. All may cause the loss of the extremity.

Because of the complex nature of the wounds, a team approach involving a trauma, a vascular, an orthopedic, and a plastic surgeon must be employed. The first priority is survival of the patient. Next, the viability of the leg must be assured with vascular reconstruction undertaken as necessary. Finally, bony fixation or stabilization must be achieved to assure adequate limb length, proper orientation, and a stable skeletal platform for soft tissue reconstruction. Open fractures of the leg present the most challenging reconstruction problems. While some wounds can be managed with skin grafts, skin flaps, or fasciocutaneous flaps, generally muscle flaps are required. These flaps have the ability to cover large areas of exposed bone, obliterate dead space, and provide a rich vascular coverage of exposed fracture sites to assist in bone healing.

In terms of available muscle coverage, the leg is divided into a proximal, middle, and distal third. Wounds of the proximal third are generally reconstructed with the medial or lateral gastrocnemius muscles, usually covered by a skin graft. Likewise, the middle third of the leg is the domain of the soleus muscle flap. Because of the lack of local muscle flaps in the distal third of the leg, free muscle transfers are usually required (Fig. 4.15). Free flaps may also be required for more proximal reconstruction when local muscles are rendered unusable as a result of trauma.

In cases where systemic disease is the cause of defects (usually ulcers) in the soft tissues of the leg, the underlying disease must first be treated. Ischemic limbs should be revascularized. When venous or lymphatic insufficiency is the underlying cause, patients should be put to bed with their extremities elevated. In addition to treating the underlying disease, infection should be treated and appropriate wound care administered. Generally, wounds that result from these diseases can be reconstructed with skin grafts. Prolonged bed rest, elevation, and, occasionally, adjuncts such as hyperbaric oxygen are necessary. In other cases, more complex reconstructive methods may be needed.

Pressure Sore Reconstruction

Pressure sores can add a significant cost and complexity to patient care. They can develop in any location but usually develop over a bony prominence. If, because of paralysis and insensitivity, debilitation, or disease, a patient lies in a given position for more than 2 hours, irreversible tissue damage will begin. The muscle and subcutaneous tissues are most susceptible to pressure damage and are closest to the bony prominences. Thus, most sores are larger at their base than at their visible surface, assuming the shape of an inverted cone. Obviously, prevention is the best treatment. Patients who are unable to turn themselves require frequent repositioning. Alternately, patients at risk can be placed on a fluidized air bed such as a Clinitron, which distributes pressure evenly throughout the body. Patients with spinal cord injuries are the most susceptible because of their insensibility in areas of pressure.

Once a pressure sore is formed, treatment is directed at caring for the wound and placing the patient on a fluidized air bed to prevent further pressure-related damage. After the wound has been debrided and is sufficiently clean, reconstruction is considered. The best candidates for reconstruction are those who are alert and cooperative enough to prevent the recurrence of pressure sores. Patients who are likely to develop pressure sores immediately after treatment should be managed with wound care alone. Likewise, patients suffering from malnutrition or other major systemic illnesses should have these problems addressed before they are considered for reconstruction.

Operative treatment is directed at *total* excision of the ulcer, removal of the underlying bony prominence, and coverage with healthy tissue. While many sores can be covered with local skin flaps, muscle flaps have been of great benefit (Fig. 4.44).

Pressure sores are most commonly located in the regions of the ischial tuberosities, sacrum, and trochanter. Less commonly, they are found at the elbows, heels, and occiput. In patients with spinal cord injuries, virtually any muscle or myocutaneous flap may be used for soft tissue coverage. Commonly used muscles include the gluteus maximus, gracilis, tensor fasciae latae, and hamstrings. However, in ambulatory patients many of these muscles are needed for ambulation and thus their function cannot be sacrificed. Also, because pressure sores may be a chronic problem, flaps should be designed, when possible, to allow their reuse if another pressure sore develops.

Head and Neck Reconstruction

Malignancy involving the head and neck, frequently intraoral squamous cell carcinoma, is by far the most

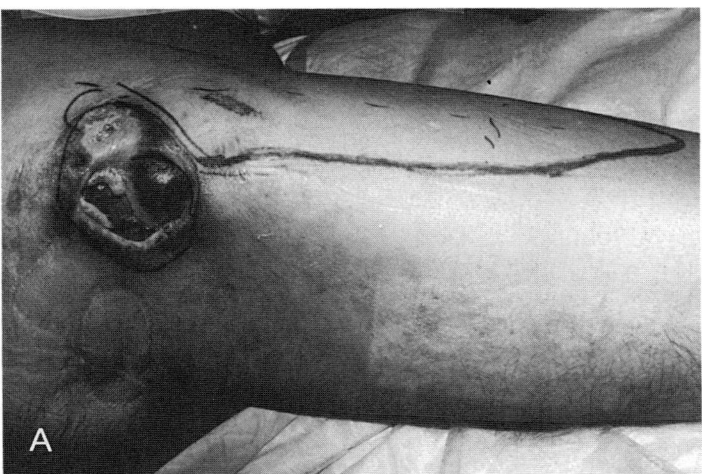

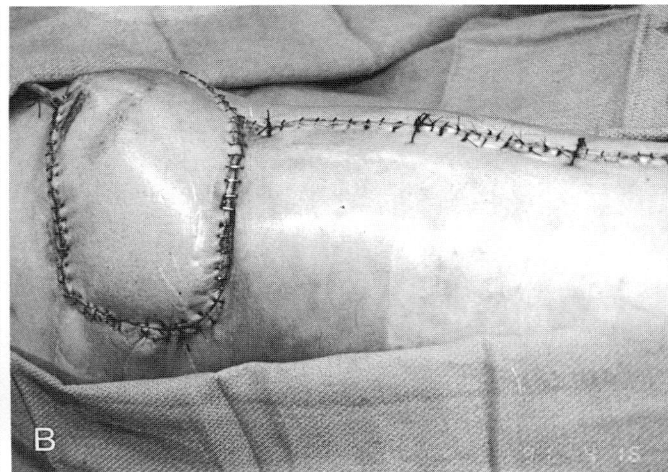

Figure 4.44. **A**, This paraplegic has developed a trochanteric pressure sore that, **B**, has been closed with a tensor fasciae latae myocutaneous flap.

common disease for which tissue reconstruction in that area may be needed. Trauma and other diseases can also produce defects that require reconstruction of the skin of the head and neck, of the intraoral mucosal lining, or of the bone—usually the mandible. In the case of cancer resection, reconstruction is usually performed at the time of tumor ablation. A number of axial pattern skin flaps have been useful in reconstructing some defects. The most commonly used is the pectoralis major myocutaneous flap (Fig. 4.45). Being based on the thoracoacromial vessels, the flap can be elevated and tunneled through the neck for use in many areas of the head. Other myocutaneous flaps have been used, such as the latissimus dorsi and the trapezius. Free flaps can also provide excellent reconstructions. Osteocutaneous free flaps, or free flaps including bone, (e.g., the radial forearm flap with a portion of the underlying radius, the iliac flap with a portion of the underlying iliac crest) may be used when mandibular reconstruction is desired.

Aesthetic Surgery

Aesthetic surgery involves improving the form of a normal structure. At times certain operations that are normally considered aesthetic are performed for reconstructive purposes, such as a rhinoplasty performed to correct the appearance of a nasal deformity resulting from trauma. All aesthetic surgery is considered elective and should be undertaken only under optimal conditions and with the patient's clear understanding of all aspects of the surgery and recovery. Since these operations are directed toward "perceived" abnormalities, extensive preoperative consultation is required to understand such perceptions and how surgery will affect them. Aesthetic surgery can be broadly divided into body-contouring surgery and surgery of the aging face. Rhinoplasty, although not performed because of problems deriving from the aging process, will be considered with these facial operations. Although the discussion below is aimed at elective aesthetic surgery, certain operations that are considered to be reconstructive will also be noted.

Body Contouring Surgery

Mammoplasty. Surgery of the breast involves changing both the shape and size of the breast. Operations aimed primarily at decreasing the size of the breast, called *reduction mammoplasty*, are reconstructive. Excessively large breasts create both physical and psychological problems. Physical problems include neck and back pain, posture-related problems, grooves in the shoulders created by bra straps, and skin problems within the inframammary fold. Psychological problems arise in adolescents who are ridiculed by their peers for having developed ample breasts at a young age. The goal of reduction mammoplasty is to decrease the size of the breast, elevate the nipple position, and preserve the blood supply to the nipple and areolar complex (Fig. 4.46). The majority of these operations leave the nipple and areolar complex attached to a pedicle of underlying breast tissue from which it receives its blood supply. Accordingly, these procedures are described by the orientation of the pedicle: inferior pedicle, superior pedicle, central pedicle, lateral pedicle, and inferior and superior pedicle. The correct nipple location must be chosen immediately preoperatively with the patient upright, at which time all skin markings for the reduction are made.

Breasts that are considered too small can be enlarged through breast augmentation (*augmentation mammoplasty*), achieved with breast implants. Implants can be placed either directly beneath the breast tissue (subglandular) or beneath the pectoralis major (subpectoral or submuscular) by various approaches in skin incisions. The implants themselves are usually made of an outer silicone shell filled with silicone gel, saline, or a combination of both. The most common problem related to implants is breast firmness, which can result

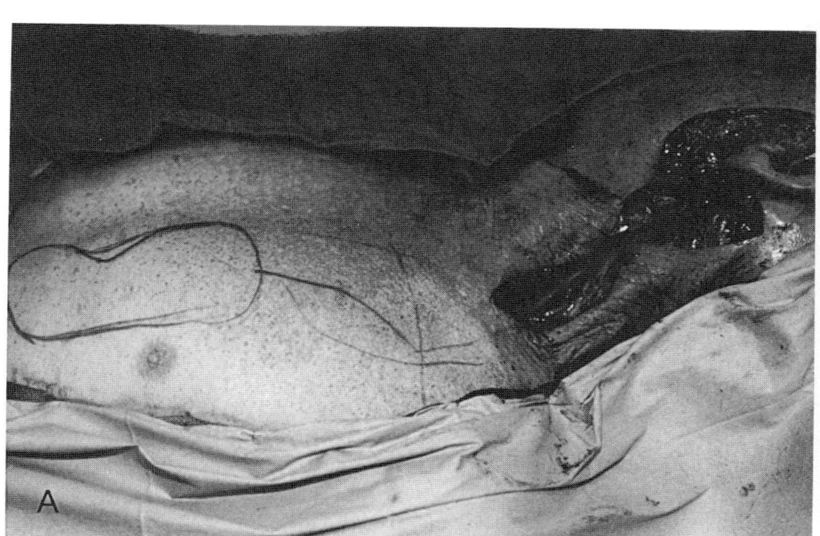

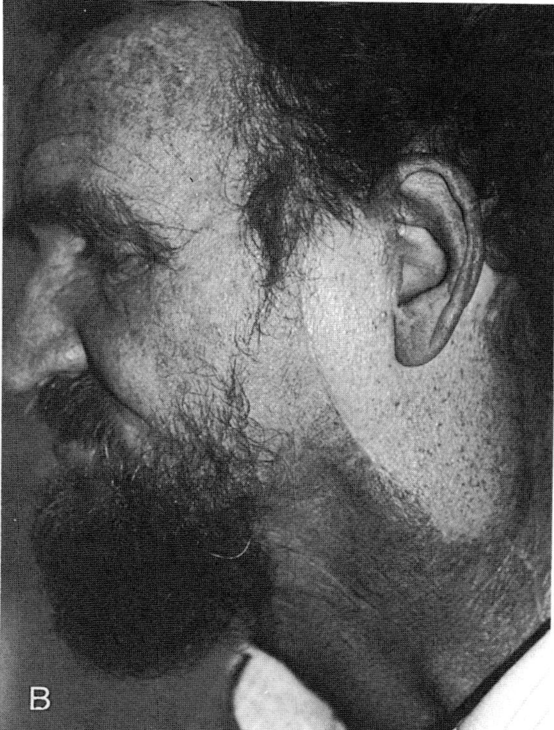

Figure 4.45. Radical resection for recurrent squamous cell carcinoma of the cheek and underlying parotid gland. **B**, Following reconstruction using a pectoralis major myocutaneous flap.

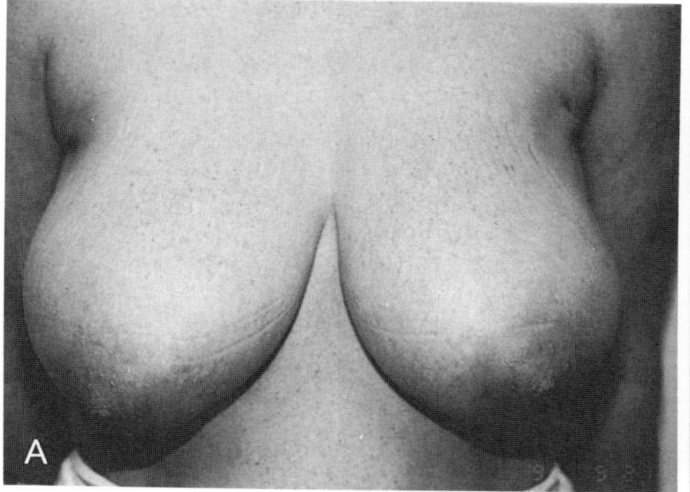

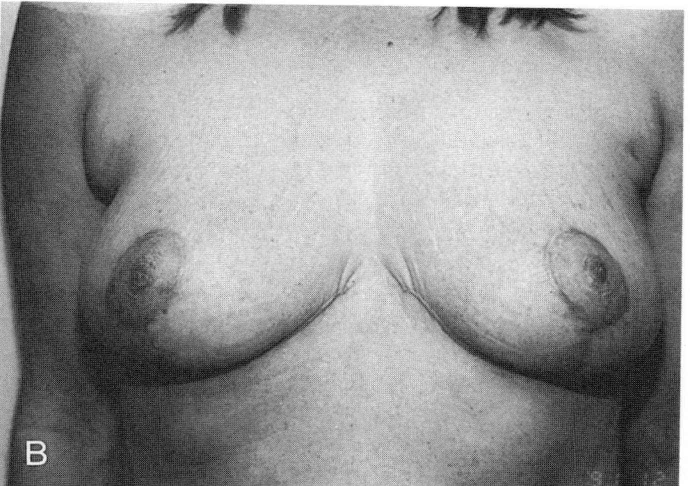

Figure 4.46. **A**, Mammary hyperplasia. **B**, After bilateral reduction mammoplasty.

from excessive scar tissue, or capsule, that normally forms around all implants. Capsular contractures may be symptomatic in 15–20% of patients, and some may require reoperation.

When breast size is adequate but shape is inadequate—because of changes resulting from pregnancy or age—a *mastopexy* or breast lift may be done. In this procedure the nipple position is elevated by an appropriate skin excision. In some patients, breast augmentation can be combined with the mastopexy (Fig. 4.47).

Abdominoplasty. Reshaping the abdominal wall generally involves the excision of abdominal skin and fat (an abdominoplasty) and the repair or tightening of the rectus abdominis muscle (repair of rectus diastasis). The latter is considered reconstructive in women because it addresses abnormalities of the abdominal wall that result from pregnancy and child bearing. Although a low abdominal incision is most commonly used, a vertical or other orientation may be required if previous surgical scars are present. In general, the goal of skin

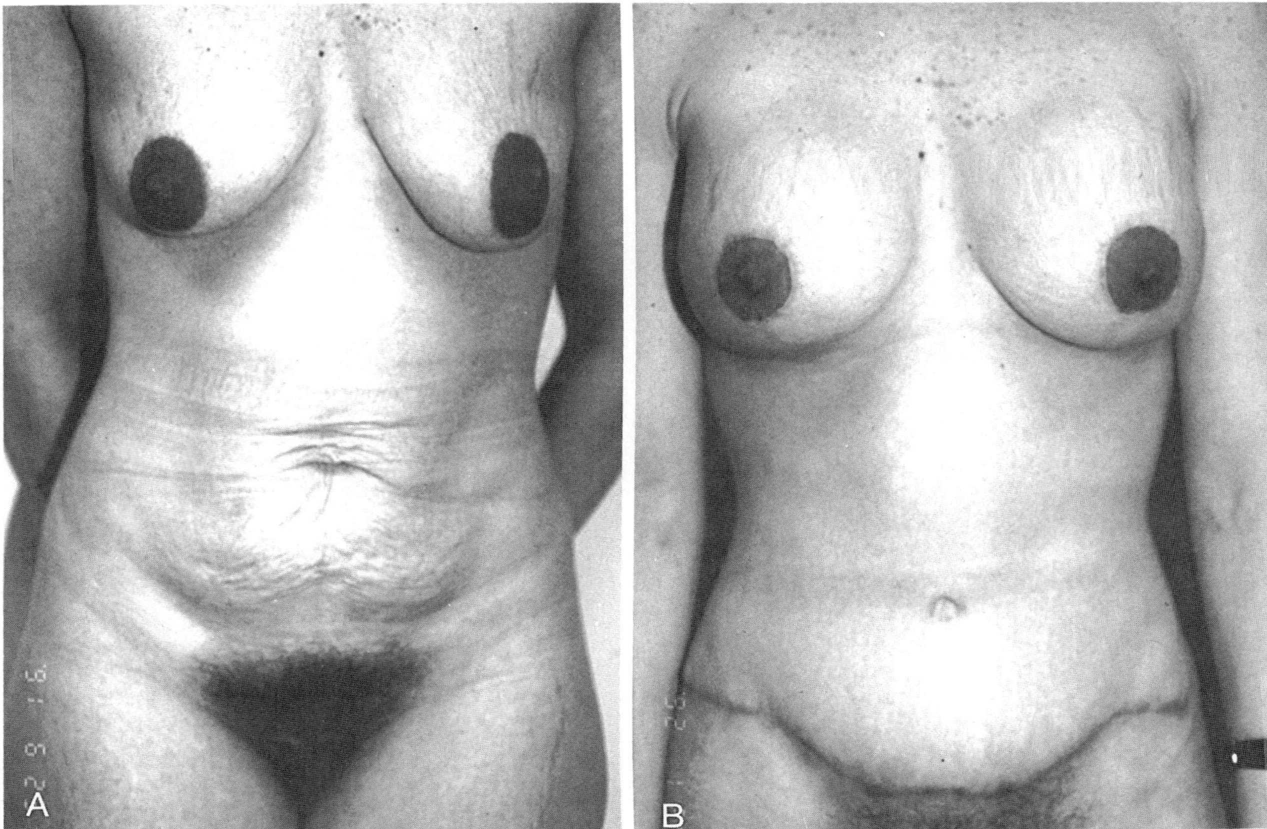

Figure 4.47. **A**, Following her childbearing years, this patient presented for an abdominoplasty and breast augmentation and mastopexy. **B**, Six months following the body contouring surgery.

excision is to remove the skin between the umbilicus and the pubic hair. The abdominal skin and fat from the underlying musculature (up to the costal margin) are elevated and the umbilicus is repositioned (Fig. 4.47).

Suction-Assisted Lipectomy. Suction-assisted lipectomy is directed at the removal of fat collections that are out of proportion to the patient's normal subcutaneous fat distribution. These procedures are not for obese patients nor are they designed for weight reduction. Rather, they should be performed on patients who are close to their ideal weight. In women, the lateral hips, thighs, legs, and abdomen are most commonly treated, while in men the hip rolls ("love handles") and abdomen are commonly suctioned.

Through small incisions, suction cannulas are introduced. When connected to two atmospheres of suction, the normally solid fat can be aspirated as a semisolid. Important technical considerations include appropriate fat removal, preservation of a normal subcutaneous fat layer, and prolonged postoperative compression (6–8 weeks).

Surgery of the Aging Face

The effects of aging are frequently seen in the skin and underlying tissue of the face, including the eyelids, forehead, and neck. A combination of factors produces these changes, including gravity, atrophy or thinning of the skin, and sun damage. While these processes are most evident in the skin, the underlying fat and musculature of the skin and neck are also affected. The signs of aging are predominantly those of sagging or ptotic skin: wrinkles and herniation of the underlying fat. The age at which these changes appear is quite variable. Some individuals in their 30s can profit from surgical correction of the aging process, particularly if they have a hereditary predisposition to early signs of aging or if they have had excessive sun damage. Generally, most patients seek such surgery in the fifth, sixth, or seventh decade of life.

Facelift. A facelift, also known as a cervicofacial rhytidectomy, is directed toward correcting the effects of aging, generally below the level of the eyes and including the neck. Areas most affected include the nasolabial folds, jaw line or jowls, and the neck. In this procedure, the skin of the face and neck is lifted up from the underlying skin and facial musculature to a variable degree by means of an incision placed in front of and behind the ear and within the hairline, and a small submental incision. Generally, a deeper layer of facial muscles and platysma is also dissected. During the operation, this deeper layer (known as the SMAS or superficial musculoaponeurotic system) is tightened, excess fat from the neck is removed, and the excessive skin is resected. The most feared complication of this procedure is injury to branches of the facial nerve that run beneath the SMAS. Other complications include bleeding and skin slough, seen mostly in cigarette smokers.

Blepharoplasty. The recontouring of the eyelids is achieved through a blepharoplasty, since these structures are changed very little by a facelift. In addition to excess skin of both the upper and lower eyelids, fat pockets within the eyelids tend to become much more pronounced with age. Fat pockets in the lower eyelids give the impression of "bags" beneath the eyes. Some patients have a strong family predisposition to lower lid fat pockets and can profit from a lower lid blepharoplasty at a young age.

For an upper lid blepharoplasty, the incision is placed within the normal eyelid crease above the eye; in the lower eyelids the incision is just beneath the eyelashes. Through these, fat from the pockets is appropriately resected, and excess skin and muscle (orbicularis oculi) is removed. Major complications result from bleeding or excess skin removal.

Rhinoplasty. Change in the shape of the nose may be sought because of either trauma or the patient's desire to improve the normal nasal profile. In cases of trauma the operation is considered reconstructive; in other cases the correction is considered aesthetic. In each case, the rhinoplasty is performed in much the same way. While this complex operation is being performed, attention must be given to the nasal airway. When this airway is obstructed, surgery on the nasal septum or turbinates may be needed.

Through incisions usually placed within the nose, the nasal cartilages and bones are exposed. These are then reshaped to give a better profile. Usual areas of patient concern are a broad nasal bridge, dorsal hump, or bulbous nasal tip. Since the nasal bones are usually cut, postoperative support is required with a splint and nasal packs.

Acknowledgment

This chapter is based in part on Plastic and reconstructive surgery: essentials for students. Chicago: Plastic Surgery Educational Foundation, American Society of Plastic and Reconstructive Surgery, 1979. Appreciation is given to the Educational Foundation of the American Society of Plastic and Reconstructive Surgeons for their assistance in the preparation of this chapter.

SUGGESTED READINGS

Green D. Operative hand surgery. New York: Churchill Livingstone, 1988.

Habal MB, Ariyan S. Facial fractures. Philadelphia: BC Decker, 1989.

McCarthy J. Plastic surgery. Philadelphia: WB Saunders, 1990.

McCraw JB, Arnold PG. McCraw and Arnold's atlas of muscle and myocutaneous flaps. Norfolk: Hampton Press, 1986.

Noone RB. Plastic and reconstructive surgery of the breast. Philadelphia: BC Decker, 1991.

Plastic and reconstructive surgery: essentials for students. Chicago: Plastic Surgery Educational Foundation, American Society of Plastic and Reconstructive Surgery, 1979.

Smith JW, Aston SJ. Plastic surgery. Boston: Little, Brown, 1991.

Yaremchuk MJ, Burgess AR, Brumback RJ. Lower extremity salvage and reconstruction. New York: Elsevier, 1989.

Skills

REPAIR OF A SIMPLE LACERATION

A patient presents with a slightly irregular 3-cm laceration overlying the right cheek parallel to the nasolabial fold. The laceration is to be excised and repaired.

Preparation and Local Anesthetic. The wound is gently cleansed with solution such as Betadine. The margins of the wound are then injected with local anesthetic (lidocaine with epinephrine). A 25- or 27-gauge needle is used for the injection so that the anesthetic is liberally dispersed intradermally and directly beneath the dermis.

Cleansing. Once the area of the wound has been properly anesthetized, the wound is irrigated with saline using a 20- or 30-mL syringe and a 21-gauge needle that allows the saline to be sprayed into the wound under some pressure. Any debris is removed.

Excision. As the margins of the wound are irregular, they are first excised in order to give a smooth edge to the laceration, facilitating a better repair. Using a No. 15 knife blade, 1–2 mm of the edges of the wound are incised. The incision is carried down through the dermis such that all irregular tissue may be excised.

Repair. The wound is repaired in layers. An absorbable suture (5-0 chromic) is used in the subdermal tissues. Simple inverted stitches are used such that the knots will be buried away from the skin edge. In placing these sutures, deeper edges of the dermis should be included in the stitch to allow the skin edges to come together and take tension off the skin itself. Next, the skin is closed with a nonabsorbable suture (6-0 nylon). Simple interrupted sutures are used, taking care to evert the skin edges. Once the repair has been completed, the wound is cleansed and dressed with an antibiotic ointment.

The patient is referred for suture removal in 5–6 days.

EXCISION OF A BENIGN SKIN LESION

A benign lesion such as a nevus or small cyst is to be excised from the forehead of a patient. Before performing this excision, you should evaluate the lines of relaxed skin tension in order to plan the long axis of the excision to parallel these. The lines may be drawn on the skin with marking pen before prepping the field.

Preparation. The field is prepared with Betadine solution. Local anesthetic (lidocaine with epinephrine) is injected intradermally around the field of excision.

Excision. An elliptical incision is made with a No. 15 blade. This incision is parallel to the lines of relaxed skin tension and is 2 to 3 times as long as the lesion is wide. The incision is then carried through the full thickness of the skin into the subdermal fat. Care is taken to completely excise any skin lesion or any lesion directly beneath the skin.

The specimen is placed in a proper container for pathologic examination. A brief clinical description of the appearance of the lesion should accompany the specimen to the pathology laboratory.

Repair. The wound is repaired in layers. Buried stitches of 5-0 chromic are used for the subdermal tissues. Simple everting stitches of 6-0 nylon are used for the skin.

The wound is dressed with an antibiotic ointment. The patient is referred for suture removal in 5–6 days. At the time of suture removal, you should review the pathology report with the patient.

EXAMINATION OF THE INJURED FACE

A patient presents with multiple facial injuries that must be evaluated. Before beginning your evaluation, you must assure that the patient's airway is secure and that the cervical spine is protected. Any areas of bleeding should be controlled by exerting pressure on them. Once the patient has been stabilized, a comprehensive evaluation of the face is undertaken.

History. Obtain a history of the accident or of the mechanism of injury. The history may be obtained from the patient, other victims or bystanders, or the paramedics. If the patient is alert, ask the patient which areas of the face hurt. Also ask whether the patient has diplopia and whether occlusion feels normal.

Inspection. Visually examine the face. Look for areas of ecchymosis and swelling. Note any asymmetries. Measure the intercanthal distance (it should be less than 38 mm). Check the occlusion. Examine the functions of the facial nerve.

Palpation. Feel for any irregular contours or step-offs of the normal bony anatomy. Begin at the top of the face, palpating each side simultaneously , and continue down to the mandible. Note any asymmetries in injured areas as compared to contralateral injured areas. Check for false motion of the facial bones, especially the maxilla and mandible. Examine the extraocular movements of the eyes to determine the presence of any entrapment. Check for anesthesia of the face.

Note any abnormal clinical findings and establish your provisional diagnosis. Obtain facial x-rays and review these with the radiologist or the plastic surgical consultant to confirm your diagnosis. If open wounds are present on the face in patients with underlying fractures, discuss with the consultant whether or not the laceration should be closed at this time or during the operative repair of the fractures.

ALLEN'S TEST

An Allen's test is used to diagnose the integrity of the ulnar or radial artery as it supplies blood to the hand. In normal circumstances, these arteries should communicate through the deep and superficial palmar arches. In circumstances where this is not the case, or when either artery has been injured, the Allen's test is of help.

The radial artery is first examined. The patient is asked to make a very tight fist. The examiner compresses the ulnar artery at the base of the hypothenar eminence. The patient is then asked to open the hand. If the radial artery is intact, the hand will be pink. If the radial artery is not intact, the hand will be blanched when the fist is opened.

The ulnar artery is examined next. The patient is again asked to make a tight fist, and the radial artery is compressed at the base of the thenar eminence. The patient is asked to open the hand. If the ulnar artery is intact, the hand will be pink. If the ulnar artery is not intact, the hand will blanch when the fist is released and will not pink up until the radial artery is released.

In most circumstances, the ulnar artery is the dominant artery to the deep and superficial palmar arches. However, there are certain circumstances and certain diseases (e.g., scleroderma) in which this is not the case.

EXAMINATION OF THE INJURED HAND

Before beginning a comprehensive examination of the hand, bleeding within the hand should be controlled with pressure. As the examination of the hand is complex, careful notation of any abnormalities found should be made.

History. Inquire about the mechanism of injury. Find out in what type of environment the injury has taken place. Ascertain the patient's hand dominance, vocation, and avocations. Ask the patient where pain is felt, where the hand is numb, and what cannot be done with the hand. Inquire about the patient's tetanus immunization status.

Inspection. Note areas of swelling and location of lacerations. Observe the normal position of all digits at rest and look for any rotational deformities of the finger.

Palpation. First ascertain that the hand is viable. Note any areas that appear to be ischemic and check for good capillary refill in all of the digits. The integrity of the ulnar and radial arteries should be confirmed using an Allen's test. A Doppler examination of these arteries and the digital arteries can also be undertaken if necessary.

Test the motor functions of the median, radial, and ulnar nerves. Also test the sensory function of these nerves. Check for anesthesia or lack of two-point discrimination in the tip of all of the digits in order to diagnose digital nerve injuries.

Examine independent flexion of each MP and IP joint. Be sure to differentiate between the deep and superficial flexors of the fingers. Examine independent extension of all MP and IP joints.

Gently palpate all the bones of the hand for any underlying bony abnormalities. Have the patient make a fist and check the alignment of the fingers.

Obtain x-rays of the hand and wrist and review these with a radiologist or hand surgeon. Ask the consultant if any lacerations should be closed and if the hand should be splinted. Administer the appropriate tetanus prophylaxis and, if appropriate, broad-spectrum antibiotics.

DRAINAGE OF A FELON

The diagnosis of a felon is made by the fusiform swelling of the pulp of the distal phalanx. The distal phalanx should be examined to determine the correct location of incisions used to drain the finger. If the abscess appears to be "pointing" on the volar pad of the finger, the incision may be made at the point. In other cases, a lateral incision along the axis of the finger should be made.

Local Anesthetic. Before any drainage is attempted, a finger block is achieved using lidocaine without epinephrine. (Epinephrine may induce permanent vasospasm of the digital arteries, which can lead to necrosis of the distal finger.) Using a 21- or smaller-gauge needle, several mL of local anesthetic are injected into the web space at the base of the affected finger on each side. Several minutes are allowed to pass to ensure that complete anesthesia has been achieved. The finger must be tested for complete anesthesia before the felon is drained. If anesthesia is not complete, more anesthetic must be injected.

Incision. The finger is then prepped and draped as a sterile field. Unless the felon is pointing through the volar fat pad, a lateral incision is made. Using a No. 11 blade, a stab incision is made from the lateral aspect of the finger into the pulp of the finger. Several mL of pus may be obtained, which should be sent for routine culture and sensitivity. It may be necessary to extend the incision completely through the pulp and out of the other side of the finger. A hemostat should be inserted and opened to ensure that any septations are broken up in order to allow complete drainage of the pus. A small piece of packing then is inserted into the finger. The finger is cleansed and an appropriate dressing is placed.

Arrangements are made for the patient to be examined the following day. At this time, the pack will be removed and the patient will be begun on twice daily soaks of the finger in warm water. The patient should be placed on broad-spectrum antibiotics to allow for coverage of *Staphylococcus aureus*. First-generation cephalosporins are probably most appropriate.

Study Questions

1. An 18-year-old female presents complaining about the appearance of a scar on her wrist from a laceration repaired 6 months ago. She thinks the scar may be a keloid. The scar is raised and reddened but does not extend beyond the boundaries of the wound. What do you recommend?
2. A 21-year-old was involved in a motor vehicle accident 4 hours ago. He struck his chin on the steering wheel and sustained an irregular 3-cm laceration. How should the laceration be repaired?
3. A 45-year-old male stumbled and lacerated his left lower leg 36 hours ago while intoxicated. Now that he is sober, he presents to you in the emergency room for treatment. The left lateral leg has a dirty, 6-cm laceration that is draining and foul smelling. How should you manage this patient and his wound?
4. While getting out of bed, a 36-year-old diabetic woman fell and lacerated her right anterior leg on a footstool. She has raised a long, proximally based skin flap in the pretibial area. You think most of the tissue is viable. How should you manage the wound to encourage healing and the viability of all of the tissue?
5. You are assisting a resident and an attending plastic surgeon on a reconstructive case, when the attending asks the residents to explain the difference between a skin graft and a skin flap. How would you respond?
6. A 53-year-old man suffered a burn to the side of his nose. The 2 – 3 cm defect now needs a skin graft. What type of graft would you use and where should you take it from?
7. What systemic conditions may interfere with successful skin graft healing? What local wound considerations may affect skin graft healing? What can you do about these?
8. What is the difference between an axial pattern flap and a random flap? Would a free flap be an axial or random pattern flap?
9. A young male is transported to your emergency room immediately following a motor vehicle crash in which he sustained injuries only to his face. He has multiple facial lacerations with underlying fractures and is bleeding significantly. Although he is not in shock, he is having difficulty maintaining an airway. Describe your initial management and evaluation of this patient.
10. A 20-year-old male college student was involved in a fight last weekend. He was told he had a blow-out fracture. How should you evaluate him to determine if he needs repair of this fracture?
11. Describe the anatomic differences between a LeFort I, LeFort II, and LeFort III fracture and how you would diagnose each of these.
12. A 32-year-old housewife sustained a cut on the volar aspect of her wrist at the base of the hypothenar eminence. The cut bled heavily at first but now has stopped. She is without sensation over her small finger and the majority of her ring finger. What do you think she has injured and how would you evaluate her?
13. In evaluating a laceration over the flexor tendons of the long finger, how can you diagnose lacerations of the superficial or deep and superficial flexors?
14. A young female slipped on the ice and fell on her outstretched right hand. She is quite tender over the anatomic snuff box, but her x-rays seem to be normal. How should you manage her?
15. A 32-year-old intoxicated male presents with a small laceration over the fifth metacarpal joint, dorsally. You suspect he may have been in a fight earlier in the evening, although he will not give you an accurate history about the etiology of his cut. What do you suspect and how should you treat him?
16. A 28-year-old female typist has been experiencing numbness and tingling in her right thumb and index finger, especially at night. What do you suspect? How can you confirm your diagnosis? How will you treat her?
17. A young mother who herself has had a cleft lip just gave birth to a child with a cleft palate. She is full of

questions. What do you tell her about the importance of the palate? In addition to a cleft palate repair, what else may the child need? If the mother and father have another child, what is the risk that this child will also have a cleft?

18. A 44-year-old woman has had a right breast biopsy that proved the presence of a 1.5-cm intraductal carcinoma. Her surgeon has recommended a mastectomy. She comes to you requesting breast reconstruction. What options are available to her?
19. A 32-year-old male sustained a point-blank shotgun blast to his left ankle when his shotgun accidentally discharged. He has sustained extensive bone loss in the ankle joint and has needed vascular reconstruction for the foot. Your orthopedic colleague, who has placed him in an external fixateur, asks you to evaluate the wound and achieve soft tissue coverage for it. What type of coverage would you select?
20. A 28-year-old obese white female presents to your office having recently heard about liposuction on a morning TV talk show. She is interested in liposuction of her abdomen, thighs, hips, and arms to help lose some weight. What do you recommend to her?
21. One of your orthopedic colleagues has referred to you a patient who complains of severe neck and back pain. She is a 23-year-old college student of medium build who wears a very large bra cup size (36 DD). What might you recommend to this woman?

5 Otolaryngology: Diseases of the Head and Neck

Toni M. Ganzel, M.D.. Serge A. Martinez, M.D., Michael B. Nolph, M.D., Welby Winstead, M.D., and Gordon T. McMurry, M.D.

ASSUMPTIONS

The student has completed a physical diagnosis course and is familiar with how to use an otoscope, nasal speculum, tongue blade for pharyngeal exam, and a laryngeal mirror.

The student knows the basic anatomy of the ear, including pinna, external auditory canal, tympanic membrane, ossicles and cochlea, and semicircular canals.

The student knows the basic auditory and vestibular neural pathways.

The student knows the anatomy of the nose, including (*a*) bony and cartilage structure and (*b*) the internal framework of the septum, turbinates, meatus, and posterior choanae.

The student knows the basic anatomy of the sinuses and the physiology of mucous clearance.

The student knows the anatomy of the oropharynx, including the tongue, palate, velopharyngeal region, tonsils, and hypopharynx.

The student knows the external support structure of the larynx, including cartilage and bony support.

The student knows the basic lymphatic drainage patterns of the head and neck.

The student understands the physiology of swallowing, phonation, and respiration.

The student knows the basic anatomy of the triangles of the neck and what structures are normally palpable in the neck.

The student knows the external landmarks for a cricothyroidotomy and tracheostomy.

OBJECTIVES

1. Differentiate between conductive and sensorineural hearing loss and identify treatable causes.
2. Compare and contrast causes of otalgia, including referred pain and lesions of the auricle, external auditory canal, and middle ear.
3. Discuss the causes, diagnosis, treatment, and complications of acute and chronic otitis media with effusion. List indications for tympanocentesis, myringotomy, and tympanotomy tube placement.
4. Classify tinnitus according to etiology and specific type.
5. Differentiate vestibular from nonvestibular causes of dizziness.
6. Describe the common risk factors for and the appropriate workup of a patient with epistaxis.
7. List the causes of nasal obstruction.
8. List the indications for surgery in acute sinusitis.
9. Discuss the pathogenesis and medical treatment of chronic sinus disease.
10. List the complications of sinusitis.
11. Describe the more common congenital, inflammatory, and neoplastic disorders of the oral cavity and pharynx. Identify malignant disorders of these structures and discuss their treatment modalities.
12. Describe the classification and causes of stridor and discuss the workup of a child with stridor.
13. List the causes and describe the workup of hoarseness.
14. List indications for endotracheal intubation, cricothyrotomy, and tracheostomy.
15. List the risk factors, workup, and three major treatment modalities of laryngeal cancer.
16. Describe the differential diagnosis, evaluation, and management of congenital, inflammatory, and neoplastic neck masses.
17. Discuss the diagnostic and management approach to a patient with penetrating neck trauma and blunt neck trauma.

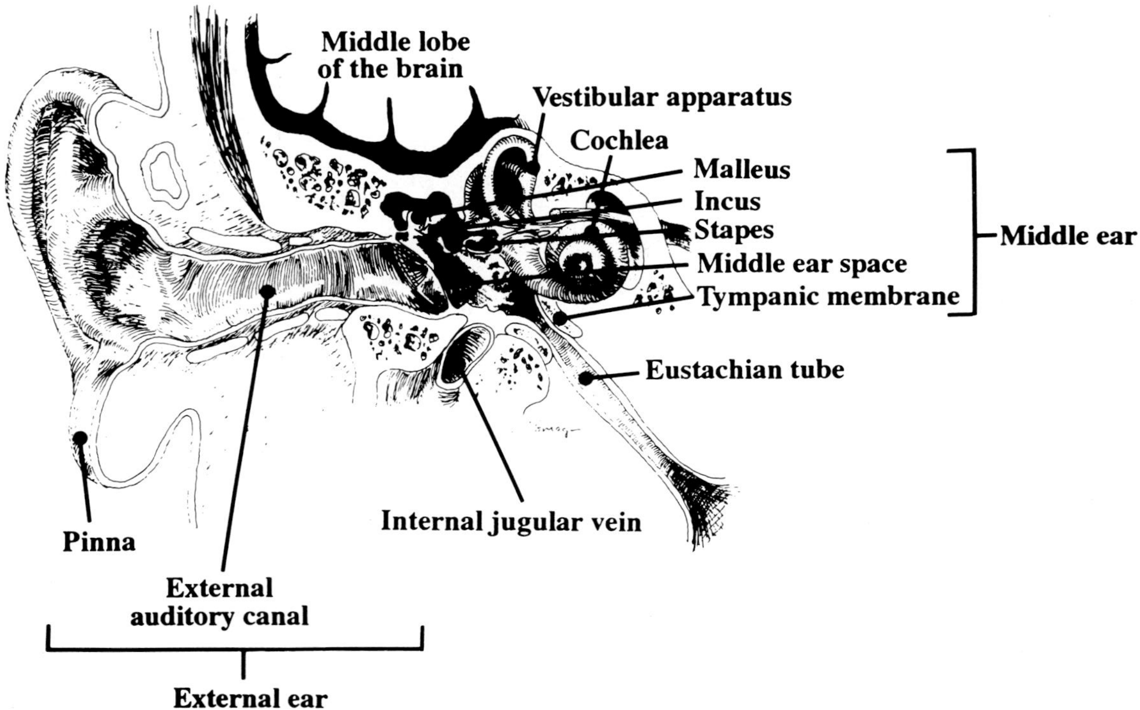

Figure 5.1. Cross-section of the ear.

The Ear, Vestibular System, and Facial Nerve

This section describes common pathological conditions of the ear, vestibular system, and facial nerve.

Anatomy

The ear is divided into the external, middle, and inner ear (Fig. 5.1). The external ear includes the auricle and the external auditory canal. The auricle has a cartilaginous framework and is shaped for collecting sound. The external auditory canal is cartilaginous in one-third of its lateral aspect and bony in two-thirds of its medial aspect. The skin of the cartilaginous external canal contains hair follicles and cerumen glands, which produce a waxy material that functions as a lubricant for the skin and as a trap for foreign particles.

The middle ear consists of the eustachian tube, eardrum (tympanic membrane), ossicular chain, and mastoid system. The eustachian tube functions to ventilate the middle ear space. Normally closed, the eustachian tube opens momentarily with swallowing, allowing equalization of negative pressure. Most middle ear diseases are related to eustachian tube dysfunction. The eardrum and ossicular chain are responsible for conducting the vibration of sound waves from the external auditory canal to the inner ear through the oval window. Through this mechanism, a relatively small, sound-produced fluctuation of the large surface of the eardrum results in larger fluctuations of the smaller stapes footplate in the oval window. The fluctuation represents a mechanical gain of about 18:1. The mastoid air cell system is more developed in some individuals than others, with some people having greater aeration of the mastoid region. Although little is known of the specific function of this system, patients in whom this system provides greater aeration have a lower incidence of middle ear disease.

The external and middle ear are closely associated with branches of cranial nerves 5, 9, and 10, with the result that pain from other sources may be referred to the ear. Patients presenting with otalgia but having no identifiable ear condition as the source should thus be evaluated for throat, temporomandibular joint, or sinus abnormalities.

The inner ear, consisting of the cochlea, semicircular canals, and internal auditory canal, is divided into the auditory and vestibular systems. The auditory system includes the cochlea and the cochlear portion of the 8th nerve, while the vestibular system includes the three semicircular canals, the utricle, the saccule, and the vestibular division of the 8th nerve. Within the cochlea are the cochlear hair cells, which pick up transmitted vibrations of sound in the inner ear fluids and transform mechanical energy into electrical impulses. These, in turn, are transmitted to the central nervous system through the auditory nerve. Within the vestibular system, each of the three semicircular canals contains hair cells that sense rotary motion of the head. Changes related to acceleration or gravity are transmitted from the hair cells of the saccule and utricle to the central nervous system through the vestibular division of the 8th nerve.

The facial nerve, lying just superior to the auditory portion of the 8th nerve in the internal auditory canal, runs from the pons in the brain stem through the middle

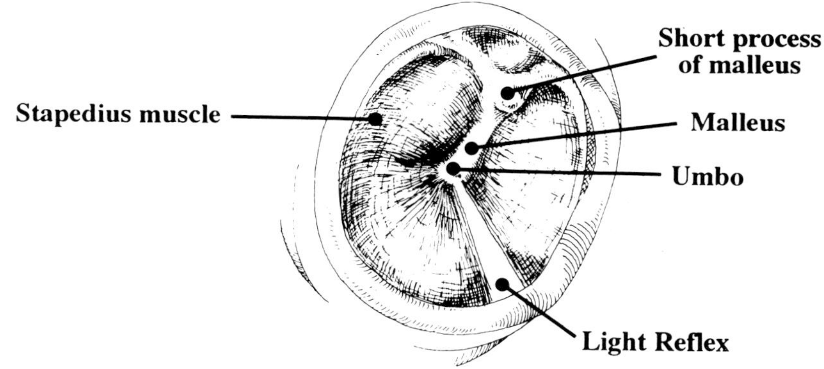

Figure 5.2. The tympanic membrane as it relates to the ossicles.

ear and emerges from the stylomastoid foramen to supply motor function to the muscles of facial expression.

Physical Examination

Examination of the ear begins with observation of the auricle. Its shape and the condition of the skin and surrounding area are noted. The external auditory canal is examined using an otoscope and the largest speculum that can fit in the ear. The external auditory canal is observed for evidence of swelling, infection, or any kind of dermatologic abnormality. Cerumen is removed to allow adequate examination. Care should be taken in removing the cerumen. The amount of cerumen produced by each patient is variable, as is the best method of removal. A small amount of hard wax in the outer portion of the ear canal is best removed with a wire loop or curette under direct vision through an otoscope. A large amount of soft wax is best removed by irrigation with warm water or peroxide if there is no perforation of the eardrum. Suctioning may also be used. Wax that is impacted against the tympanic membrane may need to be softened with peroxide drops or other over-the-counter, wax-dissolving agents such as Debrox or Cerumenex before irrigation or removal is attempted. Occasionally, the patient needs to be referred to the otolaryngologist for complete removal of the wax by means of special instruments under a microscope. A pneumatic otoscope is used to apply negative and positive pressure to the tympanic membrane to note its freedom of movement. While the eardrum is not transparent, it is translucent. In many ears one can see portions of the ossicular chain. The eardrum is observed for thickness, opacification, inflammation, and abnormal deposits such as calcium. Any unusually thin spots are noted. Perforations larger than a millimeter are quite easily seen. The eardrum should also be observed for any evidence of middle ear fluid, which may manifest as a bulge behind the eardrum or as air-fluid levels with bubbles in the middle air space (Fig. 5.2).

During the course of the examination, the patient's hearing can be assessed indirectly by noting whether the patient is able to understand normal conversational speech. Two basic tests, the Weber and Rinne, are helpful. The Weber test is performed by tapping a 512 Hz tuning fork on the heel of the hand to produce vibration and then placing it in the center of the top of the patient's head. The patient is asked whether the sound is heard better in one ear or in the center of the head. If the patient hears the sound in the center, hearing is considered to be approximately equal in both ears. If the patient hears the sound better on one side than the other, two possibilities are indicated: the patient may have a conductive hearing loss in the ear to which the tuning fork lateralizes, or a significant sensorineural hearing loss in the ear opposite the side to which the tuning fork lateralizes. In the Rinne test, the patient is asked to determine whether the tuning fork is heard louder when it is placed on the mastoid bone or when it is held approximately 2 cm from the external canal. A patient with normal hearing or sensorineural hearing loss will hear the tuning fork better when it is placed adjacent to the ear canal. A patient with a significant conductive loss will hear the tuning fork better when it is placed on the mastoid bone.

Table 5.1.
Common Causes of Hearing Loss

Conductive	Sensorineural
Otitis media	Presbycusis
Tympanic perforations	Noise-induced loss
Foreign body	Ménière's disease
Ossicular abnormalities	Acoustic neuroma
Otosclerosis	Otologic drugs
Severe external otitis	Meningitis
External canal stenosis or atresia	Sudden hearing loss

Hearing loss can be either conductive or sensorineural. A conductive hearing loss indicates a problem in the external or middle ear, while a sensorineural loss indicates one in the inner ear. Treatment of hearing loss is geared toward treating the primary cause. Most conductive losses can be treated medically or surgically, while most sensorineural losses cannot be treated except with a hearing aid. Table 5.1 summarizes causes of conductive and sensorineural losses. Patients with permanent conductive hearing losses usually respond better to hearing aids than do those with sensorineural losses.

A detailed description of vestibular system evaluation is beyond the scope of this text. However, the pa-

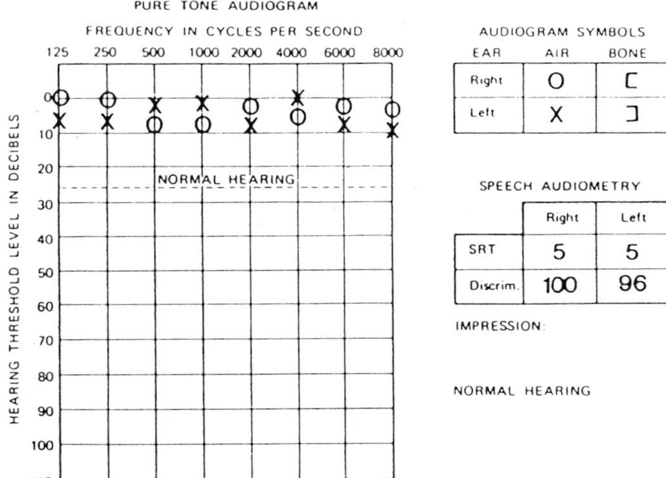

Figure 5.3. Standard audiogram report from a patient with normal hearing, good speech reception thresholds (SRT), and good word discrimination (Discrim). Sound levels are measured in decibels and recorded vertically. Different frequency sounds are recorded horizontally and measured in cycles per second (cps). Lower limits of normal hearing are indicated by the dashed line at about 25 dB.

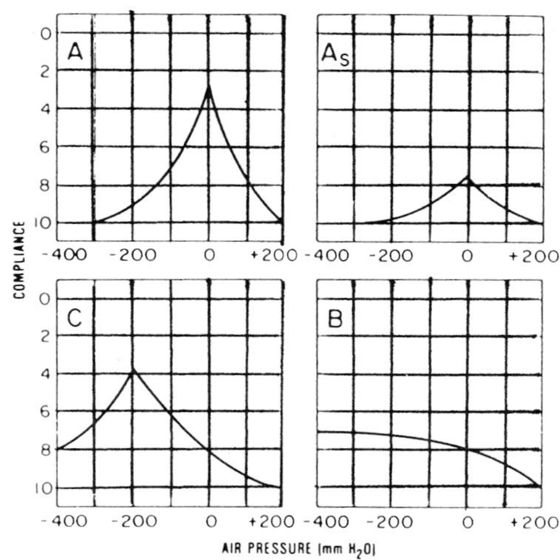

Figure 5.4. Typical patterns obtained with impedance audiometry.

tient can be observed for nystagmus with position changes quite easily, and the Romberg and tandem Romberg tests can be performed to test balance (by determining whether closing the eyes increases the unsteadiness of a standing patient). Patients suffering from significant vestibular problems at the time of examination may have positive findings on minimal evaluation.

Audiometers are used for testing hearing and can be simple or complex. Audiometry measures the patient's hearing relative to that of a normal hearing person. The resultant measurement is quantified by the decibel (dB), a logarithmic scale used to measure sound intensity. A 6 dB increase is equivalent to doubling the sound intensity. A soft whisper measures about 30 dB, conversational speech measures 40–60 dB, and a jet engine measures 140 dB. The basic components of hearing testing consist of pure tone audiometry, speech reception threshold testing, and tympanometry. Pure tone audiometry is performed by presenting a series of "beeps" at 7 different frequencies (250, 500, 1000, 2000, 3000, 4000, and 8000 Hz). The zero dB line on the audiogram (Fig. 5.3) is considered normal, and the patient's hearing levels are recorded as dB above or below the zero dB point along each of the 7 frequencies. The sound is delivered first through earphones that measure air conduction and then again through a vibrating device placed on the mastoid bone that measures bone conduction. Each is recorded. Speech reception thresholds are obtained by presenting a standard battery of words that the patient is instructed to repeat. The sound level at which the patient is able to repeat half of the words correctly represents his or her speech reception threshold (SRT). An additional test of speech audiometry measures the patient's ability to understand or discriminate words and is recorded as a percentage. Figure 5.3 represents a standard audiogram for a patient's normal hearing, good speech reception, and good word discrimination. A hearing threshold of 0–10 dB represents normal hearing, of 15–30 dB a mild loss, of 30–60 dB a moderate loss, of 60–90 dB a severe loss, and of greater than 90 a profound loss. Discrimination ability from 80–100% is considered good, 60–80% is acceptable, and less than 60% is poor.

Tympanometry measures eardrum function by means of a multichannel probe (containing a speaker, a microphone, and a transducer) that fits into the ear canal. The probe is coupled to a recording device. The transducer produces pressure changes from 400 mm H_2O of negative pressure to 200 mm H_2O of positive pressure, while the speaker delivers low frequency sound. The microphone senses the amount of sound energy reflected and records it on a tracing. Based on the tympanogram configuration, inferences can be made regarding middle ear function, presence or absence of fluid, and presence of a perforation. Figure 5.4 summarizes the common types of tympanograms seen.

Diseases of the External Ear

Infectious Diseases. The skin of the auricle and external auditory canal is subject to most common dermatologic diseases and to some that are unique to the external ear. The most common infectious disease is otitis externa, which can be localized or diffuse. The localized form is a manifestation of an abscess involving a hair follicle in the external canal. It produces pain out of proportion to findings on physical examination. Often only a small red spot is visible, but the patient will exhibit extreme pain when the ear is moved or the area is touched. The pain is a result of the inflammatory reaction involving the perichondrium and periosteum, since there is minimal, if any, subcutaneous tissue in the ear canal.

The diffuse form of otitis externa manifests with more general inflammation and pain on manipulation of the ear. Findings range from minimal inflammation and tenderness to complete closure of the ear canal with surrounding cellulitis and adenopathy. This condition is commonly described as "swimmer's ear," since often there is a history of moisture in the external canal from swimming or showering. Other etiologies are trauma to the skin produced by the patient in an effort to remove water or a foreign body from the ear canal, or perforation of the eardrum with the resulting otorrhea coming from the middle ear. Whatever the underlying cause, the skin breaks, allowing serum to mix with moisture in a warm, dark place where bacteria flourish. The most common causative agent is *Pseudomonas*, with *Klebsiella*, *Streptococcus*, and *Staphylococcus* also being frequent. Fungus may appear, but usually as a secondary growth on desquamated epithelium.

Management involves removing debris from the external auditory canal so that topical antibiotic solutions (containing neomycin or polymyxin, sometimes with steroids added) may reach the site of the infection. If the ear canal is so swollen that ear drops cannot be instilled, a small wick is placed in the external auditory canal. These wicks are commercially available or may be fashioned from gauze strips. With the wick in place, the patient is instructed to use ear drops every 2–4 hours over a 24-hour period, after which swelling usually will have subsided. During the course of management, debris should be removed frequently from the patient's ear canal. If there is marked cellulitis or inflammation involving the auricle and tissues around the ear, systemic antibiotics and steroids are generally effective. Some patients may require hospitalization so that they may be treated with intravenous antibiotics. Pain is a very significant part of the symptom complex, even in some of the relatively minor infections, and may not respond to anything short of narcotic analgesia.

A potentially lethal complication of otitis externa is malignant external otitis, which is osteomyelitis of the temporal bone caused by an invasive infection of *Pseudomonas aeruginosa*. The term *malignant* refers to the clinical course of the disease rather than to a neoplastic process. Although the complication is uncommon, it must be recognized and treated promptly to avoid the prolonged morbidity and high mortality associated with inadequate or delayed therapy. The complication usually occurs in patients who are elderly and diabetic or in those who are immunocompromised. The patient presents with persistent inflammation of the external auditory canal, accompanying pain, and development of granulation tissue in the floor of the ear canal. Because this infection does not respond to usual therapy, it must be treated aggressively with parenteral aminoglycosides or anti-*Pseudomonas* cephalosporins, in combination with surgical debridement as necessary.

Herpes zoster may involve the external ear and ear canal and result in paralysis of the facial nerve. This disease, called Ramsay Hunt's syndrome, is extremely painful. Other more common processes involving the external ear include seborrheic dermatitis, eczema, contact dermatitis, and psoriasis.

Neoplastic Diseases of the External Ear. Both benign and malignant neoplastic processes may present in the external ear. Of the benign lesions, actinic keratosis is the most common and is seen in the external ear as it is elsewhere. Lesions unique to the external auditory canal are osteomas and exostoses. They present as smooth nodules, sometimes occurring in multiples. If they produce marked obstruction or prevent the ear from cleaning itself naturally, surgical excision is indicated. Of the malignant lesions, squamous cell carcinomas, basal cell carcinomas, and malignant melanomas are the most common. They can present as an ulceration that does not heal or as an enlarging, darkly pigmented lesion on the skin of the auricle. Malignant processes can involve the cerumen glands as well. Surgical excision is indicated.

Congenital Diseases of the External Ear. Congenital abnormalities range from minor disorders of the auricular cartilage to complete absence of the auricle and external auditory canal. The most common and least severe abnormality is the absence of some of the normal folds in the auricular cartilage, leading to a condition called *lop ear*, in which the external ear protrudes from the side of the head. This abnormality can be corrected surgically. Another significant abnormality is the lack of proper embryologic development of the six small hillocks of cartilage that are precursors of the auricle itself. In some cases, the ear is markedly deformed or absent. The external auditory canal often is involved and may be very small or totally stenotic. An affected individual is likely to have middle ear abnormalities as well, even if the external auditory canal is relatively normal.

Correction of these abnormalities usually requires correction of the auricle deformity, reconstruction of the external auditory canal, and possibly reconstruction of the middle ear. Surgery involves using normal auricular cartilage and implanting sculpted rib cartilage. Correction may be quite complicated, depending upon the degree of atresia and the position of the facial nerve. The normal course of the nerve is posterior and inferior to the external auditory canal. In patients with congenital abnormalities, however, the course of the facial nerve usually is abnormal and may run through the space where the external auditory canal would normally be. If the middle ear structures are too abnormal to allow reconstruction of the hearing mechanism, then repair of the external auditory canal defect with its inherent risk to the facial nerve is contraindicated.

Other common abnormalities include preauricular cysts and/or sinus tracts, which present as small prehelical openings or pits. They result from persistence of epithelial tracts that normally would be obliterated. These tracts frequently become infected and drain, at which time they are resected surgically.

Trauma to the External Ear. Trauma to the external ear and external auditory canal can occur as thermal trauma (burn or frostbite) or as sharp or blunt injury. Tissue may be destroyed directly or the blood supply to the tissue may be damaged.

Diseases of the Middle Ear and Mastoid

Infectious and Inflammatory Diseases. Most of the infectious and/or inflammatory disease processes involving the middle ear space are secondary to eustachian tube dysfunction. When the eustachian tube does not open frequently enough to allow equalization between middle ear and atmospheric pressure, a vacuum is created as oxygen and nitrogen are absorbed into the mucous membranes of the middle ear and mastoid air cell systems. The consequence is either (*a*) increased capillary permeability and glandular activity with resultant middle ear effusion, or (*b*) retraction of the tympanic membrane with possible adherence to the ossicles and medial wall of the middle ear space. If infectious agents are present, the transudate forms an ideal culture medium leading to otitis media. If they are not present, the fluid remains sterile.

Acute Otitis Media. The most common infectious process involving the ear is acute otitis media. Next to well-baby checks, this is the most common reason children visit the doctor. By their second birthday, 75% percent of all children can be expected to have had at least 3 episodes of acute otitis media. A typical history is onset of severe pain in one or both ears, often in conjunction with an upper respiratory tract infection. In children, the infection usually is associated with pain, fever, nausea, and vomiting. Rarely, signs of meningeal irritation are present. On examination, the eardrum is red and may be bulging, with a loss of normal landmarks. Occasionally, infection results in a rupture of the tympanic membrane before the child is seen by a physician. In such cases the history is that of severe ear pain which suddenly stops as the ear begins to drain. Older children may be aware of hearing loss and may complain of a throbbing in their ears. The diagnosis is made on the basis of the clinical picture.

The most common organisms seen in acute otitis media are *Streptococcus pneumoniae* and *Haemophilus influenzae*. Antimicrobial therapy generally consists of an agent which will cover the common bacterial organisms, such as amoxicillin or trimethoprim-sulfisoxazole, or medications effective against β-lactamase-resistant organisms. Antibiotic treatment generally resolves pain within 24 to 48 hours. As normal eustachian tube function returns, fluid clears from the middle ear space within 10 days to 2 weeks. Patients must be followed until the fluid is cleared; if the eustachian tube does not begin to function, a clinically significant hearing loss can result. In preschool children such a loss can result in substantial language delay and possibly long-term learning disability. If fluid persists after 2–3 weeks, an additional course of a different antibiotic should be considered. In approximately 10% of children, middle ear effusion persists for more than 10–12 weeks. Untreated otitis media can progress to such severe complications as meningitis, brain abscess, facial nerve paralysis, and labyrinthitis, all of which require intensive medical management. Occasionally, tympanocentesis to obtain cultures is required in severely ill children or immunocompromised patients.

Otitis Media with Effusion. The second most common middle ear disease is otitis media with effusion, which may follow acute otitis media or start without apparent acute inflammation. It is related to eustachian tube dysfunction which may be anatomic or physiologic. Young infants have a more horizontally inclined eustachian tube resulting in an ineffective ability to open and close. The tubes will become more vertical and better-functioning with age. Other factors affecting eustachian tube function include edema of nasopharyngeal membranes or the eustachian tube itself from infectious or allergic processes, and anatomical abnormalities such as adenoidal hypertrophy or cleft palate. The most common culture-positive organisms involved in chronic (>3 months) otitis media with effusion are *Haemophilus influenzae* and diphtheroids. Antibiotic treatment usually is administered, but after several courses its efficacy is questionable. The majority of children will clear their effusions, but if fluid persists longer than 3 months, despite treatment, the patient should be referred to the otolaryngologist and myringotomies with placement of middle ear ventilation tubes should be considered. These allow the ear to aerate, reducing the build-up of fluid and restoring the hearing to normal. A second indication for tubes is in patients with recurrent acute otitis media (greater than 6 episodes in 6 months), in whom infection resolves with medical management but recurs within 2–3 weeks. These patients should be treated with prophylactic doses of antibiotics (daily amoxicillin or Gantrisin) after completion of therapeutic antibiotics and followed monthly. If a breakthrough otitis media develops, ventilation tubes should be considered. These tubes, staying in an average of 8–12 months, are extruded gradually as the eardrum heals beneath the tube and pushes it out. In 25% of patients, some drainage from the tubes will occur, which should be treated with both oral and topical antibiotics. In less than 1% of cases, a persistent hole is left in the eardrum, requiring eventual surgical closure. Much debate continues over the long-term effects of ventilation tubes. Once the tubes have extruded, there is no long-term protection against further fluid build-up. Hearing loss as a result of the tubes is extremely rare.

A rare type of otitis media is acute necrotizing otitis media caused by hemolytic streptococcus. In this aggressive disorder the eardrum and ossicles may both be involved. Early parenteral antimicrobial treatment is necessary.

Cholesteatoma. Cholesteatoma is a relatively uncommon but potentially serious middle ear lesion. It consists of a skin-lined cyst that develops as a result of eustachian tube dysfunction and chronic negative pressure in the middle ear. The tympanic membrane becomes retracted, and epithelial migration occurs through this retraction or through a subsequent perforation. Cholesteatomas may also be congenital, resulting from epithelial cell rests remaining in the middle ear or mastoid cavity after temporal bone formation. These lesions cause destruction from both pressure and osteonecrosis. Osteolytic enzymes in the base of the membrane of the skin cause erosion of the ossicular chain, the facial nerve canal, the cochlea, or the semicircular canals.

A patient with cholesteatoma commonly has a history of chronic and recurrent infections, and a draining ear with hearing loss. This loss may be secondary to eardrum perforation, ossicular damage, or damage to the inner ear. Facial nerve paralysis, vertigo, or intracranial abscesses may be seen. On examination, there may be a clear, serosanguinous, or purulent otorrhea and an eardrum perforation of varying size. The middle ear mucosa is inflamed and edematous polypoid tissue can be seen in the ear canal or protruding through a perforation. An audiogram will show a conductive hearing loss. Rarely, sensorineural losses occur. Congenital cholesteatomas may present with hearing loss and an opalescent mass behind the eardrum. Surgical excision is necessary, which may include a mastoidectomy and removal of the involved ossicles to prevent complications.

Congenital Lesions in the Middle Ear and Mastoid. Congenital malformations in the middle ear and mastoid range from small eardrums associated with stenotic external auditory canals to complete absence of the eardrum and middle ear space, including the ossicular chain. Middle ear abnormalities are infrequently associated with inner ear defects, because the inner ear develops earlier and has a different embryologic derivation. Deformities of the middle ear are commonly associated with deformities of the external auditory canal and the auricle itself.

Otosclerosis is an abnormality of the middle ear and occasionally of the inner ear that presents as an acquired hearing loss in young adults. The condition has a genetic predisposition and involves the growth of a small focus of spongy vascular bone over a part or all of the stapes footplate. The result is fixation of the stapes footplate, which prevents vibration and results in a conductive hearing loss of variable severity in one or both ears. It occurs in both sexes and may accelerate during pregnancy. If the cochlea becomes involved, an additional sensorineural hearing loss is produced.

While there is no medical treatment for the conductive hearing loss in otosclerosis, high doses of sodium fluoride have been used in an effort to arrest cochlear involvement. A hearing aid may be used to amplify sound to the involved ear to help restore useful hearing. Most patients, however, prefer surgical removal of the fixed stapes bone and its replacement with a small prosthesis. Hearing results are usually very good. Infrequent complications include complete loss of hearing in the involved ear or severe postoperative dizziness.

Trauma to the Middle Ear and Mastoid. The most common trauma to the middle ear is traumatic rupture of the eardrum produced by a foreign object, abrupt pressure change, or a blow to the ear. Foreign bodies, such as cotton-tipped ear swabs, sticks, or hot welding slag (from welding injuries), may injure the eardrum as well as the ear canal. Traumatic perforations raise two concerns. First, these injuries can result in damage to the ossicular chain with significant conductive hearing loss. Second, if the stapes is subluxed into the inner ear, severe sensorineural hearing loss with or without vertigo may result. When a portion of epithelial tissue is avulsed or lodged somewhere in the middle ear, cholesteatoma can result, with its potential for damage to the middle ear and mastoid cavity.

Approximately 90% of injuries heal uneventfully, unless a significant portion of the eardrum is either missing or folded (outward or inward) in such a way that regrowth cannot occur. In such situations surgical intervention may be indicated if healing is not evidenced in 3 months. A tympanoplasty graft using temporalis fascia is used to close the perforation.

Diseases of the Inner Ear and Vestibular System

The inner ear and vestibular system are affected principally by three disorders—hearing loss, vertigo, and tinnitus—and by trauma.

Hearing Loss. Inner ear hearing loss is of the sensorineural category, involving the cochlea or cochlear nerve, and is usually permanent. The loss may be congenital or acquired.

Congenital Hearing Loss. Congenital hearing loss, affecting 1 in 2000 babies born, may be either genetic (usually with a recessive mode of inheritance) or due to prenatal or perinatal conditions. These conditions include rubella, meningitis, severe jaundice, prematurity, severe hypoxia at birth, or the use of ototoxic antibiotics or other drugs in the perinatal period. Early identification is imperative, and rehabilitation with hearing aids, cochlear implants or other assisted hearing devices may maximize the communication skills of the child.

Acquired Hearing Loss. Acquired hearing loss may have many causes. The most common causes are listed in Table 5.1. Of these, presbycusis, or the hearing loss of aging, is almost universal. It begins to affect people in their 70s and goes on to affect, to some degree, 75% of those aged 80. Hearing aids can be of significant benefit. Noise-induced hearing loss is typically present as a localized loss in the mid to high frequency level of 2000 Hz. It may be caused by a sudden loud noise, such as a gunshot blast, or by prolonged exposure to industrial noise, such as that in factories. Patients should be counseled on the use of noise protection during such activities. Ménière's disease, or endolymphatic hydrops, consists of the triad of episodic hearing loss, vertigo, and tinnitus. The disease is thought to be due to an overproduction or an underabsorption of endolymph fluid, resulting in a hydrops condition of the cochlea. Medical treatment consists of a low-salt diet and diuretics. Surgical decompression or actual ablation is reserved for incapacitating symptoms that do not respond to medical treatment.

Sudden hearing loss may present at any time during adulthood and can occur within hours or days. The exact cause is unknown, but viral or vascular etiologies are theorized. Occasionally, a short course of steroids is

Table 5.2.
Common Causes of Vertigo

Vestibular neuritis
Benign postional vertigo
Viral labyrinthitis
Ménière's disease
Acoustic neuroma
Ototoxic drugs
Systemic diseases (diabetes, hypertension, thyroid)
Vascular insufficiency

Table 5.3.
Common Causes of Tinnitus

High frequency hearing loss
Ménière's disease
Aspirin ingestion (usually temporary)
Ototoxic drugs
Loud noise exposure (usually temporary)
Acoustic neuroma
Systemic diseases (diabetes, hypertension, thyroid)
Glomus jugulare (pulsatile)

of benefit, and about half of the cases will recover spontaneously.

Neoplasms of the inner ear are an unusual but important cause of sensorineural hearing loss. The most common tumor is benign and is an acoustic neuroma involving the 8th nerve. Symptoms may be subtle early in the course of tumor development; a high degree of suspicion must therefore be maintained when these symptoms are present. Since these tumors are slow-growing, their expansion is accommodated by peripheral tissues in the central nervous system. The hallmark symptom is unilateral sensorineural hearing loss with poor word discrimination, even if the sound is made loud enough. It is usually accompanied by tinnitus, or ringing in the ears. Late symptoms are severe vertigo, facial nerve paralysis, or significant hearing loss. MRI is diagnostic, and surgical excision is the treatment of choice except in cases of high anesthetic risk.

Vertigo. The second most common disorder of the inner ear is vertigo. Dizziness is a common symptom in patients but is not always otologic in origin. Spinning vertigo should be distinguished from "light-headedness," which is rarely due to inner ear causes. The most common cause of vertigo is vestibular neuritis, which is most likely an inflammatory condition. It is usually preceded by a viral upper respiratory condition. Severe vertigo usually lasts a few days, with the patient recovering gradually over a period of weeks. Treatment is supportive and symptomatic, consisting of drugs that suppress vertigo, such as Meclizine, and bed rest. Other causes of vertigo are summarized in Table 5.2.

Tinnitus. Tinnitus is the third most common inner ear disorder, usually brought on by a high frequency hearing loss. Other common causes are listed in Table 5.3. No satisfactory cure exists for tinnitus other than treating the primary cause. No medications have as yet proven effective.

Trauma. Because the inner ear is located deep in the temporal bone, it is usually protected from all but the most severe forms of trauma. Base of the skull fractures may traverse the temporal bone and damage both the vestibular and auditory mechanisms, most commonly presenting as a hemotympanum or cerebrospinal fluid (CSF) otorrhea. A conductive hearing loss usually results, which resolves spontaneously as the hemotympanum resolves or the perforation heals. Rarely, a transverse fracture may affect the cochlea and even the facial nerve. Balance disturbances as well as varying degrees of hearing loss may be observed. In most instances, the sensorineural hearing loss associated with such injuries is not recovered, but the balance system may compensate.

The Facial Nerve

Disorders of the Facial Nerve. Disorders of the facial nerve are the result of hypofunction or hyperfunction (Fig. 5.5). The most common ones result in hypofunction or paralysis, which may be partial or complete. The disorder may be caused by tumors, inflammatory processes of the temporal bone, trauma, or such vascular problems as cerebrovascular accidents. When no cause can be detected, the condition is labeled idiopathic or Bell's palsy. Research suggests that this is an inflammatory disease, possibly related to herpes simplex infection of the facial nerve. In Bell's palsy paresis usually develops in a matter of hours and may progress over a period of several days to complete paralysis. The patient may have ear pain on the involved side as well as auditory symptoms. A history of an antecedent systemic viral infection may be elicited. The most serious side effect is exposure keratitis on the involved side, leading to corneal scarring and marked impairment of vision. The application of artificial tears, ointment, and tape to keep the eye shut are measures used to protect the eye. A tarsorrhaphy may be needed. Steroids are commonly used, even though their use is controversial. Evaluation of Bell's palsy includes nerve stimulation testing when paralysis is complete. This involves placing a nerve stimulator over the area of the facial nerve just anterior to the tragus or over each of the main branches and then recording the minimal current at which the stimulation and resultant facial movement occurred. This reading is compared with that obtained from the normal side. A difference of 2.5 mA is considered significant and not as good a prognostic sign. The majority of Bell's palsies resolve spontaneously. If paralysis persists longer than 2 weeks, a magnetic resonance imaging (MRI) or computed tomography (CT) scan is recommended to rule out tumors. Surgical decompression of the facial nerve in Bell's palsy remains controversial.

Tumors of the Facial Nerve. Primary tumors of the facial nerve are rare. Almost all are benign and are either a neuroma (neurilemoma or nerve sheath tumor) or a neurofibroma (von Recklinghausen's disease). The

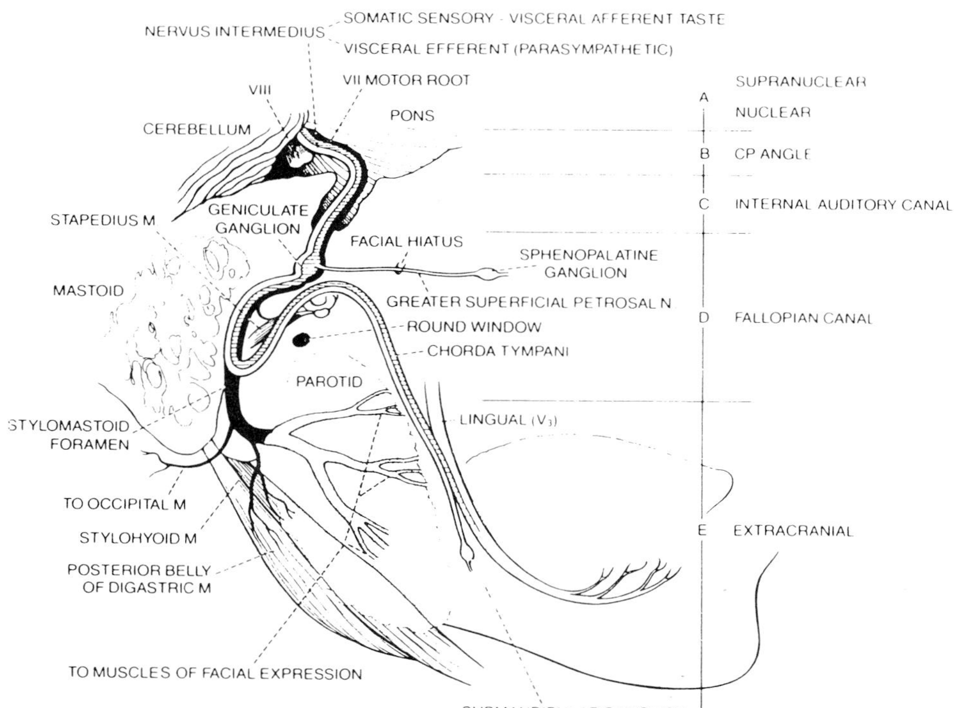

Figure 5.5. Facial nerve map.

neuroma is usually an isolated lesion that can occur at any point in the course of the facial nerve. Tumors arising in the cerebellar pontine angle may become quite large before producing symptoms. Tumors in the internal auditory canal may compress the auditory and vestibular nerves, producing corresponding dysfunction along with signs of facial nerve paresis. Tumors in the bony Fallopian canal within the temporal bone may produce symptoms of pain and paralysis before the tumor enlarges to any great degree. A neuroma of the peripheral nerve may be diagnosed by observing a palpable or visual enlargement of a mass in the region of the parotid gland.

The neurofibromas of von Recklinghausen's disease behave like neuromas, but they are generally associated with other signs and symptoms of the disease, namely café-au-lait spots and subcutaneous neurofibromas scattered around the body. These tumors may be multiple and may involve both facial nerves.

Other tumors originating in the temporal bone that may involve the facial nerve include neuromas involving the 8th nerve and glomus tumors. Metastatic disease from distant or local primary malignant tumors may also involve the facial nerve, requiring resection of the nerve. Various forms of nerve grafting and muscle tensing procedures may be needed for rehabilitation.

Malignant neoplasms involving the parotid gland, skin, or subcutaneous tissue around the ear and face may secondarily involve the facial nerve, producing paralysis. The diagnosis is made on the basis of history, radiologic studies, and imaging techniques. Both CT scan and MRI are used, with MRI being the most sensitive for lesions involving the internal auditory canal and cerebellar pontine angle. Because primary tumors involving the facial nerve are usually resected, a portion of the nerve must also be resected. If a short segment of the nerve is involved, rerouting may be possible with end-to-end anastomosis. If longer segments of the nerve are involved, a nerve graft may be necessary. Return of function is expected in most cases, along with persistent weakness.

Trauma to the Facial Nerve. The second most common cause of facial nerve paralysis is trauma. Penetrating injuries involving the side of the face, ear, or temporal bone may involve portions or all of the facial nerve. When the main trunk or one of the branches is involved, paralysis of the muscles supplied by that portion of the nerve may be seen. Transection of the nerve should be treated by immediate repair by reanastomosis or nerve grafting.

Nose and Paranasal Sinuses

Anatomy

The external dorsal structures of the nose are formed by a bony and cartilaginous framework covered externally by skin and facial muscles. The upper one-third or bony vault consists of the paired nasal bones supported by the frontal process of the maxilla and nasal process of the frontal bone. The cartilaginous vault consists of the upper lateral cartilages, which are fused to the septal cartilage medially (Fig. 5.6).

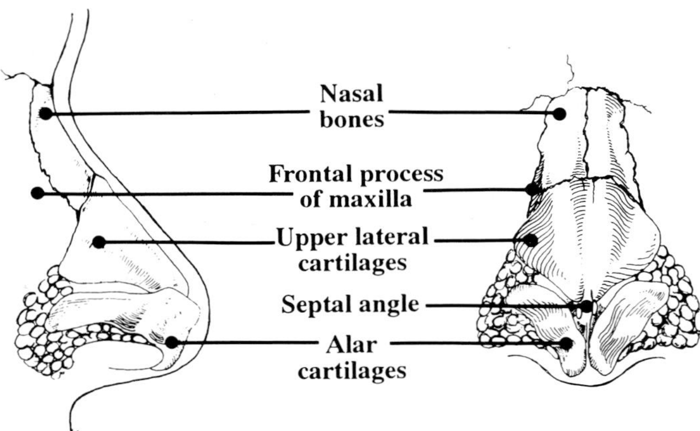

Figure 5.6. Anatomy of the nasal vault.

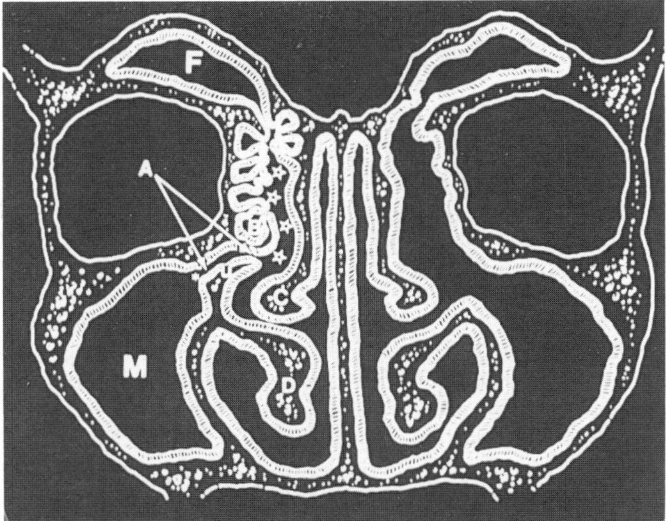

Figure 5.7. Schematic diagram of the anterior ethmoid sinus-middle meatus region (ostiomeatal complex) in the coronal projection. On the left, the middle meatus (4 stars) receives drainage from the ethmoid bulla (B) and other anterior cells. Secretions from the frontal sinus (F) must pass through the ethmoid region, and maxillary sinus (M) secretions must pass through the ostium (*) and infundibulum (A) before reaching the middle meatus. The situation after functional endoscopic ethmoidectomy is shown on the right. The uncinate process (U) has been removed, the anterior ethmoid cells opened, and the natural ostium of the maxillary sinus widened. The middle turbinate (C) is left intact. Also shown is the inferior turbinate (D).

The nasal cavity extends from the anterior nares to the posterior choanae and is divided by the nasal septum into two chambers. The roof of the nose is formed by the cribriform plate of the ethmoid bone. The lateral wall of the nasal cavity is configured by three overhanging scroll-like bones. These turbinates incompletely subdivide each nasal cavity into a corresponding meatus. Drainage from the nasolacrimal duct passes into the nose through the inferior meatus. The middle meatus, hooded by the middle turbinate, is the most complex and important region of the nose (Fig. 5.7). The ostia or drainage pathways of the anterior ethmoid, maxillary, and frontal sinuses open into the middle meatus. The anterior ethmoid sinus-middle meatus region is known as the ostiomeatal complex. The posterior ethmoid cells drain into the superior meatus and the sphenoid sinus opens into the sphenoethmoid recess, which is located immediately above and behind the superior turbinate.

The paranasal sinuses develop as evaginations from the nasal cavity during the third and fourth month of fetal life. These outpouchings pneumatize portions of the surrounding ethmoid, frontal, maxillary, and sphenoid bones in forming the respective sinuses. They maintain constant communication with the nose through ostia which persist at the original site of evagination.

Blood supply to the nose arises from both the external and internal carotid artery systems. The internal maxillary artery is the major vessel to the internal nose. Its sphenopalatine branch supplies the septum and turbinates. The anterior and posterior ethmoid arteries, branches of the ophthalmic artery, supply the ethmoid and frontal sinuses as well as the nasal roof. Kiesselbach's plexus is a highly vascular area on the anterior septum which receives blood supply from both the internal and external carotid artery systems.

Venous drainage from the nose passes via the sphenopalatine, facial, and ethmoid veins. The nose may communicate with the cavernous sinus through the pterygoid venous plexus and emissary veins. Such communication represents a potential pathway for the spread of inflammatory disease.

The nose is innervated by the first, fifth, and seventh cranial nerves, as well as by fibers from the sympathetic and parasympathetic systems.

Nasal Physiology

The nose is an integral part of the respiratory system and the organ of olfaction. It functions as a conduit for inspired air, providing variable resistance in response to changing ventilatory demands. It accounts for 50% of the total resistance to respiratory airflow. The nose also protects the lungs by conditioning inspired air: most particles and microorganisms are trapped on the mucous blanket overlying the nasal epithelium, and nearly all water soluble gases are absorbed. The increased surface area resulting from protrusion of the turbinates in the airstream facilitates temperature adjustment and humidification, so that at the nasopharynx inspired air is at 100% relative humidity and near body temperature, regardless of ambient conditions. These adjustments are accomplished by precise autonomic regulation of mucosal blood flow and nasal secretion.

Mucociliary clearance is vital in protecting the nose from disease caused by deposited particles and absorbed gases. The ciliated epithelial cells of the nasal mucosa have an intrinsic coordinated movement which results in a wave-like flow of the overlying mucous blanket. This active clearance mechanism transports secretions from the nose and paranasal sinuses posterior to the nasopharynx, where they are swallowed.

Table 5.4.
Evaluation of Nasal Disease

History
Predominant symptom(s)
Onset and duration of problem
Aggravating factors
Type and effect of prior treatment
Current medications
Known allergies/sensitivities
Topical decongestant use
Toxin exposure
Maxillofacial trauma
Prior surgery
Physical Examination
Inspection/palpation
Anterior rhinoscopy (pre- and postdecongestion)
Nasal endoscopy (flexible or rigid)
Laboratory Tests
CBC/differential
Total eosinophil count
Total immunoglobulin E/radioallergosorbent test
Skin tests
Immune profile
Nasal cytology/biopsy
Sinus puncture/aspiration
Pulmonary function test
Chest x-ray
Imaging
Plain films
CT scan
MRI

The nose also provides important information regarding the chemosensory environment. Three anatomically distinct systems are involved in chemosensation: olfaction (smell), gustation (taste), and common chemical sense (irritation). What is described as flavor of foods is the collective perception produced by stimulation of olfactory, gustatory, and trigeminal receptors. Five cranial nerves are involved in chemoreception: olfactory, trigeminal, facial, glossopharyngeal, and vagus. Olfaction, singularly innervated by the first cranial nerve, is the most vulnerable to disease. Gustation is served by the seventh, ninth, and 10th cranial nerves. The receptor cells for taste are arranged in taste buds located on the tongue, palate, oropharynx, and laryngeal mucosa. Common chemical sensation is mediated by unmyelinated fibers of trigeminal origin with free nerve endings distributed throughout the submucosa of the upper aerodigestive tract. These nerves respond to both noxious and nonirritating chemicals, providing odor sensation as well as protective reflexes.

Examination

A careful, detailed history is fundamental in evaluating nasal and sinus disease (Table 5.4). It should focus on the onset, duration, and aggravating factors for predominant symptoms. The response to current and previous therapy, surgery, or nasal trauma should be noted. Information regarding allergies, sensitivities, and current topical or systemic drug use should be elicited.

Physical examination of the nose begins with both inspection and palpation of the external dorsum for asymmetry, deviation, or collapse. The nasal cavities are relatively inaccessible, making their complete inspection difficult without the use of nasal specula or other specialized instruments. Physical examination of the sinuses is also limited by their inaccessibility. Deductions regarding their condition are best made by inspecting the region of the nose where the sinus ostia open. The application of both flexible and rigid endoscopic instruments has allowed inspection of these concealed spaces and resulted in more precise diagnosis of sinus disease.

Based on patient history and physical findings, appropriate laboratory tests are ordered. Tissue for culture and histology is obtained from individuals with unilateral signs or symptoms or from those with poor response to usual medical therapy. When unilateral disease is present, a careful search is made for a foreign body, dental disease, or malignancy.

Diseases of the Nose

The symptoms of nasal disease are nonspecific and relatively limited. Congestion, airway obstruction, and drainage are symptoms shared by a diverse group of diseases, making the evaluation of nasal problems challenging. A general classification would include epistaxis (nasal hemorrhage), structural deformity, congenital problems, neoplasms, infectious rhinitis, and noninfectious rhinitis (Table 5.5). Several clinical entities can coexist in one patient.

Epistaxis. Bleeding from the nose most commonly occurs anteriorly from Kiesselbach's plexus on the nasal septum. Anterior bleeding, usually seen in children and young adults, can be controlled by firm compression of the alar cartilages on both sides of the septum. Posterior epistaxis, more common in older adults, is often associated with arteriosclerotic cardiovascular disease, hypertension, and other systemic disorders.

The most common cause of epistaxis is trauma. Bleeding may develop following digital or penetrating injury to the nasal mucosa or from blunt external force applied to the nose that produces secondary mucosal laceration. Acute rhinitis is another common cause. Septal deviations and perforations cause excessive drying and focal inflammation of nasal mucosa, increasing the potential for epistaxis. Intranasal foreign bodies, usually seen in pediatric or psychiatric patients, should be suspected if there is unilateral purulent discharge or bleeding. Epistaxis is also an early symptom in paranasal sinus malignancy. Juvenile nasopharyngeal angiofibroma is a highly vascular, benign tumor in adolescent males which classically presents with epistaxis and nasal obstruction.

Epistaxis may also be a sign of systemic disease. Defects in coagulation secondary to anticoagulation therapy, blood dyscrasias, lymphoproliferative disorders,

Table 5.5.
Nasal Obstruction: Differential Diagnosis

Structural
- Septal deviation
- Nasal fracture/septal hematoma

Congenital
- Choanal atresia
- Dermoid cyst
- Nasal glioma
- Encephalocele

Neoplastic
- Benign
  - Nasal papilloma
  - Nasopharyngeal angiofibroma
- Malignant
  - Squamous cell carcinoma

Infectious rhinitis
- Acute
  - Vestibulitis
  - Furunculosis
  - Viral rhinitis (common cold)
  - Bacterial rhinitis
- Chronic
  - Rhinoscleroma
  - Tuberculosis
  - Syphilis
  - Leprosy
  - Fungal
    - *Aspergillus*
    - Mucormycosis
- Systemic/multisystem
  - Sarcoidosis
  - Wegener's granulomatosis
  - Polymorphic reticulosis

Noninfectious rhinitis
- Allergic rhinitis
- Nonallergic rhinitis
  - Rhinitis medicamentosa
  - Nasal polyposis
  - Hormonal rhinitis
  - Vasomotor rhinitis

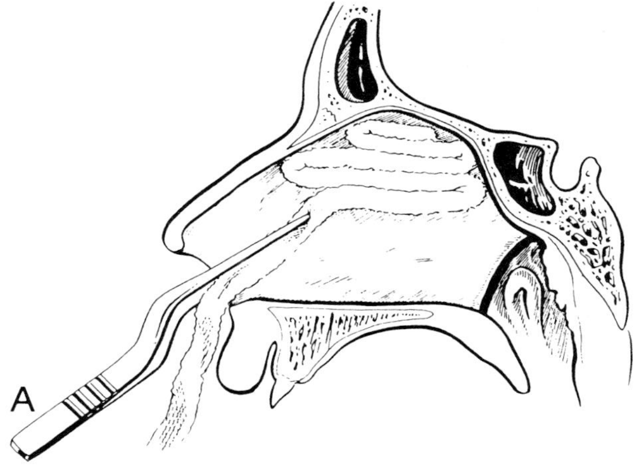

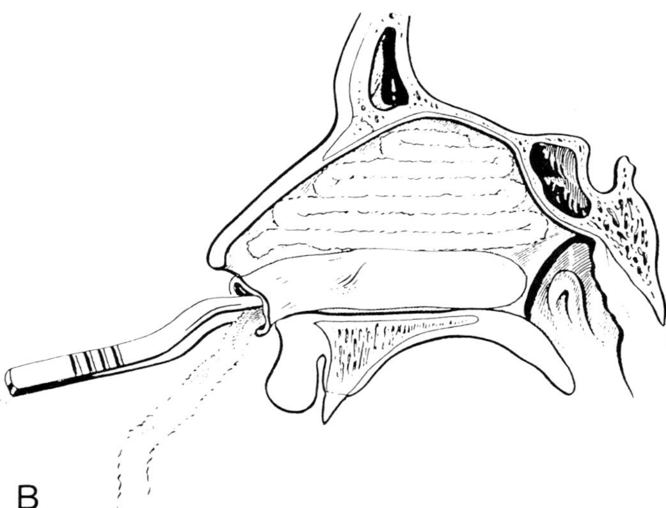

Figure 5.8. **A**, Introduction of gauze strips into the nasal cavity. **B**, Packing the nose with a finger stall.

and immunodeficiency may manifest with nasal bleeding. Hemorrhagic telangiectasia, an autosomal dominant disorder exhibiting arteriovenous malformations of aerodigestive tract mucosa, may also result in epistaxis, as these malformations rupture frequently. Individuals with this disorder have normal coagulation tests. Chronic systemic diseases predisposing to epistaxis include nutritional deficiencies and alcoholism.

Initial management of epistaxis focuses on control of acute blood loss. If the site can be identified, it is cauterized electrically or chemically with silver nitrate. If the site cannot be identified, anterior nasal packs are placed. If anterior packs fail to control bleeding or examination discloses bleeding into the pharynx, a posterior pack may be required (Fig. 5.8**A** and **B**). Posterior bleeding often is more profuse than anterior bleeding and is more common in patients over 40 years of age. A posterior pack provides a bolster against which anterior packing can be placed to tamponade posterior nasal vessels. Patients requiring posterior nasal packing need to be hospitalized. Because hypoxia is common in this group of patients, blood oxygenation is monitored by a pulse oximeter. Hypoxia is most likely due to aspiration, sedation, or poor pulmonary reserve. Humidified oxygen, prophylactic antibiotics, and bed rest are usually recommended.

If anterior and posterior packs fail to control bleeding or the patient finds them unbearable, vessel ligation may be required. Ligation provides better control the closer to the site of bleeding it is performed. Anterior and posterior ethmoid artery ligation is indicated for superior epistaxis, whereas ligation of the internal maxillary artery is performed for posterior bleeding.

Structural Rhinopathy. Septal deviation is the most common anatomical deformity causing nasal obstruction. Septal deviation may be caused by trauma or result from persistent growth after development of the nasal and palatine bones leading to lateral expansion and contortion. Symptoms of septal deviation are snoring, sleep apnea, epistaxis, facial pain, headache, or sinusitis. Septal deviation causes high velocity airflow on the side of maximum obstruction, leading to atrophic mucosal changes and localized inflammation. Surgical treatment is indicated for symptomatic disease.

Nasal obstruction is also caused by nasal fracture. In addition to bony injury, nasal trauma may result in displacement of the septum or lateral cartilages. Clinical findings in nasal fracture include edema, ecchymosis, epistaxis, abnormal mobility, crepitus, dorsal asymmetry, or palpable bony deformity. If the patient is evaluated immediately after injury, nasal bone displacement or depression may be obvious. If significant edema is present, however, it may be necessary to allow 3 to 5 days for resolution before accurate evaluation of alignment can be made. Radiographs may help exclude associated skeletal injury, while photographs better document the degree of displacement. The most frequent deformity is depression of one nasal bone and outward displacement of the contralateral bone following a lateral blow. Direct frontal blows may result in flattening and widening of the nasal dorsum. If injury is severe, forces can be transmitted posteriorly to involve the ethmoid sinus, medial orbital walls, and cribriform plate with resultant cerebral spinal fluid rhinorrhea.

Evaluation of a patient with suspected nasal fracture must include inspection of the septum for hematoma. Septal hematoma separates the septal cartilage from its nourishing blood supply in the overlying mucoperichondrium. Prompt drainage is required to prevent cartilage resorption or abscess formation that can result in loss of structural support, producing what is known as a saddle nose deformity.

Nondisplaced fractures of the nasal bones do not require reduction. Minimal deviations of the bony dorsum, with no appreciable septal displacement, are managed with closed reduction. More complex injuries and those associated with septal displacement require open reduction with repositioning of the septum to achieve satisfactory functional and cosmetic results.

Congenital Problems. Choanal atresia is a potentially life-threatening cause of airway obstruction in the neonate. Since the newborn is an obligate nasal breather, bilateral choanal atresia is a medical emergency. Diagnosis of bilateral choanal atresia is suspected in a newborn when initial feedings result in progressive obstruction, cyanosis, choking, and aspiration. The airway obstruction is temporarily relieved by crying, since that is the only time the neonate inhales through the mouth. An inability to pass a small catheter into the nasopharynx suggests this diagnosis. Confirmation of the defect is obtained by high resolution axial CT scanning. Immediate treatment includes stenting with an oral airway or endotracheal intubation if ventilatory support is needed. After the airway has been secured, the infant is thoroughly evaluated for associated anomalies. Surgery is required for definitive correction.

Neoplasms. Benign neoplasms of the nose are not common causes of nasal obstruction. When they do occur, they usually are nasal inverting papillomas, osteomas, or juvenile nasopharyngeal angiofibromas. Nasal papillomas are indistinguishable from nasal polyps on gross examination, but on close examination can be seen to have an inverted pattern of growth, rather than an exophytic growth like most polyps. Nasal inverting papillomas occur with a frequency of 1:25 that of nasal polyps. Although histologically benign, nasal papillomas are locally invasive and may have foci of squamous cell carcinoma. En bloc resection with medial maxillectomy is the preferred treatment. Osteoma is the most common tumor involving the paranasal sinuses, arising in the frontoethmoid region. Often it is an incidental finding on sinus x-ray. If it is asymptomatic, annual radiographs are sufficient to track its growth. Progressively growing osteomas are removed surgically to prevent sinus ostia obstruction, leading to mucocele formation, facial pain, or sinusitis. Juvenile nasopharyngeal angiofibroma arises in the pterygomaxillary fossa and presents with epistaxis and nasal obstruction. It occurs exclusively in adolescent males, with a mean age of 15. Diagnosis is clinical and radiographic; biopsy may cause bleeding and should not be performed. Radiographs show anterior bowing to the posterior wall of the maxillary sinus and widening of the superior orbital fissure. CT scan confirms the diagnosis. Hemorrhage following surgical excision is reduced by preoperative embolization of the internal maxillary artery. Radiation therapy is recommended if there is extensive intracranial extension or blood supply from the internal carotid system. Radiation-induced neoplasm is a legitimate concern when radiation therapy is used in a child.

Malignant neoplasms of the nose and sinus represent less than 1% of cancers. Most sinus carcinomas are advanced when diagnosed. Environmental exposure (nickel refining, woodworking) has been associated with sinus malignancy. Purulent drainage and epistaxis are the most common early symptoms. In 75 to 90% of cases, the carcinomas are squamous cell, arising in the maxillary or ethmoid sinus. Classification is based on Ohngren's line, which passes from the inner canthus to the angle of the mandible. Lesions involving the superstructure have a poor prognosis. CT and MRI scans are preferable to plain sinus films. Bony destruction on CT scan is highly suggestive of malignancy; MRI scan distinguishes secondary inflammatory sinus disease from primary malignancy. After imaging studies, a biopsy is performed to obtain histologic diagnosis. Treatment consists of a total maxillectomy combined with irradiation. Local recurrence is the most common cause of failure.

Infectious Rhinitis. Acute viral rhinitis, or the common cold, is the most common infectious disease in man. The highest prevalence is in children under 5 years. It is spread by both inhalation of infectious particles and direct contact with contaminated fingers and clothing. Following penetration of the mucous blanket in the nasopharynx, virus replication leads to desquamation of ciliated epithelial cells, peaking on the 2nd to 5th day. Viral shedding precedes the onset of symptoms, which vary significantly in severity and may include nasal stuffiness, rhinorrhea, sneezing, and airway obstruction. There may be associated cough, headache, temperature elevation, sore throat, and generalized malaise. Initial mucoid secretions are replaced by mucopurulent drainage, and secondary bacterial infection caused by resident flora develops. The disorder is self-limited with regeneration of epithelium occurring by approximately the 14th day. Rhinitis that is clinically indistinguishable from the common cold is a frequent prodromal manifestation of measles, chickenpox, and rubella.

Bacterial rhinitis is most commonly seen in children but may also develop in adults following nasal trauma or surgery. Clinically, it may be identical to the common cold. Causative organisms include *Streptococcus pneumoniae*, *Hemophilus influenzae*, and *Staphylococcus aureus*. Clinical signs which distinguish bacterial rhinitis from acute sinusitis may be subtle, with both frequently developing in a patient whose defenses have been compromised by an intercurrent viral inflammatory process. An adherent gray membrane that bleeds on attempted removal may be found. The initial clinical manifestations of chronic bacterial inflammation in the nose are nonspecific. Chronic congestion, crusting, obstruction, and drainage which respond poorly to standard medical treatment should increase suspicion. Culture and histologic examination of biopsy material are required to establish the diagnosis. Chronic bacterial rhinitis includes rhinoscleroma, tuberculosis, leprosy, and syphilis.

Fungal infections involving the nose are usually caused by the opportunistic organisms Phycomycetes (*Mucor*, *Rhizopus*) and *Aspergillus*. These normally innocuous organisms may become pathogenic in immunocompromised patients. Factors which increase risk for pathogenicity include broad-spectrum antibiotics, steroid therapy, immunosuppressive drug therapy, malignancy, diabetes, and AIDS. Rhinomucormycosis is a fulminant, invasive fungal disease that starts in the nose. The most important predisposing condition is ketoacidotic diabetes mellitus. *Mucor* thrives in acid media rich in glucose and has metabolic mechanisms to reduce ketones. The disease has a predilection for vessel invasion, resulting in thrombosis and tissue infarction. Characteristic clinical signs are bloody nasal discharge and black necrotic turbinates. Diagnosis depends upon histologic identification of the broad nonseptate branching hyphae in biopsy specimens; nasal smears are inadequate for diagnosis. Treatment requires radical surgical debridement and high-dose amphotericin B therapy.

Wegener's granulomatosis, an inflammatory but not truly infectious nasal disorder, is a multisystem disease with necrotizing granulomatous vasculitis in the upper and lower respiratory tract, focal necrotizing glomerulonephritis, and systemic angiitis. Nasal involvement, seen in 60–90% of cases, initially manifests as obstruction with purulent rhinorrhea. Diagnosis is established with mucosal biopsies that demonstrate necrotizing granuloma, vasculitis, and an intense inflammatory reaction. Systemic symptoms are usually out of proportion to nasal findings and dominated by fatigue, night sweats, cough, and migratory myalgias. An elevated erythrocyte sedimentation rate is seen in virtually all patients. Treatment includes cyclophosphamide and steroids.

Noninfectious Rhinitis

Allergic Rhinitis. Allergic rhinitis is the most common allergic disease, affecting 20% of the population. It is an immune system disease, mediated by immunoglobulin E (IgE), which is caused by hypersensitivity to inhaled particulates. The disease most commonly affects children and young adults and is often associated with reactive lower respiratory tract disease. A positive family history is found in 50% of patients. Symptoms, which may be seasonal or perennial, include rhinorrhea, nasal obstruction, sneezing, and pruritus. While bluish, edematous mucosa is suggestive, there are no rhinoscopic findings unique to allergic rhinitis. Positive skin test and elevated total and allergen-specific serum IgE levels are usually found.

Medical management begins with the identification and avoidance of offending allergens. If this measure fails to control symptoms adequately, oral antihistamine or antihistamine/decongestant combinations should be tried. Topical cromolyn sodium provides symptomatic relief by preventing the degranulation of mast cells. Topical intranasal steroid sprays are the most effective symptomatic medications.

Immunotherapy should be considered when symptoms are not controlled adequately with medication and avoidance measures. This treatment is effective only in disease caused by IgE mechanisms and usually must be continued for several years.

Nonallergic Rhinitis. Rhinitis medicamentosa is drug-induced nasal inflammation. The most common cause is abuse of decongestant nasal sprays. Topical sympathomimetic amines stimulate α-adrenergic receptors in blood vessels of the nasal mucosa, resulting in prolonged vasoconstriction. Chronic use causes vascular atony and rebound congestion. While marked erythema of the mucosa may be seen, physical findings vary. Management requires total withdrawal of topical decongestants and treatment of the underlying nasal disease which led to the use of intranasal drugs. Steroid sprays and systemic decongestants help minimize withdrawal symptoms.

Nasal polyposis is an inflammatory disease of unknown etiology. Only adults are affected; children with polyps must be evaluated for cystic fibrosis. Nasal polyps are most commonly seen in the clinical triad of polyps, aspirin sensitivity, and intrinsic asthma. Polyps are characteristically bilateral, multiple, semitranslucent masses which arise from the middle meatus and extend into the nose. Unilateral polyps should increase suspicion of neoplastic disease. Other important diagnostic possibilities include papilloma, carcinoma, glioma, or encephalocele. Initial management can include both topical steroids and a short course of systemic steroids. Surgical excision of the polyps is reserved for those patients in whom steroids are contraindicated or ineffective in restoring adequate nasal airway. Recurrence rate following surgery is 30–40%.

Hormonal rhinitis most commonly develops in association with rising endogenous estrogen levels during pregnancy. Estrogens, which cause vascular engorgement in the nose, cause the nasal congestion and obstruction occurring in the immediate premenstrual period and with the use of oral contraceptives. Hormonal rhinitis may also be seen in hypothyroidism and is caused by extracellular edema.

Vasomotor rhinitis is an alteration of nasal function of unknown etiology. It has been suggested, but not accepted, that imbalance in the sympathetic and parasympathetic tone to the nose results in the characteristic profuse watery discharge and mucosal edema. Allergy tests are negative and response to topical steroids may be suboptimal. The diagnosis of vasomotor rhinitis is made after excluding all known categories of nasal disease. Treatment is supportive.

Diseases of the Paranasal Sinuses

Acute Sinusitis. Acute sinusitis is a self-limited inflammatory process caused by bacterial pathogens. It most frequently develops as a complication of a viral upper respiratory infection (common cold) and is heralded by the onset of periorbital tenderness, facial pain, headache, fever, and purulent nasal discharge. Although there is a significant overlap of symptoms associated with rhinitis and sinusitis, the presence of pain, pressure, or headache usually indicates involvement of the sinuses. Acute sinusitis is due to ostial closure secondary to inflammatory edema from the viral upper respiratory infection. The resultant stasis of secretions leads to infection with bacteria. Common causative organisms in acute sinusitis are *S. pneumoniae*, *H. influenzae*, and *Moraxella catarrhalis*. The diagnosis is usually established on the basis of clinical findings of mucopurulent nasal drainage, inflamed turbinates, pain over the anterior face, and fever. Radiographs, reserved for confirmation, may reveal air fluid levels or opacification.

Medical therapy is begun empirically in the uncomplicated case. A 10-day course of amoxicillin (or combination erythromycin and sulfisoxazole) and a short course of topical decongestants is recommended. Supportive measures include systemic decongestants, saline nasal sprays, expectorants, humidification, warm compresses, and analgesics.

Surgical treatment in acute sinusitis is indicated if there is poor response to adequate medical therapy. Severe facial pain, orbital complications (such as periorbital abscess or orbital abscess), or acute infection in an immunocompromised patient require a drainage procedure. Aspiration and irrigation of the maxillary sinus is performed by passing a trocar through the canine fossa or inferior meatus. Antral puncture is required to obtain cultures in acute sinusitis since nasal smears correlate poorly with sinus pathogens. Acute frontal sinusitis which does not respond to 48 hours of i.v. antibiotics requires trephination and drainage to prevent intracranial extension and abscess formation.

Complications of Acute Sinusitis

Orbital Infection. Acute ethmoid sinusitis is the most common cause of orbital infection. Orbital inflammation is primarily a disease of children and young adults. Inflammation may reach the orbit by retrograde thrombophlebitis spread along the system of valveless veins connecting the sinuses and orbit or through dehiscences in the lamina papyracea. To aid diagnosis and treatment, orbital complications have been classified into five stages:

1. Preseptal cellulitis is the earliest stage of orbital inflammation, marked by hyperemia and edema of the eyelid. Because the process is restricted to tissues anterior to the orbital septum there are no signs of orbital inflammation.
2. Orbital cellulitis presents with inflammation of the orbital contents and the eyelids, as well as with chemosis, proptosis, and ophthalmoplegia.
3. Subperiosteal abscess results in severe proptosis with downward and lateral globe displacement, progressive ophthalmoplegia, and visual loss.
4. Orbital abscess is associated with complete ophthalmoplegia and rapid loss of visual acuity from ischemia or neuritis of the optic nerve.
5. Cavernous sinus thrombosis is the most advanced stage of orbital inflammation and is heralded by the development of bilateral ophthalmoplegia. Blindness, severe retroorbital pain, and signs of meningeal irritation are present.

Orbital inflammation must be treated aggressively since it poses a serious threat to both vision and life. The patient should be hospitalized and ophthalmology consultation obtained to document visual acuity, extraocular motility, and proptosis. A CT scan should be performed if clinical signs are unclear, surgical drainage imminent, or intracranial complications suspected. The most common organisms found on direct culture of abscesses at surgery are staphylococcal species, streptococci, and anaerobes. High-dose i.v. antibiotic therapy is begun immediately along with routine treatment for acute sinusitis. Surgical drainage is indicated if the patient does not improve after 24 hours of i.v. antibiotic therapy or has documented loss of visual acuity.

Osteomyelitis. Osteomyelitis develops from an acute frontal sinusitis and most commonly involves the frontal bone. Retrograde thrombophlebitis along the valveless diploic veins within the frontal bone allows direct extension from the frontal sinus mucosa to the marrow space of the frontal bone, veins of the dura, and sagittal sinus. Any patient with frontal sinusitis and severe frontal pain, tenderness, or low-grade fever should be suspected of osteomyelitis. If the avascular necrosis extends from the medullary layer through the outer cortex, a soft, fluctuant, tender mass over the frontal bone, Pott's puffy tumor, results. Penetration of the inner cortex may occur without external signs and result in an epidural abscess. A CT scan is mandatory to exclude intracranial extension. Radiographic changes of osteomyelitis may not appear for 5–7 days, at which

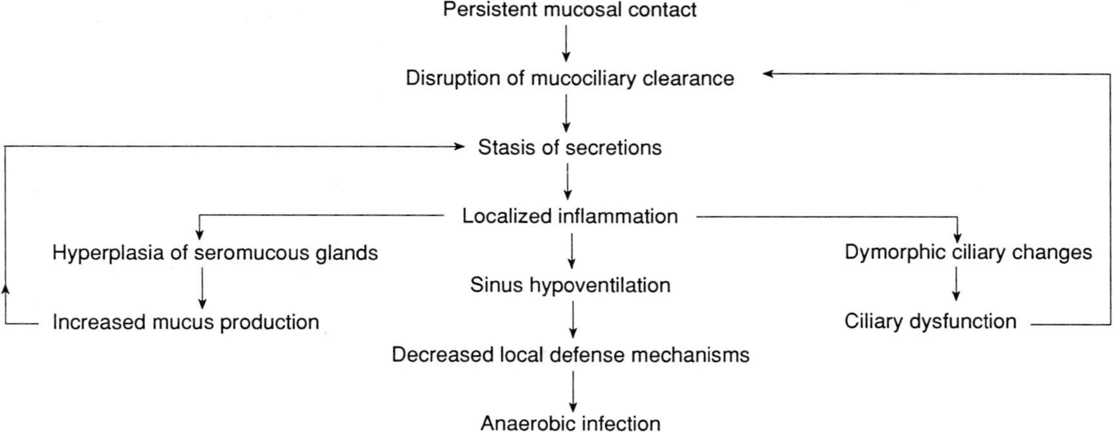

Figure 5.9. Pathophysiology of chronic sinusitis.

time a diffuse moth-eaten pattern with irregular sequestra may be seen. Staphylococcal species are the most common offending organisms. Management requires both high-dose i.v. antibiotic therapy and debridement of all necrotic bone.

Intracranial Complications. Intracranial complications are most likely to develop from inflammatory disease of the frontal sinus. Both acute and chronic frontal sinusitis may result in intracranial infection. Extension usually is along the diploic veins, but may occur through traumatic or surgical defects.

Epidural abscess, between the inner table of the frontal bone and dura, presents with severe headache and fever. A lucent, biconvex capsule may be seen on CT scan. CSF studies are normal. Management requires high-dose parenteral antibiotics, radical debridement of osteomyelitic bone, and aspiration of pus from epidural space.

Subdural empyema is a fulminant disease characterized by fever, severe headache, nuchal rigidity, and a deteriorating level of consciousness. Contrast-enhanced CT demonstrates a crescent-shaped mass, and lumbar puncture reveals a mildly elevated opening pressure, elevated protein, moderate leukocytosis, normal sugar, and negative smear and culture for bacteria. Streptococci and Bacteroides are the most common offending organisms. Antibiotic therapy and neurosurgical excision of the abscess are required, in conjunction with ablation of the offending sinus. Management includes neurosurgical irrigation of the subdural space through multiple burr holes, ablation of the offending sinus, and antibiotic therapy. The clinical signs of brain abscess develop slowly, with subtle mood or behavior changes the most common early manifestations of frontal lobe involvement. Later, depressed level of consciousness, mounting headache, and seizure are seen.

Meningitis occurs when a brain abscess ruptures into the subarachnoid space or ventricle. Meningitis may also follow sphenoid or ethmoid sinusitis, facial trauma, skull fracture, or sinus surgery. Clinical findings may be masked by previous antibiotic therapy. Fever, progressive headache, irritability, and nuchal rigidity are typically noted. Findings on lumbar puncture (LP) are elevated pressure, marked leukocytosis, high protein, decreased sugar, and positive smears and cultures. Hemolytic streptococcus and pneumococcus are the predominant organisms. Initial therapy consists of antibiotics and supportive measures. Definitive surgical drainage or repair is performed when the patient has stabilized.

Chronic Sinusitis. Chronic sinus disease is one of the most common health care complaints in the United States. It results when mucosal contact disrupts mucociliary clearance or forces closure of the sinus ostium (Fig. 5.9). Both result in stasis of secretions with localized inflammation, which in turn damages the cilia and causes hyperplasia of seromucinous glands. The cycle of chronic disease is fueled by the increased quantities of abnormally viscous mucus, along with progressive ciliary damage. Sinus hypoventilation interferes with local defense mechanisms and may lead to anaerobic infection.

Because of its multiple partitions and narrow clefts, the anterior ethmoid sinus is predisposed to ostial occlusion and mucosal contact. The anterior ethmoid sinus-middle meatus region (ostiomeatal complex) is the site of 90% of inflammatory sinus disease. Since both the maxillary and frontal sinus ostia open into the ostiomeatal complex, disease in the anterior ethmoid may result in secondary inflammation in these sinuses.

Sinus disease becomes chronic when there are recurrent bouts of acute sinusitis or when the symptoms of sinusitis persist. While the symptoms of chronic sinus disease are varied, most patients note a sensation of obstruction, facial pressure, or pain. The pain is often referred to areas supplied by the ophthalmic or maxillary division of the trigeminal nerve and characterized as dull, deep, and nonpulsatile. The clinical picture in chronic sinus disease may be dominated by nonspecific symptoms such as congestion, discharge, headache, aural pressure, sore throat, cough, generalized fatigue, or dizziness.

Predisposing factors generally can be classified into infectious diseases, noninfectious inflammatory pro-

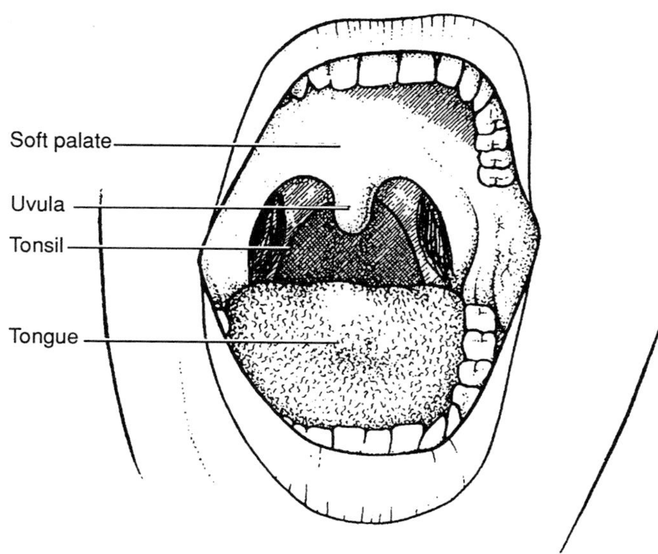

Figure 5.10. Boundaries of the oral cavity.

cesses, and structural problems. Recurrent infectious disease may be caused by ciliary dyskinesis, immune deficiency, or other systemic problems. Noninfectious inflammation includes allergy, nasal polyposis, rhinitis medicamentosa, and vasomotor disease. Structural variations that interfere with ventilation or mucociliary clearance in the ostiomeatal complex are common causes of chronic sinus disease.

In evaluating chronic sinus disease, the imaging modality of choice is a coronal CT scan. The scan allows visualization of areas hidden from endoscopic exam and displays anatomic variation that may predispose to disease, such as obstruction of the ostiomeatal complex, aeration of the turbinates (concha bullosa), and the presence of thickened mucosa in the sinuses.

The goals of medical therapy are to treat intercurrent infection, reduce tissue swelling in the ostiomeatal complex, improve mucociliary clearance, and maintain ostial patency. Antimicrobial treatment of chronic sinusitis is indicated in the presence of coexistent acute inflammation and in patients who have not received a prolonged course of a β-lactamase-resistant antibiotic. Topical intranasal steroid sprays are important adjuncts to antibiotic therapy because of their antiinflammatory effect, which helps restore ostial patency and relieves chronic symptomatology. Saline nasal sprays and expectorants enhance mucociliary clearance by reducing the viscosity of mucus. Antihistamines, on the other hand, have an anticholinergic effect, increasing the viscosity of mucus, which causes dryness and slows mucociliary clearance. Because antihistamines aggravate the underlying causes of chronic sinus disease, they should be reserved for allergic diseases.

Surgical treatment of chronic sinus disease focuses on the pivotal role of the ostiomeatal complex in the pathophysiology of disease. Using a rigid endoscope for improved visualization, the important ostia in the anterior ethmoid region are opened to establish normal ventilation and mucociliary clearance (Fig. 5.7). Determining the need for surgery in chronic sinus disease requires sound clinical judgment based on history, endoscopic findings, CT scan, and response to medical therapy. By restoring normal physiologic function in the ostiomeatal complex, endoscopic ethmoidectomy may allow secondary disease in the frontal or maxillary sinuses to clear. Surgery is indicated in patients with ostiomeatal complex pathology when symptoms are unresponsive to medical therapy. Other indications for surgery include symptomatic nasal polyps. Endoscopic surgery is contraindicated in the presence of intracranial complications of sinusitis or invasive fungal disease.

Oral Cavity and Pharynx

Anatomy

The oral cavity consists of the vestibule and the mouth cavity proper (Fig. 5.10). The vestibule is a space bounded by the lips, cheeks, gums, and teeth. The mouth cavity is bounded anteriorly and laterally by the alveolar arches, superiorly by the hard and soft palates, and inferiorly by the tongue. The tongue is the predominant organ of the mouth and plays an integral role in chewing and swallowing food. It is an essential organ of speech and is the main organ of taste. Its movements are controlled by two sets of extrinsic and intrinsic muscles, including the genioglossus, hyoglossus, chondroglossus, styloglossus, and glossopalatinus muscles, all of which are supplied by the hypoglossal nerve. Sensory innervation is supplied by both special visceral and general somatic nerve branches. The sensation of taste is transmitted from the anterior two-thirds of the tongue by the chorda tympani branch of the facial nerve. The lingual branch of the glossopharyngeal nerve supplies the posterior one-third of the tongue. General sensation is through branches of the 5th, 9th, and 10th cranial nerves.

Saliva flows into the mouth by way of ducts from three pairs of salivary glands: parotid, submandibular, and sublingual. Additional, minor salivary glands are found at the posterior portion of the tongue, palatine tonsils, soft palate, lips, and cheeks. The mouth communicates with the pharynx by way of the oropharyngeal isthmus, or isthmus faucium, which is bounded by the soft palate above, the dorsum of the tongue below, and the glossopalatine arches on each side. Just posterior to the glossopalatine arches and anterior to the pharyngopalatine arches lie the palatine tonsils. Attached to the soft palate are the levator veli palatini and tensor veli palatini muscles which raise and tense the soft palate during swallowing.

The pharynx, part of the upper digestive tract, lies posterior to the nasal cavity, mouth, and larynx (Fig. 5.11). The three major muscles of the pharynx are the superior, middle, and inferior constrictor muscles, which play major roles in the process of swallowing. The nasopharynx lies above the level of the soft palate and communicates with the nasal cavity through the

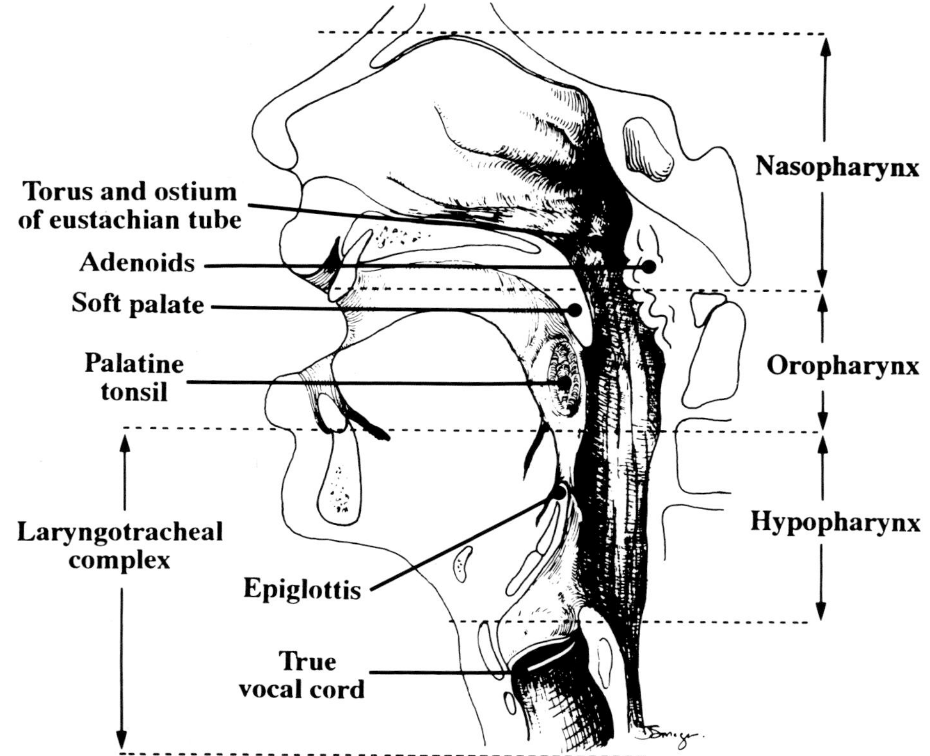

Figure 5.11. Sagittal view of pharynx, delineating landmarks of nasopharynx, oropharynx, and hypopharynx.

choanae. Opening into the lateral walls of the nasopharynx are the eustachian tubes, which allow aeration of the middle ear through the opening action of the tensor veli palatini muscles. On the posterior wall lies the adenoidal tissue.

The oropharynx extends from the soft palate superiorly to the level of the hyoid bone. It opens anteriorly to the mouth and laterally contains the palatine tonsils. The hypopharynx reaches from the hyoid bone to the lower border of the cricoid cartilage, where it narrows to become continuous with the esophagus. It communicates anteriorly with the larynx. Laterally, recesses known as the pyriform sinuses pouch out before narrowing into the esophagus.

Physical Examination

Physical examination of the oral cavity and pharynx is facilitated by ample lighting and the use of tongue blades for retraction of the cheeks and tongue. Congenital, inflammatory, or neoplastic abnormalities should be sought. Most areas of the pharynx can be inspected with mirrors, fiberoptic endoscopes, or direct vision. Digital palpation of the oral cavity and oropharynx can detect submucosal growths, and is especially important in patients at risk for malignancy, such as those who use tobacco or alcohol excessively, or who have past or family histories of aerodigestive tract carcinoma.

Diseases of the Oral Cavity and Pharynx

Benign Disorders

Congenital. The more common congenital disorders of the oral cavity include ankyloglossia (in which the tongue is bound to the mandible because of a shortened frenulum), cleft lip and/or palate, supernumerary teeth, micrognathia, cysts of the alveolar ridge or palate, lingual thyroid, and hemangiomata. If they do not obstruct the airway or interfere with swallowing, most congenital defects can be corrected surgically when the child is older. Children with cleft palates have chronic middle ear effusions, because the cleft palate interferes with the normal muscular function required for opening the eustachian tube. Children with cleft palates also tend to regurgitate liquids through the nasal cavity, and they have decreased swallowing pressures necessary for propelling boluses of food posteriorly and inferiorly. Children with Pierre Robin syndrome (mandibular hypoplasia, glossoptosis, and cleft palate) are at risk for airway obstruction secondary to posterior displacement of the tongue. Infants with this problem have lost mandibular support of the tongue and experience choking and aspiration during feeding.

Inflammatory. Inflammatory diseases of the oral cavity and pharynx are common and occur at all ages. Viral lesions of the lips and gingiva are caused by herpes simplex virus Type 1, which may also produce herpetic gingivitis, with mildly to severely inflamed mucosa that may bleed with minor irritation such as

Table 5.6.
Indications for Tonsillectomy

Recurrent tonsillitis
6–7 episodes in 1 year
3–5 episodes per year for 2 or more years
3 episodes per year for 3 or more years
Upper airway obstruction secondary to tonsillar hypertrophy
Recurrent peritonsillar abscess
Peritonsillar abscess when general anesthesia is required for incision and drainage of first abscess
Cancer

toothbrushing. Treatment is symptomatic, since no curative treatment has been developed. The most common fungal infection of the oral cavity is moniliasis or thrush, an infection caused by *Candida albicans*, with a predilection for neonates and debilitated or immunosuppressed patients. Unlike inflammation caused by viruses, however, moniliasis is treatable (with metronidazole), and most patients become symptom-free after 2–3 days on therapy.

Like the oral cavity, the pharyngeal region has extensive lymphatic tissue and therefore is susceptible to viral and bacterial infections, including pharyngotonsillitis and infectious mononucleosis. Various viruses have been identified in pharyngotonsillitis: parainfluenza, adenovirus, influenza, and Epstein-Barr. In mononucleosis, Epstein-Barr is identified as the cause, and systemic involvement includes the liver and the spleen. Occasionally, aseptic meningitis also occurs.

Streptococcal pharyngitis occurs more commonly in childhood, sometimes in conjunction with infectious mononucleosis. The infection is caused by β-hemolytic streptococcus, which can be cultured from the exudate. It is characterized by fever, malaise, cervical adenopathy, and exudative tonsillitis. Intramuscular and/or oral penicillin provides adequate treatment against the organism, but in cases where the infection recurs frequently, removal of the tonsils is necessary to eradicate the disease. β-Hemolytic streptococcus can also infect the peritonsillar region, as well as the tonsillar capsule area, resulting in peritonsillar abscess, peritonsillitis, or necrotizing tonsillitis. Adenoidal tissue can also be infected, and, in situations of chronic adenoiditis, chronic otitis media may result. Table 5.6 summarizes current indications for tonsillectomy.

Inflammation of the oral cavity and pharynx can also occur with the ingestion of caustic materials such as acid or alkalis. These lesions can be superficial or penetrating, and in the case of pharyngeal and hypopharyngeal involvement, mucosal necrosis can result in pharyngeal or esophageal perforation as well as airway obstruction secondary to mucosal edema.

Sleep apnea has recently been identified with adenoid and tonsillar hypertrophy and oropharyngeal hypotonia. During periods of sleep apnea, the respiratory pattern is disrupted and oxygen saturation drops. Snoring at night and mouth breathing are characteristic symptoms in children. Long-term systemic problems include cor pulmonale and retardation of growth. Diagnosis is made by monitoring the respiratory pattern and oxygen saturation during sleep. Treatment is based on removing the obstruction and establishing adequate airway when the patient is in a sleeping position.

Neoplasms

Benign Neoplasms. The most common benign neoplasm is the squamous papilloma, which is found in all ages and which rarely causes patient discomfort if it occurs in the oral cavity or the oropharynx. It is not premalignant and can be managed by observation or by surgical excision, depending on the discomfort it causes the patient or its suspicion for malignancy. Juvenile nasopharyngeal angiofibroma is an angiomatous lesion occurring predominantly in adolescent males. It is characterized by spontaneous bleeding, frequently following exertion, and is treated best by surgical removal.

Malignant Neoplasms. The most common malignancy of the oral cavity and nasopharynx is squamous cell carcinoma. Carcinoma of the oral cavity occurs more frequently in males and, like other head and neck carcinomas, is related to excessive use of tobacco and alcohol. Malignancies present in various ways, depending on the location of the primary lesion. Lesions of the lip usually present as exophytic or ulcerative changes in the mucosa, which are readily seen by the patient. Carcinoma of the oral cavity usually presents on the floor of the mouth, where the patient experiences a mass growing, bleeding, or, in later stages of the disease, pain. Carcinoma of the tongue typically presents as a sore area on the surface, but if the tumor originates more posteriorly in the tonsillar area, retromolar trigone, or base of the tongue, it may present with dysphagia, dysarthria, trismus, or otalgia. Some carcinomas of the pharynx (whether nasopharynx, oropharynx, or hypopharynx) may not be suspected until cervical adenopathy appears. The most common presentation of carcinoma of the nasopharynx is a palpable lymph node in the posterior triangle of the neck. Patients with this lesion may also present with middle ear effusion secondary to mechanical obstruction of the eustachian tube.

Squamous cell carcinoma is treated by surgery, radiation therapy, and—in the more extensive tumors—chemotherapy. The choice of modality is based on the patient's desires, overall systemic condition, and whether radiation therapy has been used previously in the area. Primary lesions less than 4 cm in diameter with no metastasis respond well to radiation therapy or surgery as the sole method of treatment. Lesions greater than 4 cm or those that exhibit cervical adenopathy require a combination surgery and radiation therapy. Results of studies on the effect of chemotherapy used in conjunction with the other two therapeutic modes are encouraging but not definitive.

Reconstructive techniques following radical excision of malignancies have progressed from the use of adjacent tissue (rotational flaps) to more sophisticated free grafts using microvascular anastomotic techniques. Primary closure of a defect or coverage with split-thickness skin graft is adequate for defects after small carcinomas

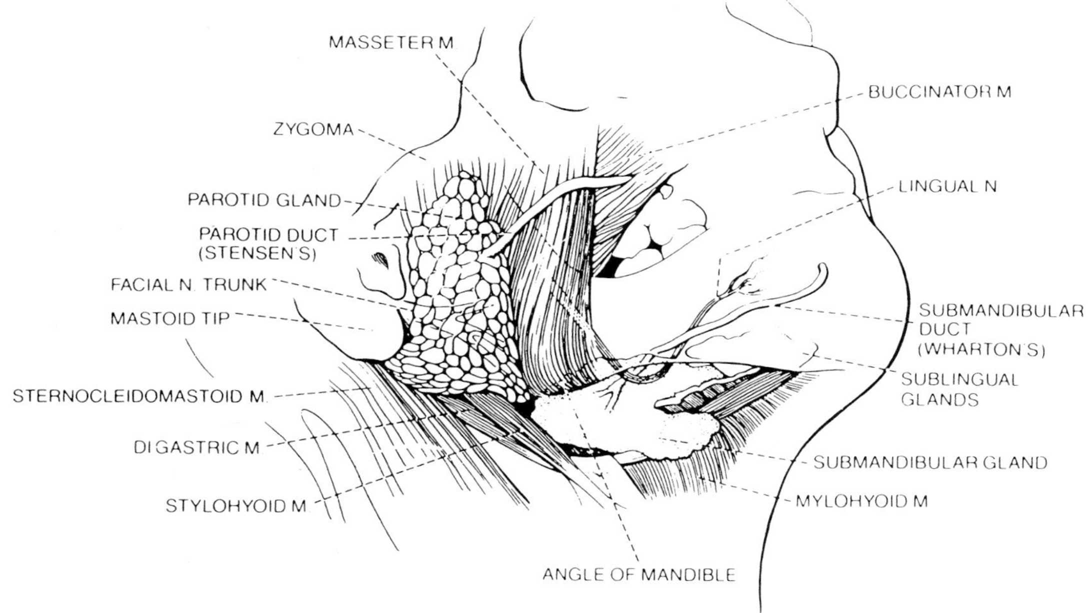

Figure 5.12. Anatomy of the parotid and submandibular glands.

have been excised. Large defects may be closed by rotation of pedicled flaps from the forehead, chest, shoulder, or temporal region. The more recent use of free, vascularized flaps has enabled the reconstructive surgeon to bring fresh tissue into a previously radiated area. Prosthetics have also come to serve a valuable role in the rehabilitation of the patient with speech, swallowing, or cosmetic defects.

The Salivary Glands

Anatomy

The major salivary glands are the parotid, submandibular, and sublingual glands (Fig. 5.12). These are paired glands and are located outside the oral cavity to which they are connected by way of ducts. The minor salivary glands are scattered throughout the oral cavity and oropharynx. They lie just deep to the mucosa and connect with the oral cavity and pharynx by way of rudimentary ducts. The major glands originate from ectoderm, whereas the minor glands derive from endoderm.

The parotid gland is the largest and lies anterior to the ear, overlying the masseter muscle. Its duct (Stensen's) arises anteriorly, approximately 1 cm below the zygoma. It traverses the masseter muscle and terminates orally in an ampulla opposite the upper second molar tooth. The most important of the multiple nerves associated with the parotid gland is the facial nerve, which exits the mastoid bone through the stylomastoid foramen and passes through the center of the gland, where it branches into the cervical, marginal mandibular, buccal, zygomatic, and temporal motor nerves. The secretomotor supply to the gland is parasympathetic from the inferior salivatory nucleus in the brain stem.

The submandibular gland, the second largest, lies in a concavity inferior to the mandible, between the anterior and posterior bellies of the digastric muscle. Its duct (Wharton's) runs anteriorly from the gland between the mylohyoid and hypoglossus muscle. It ends in an ampulla to the side of the lingual frenulum. The parasympathetic secretomotor nerve supply is derived from the superior salivatory nucleus by way of the chorda tympani nerve.

The sublingual gland, the smallest of the major glands, lies directly under the oral mucosa, forming a ridge next to the tongue. The gland empties directly into the floor of the mouth through several ducts on its superior surface. It lies close to the superior part of the submandibular gland, and minor sublingual ducts may enter into the submandibular gland. The secretomotor nerve supply is the same as that of the submandibular gland.

The sympathetic nerve supply to all of the major salivary glands is from the carotid plexus and passes to the respective glands adjacent to their arterial supply.

Physiology and Function

The salivary glands produce approximately 500 mL of saliva per day, of which 90% is secreted by the parotid and submandibular glands. Saliva acts as both a lubricant and a protective agent throughout the upper aerodigestive tract. It promotes clearing of debris and bacteria, sweeping these contaminants into the lower gastrointestinal tract. It also helps maintain oral and dental hygiene and indirectly aids in body hydration. The main digestive enzyme of saliva is α-amylase, which is important for the enzymatic breakdown of starch.

Diseases of the Salivary Glands

Inflammatory Diseases. Inflammatory diseases of the salivary glands include mumps, acute suppurative sialadenitis, parotid abscess, chronic sialadenitis, and Sjogren's syndrome. Acute sialadenitis is a nonviral infection that occurs usually in debilitated and dehydrated adults, commonly in the postoperative state. The gland becomes hard and tender, and purulent discharge can be noted from the duct. Causative organisms include *Staphylococcus aureus*, *Streptococcus pneumoniae*, and β-hemolytic streptococcus. Treatment includes hydration and appropriate antibiotics.

Abscesses of the salivary glands are treated by incision and drainage. Chronic sialadenitis is characterized by recurrent tender enlargements of the glands and is frequently associated with strictures or calculi involving the ductal system. Treatment is usually conservative, including sialogogues, massage, and antibiotics. When conservative measures are not successful, superficial parotidectomy or excision of the submandibular gland may be the most appropriate means of treatment. Sjogren's syndrome is an autoimmune disease of the salivary glands and includes xerostomia, keratoconjunctivitis sicca, and connective tissue disorders. The cause of the syndrome is unknown, but most patients exhibit hypergammaglobulinemia with elevated IgG fraction. Rheumatoid arthritis is a common characteristic, and antinuclear antibodies are present in 50% of the cases with or without clinical arthritis. Treatment of the head and neck manifestations includes local measures to counteract xerostomia and conjunctivitis. If the salivary glands are infected, antibiotic therapy is also recommended.

Neoplasms. Tumors of the salivary glands represent approximately 1% of all head and neck tumors, with 85% arising from the parotid gland. Of these, 75% are benign, while 50% of submandibular and 30% of minor salivary gland tumors are benign. Diagnostic measures taken for tumors of the salivary glands include fine-needle aspiration, sialography, scintillation scanning, CT scanning, and magnetic resonance imaging. The introduction of CT scanning and MRI over the past 15 years as well as the increased use of fine-needle aspiration for tumor information has resulted in a dramatic decrease in the use of other diagnostic techniques.

Benign Neoplasms. Benign tumors usually display painless, slow growth; tumor mobility; and secondary fibrosis or inflammation. Because of secondary infection or cystic degeneration, pain may be present but is not common. Minor salivary gland tumors usually occur on the palate but may occur anywhere in the upper aerodigestive tract. They are firm, nontender, mucosally-covered masses.

Approximately 80% of benign tumors are mixed tumors, or pleomorphic adenomas, which tend to occur in the third and fourth decades of life. Treatment consists of total removal of the submandibular gland or minor salivary gland, or superficial lobectomy of the parotid gland. Warthin's tumor occurs 6–8% of the time, primarily in the tail of the parotid gland and principally in men. It represents parotid tissue that has become incorporated into a lymph node. Treatment consists of superficial lobectomy of the parotid gland.

The most common benign parotid gland tumor in children is the hemangioma. These will usually resolve spontaneously. Surgery should be reserved for rapidly growing tumors or those that do not resolve by age 2–3.

Malignant Neoplasms. Malignant lesions of the salivary glands share many of the characteristics of their benign counterparts. However, certain signs and symptoms indicate malignancy: rapid growth, large size, tumor fixation to the overlying skin, facial nerve dysfunction, and cervical node enlargement. Children tend to have a higher rate of malignancy with salivary gland tumors.

Fine-needle aspiration allows diagnosis of malignancy in 85 to 95% of the cases. Open or partial biopsy is performed only when mucosal or skin involvement is noted. Minor salivary gland biopsy may be performed if the tumor is not accessible by fine-needle aspiration. Small tumors of the submandibular gland are best biopsied by removal of the gland.

The most common malignancy of the parotid gland is mucoepidermoid carcinoma. This tumor shows a wide spectrum of biologic behavior. Low-grade mucoepidermoid cancers usually have a favorable prognosis, grow locally, and metastasize to upper neck nodes late in the course of the disease. In the high-grade mucoepidermoid cancers, metastasis to lower neck nodes and lungs is not uncommon. Adenoid cystic carcinoma, the most common malignancy in all but the parotid gland, has a tendency to invade lymphatics and nerves. This tumor is characterized by late distant metastasis; the 10- to 20-year survival rate is poor. Other malignant tumors of the salivary glands include adenocarcinoma and squamous cell carcinoma. The primary treatment of malignancies of the salivary glands is radical removal of the tumor. Depending on the tumor grade or lymphatic involvement, cervical lymphadenectomy and/or radiation therapy may be helpful.

The Larynx

Anatomy

The larynx occupies the central compartment of the neck and has a rigid framework consisting of several cartilages and one bone, the hyoid bone, which forms the superior border of the larynx (Fig. 5.13). Within the larynx, ligamentous, tendinous, and muscular attachments from the tongue, mandible, and base of skull control the position and tension of these elements. These attachments contract during swallowing, resulting in elevation of the larynx. The largest of the cartilages, the shield-shaped thyroid cartilage, is connected to the hyoid bone by the thyrohyoid membrane, and contains a midline prominence more apparent in males

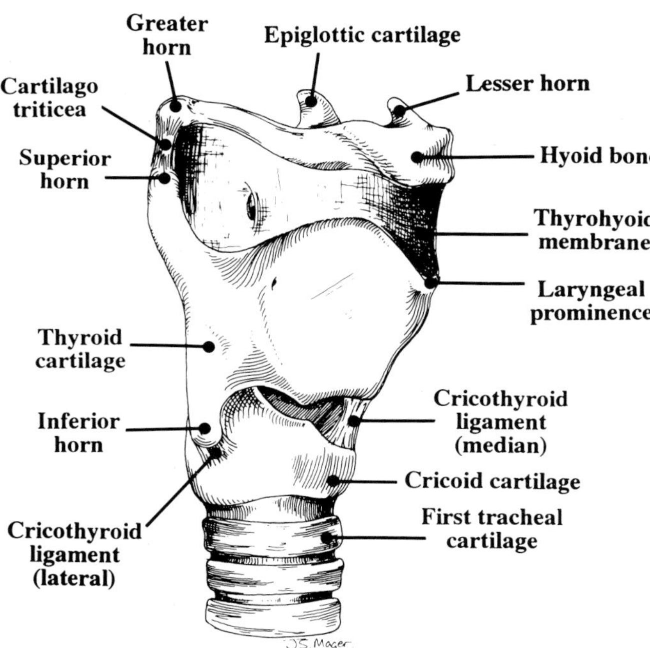

Figure 5.13. Anatomy of the larynx.

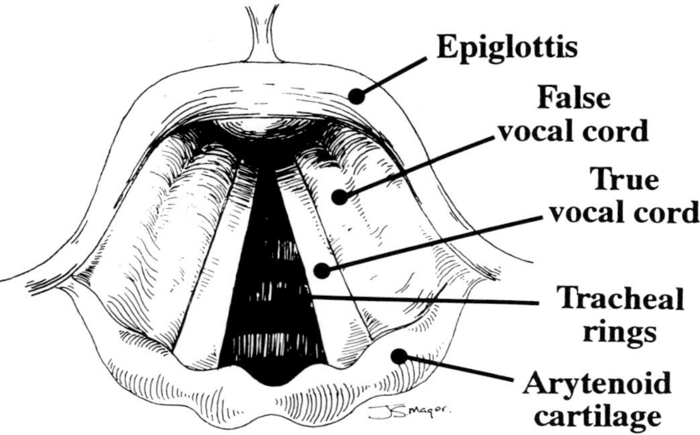

Figure 5.14. Lateral view of the larynx showing the vocal cords.

("Adam's apple"). Anteriorly, the thyroid cartilage has two superior and two inferior ala, which connect it to the cricoid cartilage by the cricothyroid membrane. The cricoid cartilage is the only complete cartilaginous ring in the larynx. The cricoid suspends the tracheal rings by membranous connections anteriorly and by a continuous membranous wall posteriorly. The remaining two cartilages are the paired arytenoid cartilages, which articulate with the thyroid-cricoid sulcus posterolaterally and the vocal ligaments anteriorly. The vocal ligaments join anteriorly at the inner surface of the midthyroid cartilage and serve to open and close the glottic niche according to contraction of the laryngeal musculature (Fig. 5.14). The epiglottis is a cartilaginous flap overlying the laryngeal inlet that closes the passage during swallowing, thus protecting the larynx from aspirated food or secretions. The muscles of the larynx are classified as extrinsic or intrinsic; the extrinsic muscles elevate and depress the larynx as a unit, while the intrinsic muscles move the vocal cords. Only one muscle, the cricoarytenoid, functions to abduct or open the vocal cords. The remainder of the intrinsic muscles serve to adduct the vocal cords, and thus close the glottic niche.

The nerve supply to the larynx derives from two branches of the vagus nerve: the superior laryngeal nerve, which provides sensory function and innervates the cricothyroid muscle, and the recurrent laryngeal nerve, which supplies motor functions to all remaining intrinsic muscles. The superior laryngeal nerve enters the larynx through the lateral thyrohyoid membrane. The recurrent laryngeal nerve courses along under the aortic arch on the left and subclavian on the right, ascending along the tracheoesophageal groove to penetrate the larynx by the posterior cricoid cartilage. The left recurrent laryngeal nerve has a longer course in the chest and thus is more susceptible to injury.

The arterial supply and venous drainage is by way of the superior and inferior laryngeal arteries and veins. These are branches of the superior and inferior thyroid vessels, respectively. Their course closely parallels the nerve supply.

Knowledge of lymphatic drainage is important, since it affects the course and treatment of malignant neoplasms. The superior drainage system drains the larynx above the level of the vocal cords to the upper deep cervical nodes, while the inferior system drains the larynx below the level of the vocal cords to the lower deep cervical nodes, pretracheal nodes, and supraclavicular nodes. The vocal cords themselves have scant lymphatic supply.

Physiology

The primary functions of the larynx are respiration, airway protection, and phonation. The glottis opens a fraction of a second before air is drawn in by the descent of the diaphragm, allowing respiration to occur. Just as opening the larynx provides an important function, so does closing the glottic niche, preventing anything but air from getting into the airway. During swallowing, the larynx elevates and the vocal cords, arytenoids, and epiglottis come together, directing food into the esophagus instead of the trachea. The third function, phonation, provides a means of communication. The voice is produced when a column of air under pressure from the lungs is forced through the vibrating vocal cords in their closed position. Pitch, loudness, and vocal quality are controlled at the level of the larynx; resonance is controlled at the level of the oropharynx and nasal cavities; and pronunciation, or articulation, is controlled by the fine motor movements of the tongue as it interfaces with the palate, teeth, and lips.

Congenital Diseases of the Larynx

Congenital anomalies of the larynx can result in abnormalities in any of its three major functions. The most common symptom is stridor, or noisy breathing.

Stridor is classified as inspiratory, expiratory, or biphasic. Inspiratory stridor localizes the problem to either the supraglottic (above the vocal cords) larynx, or the true vocal cords. Expiratory or biphasic stridor localizes the problem to the subglottic (below the vocal cords) larynx or trachea. In general, the more prominent the expiratory component, the further down the trachea is the defect.

Laryngomalacia. Laryngomalacia is the most common cause of infant stridor, accounting for 60% of all cases. In this condition, the loosely supported epiglottis and arytenoid cartilages prolapse into the glottic niche during inspiration. Laryngomalacia presents as high-pitched inspiratory stridor present from the time of birth. The stridor worsens in the supine position but rarely results in severe distress. Diagnosis is by flexible laryngoscopy with or without anesthesia, or rigid laryngoscopy with general anesthesia. The symptoms are usually self-limiting, with spontaneous resolution by 15–18 months of age. Surgical treatment is rarely indicated. Parents should be reassured but advised to avoid keeping the baby in the supine position, especially during sleep.

Supraglottic Cysts. Supraglottic cysts are another congenital cause of inspiratory stridor. Because of the large number of mucus-secreting cells of the larynx, a cyst can form, obstructing the airway. The cyst is aspirated emergently, and endoscopic marsupialization cures the condition.

Vocal Cord Paralysis. Both vocal cords can be paralyzed at birth as a result of a brainstem lesion (such as Arnold-Chiari malformation) or from an idiopathic cause. Initial treatment is a tracheostomy until the primary problem resolves or is treated. If the paralysis is permanent, vocal cord lateralization or reinnervation procedures can be done when the child is older.

Unilateral vocal cord paralysis can present as a congenital defect and is usually caused by trauma resulting from stretching the recurrent laryngeal nerve during pregnancy or delivery. Babies with unilateral vocal cord paralysis present with a hoarse cry and may have choking with feeding because of aspiration. When secondary to trauma, paralysis generally resolves during the first month of life.

Webs. Vocal cord webs are formed when normal laryngeal embryonic recanalization fails to occur. The webs are usually membranous and involve the anterior true cords. They may present as hoarseness or stridor, depending on their extent. Treatment is by endoscopic laser excision. Rarely, an open surgical repair by means of a laryngotomy is required.

Congenital Subglottic Stenosis. Congenital subglottic stenosis, if severe, presents at birth as biphasic stridor or respiratory obstruction. If the stenosis is mild it may present as recurrent croup in later infancy or as stridor after intubation for an elective surgical procedure. Like vocal cord webs, the stenosis results from an embryologic defect in the laryngeal recanalization process. Unlike webs, however, the obstruction is at the cricoid or subglottic region rather than at the vocal cords. Infants will often "grow out" of the problem, as the stenotic segment grows along with the rest of the larynx. If severe, the stenosis can be corrected by surgically incising and stenting the cricoid cartilage.

Subglottic Hemangiomas. Subglottic hemangiomas present as biphasic stridor. These vascular lesions occur in the subglottic region and are associated with cutaneous hemangiomas in over 50% of cases. They appear endoscopically as bluish lesions below the level of the cords, more commonly on the left. Infant hemangiomas tend to grow in the first 6 months and then involute spontaneously by 2–3 years of age. If the hemangiomas are large enough to obstruct the airway, they may be removed by laser excision or, after a tracheostomy has been performed, left in place until they resolve.

Tracheomalacia. Tracheomalacia presents as expiratory or biphasic stridor caused by collapse of the trachea in the anterior-posterior direction. The cartilage is often abnormally shaped and soft. Spontaneous resolution can usually be expected by age 18 months. Occasionally, surgical treatment such as tracheoplexy is required.

Inflammatory Diseases of the Larynx

The larynx is frequently involved with inflammatory processes in all age groups. Epiglottitis and croup, common in children but unusual in adults, are very different conditions that can present similarly. Because they can be life threatening, every physician should know how to diagnose and manage them. Laryngitis and vocal cord nodules are other common inflammatory diseases.

Epiglottitis. Epiglottitis is a potentially lethal inflammation of the supraglottis caused by the bacteria *Haemophilus influenzae*. The child presents with a fairly sudden (hours) onset of fever and stridor. The most common age group is 3–6 years. Physical exam reveals a child in moderate to severe distress sitting upright with head hyperextended to straighten the upper airway in an effort to facilitate air exchange. The child may be drooling and have dysphagia as well. A tongue blade must not be used to examine the child's throat, since it could produce severe laryngospasm and loss of the airway. The child should be kept calm and, if the child's condition permits, a portable lateral neck x-ray taken. If epiglottitis is revealed, the child is taken to the operating room. If the child's distress does not permit an x-ray, the child should be taken immediately to the operating room for anesthesia, direct laryngoscopy, and intubation. Oral intubation is initially done, but is often changed to a nasotracheal tube, which tends to be more stable and less likely to become displaced. In addition to an experienced anesthesiologist, an otolaryngologist or pediatric surgeon should be in attendance in the event intubation cannot be carried out and bronchoscopy and/or tracheostomy becomes necessary. Once the airway is established, cultures are taken and i.v. antibiotics effective against *H. influenzae* instituted. From the operating room the child is taken to the intensive care unit, where the nasotracheal (preferable) or orotracheal tube is kept secure while the child is placed in a croup tent. Edema usually resolves rapidly and the child can be extubated within 72 hours. Antibiotics are continued for 7–10 days. Recurrence of epiglottitis is rare.

Croup. Laryngotracheobronchitis, frequently referred to as *croup*, most commonly affects children ages 2 years and younger. It is viral in origin, affecting the subglottic larynx, but may extend the length of the trachea. The child presents with symptoms of an upper respiratory infection of a few days' duration. Over a period of several hours, the child develops a barking cough as the major symptom. Fever is usually low grade or absent. Physical exam reveals an irritable infant with mild stridor and barking cough. Lateral neck film reveals a normal epiglottis but a narrowed subglottic air column. Treatment is based on severity of symptoms. In mild cases, humidified air alone suffices. In moderate cases, racemic epinephrine treatments may be required in the emergency room. In severe cases, the child may require hospitalization with frequent racemic epinephrine treatments and i.v. or aerosol administration of steroids to decrease inflammation. Rarely the airway distress is so severe that endotracheal intubation is required to secure the airway. The edema from croup resolves more slowly than that from epiglottitis, often taking 5–7 days. Because several viruses cause croup, recurrences are common. Antibiotics are rarely required unless there is a suspicion of bacterial infection. Rarely, bacterial tracheitis is seen and is associated with a more virulent course, requiring intubation and therapeutic bronchoscopy.

Laryngitis. The most common inflammatory condition of the larynx in adults is acute laryngitis. It is usually viral in origin, presenting with hoarseness and symptoms of upper respiratory infection. Examination of the vocal cords reveals edema and erythema. The disease usually resolves spontaneously, but improvement can be expedited with humidification and voice rest. It should be emphasized that an adult with hoarseness persisting longer than 1 month needs to have an examination of the vocal cords.

Vocal Cord Nodules. Vocal cord nodules are the most common cause of hoarseness in children, although they also occur in adults. They usually are the result of localized chronic inflammation from vocal abuse. Examination reveals localized swelling at the junction of the anterior and middle one-third of the true vocal cords. Treatment should be directed toward preventing vocal cord abuse, and voice therapy can be of great benefit. While malignant degeneration is not expected, the nodules can be removed endoscopically by laser excision if they persist after vocal abuse has resolved.

Trauma

Laryngeal injuries are unusual, but they warrant discussion because the long-term sequelae are so severe. Like general neck trauma, injuries may be divided into blunt and penetrating. While penetrating injuries are readily apparent, once an airway is established blunt injuries may go unnoticed until several days later when attempts at extubation are unsuccessful. A suggested algorithm for patients presenting with laryngeal trauma is summarized in Figure 5.15.

Acquired Subglottic Stenosis. Trauma to the larynx can also occur from intrinsic sources, the most common of which is prolonged intubation. The length of time tolerated depends on the age of the patient and the basic problem necessitating intubation. Premature infants requiring intubation for ventilatory support tolerate it for prolonged periods (1–2 months) with an incidence of subglottic stenosis of less than 2–3%. The incidence is much higher in older children and adults. In older patients who have been intubated for 7–10 days and are not expected to be extubated in the following 4–5 days, a tracheostomy should be considered to prevent further subglottic damage and resultant stenosis. In subglottic stenosis there is initial mucosal damage, followed by perichondritis and chondritis of the cricoid cartilage, since the cricoid cartilage, a complete ring, cannot expand in response to injury. Once the source of irritation is removed, the cricoid lining attempts to heal itself by collagen deposition and scar formation. A tracheostomy incision is made below the level of the cricoid, thus reducing the risk of further cricoid damage.

Surgical Airways. Occasionally, a surgical airway must be established. The fastest, safest means of establishing one in adults is to perform a cricothyroidotomy, staying in the midline and assuring avoidance of vital lateral structures. Landmarks are demonstrated in Figure 5.16. Also note in Figure 5.16 the landmark differences for children and adults: children lack a cricothyroid space and thus the incision should be in the trachea. Indications for tracheostomy are airway obstruction, pulmonary physical therapy and suctioning needs, and prolonged ventilation requirements. Tracheostomy may be performed under local or general anesthesia. The technique involves a horizontal skin incision, separation of the strap muscles, and a vertical incision through tracheal rings 3 and 4. An important step is the placement of tracheal stay sutures, which are taped to the chest for 3–4 days. Since the patient with a tracheostomy tube has lost the access between the lower airway and the upper airway, the nasal functions of warming and humidifying air are lost. These functions must be provided to help keep the bronchoalveolar structures from drying out. Frequent suctioning is important, especially in the early postoperative period, to keep the secretions from plugging the tracheostomy tube. Potential early complications of tracheostomy are bleeding, pneumothorax, accidental decannulation, and cardiac arrest. Late and extremely rare complications are tracheoinnominate fistula and tracheoesophageal fistula.

Neoplasms

Benign. The most common benign tumor in children is the squamous papilloma, which can also involve the trachea and the bronchi. The papilloma is an epithe-

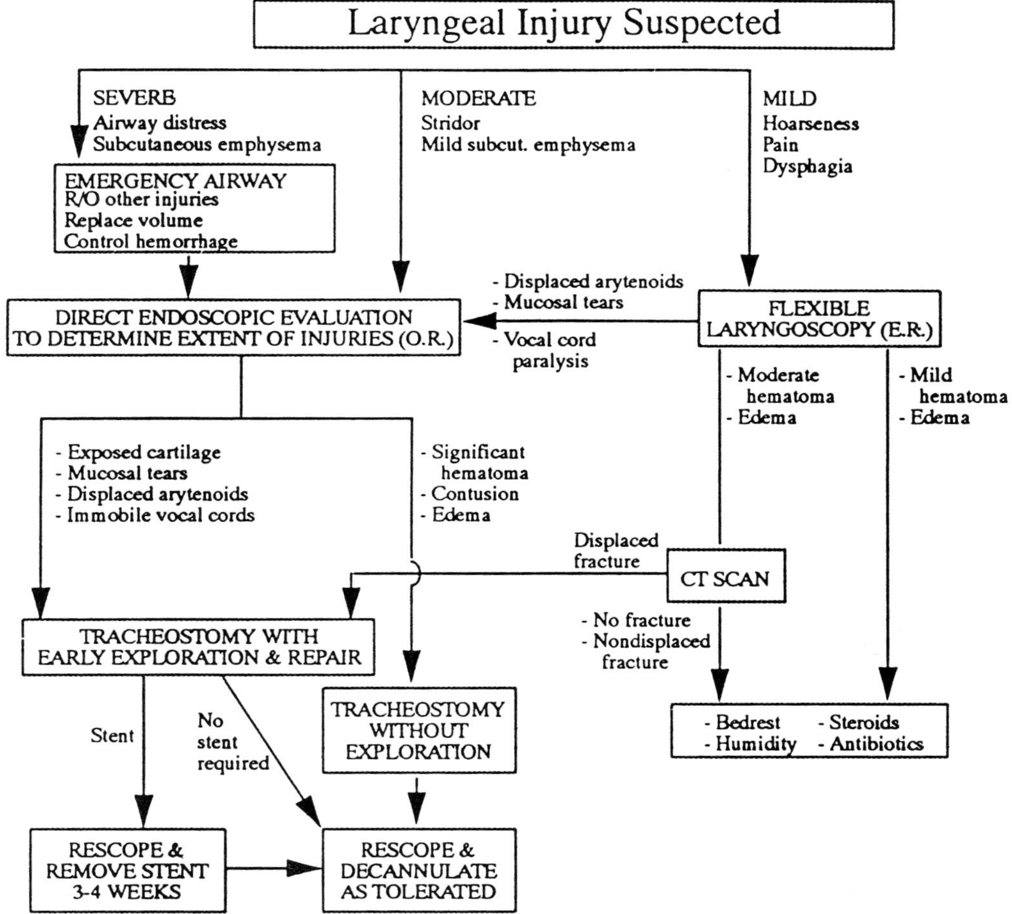

Figure 5.15. Algorithm for acute laryngeal injuries.

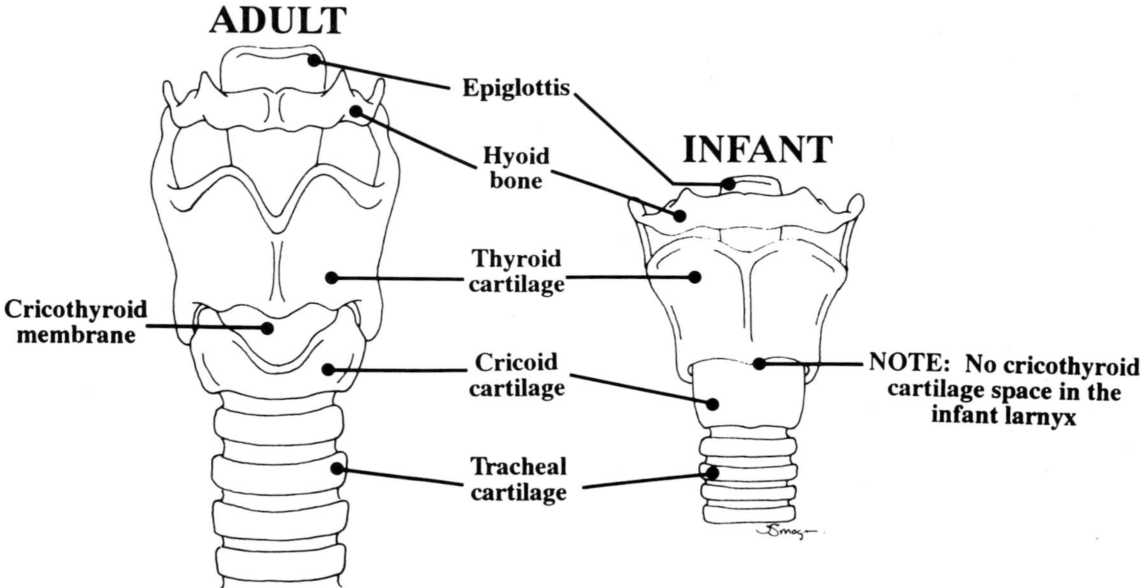

Figure 5.16. Landmarks for cricothyrotomy.

lial lesion of connective tissue covered by squamous epithelium that may be keratinized. Papillomas usually involve the anterior portions of the vocal cords, but can also involve the false cords superiorly as well as the immediate subglottic area. In children, onset usually occurs before the age of 5, and the condition can persist until late adolescence. Lesions arising in adults are not as aggressive.

Papillomas are thought to have a viral etiology and to be influenced by hormonal changes, as evidenced by their tendency to remit spontaneously around puberty. They spread by manipulation and can seed up and down the respiratory tract. These lesions were first removed piecemeal, then endoscopically, and more recently by carbon dioxide laser. Radiation therapy is detrimental rather than helpful, and a recent study has shown systemic interferon to have no long-term benefits. Antiviral agents such as acyclovir are currently being tried.

Malignant. The most common malignancy is squamous cell carcinoma. Others include sarcoma, adenocarcinoma, and metastatic neoplasms. Approximately 25% of all head and neck cancers are laryngeal. The male/female ratio is greater than 11:1. Cigarette smokers have a five times greater mortality rate than nonsmokers, and cigar and pipe smokers almost a three times greater mortality rate. The consumption of alcohol is also thought to contribute to the development of laryngeal carcinoma.

Signs and Symptoms. The most common sign of laryngeal carcinoma is hoarseness, especially with glottic and transglottic lesions. A gradual airway obstruction may be compensated for, but recurrent infections and mucosal edema will increase airway blockage. Late signs include pain on swallowing, hemoptysis, and weight loss. Patients with hoarseness that persists for more than 3 weeks should undergo mirror or fiberoptic laryngoscopy for inspection of the vocal cords. Patients presenting with hoarseness and cervical adenopathy should undergo a detailed workup even sooner.

Diagnosis. A diagnosis of carcinoma of the larynx is based on the physician's clinical assessment, noninvasive diagnostic techniques, and biopsy of the lesion. In addition to indirect mirror and fiberoptic examination of the larynx, CT or MRI scans can demonstrate the degree of involvement of supraglottic, glottic, and subglottic areas. New lesions are clinically staged according to the system proposed by the American Joint Committee on Cancer, taking into consideration tumor size and location, cervical nodal involvement, and metastasis. Patients with small tumors with no nodal involvement and no evidence of metastasis have a much greater survival rate than those with evidence of tumor spread, as would be expected.

Treatment. Primary treatment modalities include surgery, radiation therapy, or a combination of both. Chemotherapy to treat advanced stages of laryngeal cancer has not been proven to increase survival rates. For stage I or II lesions, with no cervical node involvement, either surgery or radiation therapy is expected to produce a 3-year survival rate of greater than 90%. The presence of cervical adenopathy is an indicator of a much poorer prognosis, with the size and number of nodes having an inverse correlation to the patient's survival rate. A clinical diagnosis of cervical adenopathy by either palpation, radiographic imaging, or fine needle aspiration can reduce the predicted 3-year survival rate by as much as 70%.

In determining the mode of therapy for laryngeal cancer, the size and location of the tumor, the presence or absence of cervical nodes, and the patient's own desires and physical status are taken into account. Small tumors are usually treated with radiation therapy, particularly when they involve the true vocal cords. Partial laryngectomies may be performed for small- or medium-sized lesion. These include supraglottic laryngectomies for removal of the upper portion of the larynx when the vocal cords are not involved, or vertical hemilaryngectomies when just the cord and/or the anterior commissure is involved. Total laryngectomy is recommended if the vocal cords are immobilized by tumor, if the tumor extends into the pyriform sinus through the thyroid cartilage, or if there is a recurrence of tumor following radiation therapy. Stage III or IV tumors removed surgically are also treated with radiation, either preoperatively or postoperatively.

Once laryngectomy has been performed, postoperative voice rehabilitation includes teaching the use of esophageal speech, use of an electrolarynx, or inserting a voice prosthesis through a tracheoesophageal fistula.

The Neck

Disorders of the neck consist primarily of neck masses and neck trauma. Since the neck is an exposed site, masses usually are readily apparent to patients or their families. The neck's exposure also renders it susceptible to blunt or penetrating trauma. A basic understanding of the complex embryology and anatomy of the neck is essential to the proper evaluation and treatment of clinical problems of this area.

Anatomy

For purposes of description the neck may be divided into two triangles (Fig. 5.17). The anterior triangle of the neck is bound medially by the midline of the neck, superiorly by the angle of the mandible, posteriorly by the sternocleidomastoid muscle, and inferiorly by the clavicle. The posterior triangle is bound medially by the sternocleidomastoid, superiorly by the mastoid tip and superior nuchal line, posteriorly by the trapezius muscle, and inferiorly by the middle third of the clavicle. Normal structures in the anterior triangle that can be seen or palpated include the sternocleidomastoid muscle, hyoid bone, larynx, trachea, thyroid gland, tail of the parotid gland, and submandibular gland. Deep to the sternocleidomastoid muscle in the anterior triangle lies the carotid sheath, which contains the common, external, and internal carotid arteries; internal jugular

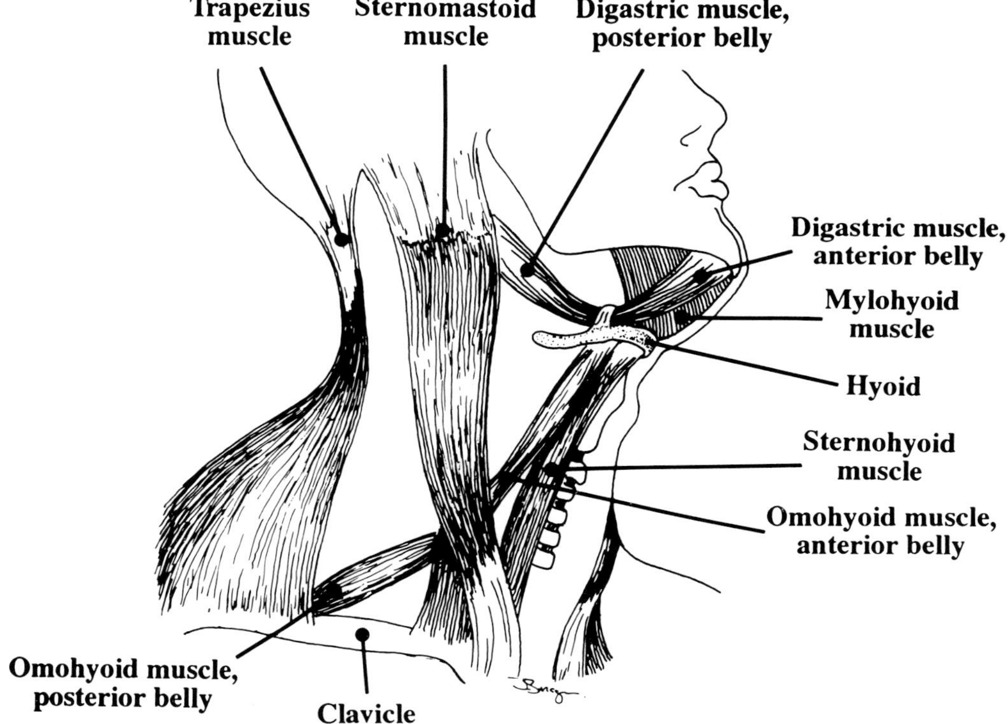

Figure 5.17. Triangles of the neck.

vein; vagus nerve; sympathetic chain; and the deep jugular lymph nodes.

Neck Masses

General Diagnostic Considerations. The patient who presents with a "lump" in the neck poses a diagnostic challenge, since a wide variety of diseases can cause a neck mass. To simplify diagnosis, neck masses are assigned one of three etiologic categories: congenital, inflammatory, or neoplastic. After a careful history and physical examination, the student should be able to assess the most likely category, and with an understanding of the most common entities in each category, should be able to carry out a systematic evaluation and appropriate treatment plan.

Age is the initial consideration in a patient being evaluated for a neck mass. Children and young adults are much more likely to have an inflammatory or congenital lesion, while older adults are more likely to have a neoplastic one. Inflammatory processes usually are more recent in onset, shorter in duration, and may have accompanying fever and symptoms related to an upper respiratory infection, such as sore throat or congestion. Neoplastic processes usually are associated with a progressively enlarging lesion, a history of alcohol and tobacco use, weight loss, and symptoms referable to the oropharynx or larynx, such as dysphagia or hoarseness. After taking a pertinent history, the physician should proceed to examine the patient's neck to determine whether the mass is a normally palpable structure or a pathologic entity. Certain features of the physical exam, such as location, size, mobility, and the presence of multiple masses, can then further delineate the most likely diagnosis. If multiple masses are present, the physician should note whether they are unilateral or bilateral and whether there is associated erythema or tenderness. A central part of the physical exam is a thorough visual inspection of all mucosal surfaces of the oropharynx and in all adults a mirror or flexible fiberoptic exam of the larynx. Palpation of the accessible mucosal surfaces or the oropharynx for masses or irregularities should also be undertaken.

Once the history and physical examination are complete, a presumptive diagnosis can be made. Various tests then help establish a firm diagnosis. Computerized tomography is highly diagnostic in determining the nature of the mass (cystic or solid), the nature of its relationship to underlying structures, and its location (within a nodal chain or a glandular structure). CT is not indicated in every neck mass evaluation, and clinical judgment must be maintained to keep its use cost effective. For those lesions involving the thyroid gland or salivary glands, radionuclide scans may be of benefit to determine degree of glandular activity or to localize the mass within the gland. Ultrasound is noninvasive and may be used to differentiate solid from cystic lesions. It is particularly useful in congenital masses. Plain radiographs of the neck are of little value, but chest radiographs should be performed on all adult patients with a neck mass, to rule out lung masses, and in children in whom there is a suspicion of lymphoma or granulomatous adenitis, to look for mediastinal masses. Useful laboratory tests include a complete blood cell count with differential, an erythrocyte sedimentation rate, and a serum test for mononucleosis.

The definitive diagnostic procedure is biopsy of the neck mass. Increasingly, fine needle aspiration has been used as part of the early evaluation of a neck mass, after the history and physical exam but before further studies. The cytologic diagnosis may be confirmed, and the ensuing workup can be more focused. Fine-needle aspiration is not to be confused with open biopsy, which is not done until the workup is complete.

Congenital Disorders. The neck is one of the most common sites for congenital disorders. An understanding of neck embryology allows prediction of the cause, location, and course of the various congenital anomalies.

Thyroglossal Duct Cysts. Thyroglossal duct cysts account for 70% of all congenital abnormalities of the neck. They present as soft, painless, persistent midline neck masses in the first or second decade of life. On physical exam, the cyst elevates with swallowing or when protruding the tongue, because of its attachment to the hyoid bone, which also elevates with those movements.

The pathophysiology of a thyroglossal duct cyst is epithelial entrapment and resultant cyst formation in the duct tract during the embryologic descent of the thyroid gland from the tuberculum impar to its final position overlying tracheal rings two and three. Before the cyst is excised, care should be taken to document the normal position and function of the thyroid gland: the cyst may contain functioning thyroid tissue. To prevent recurrent infections, surgical excision including the cyst, tract, and midportion of the hyoid bone (Sistrunk procedure) is recommended. Malignant degeneration has been reported, but is extremely rare.

Dermoid Cysts. Dermoid cysts, like thyroglossal duct cysts, present as soft, painless, persistent midline neck masses in the first or second decade of life. Unlike thyroglossal duct cysts, however, they do not elevate with swallowing, since they are not attached to the hyoid bone. Pathophysiologically, they are developmental anomalies involving pluripotential embryonal cells which become isolated and subsequently undergo disorganized growth. They are composed of ectoderm and mesoderm and often contain hair follicles, sweat glands, and sebaceous glands. The treatment of choice is complete surgical excision.

Branchial Cleft Cysts. Branchial cleft cysts usually present as persistent, painless (unless infected) masses just anterior to the middle third of the sternocleidomastoid muscle. They arise from a failure of the cervical sinus of His to obliterate. Branchial anomalies, which can involve the first through fourth arches, most commonly involve the second branchial arch. They may present as cysts, sinuses, or fistulas. The tract of a second branchial anomaly classically courses superiorly between the internal and external carotid arteries, superior to the hypoglossal and glossopharyngeal nerve. It may have an internal connection with the tonsillar fossa, a second branchial pouch derivative. These masses or tracts are subject to recurrent infection, usually in conjunction with an upper respiratory infection, and surgical excision of the cyst and/or fistula tract during a quiescent period is recommended.

Cystic Hygromas. Cystic hygromas are soft, painless, often very large multiloculated masses that are usually evident at birth or present in the first year or two of life. Pathophysiologically, they are malformations of the jugular lymphatic sac, with a failure to develop normal channels. Because of their size, their primary symptoms are compression of the larynx, trachea, and esophagus, causing stridor, dyspnea, and dysphagia. Complete surgical excision, while desirable, is often impossible. Unencapsulated, they intertwine with vital nerves and blood vessels that must be preserved. With large hygromas, multiple excisions are likely to be necessary over the course of the first several years of life. Before the lesions are excised, CT should be performed to delineate their extent and to rule out thoracic involvement.

Hemangiomas. Congenital hemangiomas, usually easily diagnosed, are developmental abnormalities present at birth. They are classified as capillary, cavernous, or mixed. They appear as bluish masses in the oral cavity, pharynx, parotid gland, or neck and generally increase in size with crying or straining. Because most hemangiomas regress spontaneously by age 5, a conservative approach is warranted. Laser surgery or excision may be of benefit in cases where hemangiomas do not resolve. Steroids have also been used with variable success.

Inflammatory Disorders. Inflammatory disorders are the most common cause of neck masses in children and young adults. Certain features are associated with inflammatory disorders: pain or tenderness, erythema, and fever. Inflammatory masses usually are recent in onset, from days to weeks, and may present with symptoms referable to an upper respiratory infection. Although salivary gland infections involving the parotid or submandibular gland may occur, most inflammatory neck masses are inflamed lymph nodes. Lymphadenitis occurs in nearly every person at some point in life, most commonly in childhood, and may be bacterial, viral, or granulomatous.

Suppurative Bacterial Adenitis. Occasionally, lymphadenitis may become suppurative, particularly in infants and children. A trial of antibiotics effective against common respiratory organisms (*Streptococcus sp., S. aureus, H. influenzae*) is indicated. If the suppurative node is superficial, fluctuation may develop because of abscess formation, and incision and drainage become necessary. Rarely, the suppurative adenitis involves one or more of the deep jugular lymph nodes. The child may appear toxemic with high fever and pronounced leukocytosis. The child will also exhibit diffuse erythema and swelling of the lateral neck. CT scan is of great benefit in diagnosing deep neck abscesses. Since these nodes and resultant abscesses are within the carotid sheath, careful incision and drainage through a lateral neck incision is indicated. If these potentially dangerous deep neck abscesses are not drained adequately, mediastinitis with a significant morbidity and mortality may result.

Viral Lymphadenitis. This nodal infection, primarily affecting children or young adults, usually is the result of a primary infectious process occurring in the vicinity of the lymphatic drainage bed of the involved node or nodes. The infection usually is found in conjunction with a viral upper respiratory infection (URI), although sometimes no primary source is identified. Since the infection tends to be self-limiting and resolves shortly after the URI resolves, antibiotic therapy generally is not indicated. However, if the nodes are tender, some otolaryngologists prescribe antibiotics for bacterial coverage.

Cat Scratch Fever. Cat scratch fever is a nonspecific granulomatous adenitis, often following a cat scratch. The lymph node from the lymphatic drainage bed in the area of the scratch becomes enlarged. Concomitant symptoms include low-grade fever, malaise, and myalgias. Granuloma formation is thought to be caused by the migration of monocytes and macrophages into an area of inflammatory or immunologic reactivity. Pathologically, the node shows multiple necrotic areas and microabscesses. A small pleomorphic bacillus has been observed within the microabscesses, and while it has been stained and visualized, it has not been cultured; the true etiologic agent remains elusive. The adenopathy may resolve spontaneously, and management usually is supportive. If suppuration occurs, needle aspiration and sometimes excision of the node are indicated.

Fungal Adenitis. Fungal adenitis is rare and when present usually occurs in compromised hosts. Fungi cause necrotizing granulomatous lymphadenitis. The condition is associated with spontaneous multiple cutaneous drainage sites. Tissue biopsy is necessary for diagnosis, and aggressive systemic treatment with antifungal agents such as amphotericin B is indicated. Surgical debridement is sometimes necessary.

Neoplasms. A firm, solid, progressively enlarging midline or lateral neck mass is most likely a neoplasm. The most common benign tumors of the neck are lipomas and neurogenic tumors. The most common malignant lateral neoplastic neck masses in children and young adults are lymphomas and rhabdomyosarcomas. In older adults, particularly those with the risk factors of alcohol and tobacco use, lateral neoplastic masses are almost always metastatic squamous cell cancer, with the primary site located somewhere in the upper aerodigestive tract. Midline neoplasms in both young and older patients usually are thyroid tumors.

Benign Tumors. Lipomas are asymptomatic masses located in the subcutaneous tissue of the neck and rarely pose a problem in diagnosis. Simple excision is all that is required. Neurogenic tumors consist primarily of schwannomas and neurofibromas. They arise from the peripheral nerve sheath of cranial nerves (such as the vagus or glossopharyngeal nerve) or the cervical sympathetic chain. They usually present as solitary lesions in the neck. Of the two neurogenic tumors, schwannomas are the more clinically benign: the individual nerve axons drape around the tumor, allowing excision of the tumor while sparing the nerve. Neurofibromas are more difficult to treat because nerve fibers pass through the tumor rather than around it: removing the tumor thus requires sacrificing the involved nerve. Patients with multiple neurofibromas should be suspected of having von Recklinghausen's disease.

Malignant Tumors. Malignant lymphomas are the most common neoplastic neck mass in children and young adults, accounting for more than 50% of cases. The masses may be bilateral, usually are nontender, and progressively enlarging. Other signs and symptoms of lymphoma include hepatosplenomegaly, abnormal chest x-ray with hilar adenopathy, and weight loss. Lymphomas are classified as Hodgkin's or non-Hodgkin's. The nodular sclerosing histologic type of Hodgkin's is the most common and is often localized to the cervical and upper mediastinal lymph nodes. Biopsy is necessary for pathologic confirmation. Treatment depends on staging, but generally consists of chemotherapy, radiation, or a combination of the two. Prognosis is stage dependent. For a more complete discussion of lymphoma, see Chapter 29, EGS2.

Rhabdomyosarcoma, usually the embryonal form, is the most common solid primary tumor of the head and neck in children. These malignant tumors of connective tissue origin most frequently involve the orbit, nasopharynx, sinuses, or neck. The diagnosis is confirmed by tissue biopsy. Once considered universally fatal, the combined treatment of surgery, radiation, and chemotherapy has significantly improved survival.

Metastatic neck masses may also be seen. A slowly enlarging, firm, solitary lateral neck mass in the older adult should be considered malignant until proven otherwise. Squamous cell carcinoma is the most common to metastasize to the neck, with the most likely primary sites being the tonsil, base of tongue, nasopharynx, or hypopharynx. Often there is a history of excessive tobacco and alcohol use, and patients may have symptoms related to their primary tumor site such as dysphagia, odynophagia, tongue pain, or airway problems. The mucosa of the upper aerodigestive tract should be examined carefully in a search for the primary tumor site. A chest x-ray should be performed to check for lung metastasis and to rule out the lung as a primary tumor site, particularly for supraclavicular masses. A CT scan can help evaluate large masses to determine their extent and relationship to the base of the skull, prevertebral fascia, and carotid artery. Fine-needle aspiration has been increasingly used as part of the early evaluation to confirm the cytology, but open biopsy is not done until the workup is complete. Diagnostic evaluation of a metastatic neck mass should also include a panendoscopy to evaluate the full extent of the tumor and to biopsy the primary lesion, if one is seen.

Treatment generally consists of radiation or surgery to the primary tumor site, depending on the site and size, and a radical or modified radical neck dissection. In 5–10% of patients with metastatic squamous cell cancer of the neck, no primary tumor can be identified on exam or endoscopy. Treatment in this group consists of a radical neck dissection with possible radiation treatment of the most likely primary tumor site. In these patients, the primary tumor will manifest itself within 2 years in 30% of patients, making regular follow-up imperative.

Thyroid Masses. Midline neoplastic neck masses usually are thyroid tumors that may be benign or malignant. They present as discrete masses or nodules rather than as diffuse enlargement. While most thyroid nodules in adults are benign, those in children are more likely to be malignant. Even though most thyroid nodules present as asymptomatic masses, the patient should be questioned regarding signs and symptoms of hyper- or hypothyroidism, dysphagia, pain, hoarseness, previous history of neck irradiation, and any other endocrine complaints. Physical exam should note size, consistency, mobility, and tenderness of the mass. If hoarseness is present, a careful laryngeal exam should be performed to evaluate vocal cord mobility. Diagnostic evaluation consists of laboratory tests, thyroid scan, and fine-needle aspiration. For a full discussion of thyroid diagnosis and management, the student should refer to Chapter 23, EGS2.

Trauma

The neck's relative exposure and lack of overlying skeletal protection renders it susceptible to trauma. Neck injuries are described according to the level at which they occur. Level one injuries occur below the cricoid cartilage; level two injuries occur above the cricoid but below the angle of the mandible; level three injuries occur above the angle of the mandible.

Injuries may be penetrating or blunt. In cases of penetrating injury, primary concerns are vascular injury, nerve disruptions, laryngotracheal disruption, and esophageal injuries. Injuries superficial to the platysma do not require surgical exploration, but most deeper injuries do. Hemodynamically stable patients with level one injuries should undergo a preoperative aortogram to rule out proximal vascular injury. If the aortogram is normal and the patient is hemodynamically stable, a contrast study of the esophagus is undertaken to rule out esophageal disruption. Even if these studies are normal, laryngoscopy, bronchoscopy, and esophagoscopy should be performed on all patients at risk for a visceral injury before the neck is explored. Patients with level two injuries may proceed directly to surgery, since all structures can be visualized at the time of surgery. Patients with level three injuries should undergo a carotid arteriogram to evaluate distal carotid injury before exploration.

Blunt injuries rarely result in vascular or esophageal injuries, but, because they may result in airway compromise from laryngeal injuries, they require prompt attention. Pain, hoarseness, and dysphagia may be seen even in the absence of fractures. Ominous signs for laryngeal fractures include stridor, subcutaneous emphysema, and loss of palpable prominence of the laryngeal cartilage. These signs necessitate visualization of the airway, CT scan in some cases, and neck exploration in others. For more detail on neck trauma, see Chapter 14, EGS2.

SUGGESTED READINGS

Adam GL, Boies LR Jr, Paparella MM. Fundamentals of otolaryngology. Philadelphia: WB Saunders, 1978.

DeWeese DD, Saunders WH, Schuller DE, Schleuning AJ II. Otolaryngology—head and neck surgery. St. Louis: CV Mosby, 1988.

Kaufman JA. Core otolaryngology. Philadelphia: JB Lippincott, 1990.

Lee KJ, ed. Essential otolaryngology. New York: Medical Examination, 1983.

Lucente FE, Sobol SM, eds. Essentials of otolaryngology. New York: Raven Press, 1988.

Wood RP II, Northern JL, eds. Manual of otolaryngology. Baltimore: Williams & Wilkins, 1979.

Skills

INDIRECT LARYNGOSCOPY

1. The patient should be sitting in an upright position facing the examiner. The patient is asked to open the mouth and protrude the tongue. The examiner gently holds the tongue out with the left hand with a gauze sponge, permitting visualization of the oropharynx. The laryngeal mirror is warmed to prevent fogging with the patient's respiration and tested on the back of the examiner's hand before introducing it into the patient's mouth. The warmed mirror is then placed against the soft palate, which is elevated into the pharynx, facilitating visualization of the larynx. The patient is asked to repeat the sound "eee" and then to take a deep breath, which allows visualization of the vocal cords in both adduction and abduction. For those patients with a sensitive gag reflex, topical spray anesthetic can be applied to the posterior pharynx (Fig. 5.11).

CRICOTHYROIDOTOMY

1. The fastest, safest surgical airway is a cricothyroidotomy. The technique involves making a skin incision directly over the cricothyroid membrane, a relatively avascular area (Fig. 5.16). The incision can be extended horizontally and spread vertically to allow the insertion of a standard tracheostomy tube. Since there is a higher incidence of subglottic stenosis associated with this procedure than with a tracheostomy, it is generally recommended to convert the cricothyroidotomy to a tracheostomy as soon as feasible.

TRACHEOSTOMY

1. Under local or general anesthesia, a horizontal skin incision is made two fingerbreadths above the sternal notch and carried down through the subcutaneous tissue. The strap muscles are identified and spread apart

in the midline, exposing the pretracheal fascia. Occasionally, the thyroid isthmus overlies the trachea at this point and it is necessary to ligate and divide it for tracheal exposure. A trach hook is placed under the cricoid to elevate and expose the tracheal rings. Stay sutures are placed in the tracheal cartilages and taped to the chest wall. They are left in place 4 to 5 days. The purpose of the stay sutures is to facilitate re-exposure of the tracheal lumen should the tracheostomy tube become dislodged and need to be reinserted before the tract becomes epithelialized. A vertical tracheal incision is made, usually between tracheal rings 2 and 3 or 3 and 4, and a tracheostomy tube is inserted. The balloon is inflated and breath sounds are checked bilaterally. The tube is sutured in and secured with trach ties around the neck. A chest x-ray is performed immediately postoperatively to check tube position and to rule out a pneumothorax.

Study Questions

1. List three treatable and three untreatable causes of conductive hearing loss.
2. What is the most common causative organism in acute otitis media? In otitis media with effusion? How are the two diseases distinguished?
3. What diagnostic tests should be performed on a patient who first presents with Bell's palsy? What percentage of patients can be expected to recover?
4. What is the diagnostic procedure of choice for a patient with a suspected acoustic neuroma?
5. How should a 20-year-old with uncomplicated acute maxillary sinusitis be managed?
6. What is the appropriate workup of a patient with chronic maxillary sinusitis (longer than 3 months)?
7. What are the risk factors for head and neck cancer? What treatment modalities are available?
8. What is the most common cause of unilateral foul-smelling nasal drainage in a 3-year-old?
9. What diagnostic test must be performed prior to surgical removal of a soft midline neck mass in a child and why?
10. What is the most common cause of subglottic stenosis? How can it be prevented?

6 Cardiothoracic Surgery: Diseases of the Heart, Great Vessels, and Thoracic Cavity

Norman J. Snow, M.D. John R. F. Guy, M.D.
Richard H. Feins, M.D.,
and Michael L. Spector, M.D.

ASSUMPTIONS

The student understands heart, lung, chest wall, and mediastinal anatomy.

The student knows cardiovascular and pulmonary physiology.

The student has learned to perform cardiac and pulmonary physical examinations.

OBJECTIVES

1. Assess a list of typical hemodynamic measurements (including central venous pressure (CVP), pulmonary arterial pressure (PAP), pulmonary artery wedge pressure (PAWP), and cardiac output) in a normal patient as well as one with hypovolemic shock, cardiac tamponade, or acute myocardial infarction.
2. Discuss the advantages of, indications for, and possible complications of a central line versus a Swan-Ganz catheter.
3. Discuss and understand the unique contributions of extracorporeal circulation and myocardial preservation techniques to cardiac surgery.
4. List the risk factors and common clinical symptoms in a patient with ischemic heart disease and discuss the differential diagnosis.
5. List treatment options for patients with ischemic heart disease.
6. Describe the indications for surgical intervention in a patient with ischemic heart disease.
7. Describe the complications of a myocardial infarction.
8. Explain the physiologic benefits of intra-aortic counter pulsation as well as its complications and contraindications.
9. State the clinical indications for aortic, tricuspid, and mitral valve replacement.
10. List the American Heart Association indications for prophylactic antibiotics in patients with heart disease.
11. Discuss the common congenital cardiac abnormalities, including patent ductus arteriosus, tetralogy of Fallot, coarctation of the aorta, septal defects, transposition of the great vessels, and stratify them according to cyanotic or acyanotic presentation.
12. Describe the appropriate management of acute cardiac tamponade.
13. List the indications that necessitate pacemaker insertion.
14. Describe the evaluation, treatment, and complications of treating traumatic transection of the great vessels.
15. Describe the evaluation and treatment of aortic dissection.
16. Describe the clinical manifestation, anatomy, and therapy for thoracic aortic aneurysms.

17. Compare and contrast the management and prognosis of metastatic versus primary lung malignancies.
18. List the most common sources of malignant metastases to the lungs.
19. Create an algorithm for the evaluation of a patient with a solitary pulmonary nodule on chest x-ray.
20. Discuss the common risk factors and clinical symptoms in lung cancer.
21. Identify conditions that preclude curative surgical resection for lung cancer.
22. Describe cardiac and pulmonary assessments that need to be performed to determine the patient's tolerance for thoracic surgery.
23. Describe the surgical approach to lung cancer as dictated by location of the lesion.
24. Describe the most common diagnostic procedures used to evaluate chest wall and mediastinal lesions.
25. Describe the common tumors of the anterior, posterior, and superior mediastinum.
26. Describe the differential diagnosis of hemoptysis and outline initial evaluation and therapy.
27. Describe the common causes of pleural effusion and distinguish between transudate and exudate.
28. Discuss the etiology and management of lung abscess and empyema.
29. Describe the clinical manifestations and treatment of pneumothorax, tension pneumothorax, and massive hemothorax.
30. Define flail chest and discuss appropriate management of this condition.

The Heart

The heart, a hollow, muscular organ, provides the physical force necessary to deliver oxygen-rich blood to the body and return oxygen-poor blood to the lungs. The anatomy of the normal heart is well suited for this task, since blood destined for the lungs is kept separate from blood destined for the periphery. The atria, receiving blood from the peripheral and central circulation, allow its passage through one-way atrioventricular valves (tricuspid on the right and mitral on the left) into the primary pumping chambers or ventricles. The left ventricle, which must deliver blood against systemic vascular resistance, is more muscular than the right, which delivers blood to the lower-resistance pulmonary circuit. The heart is an end organ itself, receiving its circulation from the epicardial coronary arteries arising from the sinuses of Valsalva distal to the aortic valve. As an end organ, it may be affected by physiologic disturbances that affect peripheral organs. Similarly, the heart's ability to provide blood to the periphery may be adversely affected by any interruption of the circulation to the heart, such as defects of the atrial or ventricular septum, valvular incompetence or stenosis, or coronary artery obstruction.

Assessment of Cardiac Function

Despite the introduction of sophisticated physiologic measurements near the turn of the century, assessment of cardiac function has until recently been made using simple clinical parameters. Assessments of blood pressure, urine output, skin color and texture, mental status, and heart rate have been used to measure circulation. Unfortunately, these measurements do not always reflect changes in cardiac function until deterioration has occurred, sometimes irreversibly. Earlier detection of myocardial dysfunction has become possible using more sophisticated, invasive measurements, and this permits pharmacologic and mechanical intervention to halt deterioration.

A catheter placed in a central vein proximal to the thoracic inlet monitors central venous pressure, which is useful in detecting compromised left ventricular function in patients not otherwise known to have heart disease. While the CVP does not measure left heart function directly, it measures the ability of the right heart to deal with a volume load delivered by systemic veins. Central venous pressure measured electronically with a transducer is more reliable, since the "mean" measurement more nearly approximates the true pressure in the right atrium. The oscillations in a water manometer are frequently too slow to give a true index of the actual pressure. A record of changes in CVP over time is more useful than an isolated measurement. When there is evidence of intrinsic cardiac disease, the response of the left heart will likely differ from that of the right, and a single CVP measurement will probably over- or underassess the dysfunction. Furthermore, any clinical derangement that affects pulmonary vascular resistance may alter the CVP without actually altering cardiac function.

A flow-directed pulmonary artery catheter reflects the left ventricular end-diastolic volume component of cardiac output (Figs. 6.1 and 6.2). Because left ventricular muscle contractile force is proportional to myocardial fiber stretch, the greater the volume of blood within the ventricle at the end of diastole, the greater is the force of contraction and therefore of cardiac output. Since rapid bedside methods of measuring end-diastolic volume are not available, measurements of reflected left ventricular end-diastolic pressure are used. A catheter placed in a small, end, unobstructed pulmonary artery reflects pressure in the left ventricle at the end of diastole when the mitral valve is open. This pressure is called the pulmonary capillary wedge pressure, and it is used as a guide to the volume status or "filling pressure" of the heart. At that moment, there is free communication between the left ventricle and the small pulmonary capillary. The translation of left ventricular end-diastolic volume into a clinically useful pressure measurement assumes that compliance of the ventricle remains constant. However, such is not always the case. Certain clinical conditions, such as left ventricular hypertrophy or acute myocardial infarction that acutely alters left ventricular compliance, will change the relationship between left ventricular end diastolic volume and pressure.

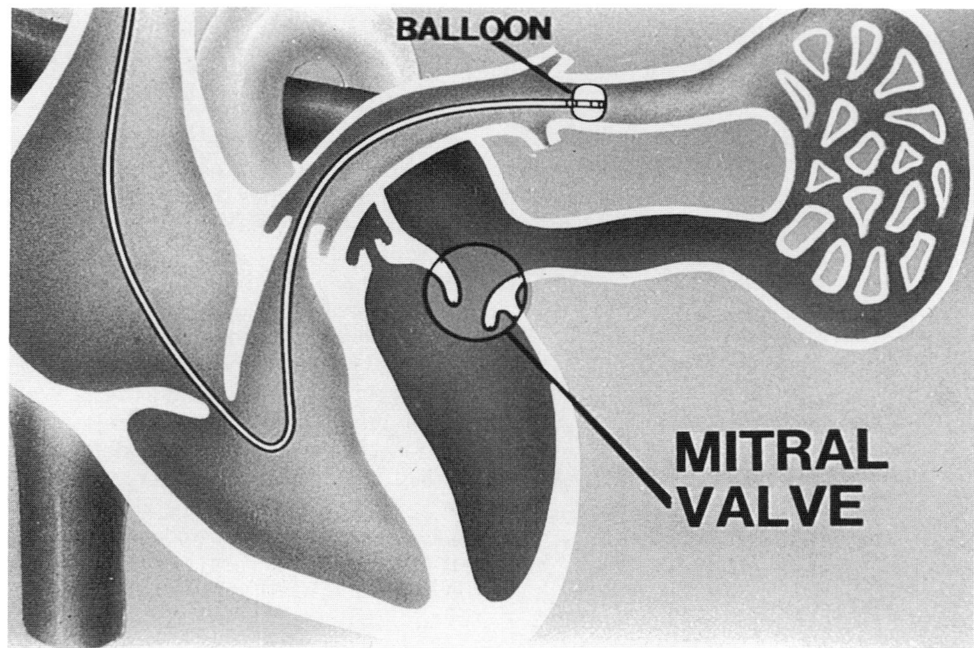

Figure 6.1. A flow-directed pulmonary catheter in place.

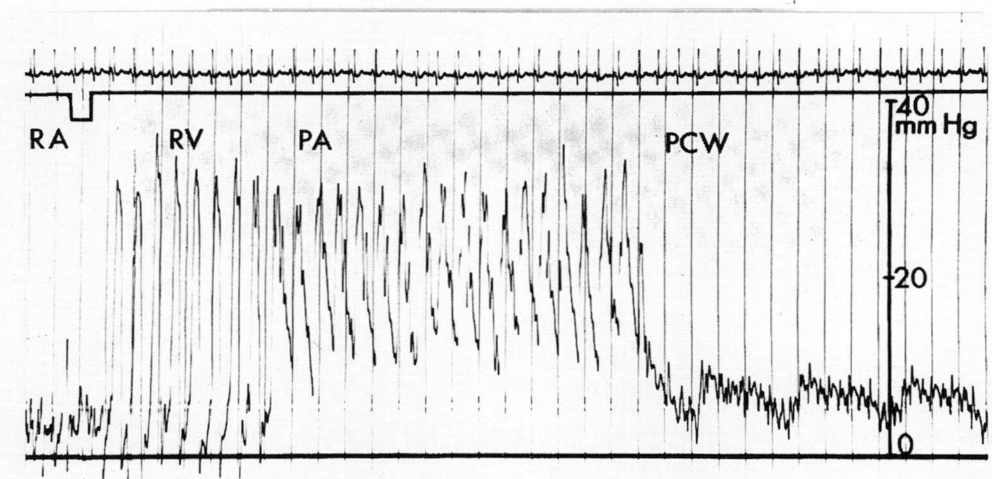

Figure 6.2. Tracings from a flow-directed pulmonary artery catheter.

Sophisticated thermodilution computer techniques using a thermistor-tipped catheter can be used to calculate cardiac output, systemic vascular resistance, and pulmonary vascular resistance. These calculations are combined with CVP and pulmonary artery wedge pressure measurements to assess cardiac function. Adding a fiberoptic system capable of real-time, on-line measurement of oxygen tension allows further discrimination in such assessment. The mixed venous oxygen tension (SVO_2) reflects cardiac index and oxygen delivery as long as hemoglobin levels and oxygen extraction (metabolic activity and work) are accounted for. A decrease in SVO_2 can be caused by a decrease in cardiac output, a decrease in hemoglobin levels, or an increase in the amount of oxygen extracted at the cellular level. Careful assessment is necessary in order to decide which variable is operational in any given patient scenario. The mixed venous oxygen saturation, although affected by hemoglobin concentration, has become a clinically useful tool for moment-to-moment assessment of cardiac function. Table 6.1 provides the basic formulae used for the assessment of myocardial function based on measurements available in an intensive care unit.

A patient in hypovolemic shock usually is diagnosed by clinical signs (trauma, hemorrhage, vomiting, diarrhea, dehydration) and simple bedside measurements (assessment of mucous membranes, skin turgor, urine output, blood pressure, pulse rate). However, when clinical indicators are equivocal, invasive measurements demonstrating low PAWP, CVP, and cardiac index usually confirm a low circulating volume. Appropriate therapy is transfusion with blood products or balanced elec-

Table 6.1.
Assessment of Myocardial Function

Function	Normal Values
Arterial Blood Pressure	120/80 mm Hg
Mean Arterial Pressure (MAP) $\frac{\text{pulse pressure}}{3}$ + diastolic blood pressure	70–90 mm Hg
Heart Rate	60–100 beats/min
Central Venous Pressure (CVP)	2–8 mm Hg
Pulmonary Artery Pressure (PAP)	25/10 mm Hg
Pulmonary Wedge Pressure (PWP)	6–12 mm Hg
Cardiac Index (CI)	2.5–3.0 L/min/m^2
Systemic Vascular Resistance (SVR) $\frac{\text{MAP} - \text{CVP} \times 80}{\text{CO}}$	900–1200 dyn/sec/cm^{-5}
Peripheral Vascular Resistance (PVR) $\frac{\text{PAP (mean)} - \text{PWP} \times 80}{\text{CO}}$	150–250 dyn/sec/cm^{-5}
Stroke Volume (SV) $\frac{\text{CO}}{\text{Heart Rate}}$	60–70 mL/beat
Stroke Index (SI) $\frac{\text{SV}}{\text{BSA (body surface area)}}$	35–45 mL/beat/m^2
Left Ventricular Stroke Work Index (LVSWI) SI × MAP × 0.014	51–61 g/min/m^2
Arterial O_2 Content (CaO_2) = % Sat (Hb × 1.39) + 0.003 (PaO_2)	18–20 mol/dL
Arterial O_2 Delivery (DO_2) = CI × CaO_2	550–600 mol/min/m^2
Mixed Venous O_2 Sat (SVO_2)	55–70%

trolyte solutions using both clinical and invasive measurements to gauge patient response.

Generally, patients with heart failure because of either chronic conditions, such as valvular heart disease, or acute problems, such as acute myocardial infarction, have elevated PAWP because of inadequate myocardial pump function and diminished cardiac index. However, the caution regarding integration of myocardial compliance, wedge pressure, and cardiac index is frequently forgotten in the setting of acute cardiac dysfunction. For example, a patient with an acute myocardial infarction who has a cardiac index of 1.8 L/min/m^2 and a wedge pressure of 6 mm Hg is hypovolemic. That patient's edematous infarcted myocardium may require filling pressures in excess of the "normal" wedge pressure of 12–15 mm Hg in order to stretch the myocardium sufficiently to generate adequate cardiac output. Conversely, another patient with an acute myocardial infarction may have a cardiac index of 1.8 L/min/m^2 but a wedge pressure of 25 mm Hg. That patient is clearly in pulmonary edema and will benefit from a reduction in the filling pressures of the left ventricle to allow improved coronary perfusion of the critical areas of subendocardial myocardial muscle mass. According to the law of Laplace, the wall tension is directly proportional to the radius; a dilated left ventricle will therefore experience subendocardial perfusion deficits based on transmyocardial pressure gradients within the coronary circulation. Reducing the radius of the left ventricle with pulmonary vasodilators (morphine, nitroglycerin), diuretics (furosemide), or phlebotomy (actual or rotating tourniquets) will increase subendocardial perfusion and therefore overall cardiac function.

Although invasive monitoring devices provide valuable information, they can cause complications. Depending upon the site of insertion, a central venous cannula can cause hemorrhage and pneumothorax. In an acutely deteriorating critically ill patient, it is not unusual for proper insertion techniques to be circumvented. The safest approach to introducing a pulmonary artery flotation catheter is a posterior superior approach to the right internal jugular vein. In this approach the introducer needle is never in contact with the pleura. Lower jugular or subclavian approaches are more likely to cause pneumothorax; they must be used especially cautiously in patients with blood dyscrasias and clotting abnormalities, since direct pressure cannot be applied to the subclavian vein or the internal jugular vein beneath the clavicle. In these patients, the high cervical approach to the central veins or the temporary use of the femoral vein is recommended. Perforation of the pulmonary artery with massive hemoptysis has been reported following insertion of pulmonary artery catheter. In addition, cardiac arrhythmias can occur when the catheter is passed through the right ventricle. Infectious endocarditis also is a potential problem, especially when the catheter is in place for more than 3 days. Catheter sites should be rotated at 72-hour intervals, since the incidence of infectious complications seems to increase after 3 days.

Additional, noninvasive means of assessing cardiac function include radionuclide scanning and echocardiography. Multiple gated acquisition (MUGA) scans will demonstrate ejection fractions quite accurately and therefore can categorize cardiac function (Fig. 6.3). A stress-thallium examination will demonstrate electrocardio-

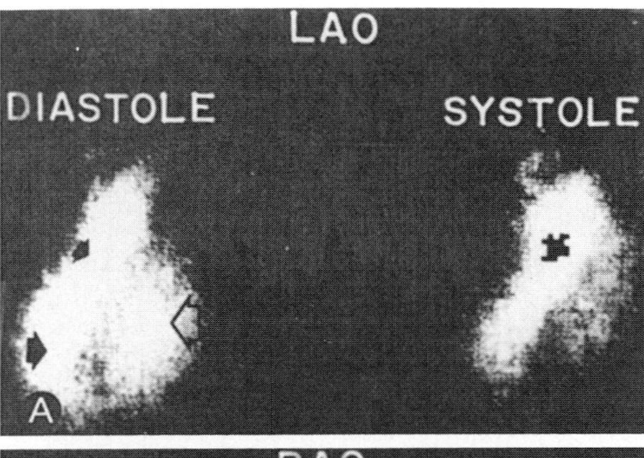

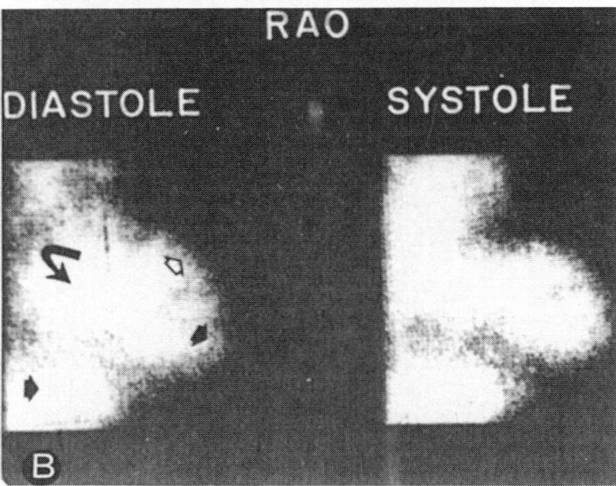

Figure 6.3. **A**, Gated radionuclide angiocardiography in the left anterior oblique projection. The systolic image in the upper right shows strong uniform contraction of the left ventricle. Lower arrow = right ventricle; upper arrow = pulmonary artery; open arrow = left ventricle. **B**, Diffuse asynergy with little difference in intensity and size of the left ventricular contour between the systolic and diastolic images on right anterior oblique projection. There is superimposition of right and left ventricles over their basal aspects (curved arrow). Left arrow = liver; right arrow = apex of left ventricle; open arrow = anterior wall.

graphic changes of ischemia if present and graphically locate the ischemic myocardium by absence of tracer images in the ischemic area (Fig. 6.4). Resting echocardiography easily shows regional wall motion abnormalities consistent with ischemia or infarction, and allows estimating valvular dysfunction, pulmonary artery pressures, and chamber size. For patients with normal resting valves, an inotropic challenge with dobutamine may unmask ischemic myocardium (Fig. 6.5).

Cardiopulmonary Bypass and Myocardial Protection During Surgery

The ability to perform surgery upon the heart and great vessels awaited the development of a method to support the circulation and respiration so that reparative operations could be performed on the heart itself. In the 1930s Dr. John Gibbon began work on a technique of circulatory support to allow pulmonary embolectomy, a procedure he felt was inadequately dealt with by the closed techniques of Trendelenburg. In the early 1950s, cooperation between Gibbon, IBM Corporation, the University of Minnesota, and the Mayo Clinic produced the first clinically successful pump oxygenators. The first successful case of open heart surgery, reported from Gibbon's hospital in 1953, entailed the use of the pump oxygenator for the repair of a secundum atrial septal defect in a young girl. Numerous failures had occurred before this case; the mortality rate for early open heart surgery approached 40 to 50%. Over time, biomechanical improvements have brought safer cardiopulmonary bypass into the clinical arena.

The components of the "heart-lung machine" include both a pump to supplant the heart and a means of oxygenating the blood to supplant the lungs. Numerous designs have been tried; today, the roller pump and the vortex pump are the devices most frequently used. Early oxygenators placed a film of blood across a screen. A direct oxygen-blood interface ensued, resulting in oxygenation at the surface of the film. These screen oxygenators were the first clinically used heart-lung machines. Subsequent developments included the bubble oxygenator, in which gas is bubbled through the blood, again with a direct blood-gas interface occurring, resulting in oxygenation of the blood cells. Further research has resulted in the use of membrane oxygenators, which, like the human lung itself, interpose a semipermeable membrane between the blood and gas, thus preventing electrochemical damage to the blood elements at the blood-gas interface. Studies have shown that the use of membrane oxygenators is somewhat less traumatic to the blood and its coagulation properties than the use of bubble oxygenators.

Blood is withdrawn from the venous circulation either through a single cannula in the right atrium or through separate cannulae in the inferior and superior venae cava, then passed through the oxygenator, at which time oxygen levels are replenished and carbon dioxide is removed. With the use of the appropriate pump mechanism, blood is reintroduced into the circulation by way of either the ascending aorta or the femoral artery. Mild, moderate, or deep hypothermia is often induced, since metabolic demands are diminished at lower temperatures. The metabolic derangements associated with abnormal flow states occurring during cardiopulmonary bypass are thus minimized.

The optimal environment for working on the heart includes a quiet, bloodless field. Cardiac activity is stopped and coronary circulation occluded. In the 1950s cardiac arrest was induced with high levels of potassium. Those levels proved too high, resulting in myocardial damage and fibrosis, which in turn led to congestive heart failure. The technique was reintroduced with modifications in 1970, and since then has been the technique of choice. Cardioplegic arrest is now usually achieved by (*a*) injecting an electrolyte solution, often with a high potassium content (20–25 mEq/L), to eliminate the concentration gradient of potassium and thus induce electrochemical paralysis of myocardial cellular function, and (*b*) inducing profound hypothermia to minimize metabolic demands during the time of ischemic arrest.

Cardiopulmonary bypass is instituted with right atrial or bicaval cannulation and occasional venting of either the pulmonary artery or the left atrium.

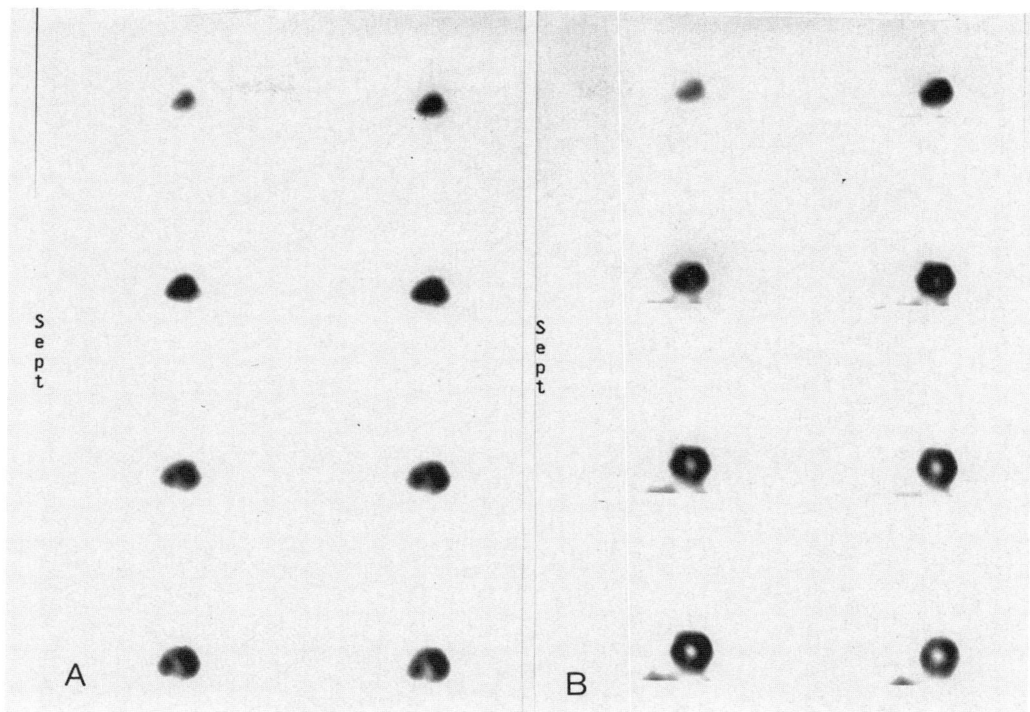

Figure 6.4. Stress-thallium examination. **A**, Resting images with uniform tracer presence. **B**, Exercise images demonstrate inferior ischemia by a "gap" in tracer presence at the "6 o'clock" position due to coronary artery occlusion in the inferior distribution.

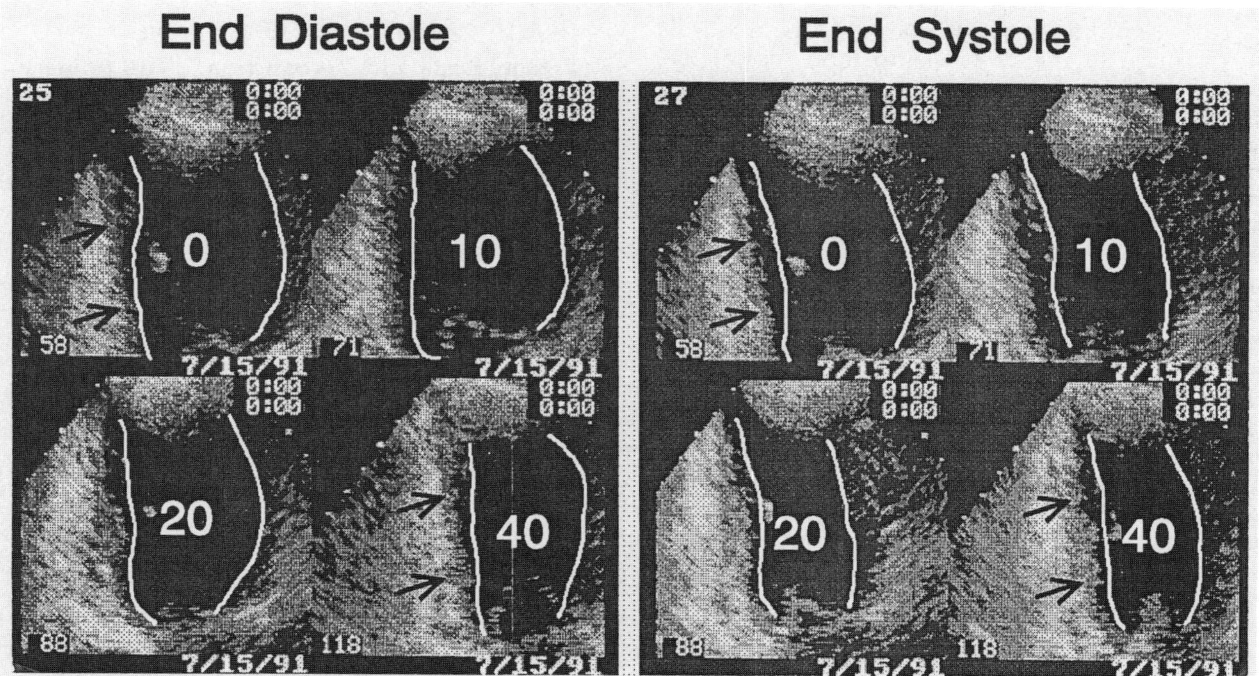

Figure 6.5. Dobutamine stress echocardiogram from a patient with prior inferior wall myocardial infarction. End diastolic and end systolic frames from the apical two-chamber left ventricular view are presented. End diastolic and end systolic screens are divided into four quadrants, with representative images at four dobutamine doses: 0, 10, 20, and 40 mcg/kg/min. Note decreasing chamber size with augmenting dobutamine stress. The inferior wall, indicated by black arrows, is akinetic at rest and remains akinetic at 40 mcg/kg/min dobutamine. At intermediate doses, there is no evidence for enhanced inferior wall systolic thickening, while the anterior wall, seen contralateral to the inferior wall, augments systolic motion with increasing dobutamine levels. Anatomically, the inferior wall should show extensive scar formation, with very little functioning or viable myocardium. Such a region would not respond favorably to revascularization.

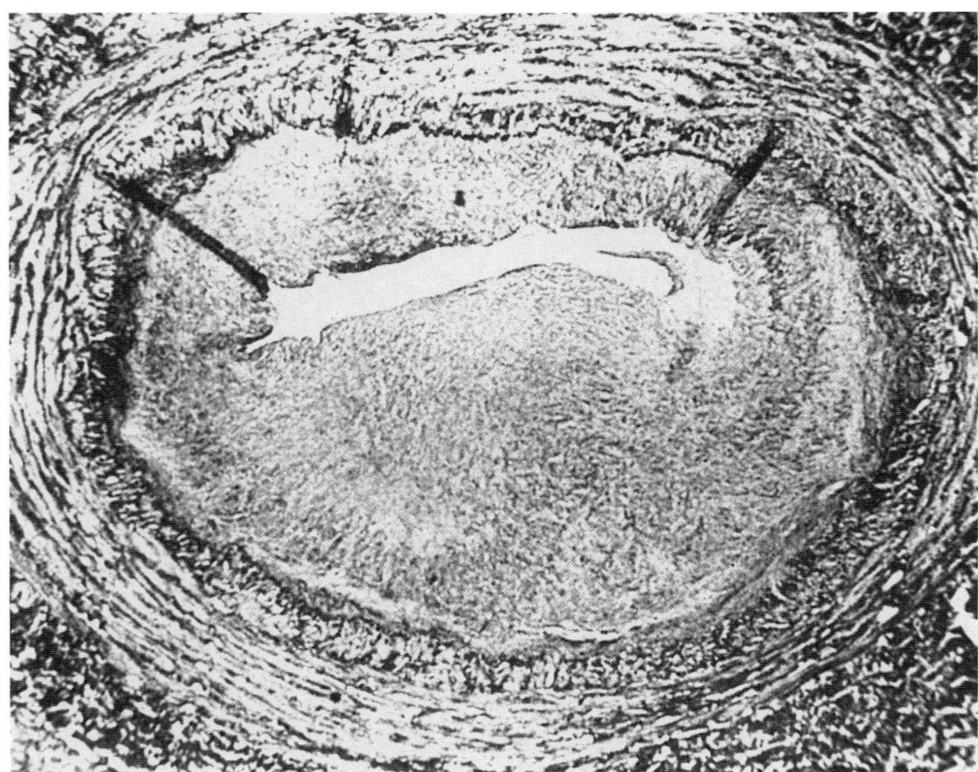

Figure 6.6. Atherosclerotic obstruction of a coronary artery resulting in marked reduction of blood flow to affected heart muscle.

Aortic cross-clamping, intra-aortic antegrade cardioplegia proximal to the cross clamp, and topical hypothermic agents (such as iced saline or slush) facilitate the operation. The composition of the cardioplegic solution varies among institutions but most often consists of either a crystalloid or blood carrier, a buffer to antagonize the ischemic acidosis, and a substance such as mannitol to render it hypertonic to the myocardial cell in order to minimize edema. Various modifications of this solution can be used for cardioplegia induction and reperfusion. To overcome the heterogeneous distribution of antegrade cardioplegia due to coronary artery stenoses, cardioplegic solution has been instilled in a retrograde fashion via the coronary sinus. Because the coronary venous system has no valves and is not subject to atherosclerotic obstruction, the homogeneous distribution of the cardioplegia is more certain, and uniform cooling as well as superior cardioplegic arrest have been enhanced by this technique.

Periods from 1–3 hours of ischemic cardioplegic arrest have been well tolerated, and cardiac activity resumes after normal perfusion is restored. There is evidence that any damage caused during the reperfusion state following ischemic arrest can be aggravated by various electrochemical elements such as oxygen-free radicals and that free-radical scavengers can improve cardiac performance following ischemic arrest. New techniques in warm, continuous, hyperkalemic cardioplegia may actually provide a warm "aerobic" arrest and further improve postoperative cardiac performance.

Ischemic Heart Disease

Pathogenesis and Recognition. The primary cause of ischemic heart disease is atherosclerotic plaque formation on the walls of the epicardial coronary arteries, resulting in diminished blood flow to the heart muscle (Fig. 6.6). Although the precise etiology of atherosclerosis is not understood, common risk factors include a genetic predisposition, diet, lack of exercise, stress, smoking, diabetes, and hypertension. Because cardiac dysfunction may not be apparent until the demand for oxygen increases with exercise, the level of exercise at which cardiac symptoms occur mirrors myocardial oxygen demand and therefore the severity of the disease. Angina pectoris, or chest pain of cardiac origin, is the most common symptom and is described as a pressure, squeezing, or heavy weight on the chest. The sensation may be located in the anterior or left precordium, or it may radiate to the jaw and down the left arm. Angina symptoms are striking and easily recognizable. To assess the severity of the disease, it is important to question the patient about the inciting event, the length of time the pain has persisted, and the level of exercise at which it was initiated. Angina occurring at rest or with minimal exercise denotes a patient at higher risk for sudden cardiac events than one who has angina with maximal exertion.

Less common causes of coronary ischemia include aortic stenosis and insufficiency, inflammatory diseases of the aorta, and congenital malformations of the coronary arteries. Rarely, coronary emboli produce cardiac ischemia. Acute ischemic heart failure, or "flash pulmonary edema," is an anginal equivalent, as is syncope, profound fatigue, and cardiac arrhythmias. Ischemic cardiac dysfunction resulting in transient pulmonary edema may not be associated with typical chest pain and therefore may be confused with heart failure from other causes. If heart failure is reversed quickly by antianginal therapy, it is ischemic in origin. Causes of pain that can simulate coronary ischemia include heartburn secondary to reflux esophagitis, musculoskeletal chest wall pain, thoracic outlet syndrome, and pain associated with inflammatory or neoplastic chest wall lesions. Pericarditis and pleuritis can also mimic angina. In most instances, cardiac and noncardiac causes of pain can be distinguished by such means as chest x-ray, electrocardiogram, and computed tomography of the chest.

Symptomatic patients undergo a variety of increasingly sophisticated investigations in order to confirm the diagnosis of ischemic heart disease. The resting electrocardiogram may display evidence of myocardial infarction or ongoing cardiac ischemia by ST- and T-wave changes and by QRS morphology. Electrocardiographic signs of myocardial cellular injury are caused by the inability of the affected myocytes to repolarize normally. S-T segment elevation is the surface electocardiogram (ECG) manifestation of such an injury. Q waves generally indicate myocardial cellular necrosis due to inability of these dead cells to become electrically excitable. T wave inversions and Q-T prolongation may reflect ongoing cardiac ischemia due to delayed repolarization. The electrocardiogram may also be normal when the heart is in the resting state. Physiological provocation of coronary ischemia is probably the cornerstone of diagnosis. A stress electrocardiogram using simple ambulatory exercise or bicycle/arm ergometry demonstrates the onset of coronary ischemia and allows correlation between ischemia and the level of exercise necessary to produce it. Similarly, radionuclide angiography with thallium can demonstrate areas of reversible hypoperfusion indicative of cardiac ischemia. Stress echocardiography delineates regional wall motion abnormalities resulting from ischemia.

The decision to proceed with more invasive testing depends upon the index of clinical suspicion, the severity of the disease, and the concern over impending cardiac events such as myocardial infarction. Invasive testing is recommended for symptomatic patients with high risk clinical indicators, such as ischemic abnormalities on the electrocardiogram, ST depression during exercise testing, concomitant peripheral vascular disease, age and smoking history, and family history of atherosclerotic heart disease.

At present the most accurate diagnostic modality for defining the anatomy, physiology, and prognosis of coronary artery disease is cardiac catheterization with coronary angiography. Catheters to measure pressures or to inject contrast material are introduced either through a surgical cut down on the brachial artery (Sones technique) or percutaneously through the femoral artery (Judkins technique). Both are safely and routinely performed in patients with severe disease and can give a precise definition of coronary artery anatomy and ventricular function. Coronary anatomy is commonly discussed in terms of three major coronary arterial systems: the right coronary artery, the left anterior descending coronary artery, and the circumflex coronary artery. Obstruction of the left main coronary artery carries with it a significantly worse prognosis because of the inclusion of both the circumflex and anterior descending systems within its watershed. A 50% stenosis of a coronary artery visualized in two planes usually constitutes a hemodynamically significant lesion and is commonly associated with a 75% reduction in cross-sectional area. Studies of the natural history of coronary artery disease have demonstrated that the prognosis worsens as the disease increases from one to three vessels (Fig. 6.7).

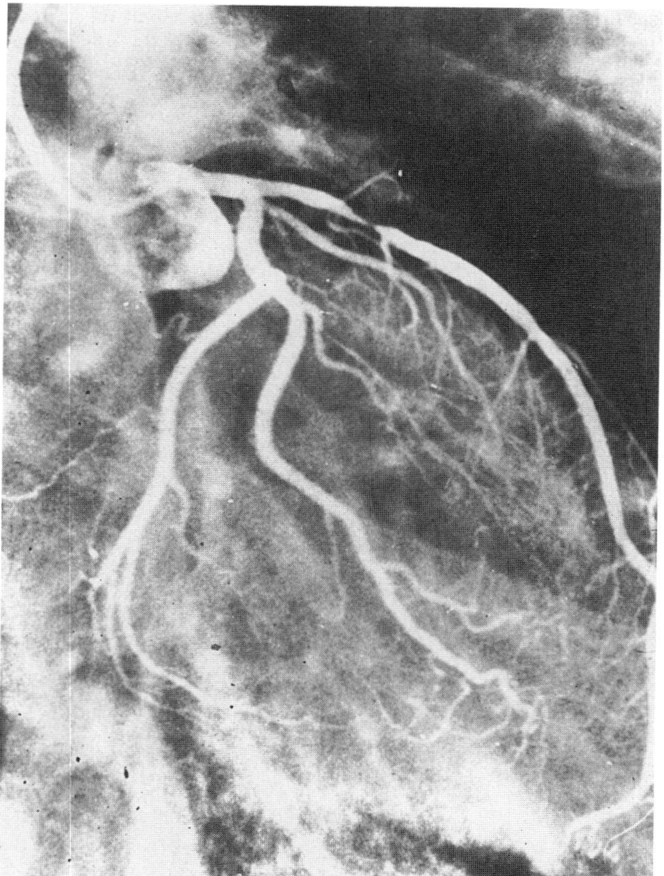

Figure 6.7. Coronary angiography demonstrating obstruction in the proximal left anterior descending artery.

Other information obtainable by cardiac catheterization includes an estimate of left ventricular function, evidence of valvular heart disease, and the amount of myocardium served by each coronary artery vessel. It is not enough to denote single-, double-, or triple-vessel disease without allowing for variations in amount of myocardium served by each vessel. For example, high-grade stenosis of a nondominant right coronary artery would not constitute an indication for coronary revascularization, but high-grade stenosis of a large, dominant right coronary artery (especially in the presence of anterior descending obstructive disease) would constitute a surgical emergency because of the amount of myocardium in jeopardy. Left ventricular dysfunction (a cardiac index of less than 2 L/min/m^2 and an ejection fraction of less than 40%) has a measurable and significant effect on prognosis, both with and without surgical revascularization. Most studies have demonstrated a reduced survival with this dysfunction and higher operative risks as well.

Treatment and Indications for Surgery. Symptoms of angina pectoris can be treated by modifying physical activity to diminish myocardial oxygen demand and by taking medications such as β-blockers, calcium channel blockers, and nitrates. While the medications have no direct effect on coronary artery obstruction, they can be used to manage patients with mild, chronic stable angina. The onset of more severe angina indicates the need for eventual surgical intervention. Direct myocardial revascularization is recommended for patients exhibiting the following: (*a*) angina unresponsive to medical therapy; (*b*) unstable anginal syndromes such as accelerated, preinfarction, or postinfarction angina; (*c*) certain anatomically critical stenoses such as occlusion of the left main coronary artery; and (*d*) complications of myocardial infarction such as ischemic pulmonary edema, ventricular septal defect, papillary muscle rupture with mitral regurgitation, rupture of the heart, and ventricular aneurysm formation with attendant heart failure or arrhythmias.

In selected instances, percutaneous transluminal coronary angioplasty (PTCA) can be substituted for surgery to dilate coronary stenosis. In this procedure, a balloon placed fluoroscopically across a coronary stenosis is inflated to pressures of 1–5 atm to either compress or crack atherosclerotic plaque. Luminal diameter is increased, thereby restoring coronary blood flow. Restenosis rates may reach 25–30% at 6 months, but repeat angioplasty can be performed successfully. Certain anatomic characteristics, such as eccentricity of the lesion, calcification, or presence at a bifurcation, may contraindicate PTCA. Surgical standby is often provided for angioplasty, since occlusion or coronary artery dissection with thrombosis may occur acutely with profound cardiovascular consequences. Emergency surgery is performed in cases of catastrophic collapse, with salvage occurring in most cases. Patients with more than two significant lesions usually undergo coronary bypass surgery.

The results of direct surgical coronary artery revascularization are excellent. Between 75 and 90% of patients are immediately relieved of angina, and between 50 and 66% of patients remain free from angina at 5–10 years. At varying intervals following surgery, angina may recur as grafts close and atherosclerotic disease progresses. Secondary and tertiary coronary revascularization can be accomplished at morbidity and mortality rates only slightly higher than those of the original operation.

The choice of the graft conduit plays an important role in the long-term success of the operation. Internal thoracic artery (internal mammary artery) patency rates have been well above 90% at 5 years, and on follow-up patients have shown relief from cardiac symptoms. Saphenous vein graft patency rates, on the other hand, have been shown to diminish to 50–65% at 10 and 15 years. The added operative time to harvest and use internal mammary arterial grafts is significantly outweighed by superior clinical results.

Postoperative Care. With careful monitoring, postoperative complications can often be anticipated and therefore prevented. Patients selected for coronary revascularization are among the most critically ill and in many instances would not be considered for noncardiac surgery. However, sophisticated invasive techniques have allowed moment-to-moment assessment of cardiac and pulmonary function to permit intervention before catastrophic decompensation. An example of the value of such monitoring is the use of a catheter to measure PAWP in a patient whose blood pressure demonstrates a steadily downward trend, but whose urine output remains high because intravenous mannitol is being infused. The catheter would show the wedge pressure to be low, indicating the patient was hypovolemic and in need of a transfusion. Without this monitoring device it would be uncertain whether the patient was experiencing primary cardiac failure, cardiac tamponade, or hypovolemia. Intervention before decompensation has been possible in many instances, thereby avoiding cardiac arrest and sudden death early in the postoperative period.

Low Cardiac Output. Low cardiac output can be analyzed in terms of preload, cardiac contractility, and afterload. Transfusion of the hypovolemic patient is an example of preload manipulation to optimize cardiac output. Contractility is manipulated by the use of various pharmacologic agents that have inotropic activity, such as β_1-adrenergic. It is important to distinguish between β-adrenergic receptors that have inotropic activity and are therefore used to increase contractility of the myocardium, and vasopressors, which merely raise blood pressure by constricting peripheral vasculature and have no effect on cardiac contractility. Blood pressure may be normal, but if the cardiac index is inadequate, systemic perfusion will likewise be inadequate and a profound metabolic acidosis may ensue. The afterload or peripheral vascular resistance, commonly reflected in the systolic and diastolic blood pressures, represents an impedance to left ventricular ejection. Reducing systemic vascular resistance by vasodilators such as sodium nitroprusside and nitroglycerin may have a profoundly favorable effect on cardiac output by minimizing physiologic obstruction to left ventricular outflow.

When pharmacologic intervention fails to improve myocardial function, mechanical circulatory assistance is used. An intra-aortic balloon pump is placed in a retrograde fashion, usually through the femoral artery to a position just distal to the left subclavian artery in the descending thoracic aorta. (The intra-aortic balloon has also been placed at the time of cardiac surgery by introducing it into the ascending aorta.) Inflation and deflation of the balloon is timed to either the electrocardiogram or the pressure wave of the arterial pulse. The balloon maximally inflates during diastole and deflates during systole. In this way diastolic pressure is increased in order to maximize coronary blood flow, and systolic pressure is reduced because of a "pressure sink" distal to the aortic valve. Following this procedure, prompt improvement in cardiac output and peripheral organ perfusion usually occurs.

Because complications following this procedure may be significant, judgment in using the intra-aortic balloon must be made in each case. Vascular complications secondary to dislodgement of atheromatous plaques may result in distal limb ischemia. Occlusion of the iliofemoral outflow system may cause leg ischemia, necessitating debridement, fasciotomy, or even amputation. Femoral-femoral cross-over grafts are indicated when balloon pumping is necessary in spite of the ischemia. Occlusion of such vessels as celiac, mesenteric, or spinal arteries may result in catastrophic visceral ischemia. Some complications can be repaired surgically, while others—such as spinal cord ischemia—can not. Contraindications to the procedure include aortic insufficiency and the inability to pass the balloon transfemorally.

Other mechanical assistance devices include prolonged temporary cardiopulmonary bypass and left ventricular assist devices (LVAD). More permanent devices are used only as a bridge to cardiac transplantation in the event of irreversible myocardial failure.

Valvular Heart Disease

The treatment of valvular heart disease reflects the evolution of cardiac surgery itself. As artificial heart valves have been invented, refined, perfected, and discarded, comparisons have been made between the natural history of valvular pathology and the clinical course of patients receiving prostheses. Between 1961 and 1990 opinions changed regarding surgical intervention for valvular pathology. Recent, noninvasive methods of measuring cardiac function, such as echocardiography and radionuclide angiography, have provided much useful information on how cardiac disease behaves and what effect interventions have on it.

Aortic Valve Disease. Aortic valve disease is generally a slow, progressive process, resulting from either a congenitally bicuspid (two-leaflet) valve or senile, calcific degeneration. It rarely is rheumatic in origin. As the leaflets calcify and become immobile, resistance to left ventricular outflow ensues, increasing left ventricular systolic pressure. This pressure overload on the left ventricle induces a compensatory hypertrophy of muscle mass. While the process may not cause symptoms for prolonged periods, ultimately it leads to decompensation and dilatation with left ventricular failure. Symptoms such as heart failure, angina, or syncope signal the end of the quiescent phase. A rapid decline and early death follow unless the patient is treated urgently.

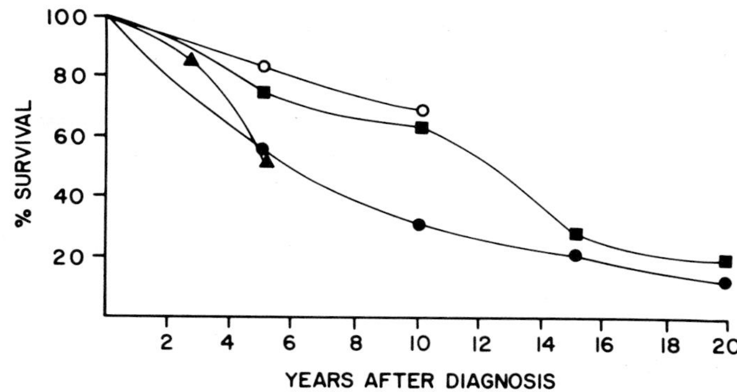

Figure 6.8. Natural history of mitral stenosis. Black square = data of Rowe JC et al. Black circle = data of Oleson KH. Black triangle = data of Munoz S et al. White circle = data of Rapaport E.

Aortic regurgitation is caused by failure of the leaflets to coapt because of annular dilatation (Marfan's syndrome) or valvulitis leading to retraction of leaflet substance (rheumatic fever). Leaflet destruction from trauma or infection also causes insufficiency. Volume overload of the left ventricle follows, leading to chamber dilatation to accommodate the regurgitant volume. Acute insufficiency of the aortic valve occurs with infective endocarditis or trauma and is generally catastrophic, producing acute fulminant heart failure requiring emergency operation. Symptomatic patients with stenosis or insufficiency should be offered surgical replacement of the valve. Asymptomatic patients may undergo valve replacement if measurements of left ventricular function (echocardiography, nuclear angiography, catheterization) demonstrate abnormal or deteriorating function as measured by ejection fraction or diastolic volumes and chamber size. Because failing or abnormally decompensated ventricular function raises operative risks and long-term outcome, such patients should undergo surgery prior to significant deterioration.

Mitral Valve Disease. The predominant cause of mitral stenosis is rheumatic valvulitis and its sequelae. Since surgical repair or replacement of the mitral valve was the first operation performed by cardiac surgeons, much attention has been devoted to the natural history of mitral stenosis. Before surgery was widely performed, patients deteriorated inevitably; mortality at 20 years was 70–90% (Fig. 6.8).

The pathophysiology of mitral stenosis includes left atrial hypertension with resultant pulmonary congestion, right heart overload, and signs of dyspnea, edema, and fatigue. The predominant adverse effects are incurred by the right ventricle, since the left ventricle is "protected" by the stenotic valve. Atrial dilatation often results in chaotic atrial dysrhythmias, producing relative stasis of blood and development of intracardiac thrombi, which may eventually embolize to any systemic vascular bed, especially to the cerebral, renal, or iliofemoral systems. Rheumatic valvulitis leads to valvular thickening, commissural fusion, and subvalvular obstruction resulting from fusion and foreshortening of the chordae tendineae.

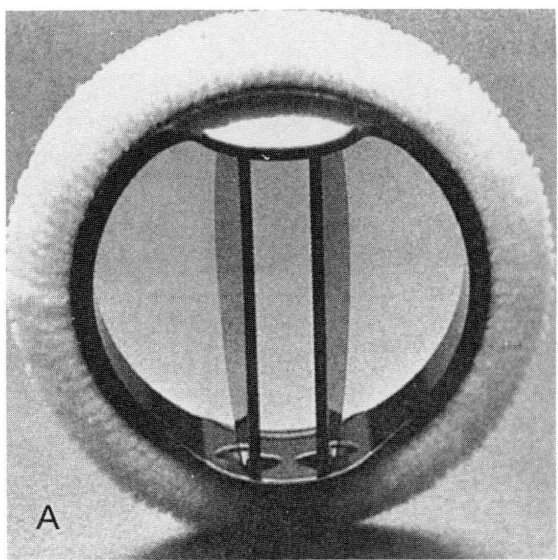

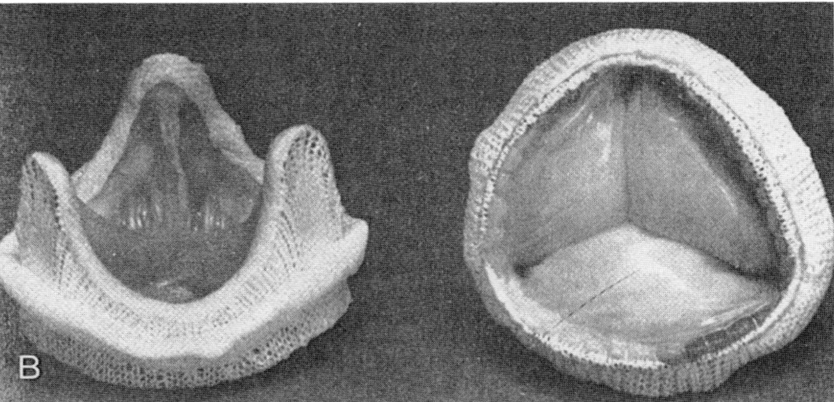

Figure 6.9. Valve prostheses. **A**, Mechanical prosthesis—bileaflet St. Jude. **B**, Bioprosthesis—porcine.

Causes of mitral regurgitation include rheumatic heart disease, myxomatous degeneration with and without prolapse, endocarditis, and ischemic heart disease with papillary muscle infarction or ischemia. Most patients with mild mitral regurgitation are stable or asymptomatic for long periods of time. The onset of symptoms heralds an acceleration of progressive and inevitable disability. Mitral regurgitation adversely affects left ventricular function, while mitral stenosis "protects" it. Patients with regurgitant mitral valve lesions have increased morbidity and mortality rates because of the effects of left ventricular dysfunction. Since the preload is increased and the afterload is decreased with mitral regurgitation (blood is ejected retrograde into the low pressure left atrium), the ejection fraction is artificially elevated and does not reflect the true contractive state of the left ventricle. Echocardiographically determined end systolic and diastolic dimensions may be more accurate in this regard.

Indications for surgery include symptomatic congestive heart failure with stenosis or insufficiency of the mitral valve, as well as deteriorating left ventricular function indices with mild or moderate symptoms. Symptomatic improvement, operative risk, and longevity are enhanced by valve surgery prior to severe left ventricular dysfunction.

Tricuspid Valve Disease. Most tricuspid valve problems arise from infection or left-sided valve lesions leading to right heart dilatation. Infective endocarditis of the tricuspid valve is most frequently encountered in patients who have bacteremia as a result of intravenous drug abuse or in those who have had long-term intravenous access lines. These patients also are susceptible to septic pulmonary emboli and infarction. Persistent bacteremia, sepsis, or emboli are the principal indications for surgery. Valvulectomy is the procedure of choice, since it is well tolerated in the absence of pulmonary hypertension and since prostheses in these patients are usually the site of reinfection.

Table 6.2.
Comparison of Prosthetic Heart Valves

	Mechanical Valves	Bioprosthetic Valves
Durability	+ +[a]	+/−[b]
Thromboembolism	−	+
Obstruction in small sizes	+	−
Calcification with age	+	−
Calcification with dialysis	+	−

[a]A plus sign (+) indicates the valve compares favorably.
[b]A minus sign (−) indicates the valve compares unfavorably.

In some cases, right ventricular dilatation may cause the tricuspid annulus to dilate, rendering a valve incompetent in the face of normal leaflets. Because correction of the left-sided mitral or aortic lesion may still leave the patient hemodynamically compromised, some form of annuloplasty (shrinking) of the tricuspid annulus is necessary to allow the leaflets to coapt and thereby become competent.

Valve Prostheses. Although numerous valvular prostheses have been designed and manufactured since 1962, two types are available today: mechanical prostheses and bioprostheses.

Mechanical prostheses are constructed of metal, plastic, and cloth, and have some form of occluder (or leaflet) that opens during systole and closes during diastole to prevent regurgitation. The occluder may take the shape of a round ball (the Starr-Edwards valve), a single tilting disk (Bjork-Shiley), or a bileaflet configuration (St. Jude prosthesis, see Fig. 6.9**A**). Leaflets are usually constructed of a highly polished pyrolite carbon material that is thromboresistant and durable. The skeleton for the valve is a strong, lightweight metal such as titanium. Some prostheses use newer plastics. The sewing

Table 6.3.
Classification of Hemodynamic Alterations in Congenital Heart Disease

Pulmonary Blood Flow	Acyanotic	Cyanotic Right-to-Left Shunt
Increased	Left-to-right shunts	Admixture lesions
	Atrial septal defect	Transposition of great arteries
	Patent ductus arteriosus	Truncus arteriosus
	Ventricular septal defect	Total anomalous pulmonary venous connection
Normal	Obstructive lesions	None
	Aortic stenosis	
	Pulmonary stenosis	
	Coarctation of aorta	
Diminished	None	Intracardiac defect and obstruction to pulmonary blood flow
		Tetralogy of Fallot
		Tricuspid atresia
		Ebstein's malformation

ring is made of Dacron and becomes incorporated within the valve annulus. The advantages of mechanical prostheses are durability, availability, and an engineering design that permits adequate flow in smaller sizes. Their disadvantages are that they are thrombogenic, requiring permanent anticoagulation, which in the older age population predisposes to risks of hemorrhage after minor trauma.

Bioprosthetic valves are fabricated from either homograft or xenograft materials. Homograft valves are harvested from fresh cadavers and treated with antibiotics as well as chemical sterilization with glutaraldehyde fixation calculated to minimize structural damage to the valves. The donor source for such valves is limited, however, and appropriate sizes are not universally available. Xenograft valves are generally porcine; the leaflets are mounted on artificial stents of either metal or plastic and covered with the appropriate cloth material (Fig. 6.9**B**). These valves are much more readily available and almost all sizes and configurations are kept on the shelf. Smaller sizes are more obstructive because a portion of the graft is occupied by the mechanical process of mounting it on the stent. Mitral homografts or xenografts do not require anticoagulation unless other indications exist, such as a history of thromboembolism, dilated atria, or atrial fibrillation. Bioprosthetic valves in the aortic position seldom require permanent anticoagulation.

Bioprostheses are used in patients over the age of 70 or in those for whom anticoagulants are contraindicated because of recalcitrant gastrointestinal bleeding, blood dyscrasias, or sensitivity to anticoagulants. Their durability has been questioned, with some studies demonstrating that as many as 30% of these valves degenerate at 7 to 10 years. They are not used for patients expected to live more than 10 years. Degeneration involves calcification: the leaflets become brittle, break, and crack, resulting in valvular insufficiency and valvular stenosis.

Homograft valves are particularly useful for patients with complex reconstructive problems of the aortic root and left ventricular outflow tract, since the valve is supplied in continuity with the outflow tract. Conditions that require avoiding foreign materials, such as infective endocarditis and annular abscess and erosion, are particularly well suited to the use of the homograft valve. This valve has shown to have been a durable prosthesis (lasting approximately 10 years) in several short- to long-term follow-up studies.

The decision to recommend valve replacement requires balancing the natural history of the disease with the risks of the prosthesis or repair. Valve replacement is not curative; it merely substitutes one disease (a prosthesis) for another (the valve lesion). Common sequelae of valve replacement include thromboembolism (2 to 6%), mechanical failure, prosthetic endocarditis (1 to 2%), and bioprosthetic deterioration (30% at 10 years). In contrast to valve replacement, valve repairs, especially for mitral stenosis and regurgitation, are safe, effective, and durable when properly performed.

Choice of a valve substitute, whether mechanical or bioprosthetic, must take into account risks of anticoagulation, patient age, comorbidity, and ability to follow medical regimens (Table 6.2). Mechanical valves are chosen for most patients except those who are over 70, very young, on dialysis, or unable to maintain medical follow-up. Despite its likelihood of degeneration and the need for reoperation, a bioprosthesis is also recommended for women of childbearing age because of the harmful effects of anticoagulants on a fetus.

Antibiotic Prophylaxis. Antibiotic prophylaxis for patients with heart disease has been problematic for many reasons. It is unclear whether it is completely effective in preventing endocarditis, it is unclear how many patients are at risk of developing endocarditis with bacteremia, and it is unclear which regimens are most effective. Bacteremia occurs after tooth extraction, periodontal surgery, tooth brushing, urological manipulation, endoscopic procedures on the bronchial and gastrointestinal systems, and normal obstetrical delivery. Recommended antibiotic regimens are related to the particular prophylaxis desired (Table 6.3).

Antibiotic prophylaxis must be considered in patients with prosthetic heart valves, since foreign materials often serve as a nidus for blood-borne infections. Prophylaxis should be tailored to the individual risk factors. For example, patients with artificial valves undergoing dental manipulations should receive antibiotics

Table 6.4.
Antibiotic Prophylaxis for Patients with Heart Disease

Procedure	Valvular Heart Disease/Congenital Heart Disease	Prosthetic Heart Valves
Dental procedures or surgery	Parenteral plus oral penicillin (vancomycin or erythromycin for penicillin-allergic patients) or Penicillin and streptomycin	Penicillin and streptomycin or vancomycin
GU, GI, surgery or endoscope	Ampicillin and aminoglycoside or Vancomycin and aminoglycoside	
Cardiac surgery	Cefazolin—short-term or Cefazolin and aminoglycoside (vancomycin can be used in penicillin-allergic patients)	

(such as penicillin) known to be active against oral anaerobes and microaerophilic organisms. Patients undergoing manipulation of the urinary tract should receive antibiotics known to be active against common urinary pathogens. Similar applications should be followed for surgery on lungs, extremities, and gastrointestinal tract. Prophylaxis against rheumatic fever should continue as before, since the purpose is to prevent reinfection with the ubiquitous streptococcal organisms.

Congenital Heart Disease

Congenital heart defects occur in 1:125 live births. To aid in determining the type and timing of surgical intervention, heart defects are classified according to the amount of oxygenated blood delivered (cyanotic versus acyanotic) and the amount of pulmonary blood flow allowed (Table 6.4). In cyanotic heart defects less oxygenated blood is delivered to the body. Intervention is indicated when the oxygen saturation falls below 80%, or the hematocrit rises above 60%. (Chronic hypoxia causes an increase in the hematocrit, thus increasing the risk of stroke.) Increased pulmonary blood flow has both an acute and a chronic effect on the patient. If the pulmonary flow is great enough, acute effects are pulmonary edema and congestive heart failure, Surgical intervention is indicated if the condition cannot be treated medically or the patient fails to thrive. Surgery is also indicated to correct chronic increased pulmonary blood flow, a condition leading to irreversible pulmonary hypertension.

Acyanotic Patients

Ventricular Septal Defect. The most common congenital heart defect, ventricular septal defect (VSD) is an abnormal communication between the right and left ventricles. It is classified according to location. If it is under the pulmonary annulus, it is classified as supracristal; if in the membranous septum, it is perimembranous; if in the muscular septum, it is muscular; if adjacent to the tricuspid valve at the inlet septum, it is atrioventricular (A-V) canal (Fig. 6.10). The defect is an acyanotic lesion with increased pulmonary blood flow.

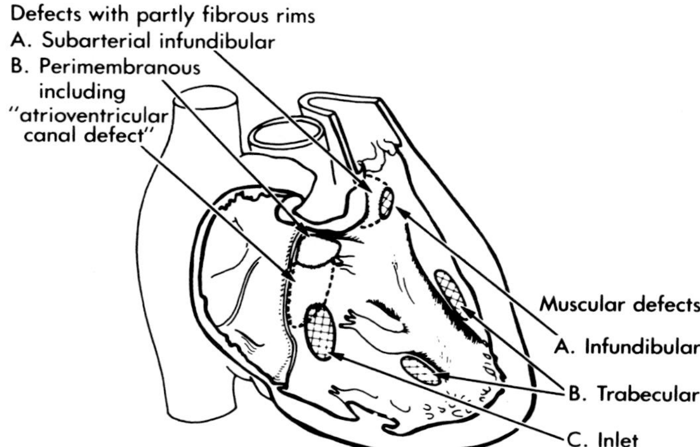

Figure 6.10. Classification of VSDs according to their location within the septum.

The increased left-to-right shunt is related to the degree of pulmonary vascular resistance. Irreversible pulmonary hypertension can occur by 1 year of age in the nonrestrictive ventricular septal defect. Fortunately, 50–80% of ventricular septal defects close spontaneously within the first 2 years of life. Surgical intervention is indicated in any infant less than 6 months of age if congestive heart failure is not controlled by medical management. If by 12 months of age the ventricular septal defect is still nonrestrictive and pulmonic pressure remains greater than two-thirds of systemic pressure, surgical intervention is indicated. Closure is also indicated in children who maintain a shunt fraction of greater than 2:1 beyond 4 years of age.

Most ventricular septal defects can be closed using a cardiopulmonary bypass. However, a palliative procedure of pulmonary artery banding to decrease pulmonary blood flow is indicated in infants with multiple ventricular septal defects, infants with multiple associated defects, or infants too ill to undergo a primary corrective procedure. In patients over 1 year of age, closure can usually be performed through the atrium or the pulmonary valve, thereby avoiding a ventriculotomy

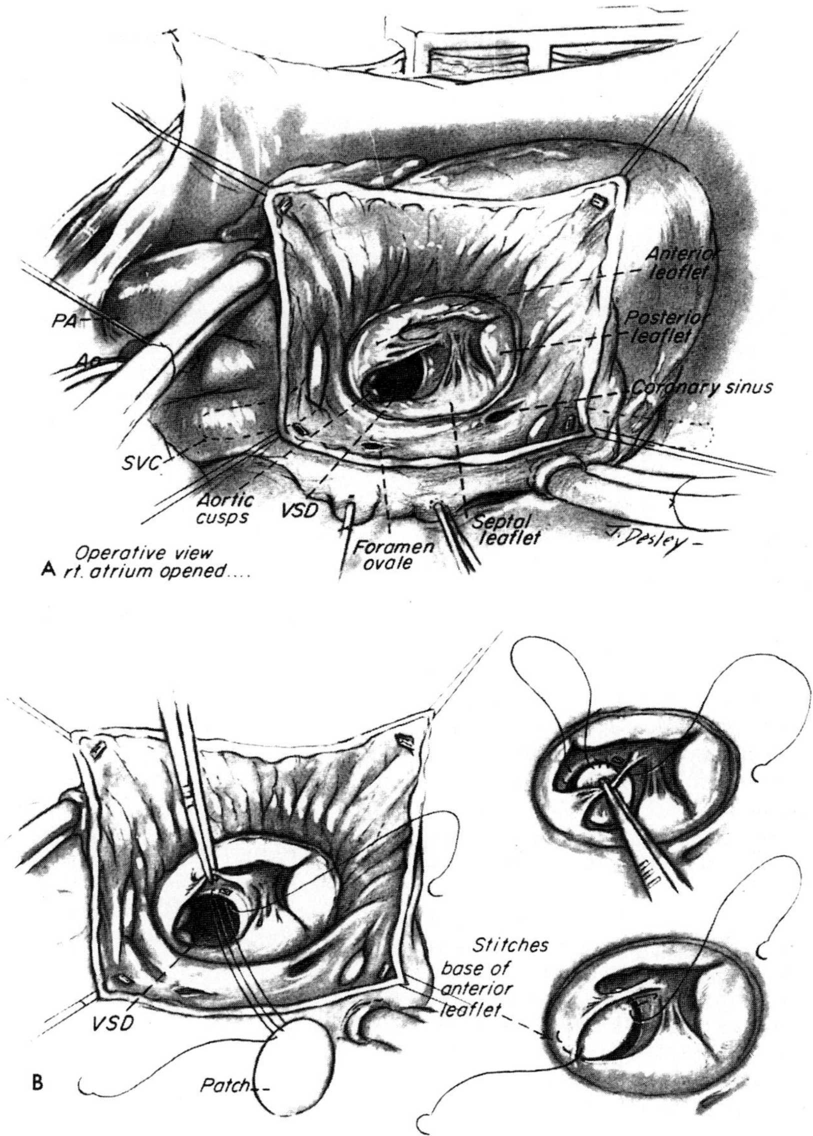

Figure 6.11. Closure of ventricular septal defect through the tricuspid valve.

(Fig. 6.11). Major complications are low output syndrome and complete heart block. Heart block may be produced by the sutures with which prosthetic patches are sewn into place to obliterate the defect. The conduction system (A-V node, bundle of His, and right bundle) is found along the rim of the defect and may be damaged by sutures placed too deeply. The incidence of recurrence is less than 1%.

Patent Ductus Arteriosus. The second most common congenital heart defect, patent ductus arteriosus, is acyanotic with increased pulmonary blood flow. During fetal life, the ductus arteriosus conducts desaturated blood from the pulmonary artery to the aorta, bypassing the lungs. Within hours to days after birth, the ductus normally closes spontaneously. If the ductus remains patent, the low pulmonary vascular resistance allows reversal of blood flow so that saturated blood from the aorta floods the pulmonary artery increasing its overall flow. Especially in premature infants, this increased flow can lead to early congestive failure. Pulmonary hypertension may occur by the second decade of life. Other complications include aneurysm formation or infective endarteritis. If left untreated, these patients have half the normal life expectancy.

Although the patent ductus may close at any time, it is unlikely to do so after the age of 1 year. If used within the first several weeks of life, indomethacin, a drug that acts on smooth muscle fibers, will close the ductus. Surgical ligation is indicated when significant heart failure persists or the ductus remains patent beyond 3–6 months of age. Ligation is performed through a fourth interspace posterolateral thoracotomy. Ligation with multiple ties is routine, although division and oversewing the ends may be indicated for a wide, short ductus. Mortality rates are below 0.5%.

Atrial Septal Defects. An atrial septal defect, the third most common congenital heart problem, is an acyanotic lesion with increased pulmonary blood flow. Because of greater compliance in the normal right ventricle, the direction of blood flow through the atrial septum is from left to right. Rarely in infancy is the shunt large enough to produce congestive heart failure or failure to thrive. Most children remain asymptomatic, but may develop fatigue, right-sided failure, pulmonary vascular disease, and arrhythmias. The average life expectancy in the untreated patient is 45 years of age.

Types of atrial septal defects include the incompetent foramen ovale, the secundum atrial septal defect, the primum atrial septal defect, the sinus venosus defect, and the unroofed coronary sinus. Elective surgical repair is usually performed at 3–5 years of age as prophylaxis against late pulmonary hypertension. Repair usually is accomplished using cardiopulmonary bypass through a median sternotomy or right fifth interspace anterior thoracotomy. Primary suture is possible in most patients with a secundum atrial septal defect; a pericardial or Dacron patch is required for primum and sinus venosus defects. Mortality is less than 2%. Postoperative complications are sick sinus syndrome, primarily associated with the sinus venosus defect, or complete heart block, primarily associated with the repair of the primum atrial septal defect, since the conduction system travels along the rim of the defect and may be damaged by sutures used to anchor the patch used to obliterate the shunt. Although right ventricular function may not return totally to normal, most patients are asymptomatic.

Coarctation of the Aorta. The sixth most common congenital heart defect, coarctation of the aorta is an obstructive lesion in the descending aorta, usually just distal to the left subclavian artery. This acyanotic lesion has normal pulmonary artery blood flow. Left-sided failure from the obstruction occurs eventually in all affected patients. The defect may present early in life, especially when associated with such other defects as ventricular septal defect or severe aortic stenosis. Other complications include stroke, aneurysm formation, subacute bacterial endocarditis, and paralysis. The average life expectancy of a patient with coarctation of the aorta is 35 years.

Whenever significant heart failure is present, surgical intervention is indicated. Otherwise, the repair should be performed electively at age 3 to 5. The repair is best managed by either a subclavian flap arterioplasty or coarctation segment resection with end-to-end anastomosis. Because coarctation recurrence in the young infant is as high as 25%, surgery is deferred if possible until after the patient is 3 years of age and the aorta has grown to 55% of its expected size. A lesion repaired at this age has a recurrence rate of less than 2%. Surgery is performed through a posterolateral fourth interspace incision. Operative risks for older children are quite small. Paraplegia is a potential complication in about 4–6% of patients. Paradoxical hypertension occurs commonly in the postoperative period and requires treatment if blood pressure is greater than a mean of 100 mm Hg. Late hypertension can occur in as many as 25% of patients.

Cyanotic Patients

Tetralogy of Fallot. The fourth most common congenital heart defect, tetralogy of Fallot is a cyanotic lesion with decreased pulmonary blood flow. Its four components are ventricular septal defect, pulmonary stenosis, right ventricular hypertrophy, and overriding of the aorta. The degree of cyanosis is related to the degree of pulmonary stenosis with its associated right-to-left shunt. Stenosis may be so mild that patients remain acyanotic (the pink tetralogy), or it may be so complete as to cause pulmonary atresia. Cyanosis may also be significantly increased during episodes of "spelling" during Valsalva-type maneuvers (crying, squatting, or grunting resulting in diminished pulmonary blood flow), which carry a 10% mortality rate if frequent and recurrent. Patients with uncorrected tetralogy are at risk for strokes, brain abscesses, and bacterial endocarditis. The diagnosis is suspected on chest x-ray, when there is loss of pulmonary vasculature and the typical "coeur en sabot" shape of the cardiac silhouette. The ECG will show right ventricular hypertrophy, and echocardiography demonstrates a ventricular septal defect and overriding aorta. Treatment of the defect has gradually been changing. The more conservative approach reserves total repair for patients over 1 year of age with adequate sized distal pulmonary arteries. Currently, however, some institutions recommend total repair at any age. Neonates or infants with very small pulmonary arteries and severe cyanosis require a palliative procedure. The most common one is a Blalock-Taussig shunt, a direct connection between the subclavian artery and the pulmonary artery to increase pulmonary blood flow. A modified Blalock-Taussig shunt consists of a Gore-Tex conduit between the subclavian artery and the pulmonary artery. Other systemic-to-pulmonary shunts include the Waterston shunt, a connection from the ascending aorta to the right pulmonary artery, and the Potts shunt, a similar connection from the descending aorta to the left pulmonary artery. These last two are rarely used because of possible pulmonary artery distortion and inadequate control of blood flow to the lungs. Occasionally, a Gore-Tex shunt from the central aorta to the pulmonary artery is used. When the patient is deemed to have adequate pulmonary artery size, complete correction is accomplished through a sternotomy and cardiopulmonary bypass. The ventricular septal defect is closed with a prosthetic patch, and the right ventricular outflow tract is widened. An outflow tract patch is used to enlarge the hypoplastic right ventricular infundibulum; it may be extended through the annulus and beyond to the right or left pulmonary arteries. Relief of the pulmonic obstruction is imperative, and right ventricular pressures should be lowered to less than two-thirds systemic pressure. Complica-

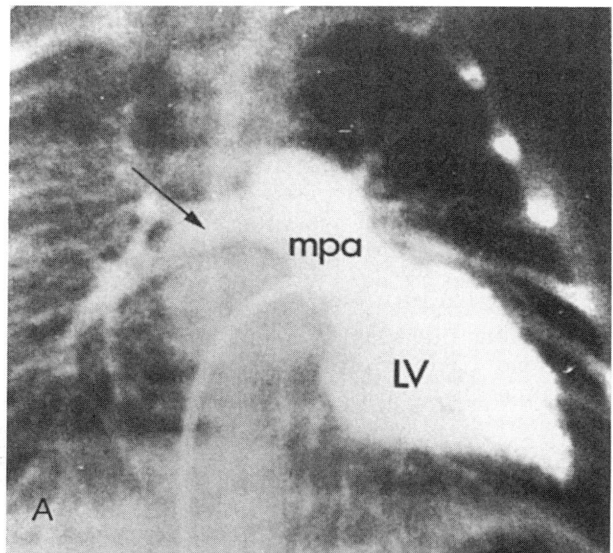

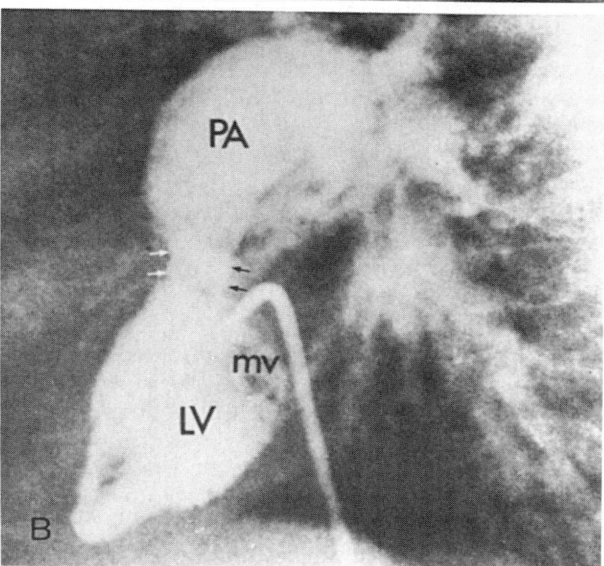

Figure 6.12. Angiograms demonstrating transposition of the great arteries, in which the left ventricle empties into the pulmonary artery.

tions of surgery include bleeding, heart block, or low cardiac output syndrome. Mortality is approximately 3–5%.

Transposition of the Great Arteries. Transposition of the great arteries, the fifth most common defect, consists of an atrial-ventricular concordance with a ventricular-arterial discordance. The right ventricle empties into the aorta and the left ventricle empties into the pulmonary artery. This lesion is cyanotic with increased pulmonary blood flow (Fig. 6.12). Because the defect consists of two parallel circulations, survival of the infant depends on intracardiac mixing. Affected infants have severe cyanosis in the first days of life. Without treatment, 50% will be dead by 1 month and 80% by 1 year. Patients initially can be treated with prostaglandins to increase pulmonary blood flow through the ductus arteriosus. A palliative balloon septostomy enlarges the atrial septal defect and increases mixing.

Therapy for transposition of the great arteries has changed significantly over the last several years. In the past, an intra-atrial repair (either a Mustard or Senning procedure) was performed on infants 3–6 months of age. Redirection of venous blood by a baffle of cloth or pericardium allowed the "blue" venous blood to flow from the inferior and superior venae cavae underneath the baffle to the mitral valve. Blood would flow from the left ventricle to the pulmonary arteries and return oxygenated by way of the pulmonary veins. It would then be directed from the pulmonary veins through the tricuspid valve to the right ventricle and out the aorta to the body. Overall survival rate with this surgical procedure was excellent, with mortalities less than 5%. However, because of such complications as arrhythmias, ventricular failure, and baffle obstruction, another procedure has come into favor. In the Jatene procedure, infants are corrected within the first 2 weeks of life by switching the pulmonary artery with the aorta and by translocating the coronary arteries to the neo-aorta. When performed by an experienced surgeon, this procedure carries a risk of less than 10%.

Tricuspid Atresia. Tricuspid atresia, constituting 3% of congenital heart defects, is the absence of the right atrioventricular connection. Usually, it is a cyanotic lesion, although some patients have a ventricular septal defect that allows shunting of blood to the pulmonary artery. Pulmonary artery flow may be increased with large ventricular septal defects, it may be normal with infundibular stenosis, or it may be decreased when the ventricular septal defect is severely restrictive. In infants with increased pulmonary blood flow, pulmonary artery banding is performed in the first few months of life. In children with restricted blood flow, a systemic-to-pulmonary artery shunt usually is performed within the first year of life. Subsequent palliation may be indicated depending on ventricular function and pulmonary artery connection. For patients of 1–2 years of age, a cavopulmonary or Glenn shunt, a venous shunt from the superior vena cava to the right pulmonary artery, can be performed. For patients over 2 years of age, a Fontan procedure is performed in which the right atrium is connected directly to the pulmonary arteries, allowing all venous blood to flow directly to the pulmonary arteries, bypassing the ventricle. Mortality for this last procedure is approximately 10%.

Pericardial Disease

The purpose of the pericardium is unclear, since its removal is not accompanied by any serious sequelae. However, it is thought to provide some important functions. It is a very strong fibrous sac that prevents acute dilation of the heart, which is detrimental to cardiac function. Chronic dilation is possible when caused by slow increments in cardiac size and accumulation of pericardial effusions, but acute dilation is not possible. The pericardium also limits the lateral and vertical mobility of the heart within the mediastinum, thus preventing hemodynamic sequelae such as torsion or kinking of the great veins.

The pericardium may be involved with inflammatory traumatic or neoplastic conditions, in addition to rarely encountered malformations. Pericarditis (pericardial inflammation) may be primary or secondary. Common causes of exudative pericarditis are bacterial, mycobacterial, or viral infections; acute myocardial infarction; and uremia. The exudate may be effusive (thin fluid) or purulent (viscous fluid). Nonspecific benign pericarditis usually causes chest pain, fever, and/or a pericardial friction rub. Shortness of breath, a dry, hacking cough, and relief obtained by leaning forward are often seen. Electrocardiographic changes (ST elevations) may be confused with myocardial ischemia. Exclusion of other forms of pericarditis assures the diagnosis, and its course is usually harmless and self-limiting. Salicylates, ibuprofen, or steroids may be useful for treating the symptoms and limiting the effusion.

Purulent pericarditis results from direct contamination of the pericardial space, as in penetrating trauma, or as a result of bacteremia from pneumonia, osteomyelitis, or other bacterial infections. Marked symptomatology with chest pain, fever, and systemic toxicity are usually seen. Rapid pericardial fluid accumulation and tamponade are often encountered. Appropriate antibiotic coverage and surgical drainage of the pericardium offer the best chance for cure. Tuberculous pericarditis should be treated as early as possible, since the fibrosis that follows mycobacterial infection can result in constrictive pericardial disease, which dramatically diminishes myocardial function.

Cancer may cause pericardial effusion in one of two ways: either by direct metastatic pericardial tumor implantation with resultant fluid production, or by neoplastic lymphatic obstruction preventing pericardial fluid clearance. In either case, the extent of systemic disease determines the ultimate outcome. The prognosis is usually poor. However, relief of tamponade may provide excellent palliation and may be accomplished by pericardiocentesis or surgical pericardiostomy with tube drainage. Occasionally, sclerosing agents are instilled to prevent recurrence of effusion. If drainage is complete and parietal and visceral pericardium are apposed, however, the recurrence rate approaches zero.

Hemopericardium secondary to trauma is considered the hallmark of cardiac injury requiring surgical exploration. The usual criteria for hemopericardium with tamponade, such as pulsus paradoxus, muffled heart tones, and jugular venous distension, are often unreliable in the acute trauma setting, and a high false-negative rate has been noted in several centers. Therefore, we have resorted to surgical subxiphoid pericardiotomy for any suspected blunt cardiac injury or for any penetrating precordial injury with wounds entering or exiting in an area from the clavicles to the hypochondrium, medial to the nipple line. When hemopericardium is found, the incision is readily converted to a median sternotomy for optimal exploration and cardiorrhaphy, if indicated. A high percentage of patients with hemopericardium are found to have significant injury, thus justifying this approach. A negative exploration is well tolerated in this patient population.

Patients with cardiac tamponade exhibit a classical hemodynamic picture consisting of diminished cardiac output secondary to restricted diastolic filling because of high intrapericardial pressures exerted on the heart muscle. A typical profile demonstrates elevated right atrium, right ventricle, and pulmonary artery wedge pressures, as well as a unique equalization of the same three diastolic pressures. Equalization of CVP, pulmonary artery diastolic pressure, and pulmonary artery wedge pressure are classic signs of cardiac tamponade. Treatment begins with a high index of suspicion based on clinical signs and physical findings. Echocardiography will show effusion, if present, and other signs of tamponade, such as diastolic collapse of the right atrium and a leftward shift of the ventricular septum. Effusion without other signs is less compelling evidence of tamponade. Immediate pericardiocentesis via a subxiphoid route is preferred and can be accomplished at the bedside using materials available in a commercial package. For continued drainage, an intrapericardial catheter is placed using a Seldinger guide wire technique. Following pericardiocentesis, surgical pericardial drainage may be accomplished electively by either the subxiphoid extrapleural approach or transthoracically by a left 4th or 5th interspace thoracotomy.

Pericardiostomy, sometimes referred to as a "pericardial window," may be used to effect pericardial drainage. The term window originally referred to the creation of an opening from the pericardium into the pleural space to allow resorption of the fluid by the relatively large pleural surface. However, this "window" often closed early after operation, becoming obliterated by lung and fibrin, necessitating more long-lasting drainage. Subxiphoid pericardiostomy is now performed by incising the midline abdominal structures between the xiphoid and halfway to the umbilicus. The peritoneum is not entered. The diaphragmatic fibers are bluntly dissected from the inferior pericardial surface, which is incised. The fluid is evacuated, and a tube is placed within the pericardial cavity and connected to suction for 5 days. This technique assures apposition of the parietal and visceral pericardial surfaces and seems to prevent recurrence in nearly every case.

Pacemakers

Cardiac pacemakers use electrical power to substitute for an abnormal cardiac conduction system in order to preserve an adequate heart rate or atrioventricular synchrony. Pacemakers consist of:

1. A power source—usually lithium-based and of varying size and composition
2. Circuitry—sophisticated analytical electronics to insure variability in rate, power applied, sensing capabilities, telemetry, and all parameters within the system

3. Housing—hermetic sealing of the electronics to prevent body fluids from leaking into the battery and thereby disabling the circuit
4. Electrode—the conducting mechanism from the power source and circuitry to and from the myocardium; may be unipolar or bipolar; the stimulating electrode is always "negative" (cathodal stimulation principle).

Candidates for pacemaker insertion include all patients with correctable symptomatic arrhythmias and those with other conduction abnormalities that may intermittently lead to sudden death. A partial list of pacemaker indications includes:

1. Complete heart block
2. Mobitz II second-degree heart block
3. Bradycardia associated with syncope, dizziness, seizures, confusion, heart failure (correlation of symptom and bradycardia is needed)
4. Bradycardia as a consequence of necessary drug therapy for which there is no alternative
5. Bradycardia associated with symptomatic supraventricular tachycardia or malignant ventricular arrhythmias
6. Bifascicular or trifascicular heart block with syncope
7. Complete heart block following myocardial infarction

In order to simulate normal cardiac electrophysiologic activity, the pacemaker must be able to sense intrinsic cardiac electrical activity, integrate that activity into a preprogrammed algorithm, and then dispense appropriate electrical discharges to one or both cardiac chambers. Patients with complete heart block, for example, have atrial electrical discharges (P waves) at appropriate rates, but because they are not conducted to the ventricles and do not incite sequential ventricular contractions, atrioventricular synchrony is lost. The pacemaker must conduct the atrial activity (P wave) through its atrial electrode to the generator for analysis and then, at appropriate programmed intervals, stimulate a ventricular contraction through the ventricular electrode. It must also, therefore, sense the absence of the ventricular activity following the P wave.

Pacemakers may be used in the atrium or ventricle alone, or may be dual chamber devices with sensing and pacing capabilities in both chambers. Pacemakers are classified according to a three-letter code (with some modifiers):

1. First letter is chamber paced: A = atrium, V = ventricle, D = both
2. Second letter is chamber sensed: A = atrium, V = ventricle, D = both
3. Third letter is function: I = inhibited, T = triggered, D = both, O = neither.

Thus, a simple ventricular demand pacemaker, which is inhibited when it senses an intrinsic beat, is classified as VVI. An atrial pacemaker with similar function is AAI. A dual chamber pacemaker performing both sensing and pacing in both chambers mimicking normal atrioventricular electrophysiology is DDD.

Thoracic Aorta and Great Vessels

The thoracic aorta and the "great vessels" (innominate, intrathoracic carotid, and subclavian arteries) are subject to the same pathology as blood vessels elsewhere: atherosclerosis, trauma, and inflammatory diseases. The size and propensity for exsanguinating hemorrhage, as well as visceral ischemia, render recognition of the disease processes of these vessels extremely important.

Trauma

Transection of the aorta and great vessels is a potentially life-threatening injury. It is caused by deceleration forces that occur upon impact. Motor vehicle accidents and motorcycle trauma are the most frequent causes, and young people are most affected. Because surrounding pleura, adventitia, and mediastinal tissues often contain the false aneurysm and blood flow occurs normally, there may be no immediate physiologic consequences of great vessel transection. Many patients die at the scene due to rapid exsanguination, but for those who survive initially, physiologic derangement may be absent or delayed in onset. Surviving patients nearly always sustain tears distal to the left subclavian artery, while tears just above the aortic valve are uniformly fatal. These tissues give way over time, however, resulting in exsanguinating hemorrhage and death in 95% of patients. Approximately 5% of patients form chronic false aneurysms, which are noticed months to years later as they expand. Since there are few immediate physiologic consequences of an aneurysm, a heightened awareness of the possibility of this injury must exist when treating trauma patients. Knowing the mechanism of injury is therefore important. History of a decelerating injury or a fall from a great height should prompt a search for the injury as soon as possible. The chest x-ray remains the most important screening tool. Radiologic findings on a supine anterior-posterior (AP) portable chest x-ray include widening of the mediastinum to more than 8 cm at the level of the aortic knob, an apical pleural cap indicating the presence of an extrapleural mediastinal hematoma at the apex of the right hemithorax, loss of the contour of the aortic knob and aortopulmonary window, depression of the left main bronchus, and rightward deviation of a nasogastric tube indicating displacement of the esophagus. It is important to realize that all of the findings on the chest x-ray indicate the presence of a mediastinal hematoma and are not specific for great vessel injury. The trauma surgeon must distinguish between great vessel injury, which requires immediate treatment, and mediastinal hematoma, which does not. The latter is largely the result of injury to small arteries and veins in the mediastinum. An aortogram is best for delineating aortic trauma (Fig. 6.13). Computed tomography (CT) scans have been associated with a high false-negative rate, unac-

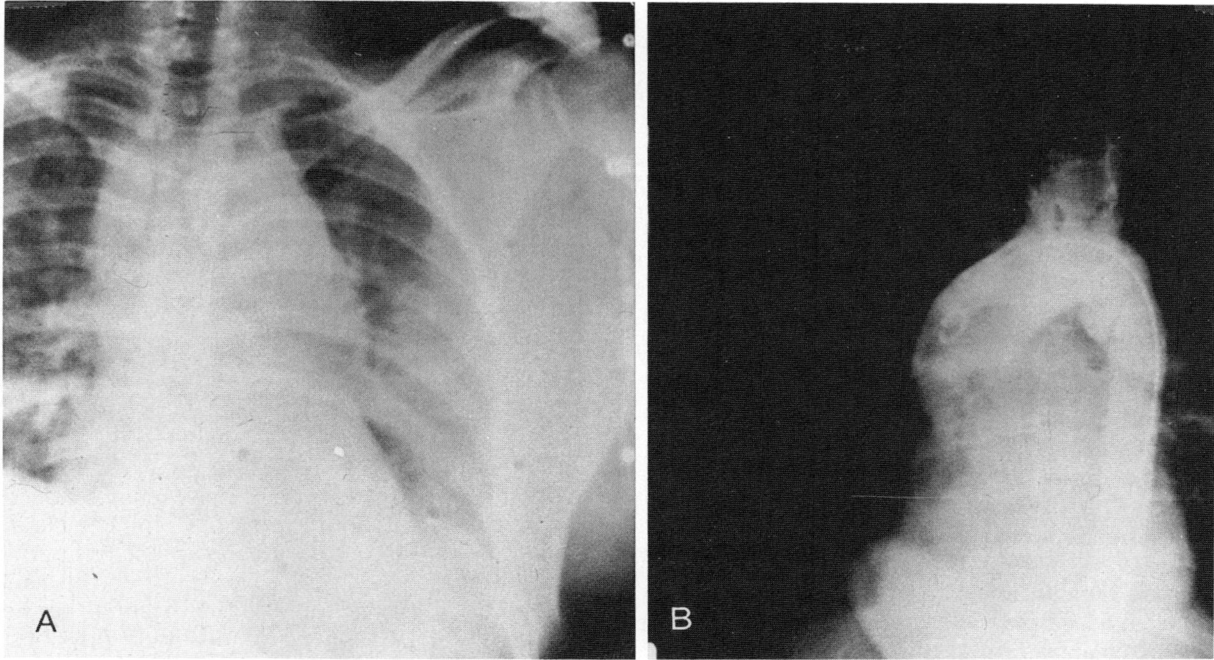

Figure 6.13. Transection of the thoracic aorta. **A**, Chest x-ray showing signs of mediastinal hematoma (see text). **B**, Aortogram demonstrating false aneurysm distal to the left subclavian artery.

ceptable in this highly lethal injury. Additionally, a scan may delay the aortogram, which may show an injury that mandates immediate surgery.

Treatment of this injury depends on its extent. Partial disruptions can be repaired using simple suture techniques, avoiding the use of prosthetic grafts. Most patients, however, incur total transection of the aorta with retraction of the edges for a distance of 2–6 cm. Interposition of a prosthetic graft is usually necessary. Graft interposition requires cross-clamping of the thoracic aorta, usually between the left subclavian and left carotid arteries proximally, and distally just beyond the aortic tear. Problems generated by cross-clamping include proximal hypertension and inadequate flow to the visceral arteries distal to the clamp. Surgical approaches have included a "clamp and sew technique," which usually suffices if there has been no preoperative hypotension and if the cross-clamp time can be held to approximately 30 minutes. Other techniques include left atrial-femoral bypass utilizing a pump and an oxygenator to provide distal perfusion. Heparin-bonded plastic shunts can be placed proximal and distal to the area of clamping to provide flow to the lower body. Shunts of sufficient size (9 mm) must be used if adequate flow is to be maintained. Contraindications to heparinization, and therefore femoral-femoral bypass with an oxygenator, include severe head trauma and massive retroperitoneal injury.

Complications in treating thoracic aortic injuries are spinal cord ischemia and renal ischemia. Because it is uncertain which segment of the aorta gives rise to the anterior spinal artery (of Adamkiewicz), the danger exists of creating spinal cord ischemia during aortic cross-clamping; this occurs in 5–15% of cases. Perfusion of the lower body should be protective; however, the actual incidence of spinal cord ischemia does not seem to vary with the technique of spinal preservation. Renal failure is unusual following these operations if the patient is adequately rehydrated, mannitol is used, and hypotension and acidosis are avoided after the aorta is unclamped. Since the recurrent laryngeal nerve courses through the exact location of aortic injury around the ligamentum arteriosum, care should be taken to seek out the nerve and protect it if possible. Loss of the recurrent laryngeal nerve may predispose to airway compromise postoperatively due to vocal cord paralysis. Long-term sequelae are few if there are no early perioperative complications. Occasionally, false aneurysms form at the anastomotic sites. These can be minimized by using monofilament and nonabsorbable sutures.

Great vessels other than the aorta may be injured. Aortography should always include the origins of the brachiocephalic trunks, since overlooking injuries to these vessels could result in stroke and extremity ischemia. Often, intimal flaps are produced, which eventually lead to thrombus formation or occlusion of the artery. Repair techniques for these vessels are similar to those of the thoracic aorta except for the incisions used. Innominate artery injuries are approached through a median sternotomy with extension into the base of the right neck. Similarly, left common carotid or subclavian injuries may be approached through a sternotomy for proximal control with extension into the left neck or left hemithorax for distal exposure. Bypass techniques are seldom necessary for brachiocephalic injuries, and sequelae are few.

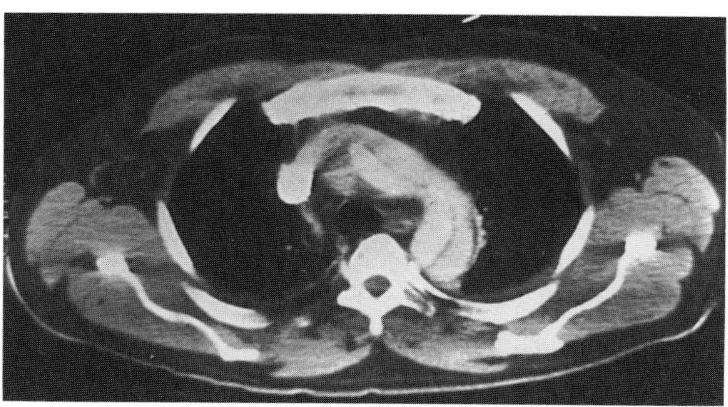

Figure 6.14. CT scan with contrast demonstrating true and false lumens with intervening intimal flap in the aortic arch.

Degenerative

Aortic dissection, formerly called dissecting aortic aneurysm, is a tear in the intima of the aorta resulting in a dissecting hematoma between the intima and media of the vessel (Fig. 6.14). This dissecting hematoma may occlude and compromise visceral circulation (such as coronary, carotid, or splanchnic vessels), or it may rupture into the pleura or peritoneum causing exsanguinating hemorrhage. The underlying pathogenesis is an abnormal aortic intima caused either by atherosclerotic plaques with hemorrhage or by cystic medial degeneration of the vessel because of a connective tissue disorder. The patient describes an excruciating "tearing, ripping" pain—the worst pain imaginable—usually beginning in the precordium and radiating through to the back and flanks. The pain can be confused with the pain of coronary ischemia, but careful questioning can usually elicit the difference between the chest pressure of angina and the tearing quality of aortic dissection pain. A normal ECG and abnormal chest x-ray demonstrating a widened mediastinum may help in differentiating aortic dissection from angina or myocardial infarction. The diagnosis may be confirmed by echocardiogram, transesophageal echocardiogram, CT scan, or angiography.

The classification of aortic dissection depends upon its anatomic location. Recent classification methods from Stanford University term all dissections involving the ascending aorta, regardless of origin, Type A, requiring immediate surgical intervention. Those confined to the descending thoracic aorta distal to the left subclavian artery are Type B and may be treated operatively or nonoperatively. The rationale for this treatment algorithm stems from the fact that retrograde dissection into the ascending aorta may lead to rupture within the pericardial cavity, immediate tamponade, and death. Outcome of patients treated nonoperatively with Type A dissections is dismal and therefore urgent surgery is mandatory. On the other hand, patients with dissection of the descending thoracic aorta, in the absence of visceral artery occlusion, may be treated nonoperatively with drugs that diminish the force of left ventricular contraction and therefore minimize the force propelling the dissecting hematoma. Such drugs include antihypertensive agents such as sodium nitroprusside or hydralazine, and a β-blocker that diminishes the force of left ventricular contraction. Additional antihypertensive agents may be added as necessary. Patients who are treated nonoperatively must be monitored closely in the intensive care unit and frequent measurements taken of arterial blood pressure, urine output, and central venous and pulmonary artery pressures. A change from a nonoperative course to surgery would be indicated for visceral artery occlusion (such as splanchnic ischemia), enlargement of the dissection based upon CT or chest x-ray, unremitting and uncontrollable pain, or evidence of leakage of the dissection into the pleural space with resultant hemothorax.

Operative techniques are similar to those used for traumatic aortic transection in terms of bypass, blood salvage, and perfusion of the lower body. Because the aorta is friable, methods to bolster suture techniques and graft interposition often must be employed. Pledget material to distribute the force of the sutures and to prevent their tearing through the aortic wall are also usually necessary. Operative mortality is 5–20%, with dissection at a site distal to the original tear commonly being the cause of death.

Aneurysm

Atherosclerotic aneurysms, as well as posttraumatic and infectious aneurysms, may affect the thoracic and abdominal aorta. Recognizable symptoms, such as chest and back pain caused by enlargement of the aneurysm against the vertebral column, or discovery on a routine chest x-ray are common presentations. The indications for surgery include symptomatic aneurysms, enlarging aneurysms, aneurysms more than 5 cm in diameter, or leaking aneurysms. Bypass and perfusion techniques are similar to those described previously and vary with the location of the aneurysm. Aneurysms in the ascending aorta and aortic arch are approached through a median sternotomy and necessitate femoral artery perfusion. The patient is often placed in hypothermic total circulatory arrest as a protective mechanism both for the brain and for the viscera. Numerous grafting and repair techniques have been developed; most include resection and grafting of the aneurysmal tissue with Dacron grafts.

Thoracic Cavity

Neoplasms

Lung Cancer. Lung cancer is the most common cause of nondermatological cancer in North America, accounting for one-fifth of all new cancers and one-third of all cancer deaths per year. More than 85% of lung cancer patients have a very strong smoking history. Other patients develop lung cancer from exposure to radioactive materials, including asbestos dust and fluorspar. Smokers with occupational exposure to radi-

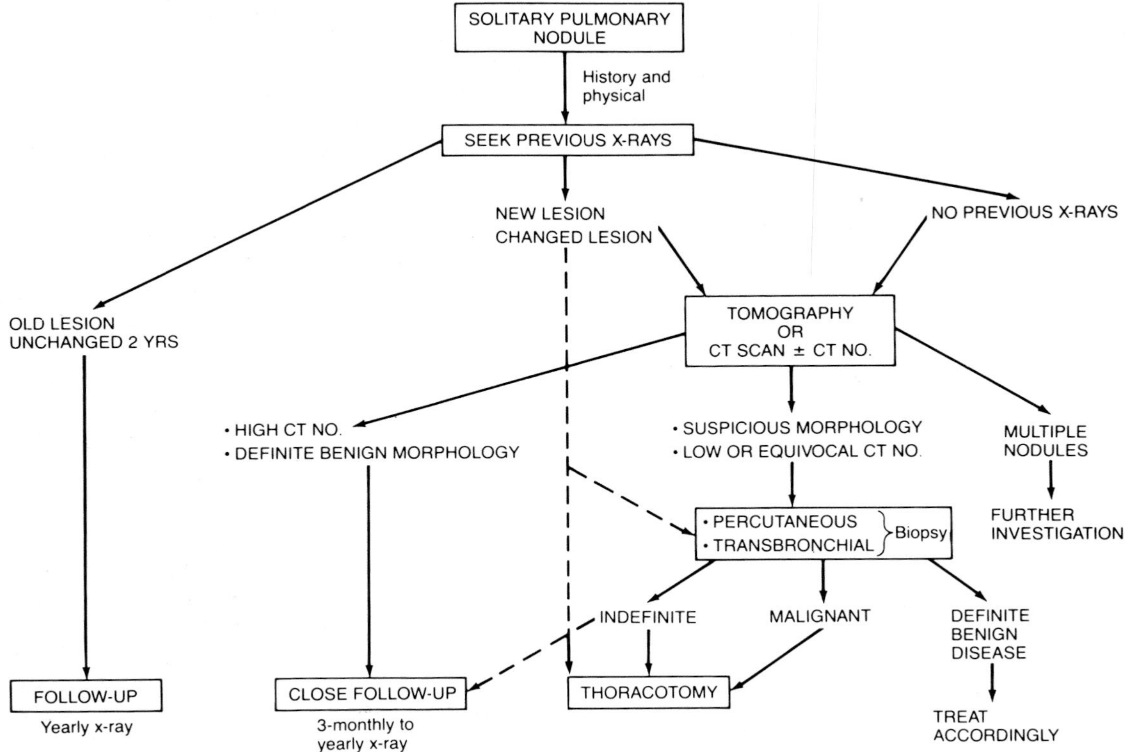

Figure 6.15. Management plan for assessment of patients with asymptomatic solitary pulmonary nodule.

oactive materials are at increased risk of developing lung cancer.

Cancers of the lung are primary or secondary. Primary lung cancer begins at the cellular level and progresses from dysplastic changes to in situ changes to frankly invasive carcinoma. It develops from two distinct cell lines:

1. Large cell lines, e.g., squamous cell carcinoma, adenocarcinoma, and mixed cell type
2. Small cell lines, e.g., "oat cell" carcinoma, intermediate cell type, mixed cell type

Information regarding cell type is obtained from a variety of diagnostic procedures, including cytological evaluation of sputum, bronchial washings, and histological and cytological evaluation of tumor tissue obtained by direct or transpulmonary biopsy (either through the bronchus or through the chest wall by fine-needle aspiration). Identifying the originating cell line is important in determining treatment. Because tumors from the small cell line tend to metastasize earlier, patients present with disease that needs to be managed systemically (with a combination of chemotherapy and radiotherapy) rather than surgically. However, surgery may play a role in selected early lesions without evidence of metastasis. Patients with neoplasms of large-cell origin are always evaluated with resection in mind, since surgical extirpation offers the best chance for cure.

Secondary lung cancers result from metastasis of lesions elsewhere in the body, usually from the breast, the gastrointestinal system, the genitourinary tract, or soft tissue. Surgery is rarely an option because there is usually evidence of other distant metastatic lesions. However, in selected cases surgical removal of solitary or well-localized metastatic lesions in the lung is justified by improvement in survival rate. While development of metastatic lesions to the lung carries a generally poor prognosis, aggressive combination therapy can produce long, disease-free intervals and in some cases improve survival rate.

Presentation. The presentation of lung cancer is varied. Approximately 5% of patients are asymptomatic and a lesion is discovered incidentally by chest radiographs performed for health or insurance examinations. Because the yield is low, particularly in nonsmokers, routine screening chest x-rays are generally not recommended. If radiographs demonstrate a solitary pulmonary nodule or "coin lesion," a workup is required in order to formulate a management plan (Fig. 6.15). The importance of previous x-rays cannot be overstated, since knowledge of prior lesions and estimates of their growth rate greatly affect management decisions. Stable lesions are usually benign. New masses and those demonstrating enlargement must be presumed malignant until proven benign.

The remaining 95% of patients are symptomatic, with signs and symptoms that can be categorized according to whether they are bronchopulmonary, extrapulmonary, metastatic, nonspecific, or nonmetastatic (Table 6.5). Extrapulmonary signs and symptoms often herald the presence of advanced disease. Paratracheal lymph node metastases may produce hoarseness result-

Table 6.5.
Signs and Symptoms in Patients with Lung Cancer

Category	Sign or Symptom
Bronchopulmonary	Cough
	Chest pain
	Dyspnea
	Hemoptysis
Extrapulmonary	Superior vena caval obstruction
	Hoarseness (recurrent nerve invasion)
	Pleural effusion
Metastatic	Neurological
	Skeletal
	Visceral
Nonspecific	Weight loss
	Anemia
	Fatigue
Nonmetastatic	Dermatological
	Endocrine
	Vascular
	Neurogenic
	Metabolic
	Hematologic
	Skeletal

ing from involvement of the recurrent laryngeal nerve on the left side. Superior vena caval obstruction may occur with right-sided nodal enlargement or direct invasion. Pleural effusion may result from metastatic disease in the pleura or from pneumonia or lymphatic obstruction. If no malignant cells are present in the effusion, metastatic disease can be ruled out and surgery can be performed. Neurological and skeletal symptoms usually represent metastases, and a thorough search for these deposits must be undertaken using CT scans of the brain and abdomen as well as bone scans. Nonmetastatic symptoms or "paraneoplastic syndromes" occur in a small percentage of patients and may be very early signs of a primary lung cancer; these include inappropriate ADH secretion and hypercalcemia.

Management. Once the possibility of bronchogenic cancer is raised, the physician must define a management plan that depends on a precise diagnosis, the stage of the disease, and the ability of the patient to undergo operative treatment. Three questions are asked rhetorically:

1. What is the diagnosis?
2. Can the patient undergo an operation?
3. Can the patient tolerate the maximally anticipated lung resection?

The diagnosis of bronchogenic carcinoma is confirmed by bronchoscopy or percutaneous needle biopsy. Flexible or rigid bronchoscopy visualizes proximal tumors, and direct biopsy (or washings and brushings) can effect a precise diagnosis in over 90% of patients. Even peripheral lesions not directly visible endoscopically can be biopsied with fluoroscopic guidance into the appropriate bronchopulmonary segment. Lesions not amenable to bronchoscopic biopsy are evaluated by percutaneous needle biopsy guided either by fluoroscopy or CT scan. Cytologic analysis is performed even though some needles yield only a small histologic specimen. In most patients, needle biopsy results properly guide clinical management.

Judgments must be made regarding comorbid conditions such as age and any cardiac, renal, hepatic, or neurological conditions that may adversely affect operative risk. Occasionally, corrective surgery such as coronary bypass must be performed, either before or during pulmonary resection. Assessment of overall physical and social status requires experience and judgment; single diseases, laboratory values, or social problems seldom preclude surgical intervention in lung cancer.

Various assessments need to be performed preoperatively to determine the patient's tolerance for the proposed procedure in terms of cardiac and pulmonary function (see Figs. 6.16 and 6.17). Cardiac reserve is of foremost importance and is evaluated by history, physical examination, electrocardiogram, and sometimes stress testing. Occasionally, staged or simultaneous coronary revascularization is recommended. Pulmonary reserve is estimated by history, physical examination, and exercise testing. Numerical evaluation is best done by pulmonary function tests, measurement of arterial blood gas levels, and sometimes selective ventilation perfusion scanning. Spirometry evaluates a number of components of the inspiratory and expiratory phases of respiration and is used to measure the volume of gas expired within a specific period of time (forced expiratory volume—FEV), usually within the first second (FEV_1). This value can be expressed as an absolute volume of gas or as a percentage of the predicted normal value for that individual based on sex, age, height, and weight. The FEV_1, usually reduced in patients with obstructive pulmonary disease, is extremely helpful in identifying patients at high risk for pulmonary resection. It is estimated that the FEV_1 has to be greater than 800–1000 mL to avoid chronic respiratory insufficiency after surgery. Another value, maximal voluntary ventilation (MVV), is crucial to assessing patients' ability to tolerate pneumonectomy.

Measurement of arterial blood gases also is important in predicting pulmonary reserve. The concentration of carbon dioxide in the blood (PCO_2) gives an indication of the adequacy of alveolar ventilation. Evidence of carbon dioxide retention, particularly after exercise, would preclude pulmonary resection. Generally, a PCO_2 greater than 50 mm Hg contraindicates resection. Interpretation of the oxygen concentration in the blood (PO_2) is more difficult. However, it is felt that a PO_2 of less than 50 mm Hg (or 90% saturation) is usually associated with such severe restriction that pulmonary resection is not feasible. In certain instances, further preoperative tests are performed, including studies of regional ventilation and pulmonary circulation.

Staging. Staging refers to the determination of tumor size and spread. The most widely used classification is the TNM system of the American Joint Committee for Cancer Staging and End Results reporting. T refers to the size and location of the tumor, N to the

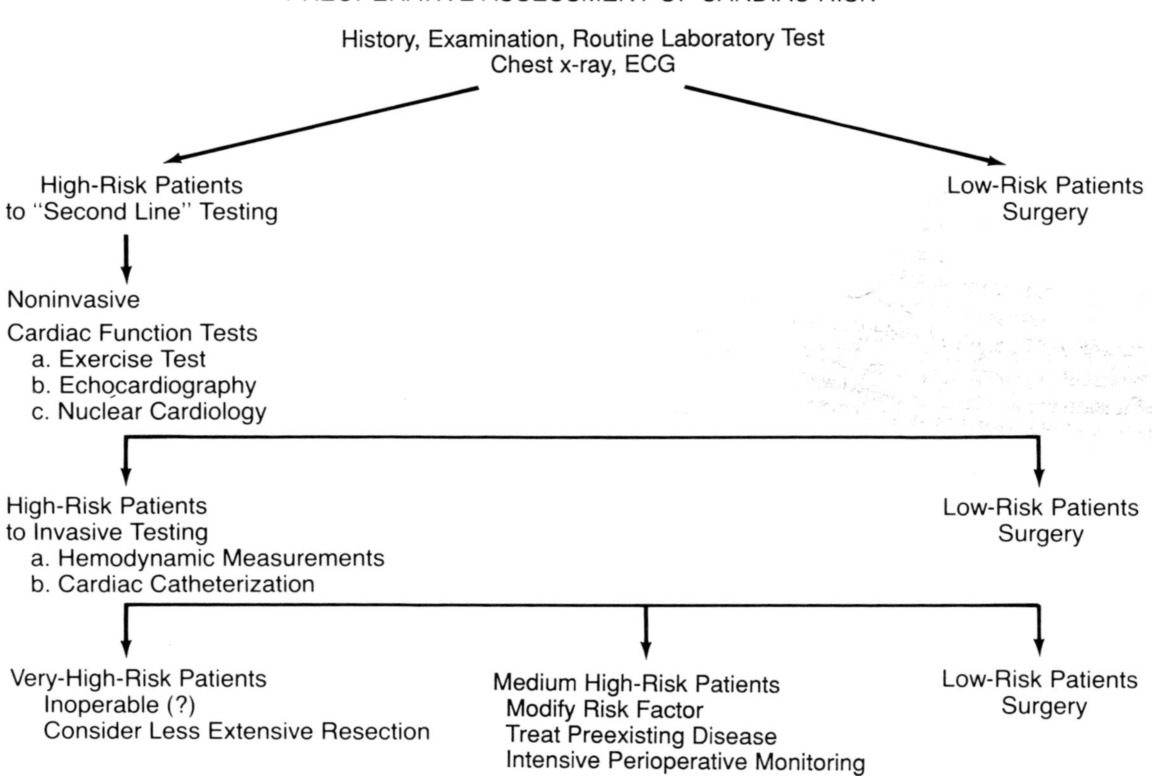

Figure 6.16. Preoperative assessment of cardiac risk.

presence and location of lymph node metastases, and M to the presence or absence of distant metastases. TNM classification allows the surgeon to provide a stage grouping for the patient (Table 6.6), and it is upon this stage that statistical prognostication can be made for large numbers of patients.

The tumor is located by direct observation through rigid or flexible bronchoscopy and radiological evaluation, including conventional radiography and CT scanning. Tumors at or near the carina are, with rare exception, not considered resectable. Their proximity to vital structures can be ascertained by CT scanning with contrast and bronchoscopy. Patients with a tumor limited to the ipsilateral hemithorax with no evidence of mediastinal lymph node metastases and no involvement of other vital structures are considered surgical candidates. Figure 6.18 lists the types of resection indicated according to whether the tumor is stage I, II, or III.

The search for metastatic disease in a patient with lung cancer must be as complete as possible before that patient undergoes pulmonary resection. Pulmonary resection that leaves malignancy behind is not only fruitless but dangerous. The search is conducted by means of history, physical examination, and such investigations as nuclear scans of the brain, bone, and liver. Although these scans help determine the presence of metastatic disease, their relative insensitivity has given way to newer techniques. CT scanning assists not only in discovering metastases but in determining the presence of enlarged mediastinal lymph nodes. These nodes are the initial metastatic sites of bronchogenic carcinoma that spreads by way of the bronchopulmonary lymphatics. A suspicion of lymph node involvement should be confirmed by biopsy, not x-ray. The hilar and paratracheal lymph nodes are biopsied at mediastinoscopy and subjected to microscopic and histochemical evaluation. The presence of metastases at these nodes reduces the surgical cure rate to a level at which few centers attempt surgical resection.

Surgical Treatment. Surgical treatment is indicated once a patient has been deemed operable and the tumor resectable. The patient's operability depends on cell type, cardiac and pulmonary reserve, and underlying medical conditions. The tumor's resectability depends on whether it has metastasized or invaded vital organs and whether the surgeon can grossly remove all malignant cells. Generally, stage I and some stage II tumors can be resected completely. Extensive resection can be accomplished by ligating pulmonary vessels within the pulmonary cavity to circumvent hilar involvement with the tumor and by excising segments of chest wall, provided complete tumor removal is anticipated.

Patients should have the anatomical resection that removes the tumor completely yet leaves enough lung tissue to permit satisfactory respiration. Resections may be of a segment (segmentectomy), a lobe (lobectomy), or the whole lung (pneumonectomy). If the lesion is peripheral, then a lesser resection such as a wedge resection may be possible. When the lesion is more proximal, lobectomy or pneumonectomy is necessary for

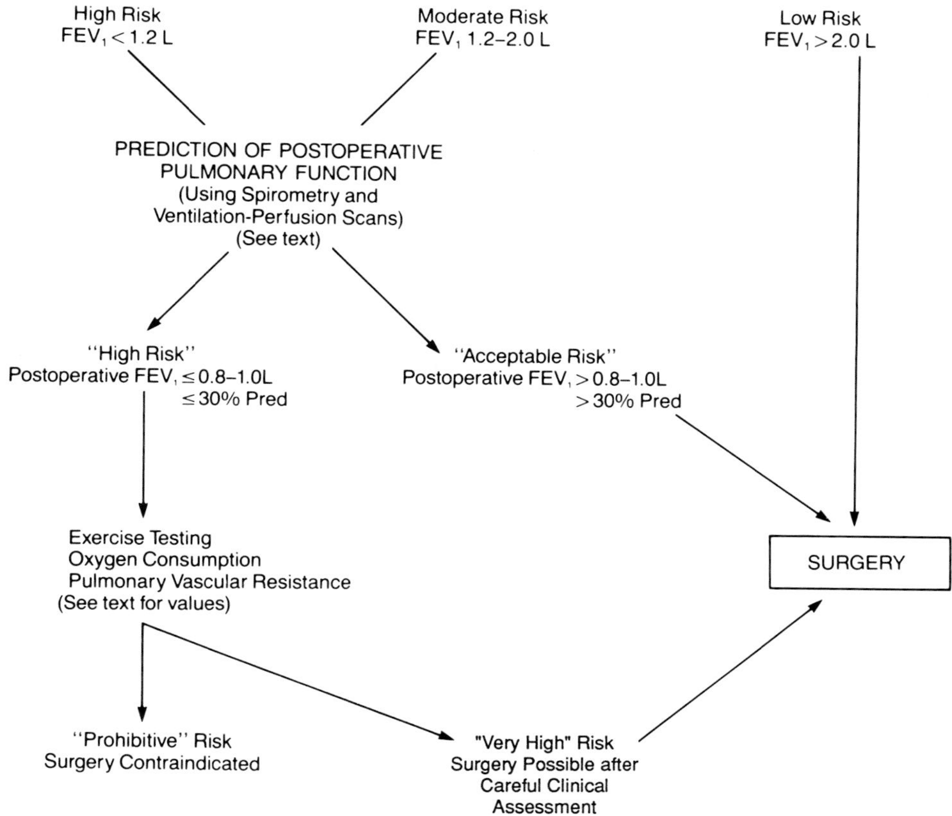

Figure 6.17. Preoperative assessment of respiratory risk.

complete extirpation. More complex operations have become possible with the advent of bronchoplastic procedures and reconstruction of the tracheobronchial tree.

Surgical resection for large-cell lung cancer can be extremely beneficial: the approximate risk of resection is 2 to 5%, depending on the extent of the resection and the age and underlying condition of the patient (Table 6.7). The long-term survival of patients undergoing pulmonary resection depends on the stage of the tumor and its cell type. Patients with a well-differentiated squamous cell carcinoma that is completely resected have a 60–70% chance of 5-year survival. Patients with more advanced or less well-differentiated tumors carry differing prognoses (Table 6.8). Because only those lung cancer patients undergoing pulmonary resection have a chance for long-term survival, however, the physician must identify as many patients as possible with a cancer lending itself to resection.

Chest Wall Tumors

Half of all chest wall tumors are primary, and of these 60% are malignant. The other half are metastatic, usually arising from lung, thyroid, gastrointestinal, or genitourinary tumors. Both kinds usually present as enlarging chest wall masses, with malignant lesions more often being painful. The most common malignant tumor is chondrosarcoma, and the most common benign tumor is fibrous dysplasia (Table 6.9).

Any chest wall tumor should be considered malignant until proven otherwise. A careful history and physical examination searching for potential sources of metastatic disease should be performed. Posterior-anterior (PA) and lateral chest x-rays are followed by a CT scan of the chest to localize the tumor, determine if it is solitary, and assess underlying lung parenchyma and mediastinal structures. All patients should undergo a bone scan to determine other sites of osseous involvement.

Treatment of chest wall tumors has changed in recent years. Previously, the fear that a subtotal or incisional biopsy would adversely affect survival led to the recommendation of a total wide excision for all chest wall tumors. It is now clear, however, that an incisional biopsy does not adversely affect survival. Thus, if the tumor is small, complete removal at a single operation should be performed as the biopsy procedure.

With the exception of plasmacytoma, which should be treated as systemic myeloma, most solitary primary tumors should be removed with a wide excision encom-

Table 6.6.
New International Staging System: TNM Classification and Stage Grouping

Primary Tumor (T)	
T0	No evidence of primary tumor.
Tx	Tumor proven by the presence of malignant cells in bronchopulmonary secretions but not visualized roentgenographically or bronchoscopically, or any tumor that cannot be assessed as in a retreatment staging.
T1S	Carcinoma in situ.
T1	A tumor that is 3.0 cm or less in greatest dimension, surrounded by lung or visceral pleura, and without evidence of invasion proximal to a lobar bronchus at bronchoscopy.[a]
T2	A tumor more than 3.0 cm in greatest diameter or a tumor of any size that either invades the visceral pleura or has associated atelectasis or obstructive pneumonitis extending to the hilar region. At bronchoscopy, the proximal extent of demonstrable tumor must be within a lobar bronchus or at least 2.0 cm distal to the carina. Any associated atelectasis or obstructive pneumonitis must involve less than an entire lung.
T3	A tumor of any size with direct extension into the chest wall (including superior sulcus tumors), diaphragm, or the mediastinal pleura or pericardium without involving the heart, great vessels, trachea, esophagus, or vertebral body, or a tumor in the main bronchus within 2.0 cm of the carina without involving the carina.
T4	A tumor of any size with invasion of the mediastinum or involving heart, great vessels, trachea, esophagus, vertebral body or carina or presence of malignant pleural effusion.[b]
Nodal Involvement (N)	
N0	No demonstrable metastasis to regional lymph nodes.
N1	Metastasis to lymph nodes in the peribronchial or the ipsilateral hilar region, or both, including direct extension.
N2	Metastasis to ipsilateral mediastinal lymph nodes and subcarinal lymph nodes.
N3	Metastasis to contralateral mediastinal lymph nodes, contralateral hilar lymph nodes, and ipsilateral or contralateral scalene or supraclavicular lymph nodes.
Distant Metastasis (M)	
M0	No (known) distant metastasis.
M1	Distant metastasis present. Specify site(s).
Stage I	
T1SN0M0	Carcinoma in situ.
T1N0M0	Tumor that can be classified T1 without any metastasis to the regional lymph nodes.
T1N1M0	Tumor that can be classified T2 with metastasis to nodes or distant metastasis.
T2N0M0	Tumor that can be classified T without any metastasis to nodes or distant metastasis.
Stage II	
T1N1M0	Tumor classified as T2 with metastasis to the lymph nodes in the ipsilateral hilar region only.
Stage IIIA	
T3N0	Tumor classified as T3 with no nodes.
T3N1	Tumor classified as T3 with ipsilateral hilar nodes.
T1–3N2	Tumor classified as T1, T2, or T3 with metastasis to ipsilateral mediastinal nodes or subcarinal nodes.
Stage IIIB	
Any T1N3	Any size tumor with metastasis to contralateral, supraclavicular, or scalene nodes.
T4, Any N	Tumor invading heart, great vessels, esophagus, or vertebral body or carina or presence of malignant pleural effusion.

[a]The uncommon superficial tumor of any size with its invasive component limited to the bronchial wall, which may extend proximal to the major bronchus, is classified as T1.
[b]Most pleural effusions associated with lung cancer are due to tumor. There are, however, some few patients in whom cytopathologic examination of pleural fluid (on more than one specimen) is negative for tumor, and the fluid is nonbloody and is not an exudate. In such instances in which these elements and clinical judgment dictate that the effusion is not related to the tumor, the patient should be staged as T1, T2, or T3, excluding effusion as a staging element.

passing involved soft tissue, rib cage, sternum, and underlying lung or pericardium. Margins of 2 to 4 cm are recommended. Chest wall defects of 5 cm or more in diameter anteriorly or 10 cm posteriorly should be reconstructed using synthetic mesh for bony thorax and muscle pedicle flaps (most commonly from the latissimus dorsi) to cover soft tissue defects. Patients with Ewing's sarcoma, osteogenic sarcoma, or soft tissue sarcoma are also candidates for postoperative radiation therapy, chemotherapy, or both.

Mediastinal Tumors. A large number of benign and malignant tumors, both primary and metastatic, can present in the mediastinum. While most tumors are first found on standard PA or lateral chest x-ray, CT scanning is essential to localize the tumor accurately. MRI does not have significant advantages over CT scan except in posterior paraspinal tumors.

Mediastinal tumors are approached according to their location (Fig. 6.19). The anterior mediastinum is defined by an imaginary line extending along the anterior wall of the trachea down over the anterior pericardium. The posterior mediastinum is defined by an imaginary line from the anterior border of the vertebral bodies to the costovertebral sulci. The middle mediastinum is the space in between. Tumors occur most often in the anterior mediastinum and least often in the middle mediastinum.

The most common anterior mediastinum tumors are thymoma, substernal thyroid, teratoma (germ cell tu-

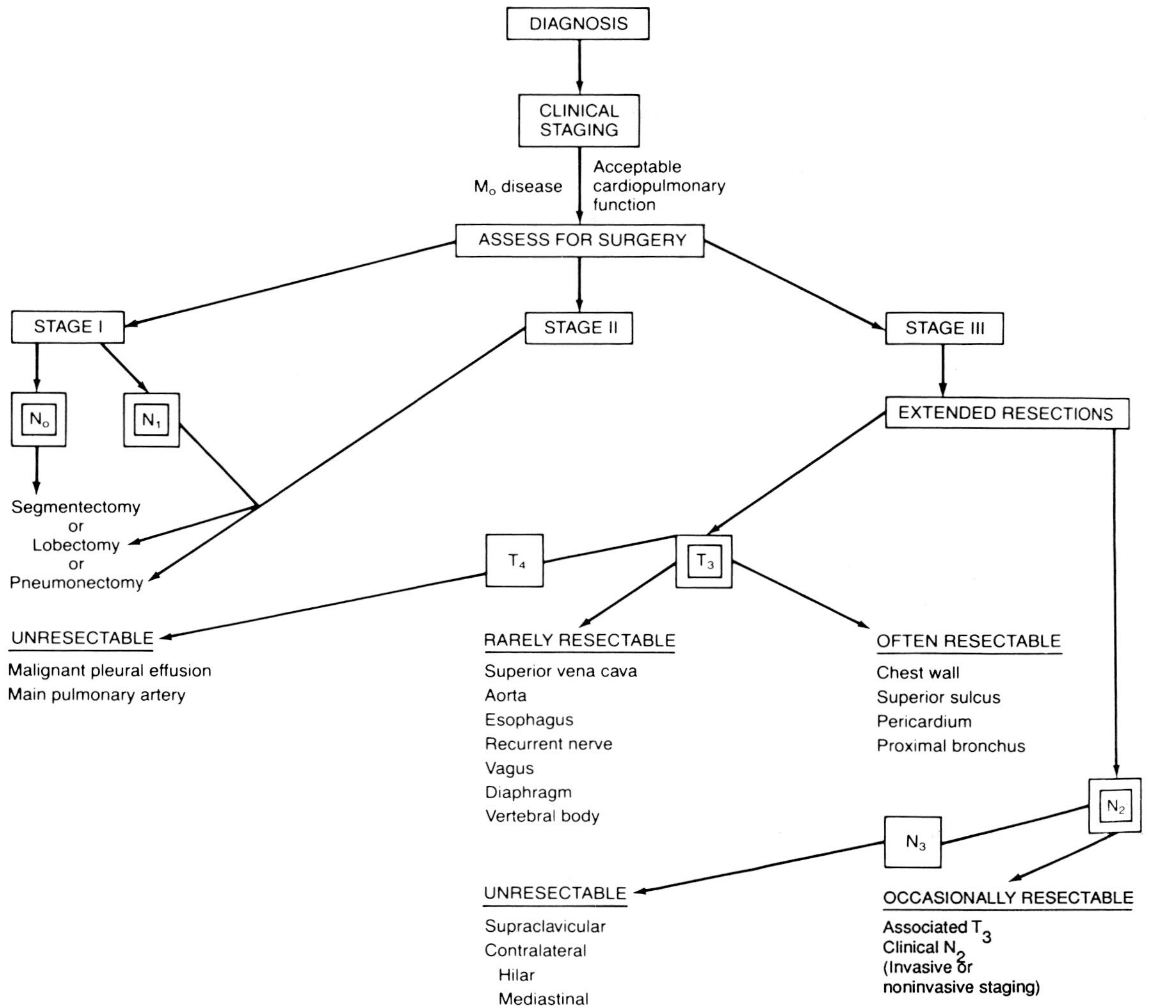

Figure 6.18. Staging of lung cancer to assess resectability.

Table 6.7.
Postoperative Mortality Following 2220 Pulmonary Resections for Lung Cancer

Type of Resection and Age of Patient	Number of Resections	30-Day Mortality (Percentage)
All resections	2220	3.7
Pneumonectomy	569	6.2
Lobectomy	1508	2.9
Segmentectomy or wedge resection	143	1.4
60 years	847	1.3
60–69 years	920	4.1
70 years	443	7.2

mors), and lymphoma. Symptoms in patients with malignant lesions include chest pain, dyspnea, fever, chills, and cough. Patients with benign lesions usually are asymptomatic, and the lesions are found only on routine chest x-ray. A careful history and physical exam can give clues as to the type of tumor present. A lymphoma can cause night sweats, weight loss, and peripheral adenopathy. A mediastinal germ cell metastasis can appear as a testicular mass. A thymoma can cause symptoms of myasthenia gravis. A substernal thyroid tumor often partially compresses the trachea, one of the few tumors to do so. Excision is the best treatment except for lymphoma, which usually requires anterior mediastinotomy to make the diagnosis if no extramediastinal adenopathy exists. Almost all substernal thyroids can be removed through a cervical incision. Resection of all other anterior mediastinal tumors is best approached by median sternotomy.

The most common masses in the middle mediastinum are metastatic lymph nodes from lung cancer and

Table 6.8.
Analysis of Survival According to Stage and Histology from the Lung Cancer Study Group[a]

Stage	Subset	Cell Type	4-year Survival (Percentage)
I	T_1N_0	Squamous cell	85
		Adenocarcinoma	72
	T_1N_1	Squamous cell	80
		Adenocarcinoma	63
	T_2N_0	Squamous cell	65
		Adenocarcinoma	60
II, III		Squamous cell	37
		Adenocarcinoma	25

[a]Postoperative mortality is excluded.

Table 6.9.
Chest Wall Tumors

Benign	Malignant
Fibrous dysplasia	Chondrosarcoma
Chondroma	Osteogenic sarcoma
Osteochondroma	Plasmacytoma
Eosinophilic granuloma	Ewing's sarcoma

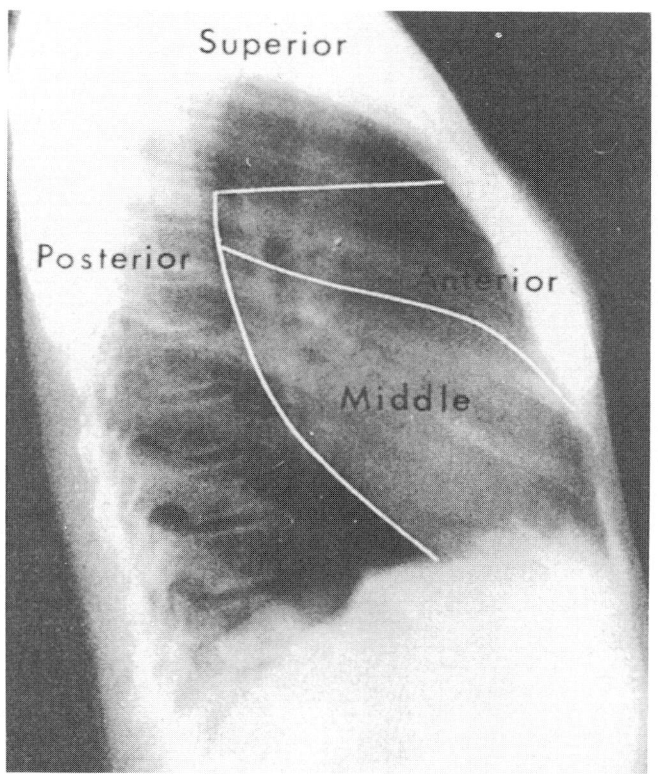

Figure 6.19. Lateral film of the chest showing the anatomic divisions into four subdivisions of the mediastinum.

enterogenous cysts. (The evaluation of mediastinal adenopathy in order to stage bronchogenic carcinoma is discussed under lung cancer.) Asymptomatic mediastinal adenopathy can also be a manifestation of sarcoidosis and can be diagnosed by mediastinoscopy. Middle mediastinal cysts (bronchogenic, esophageal, and pleuropericardial) should be removed by lateral thoracotomy to rule out a malignancy presenting with similar radiographic findings.

The most common tumors of the paravertebral sulci are of neurogenic origin: neurilemomas, neurofibromas, ganglioneuromas, and neuroblastomas. Tumors in this location must be evaluated by MRI for extension into the spinal canal. If they extend into the canal, a combined neurosurgical-thoracosurgical approach is essential to insure complete removal. Failure to remove the spinal canal component has resulted in paralysis years later, as the residual tumor slowly grows and presses against the spinal cord.

Other Diseases

Hemoptysis. Over the last 20 years the principal causes of hemoptysis have changed from tuberculosis and bronchiectasis to bronchitis and cancer. Today, bronchitis accounts for approximately 50% of hemoptysis, tumor 19%, tuberculosis 7%, and bronchiectasis 1%. Most hemoptysis is now treated nonoperatively with sedation, humidification, antitussives, antibiotics, and bed rest.

Any patient with persistent, recurrent, or massive hemoptysis should undergo a thorough workup. If hemoptysis is not massive (<600 mL/24 hours), the workup can be done electively; if it is, the patient requires immediate diagnostic and therapeutic intervention. In approximately 90% of cases, PA and lateral chest x-rays followed by bronchoscopy reveal the cause of hemoptysis. Early bronchoscopy for lateralization is helpful when sudden deterioration occurs and operative intervention is indicated. CT scan offers little additional help in managing patients acutely. If bleeding is massive, an aortogram with bronchial arteriography facilitates management, since in 95% of patients with life-threatening hemoptysis the cause originates in the systemic bronchial circulation. Bronchial arteriography can be combined with bronchial arterial embolization to control hemoptysis temporarily.

Patients with severe hemoptysis require emergency intervention to prevent asphyxiation secondary to aspiration of blood into the "normal" lung. If the side containing the lesion is known, the contralateral main bronchus is intubated and the contralateral lung elevated. Bronchoscopy is done with the rigid bronchoscope, and a Fogarty venous occlusion catheter (#4 to #8) is used to occlude the main bronchus, thereby isolating the normal lung from contamination and aspiration. A double lumen endotracheal tube can also be placed to isolate one lung from the other. A 2.9-mm diameter pediatric flexible bronchoscope is passed down each side of the tube selectively to help determine which side is bleeding.

A potential cause of hemoptysis in patients with indwelling pulmonary artery catheters is rupture of the pulmonary artery, occurring most frequently when the

Table 6.10.
Tests to Differentiate Transudative from Exudative Fluid

Test	Exudate	Transudate
Protein (g/dL)	>3.0	<3.0
Pleural fluid/serum protein (g/dL)	>0.5	<0.5
LDH (IU/L)	>200	<200
Pleural fluid/serum LDH (g/dL)	>0.6	<0.6

Table 6.11.
Common Causes of Pleural Effusion

Transudates	Exudates
Congestive heart failure	Infection
Cirrhosis	Malignancy
Hypoalbuminemia	Chylothorax
Nephrotic syndrome	Tuberculosis

catheter is inserted or repositioned. Patients at highest risk are those with pulmonary hypertension or those who are elderly. Management is directed toward evacuating aspirated blood and preserving ventilation. If this is done, the bleeding usually stops on its own. To help ascertain the side of injury, the pulmonary artery catheter should not be removed before a chest x-ray is performed. Rarely, pulmonary resection is necessary to control bleeding, but the mortality rate is high.

Determining the site of bleeding can be difficult. Blood can collect throughout the endobronchial tree such that at bronchoscopy it appears to be coming from multiple segmental orifices. Blood may also be coming from sources other than those identified on chest x-ray. Since treatment of the contralateral lung is nearly impossible through a lateral thoracotomy, it is essential that the correct side from which the bleeding originates be determined before surgery. Diligent bronchoscopy, use of occluding Fogarty catheters, bronchial angiography, and sometimes repeated bronchoscopies may be necessary.

Surgical treatment is based upon the etiology of the hemoptysis. In benign disease as little lung tissue as possible should be resected. In malignant disease more extensive resection is necessary for any potentially curable malignancy. In recent years, the photocoagulating properties of the yttrium-argon-garnet (YAG) laser have been used to treat hemoptysis from proximal endobronchial tumors. If not massive, bleeding is controlled immediately. Laser bronchoscopy is performed with a rigid bronchoscope because of significantly better airway control and suction capability.

Pleural Effusion. Pleural effusions (fluid in the pleural space) are divided for diagnostic and therapeutic reasons into two types: transudates and exudates. Transudates originate from some external cause that upsets the normal balance of fluid secretion and absorption in the pleural space, causing it to collect in the chest. Congestive heart failure, cirrhosis, and atelectasis are common causes. Exudates are caused by primary disease processes of the pleural space, such as malignancies exuding fluid or blocking lymphatic channels to create fluid.

Symptoms of pleural effusions include shortness of breath, pleuritic pain, and a sense of fullness in the chest. Dullness to percussion and decreased breath sounds are present on physical examination. Thoracentesis is the primary diagnostic procedure. The extracted pleural fluid is analyzed as to whether it is transudative or exudative (Table 6.10). A Gram's stain and cultures (including those for tuberculosis and fungus) should be performed. As much fluid as possible is removed to allow subsequent x-rays to detect hidden lesions.

Treatment of pleural effusion depends on its etiology (Table 6.11). Transudates should be treated by addressing their underlying cause, such as congestive heart failure or ascites. Rarely is chest tube drainage of transudates necessary. Exudates, on the other hand, require chest tube drainage, particularly if malignancy is the cause, because malignant effusions invariably recur after thoracentesis. Pleural space drainage with a chest tube and instillation of a chemical sclerosing agent (such as bleomycin, tetracycline, and talc) prevent reaccumulation 60–80% of the time. The underlying lung must fully reexpand to allow apposition of the visceral and parietal pleura.

Lung Abscess. With the increase in numbers of immunocompromised patients, the incidence of lung abscess has begun to rise. A lung abscess should be suspected in any patient with a fever and an air-fluid level within the parenchyma on chest x-ray. Differentiation between lung abscess (a parenchymal process) and empyema (an extraparenchymal pleural process) may be difficult but can usually be made by CT scan. The most common etiology of lung abscess is aspiration of stomach contents, often associated with excessive alcohol abuse and loss of consciousness. Persistent pneumonia can evolve into a lung abscess as can pulmonary infarction from both infected and noninfected clots. A bronchial neoplasm or an aspirated foreign body may also be the cause and should be excluded by flexible bronchoscopy.

Treatment consists of prolonged antibiotic therapy and vigorous respiratory physiotherapy. A lung abscess caused by aspiration usually involves organisms of the upper respiratory tract, such as *Staphylococcus* sp., fusiform bacilli, α-hemolytic streptococcus, and *Bacteroides fragilis*. For these organisms, high-dose penicillin (3 million to 20 million units/day) is usually satisfactory. Immunocompromised patients may harbor Gram-negative organisms, such as *Pseudomonas*, *Proteus*, *Escherichia coli*, and *Klebsiella*. Until the pathogen can be identified, broad-spectrum antibiotics are indicated.

In almost all patients with a lung abscess, bronchoscopy is indicated to obtain reliable cultures, promote drainage, and rule out an endobronchial lesion. Surgery is not indicated unless the patient continues to be septic, has an enlarging cavity despite adequate antibiotics, or has a resectable endobronchial carcinoma. In good-risk patients lobectomy can be performed; in others tube drainage is preferable. Several studies have shown that lung abscesses treated with an accurately placed

Table 6.12.
Criteria for Chest Tube Drainage

Organisms identified on Gram's stain	
pH	<7.1
Glucose	<40 mg/dL
LDH	>1000 IU/L

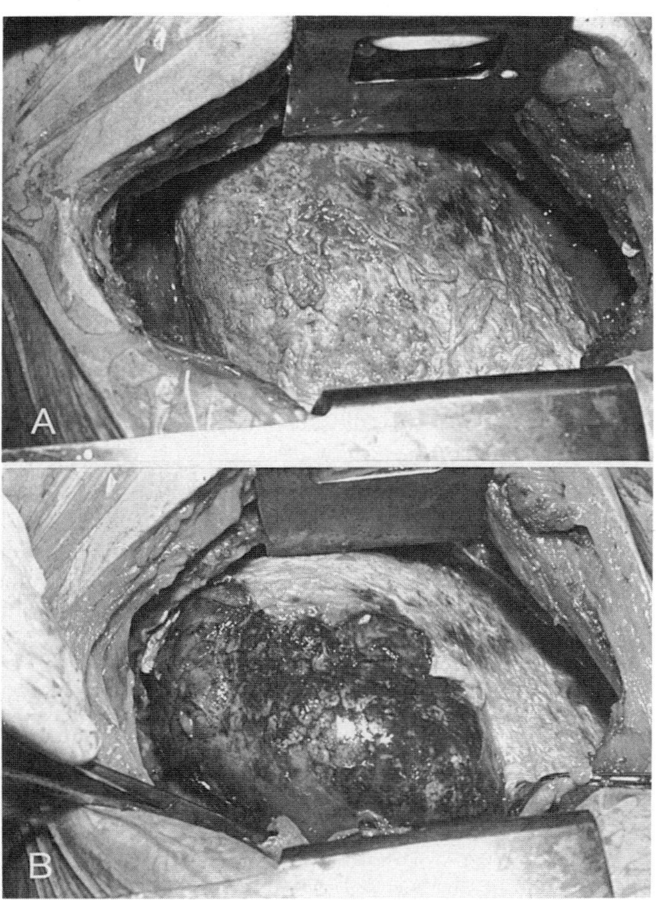

Figure 6.20. **A**, Lung trapped by exudative "rind." Note space between lung and chest wall. **B**, Partial decortication with lung released from entrapment and beginning to expand.

tube will heal with time, allowing extrusion of the tube or replacement by excision of one or more ribs. The resulting cavity usually heals secondarily, while the patient is under outpatient observation over several weeks to months.

Empyema. Empyema, an infected pleural effusion that may require drainage, occurs most frequently in conjunction with an underlying bronchopulmonary infection. The fluid may not culture organisms, particularly if the patient has been receiving antibiotics. Fluid meeting drainage criteria on thoracentesis (Table 6.12) should be drained with a fairly large (36 French) chest tube to avoid occlusion from thick fluid or particulate matter. The tube can be removed once the space is evacuated, the lung reexpanded, and fluid is no longer purulent. Occasionally, the tube is left for 10–14 days, then opened to air and extruded over 2–3 weeks. Before the tube is extruded, the fluid in the water seal chamber should have stopped fluctuating (indicating obliteration of the pleural space) and the lung should remain expanded with the tube opened to air, thus ensuring pleural adhesions and continued lung expansion.

Complex empyemas often require further procedures. If the fluid is loculated or pocketed off within the chest, several chest tubes may be necessary to effect drainage. On occasions when a chest tube only partially drains a space, two alternatives exist. The first is to allow the lung to stick to the chest wall elsewhere and remove several short segments of ribs to open the cavity and allow drainage (rib resection and drainage). If a bronchopleural fistula does not exist, the cavity is irrigated and left to close secondarily over several months. If a fistula does exist, the wound is dressed on the surface and periodically wiped out with gauze. This cavity too will often close secondarily, but may require closure later with a muscle pedicle flap. Rib resection is the procedure of choice for patients who are either very ill or poor surgical candidates. The second alternative for patients with a partially drained space with lung entrapment is decortication. A thoracotomy is performed and the visceral pleural peel trapping the lung is removed, allowing the lung to reexpand (Fig. 6.20). If the underlying lung parenchyma is reasonably healthy, the lung will reexpand, the space will be obliterated, and chest tubes can be removed after drainage has decreased, usually within 5–7 days. Decortication has the advantage of restoring lung function and allowing the patient to be discharged without chest tubes.

Obliteration of the pleural space is the single most important principle guiding therapy for empyema. Once synthesis between parietal and visceral pleural surfaces has occurred, resolution is all but insured. This can be accomplished by decortication, which will allow the lung to expand to fill the hemithorax. If lung expansion is not possible (either because of parenchymal disease or absence by resection), then the chest wall is allowed to fall in to meet the lung by excision of the ribs with a thoracoplasty.

Pneumothorax. Pneumothorax is the partial or total collapse of the lung from air collecting in the pleural space, thus eliminating the negative intrapleural pressure that counteracts the elastic recoil of the lung and prevents lung collapse.

Spontaneous Pneumothorax. Spontaneous pneumothorax occurs for no apparent reason (primary) or is caused by underlying lung pathology (secondary). Most frequently it occurs in tall, thin patients and is associated with the spontaneous rupture of an apical emphysematous subpleural bleb. The diagnosis is readily made on chest x-ray, with care being taken to differentiate a pneumothorax from an area with no lung markings secondary to a giant bulla. Old x-rays may be the only way to readily distinguish one from the other.

A pneumothorax is best described by the distance between the chest wall and lung rather than by percentage of lung collapse. The latter method has significant observer variability and does not involve three-dimensional considerations. A small pneumothorax, 2–4 cm from the apex and nearly out to the side, usually can be watched if the patient is reliable and comfortable. About 1% of the air in the pleural space will be reabsorbed each day.

A large pneumothorax or one causing significant patient discomfort requires a chest tube. The tube is placed in the fourth or fifth interspace in the midaxillary line, unless the pneumothorax is loculated and/or the pleural space is compartmentalized by adhesions. In such cases, the tubes are directed into the appropriate pockets of air. When anesthetizing the patient with local anesthesia, the needle should be passed into the pleural space to ascertain that air can be freely aspirated. If air cannot be aspirated, either the diagnosis or location of the pneumothorax should be reassessed. If the diagnosis is confirmed by needle aspiration, blunt dissection with a hemostat clamp through the muscles and over the top of the rib into the pleural space allows easy placement of the tube. For spontaneous pneumothorax, a 28-French tube is large enough. Placement of the tube by trocar is no easier and carries the risk of injuring the underlying lung. The chest tube should be placed to water seal or, preferably, to -20 to -30 cm H_2O suction. A lung that reinflates rapidly may cause significant transient pain requiring analgesia. The chest tube can be removed 48 hours after the air leak has stopped.

Surgical treatment should be considered for patients who have an air leak persisting for more than 7–10 days, recurrent pneumothorax, bilateral simultaneous pneumothoraces, or high-risk occupations. Surgery consists of thoracotomy through an axillary incision or a small latissimus-sparing incision, closure, and exclusion of the ruptured bleb or any other large blebs with the surgical stapler and mechanical pleurodesis. Pleurodesis, the creation of a fibrous adhesion between the visceral and parietal layers of the pleura, is accomplished by rubbing the parietal pleura with dry gauze to create an inflammatory reaction, which, when coupled with complete lung expansion, assures obliteration of the pleural space and prevents recurrence of pneumothorax. Mechanical pleurodesis is preferred over pleurectomy (removal of the pleura) because of a much lower complication rate. A new surgical procedure currently undergoing evaluation consists of thoracoscopy, lysis of adhesions, and scleroses.

Traumatic Pneumothorax. Blunt or penetrating injuries or pneumothorax secondary to high pressure ventilation is treated with prompt chest tube drainage, which should be continued for 48 hours after the air leak has stopped.

Tension pneumothorax, a life-threatening condition, develops when air escapes into the pleural space with no way of exiting. The increased tension in the space causes the trachea and mediastinum to shift to the opposite side and the diaphragm to be displaced downward. Shifting of the mediastinum can result in significant decrease in venous blood return to the heart and cardiovascular collapse. Emergency treatment centers on allowing the air under tension to escape, converting a tension pneumothorax to an ambient pneumothorax, which is not life threatening. If a tube thoracostomy cannot be performed immediately, a large-bore needle is inserted to relieve pressure and restore cardiac and respiratory function.

Hemothorax. Hemothorax, the collection of blood within the pleural space, is most often caused by trauma. Physical findings include dullness to percussion and reduced breath sounds. The diagnosis is confirmed by x-ray in most instances, but often tube thoracostomy is performed on clinical suspicion alone. Sources of intrapleural blood include the lung, intercostal vessels, chest wall musculature, heart, great vessels, and abdomen through rents in the diaphragm. Nontraumatic hemothorax can arise from vascular adhesions torn during thoracentesis or from pneumothorax as the lung falls away from the chest wall. Anticoagulants magnify the significance and size of hemothorax. Three major derangements are associated with hemothorax: hypovolemia from blood loss, compromised ventilation in the blood-filled pleural cavity, and compromised circulation from a tension hemothorax (similar to a tension pneumothorax).

Treatment centers on relieving the physiological abnormalities and treating the cause. Tube thoracostomy simultaneously relieves the compressed lung, restores normal intrapleural and therefore ventilatory dynamics, and allows assessment of bleeding rate and magnitude. Operative therapy is guided by rate of bleeding and its presumed or actual source. A decreasing bleeding rate of 200 mL/hr, 150 mL/hr, to 100 mL/hr permits for nonoperative observation, while an increasing rate of 200 mL/hr, 250 mL/hr, to 300 mL/hr indicates the need for thoracotomy. Pleural blood salvage and autotransfusion are safe and should be used whenever possible. If surgery is indicated, lateral thoracotomy usually suffices and ligation or repair of the bleeding sources normally is straightforward and simple. Commonly encountered bleeding sources are intercostal or internal mammary arteries and veins. Rarely are sophisticated adjuncts, such as heart bypass, necessary.

Flail Chest. A flail chest occurs when one rib is fractured at two sites, disrupting the stability of the chest wall: on inspiration the segment of the chest wall involved moves inward instead of outward. This movement, termed paradoxical respiration, has been thought to cause respiratory failure. Such failure is more likely due to the underlying pulmonary contusion and/or from inadequate ventilation efforts as a result of splinting from pain. Patients may be managed without mechanical ventilation provided the injury to the underlying pulmonary parenchyma is not severe or extensive and adequate pain management is achieved by systemic, epidural, or local analgesia. The encouragement of rigorous pulmonary physical therapy and suctioning to prevent atelectasis and to expectorate secretions is essential. Patients who have inadequate spontaneous minute ventilation for whatever reason will require intubation and mechanical ventilatory support until the fractures stabilize, the underlying parenchymal injury heals, or pain control becomes possible. Surgical stabilization of flail segments has been used by some surgeons but is not commonly needed with sophisticated intensive care units.

SUGGESTED READINGS

Grillo HC, Austen WC, Wilkens SW, Mathisen DJ, Vlahakes GJ. Current therapy in cardiothoracic surgery. Toronto: BC Decker, 1989.

Kirklin NJ, Barratt-Boyes. Cardiac surgery. New York: John Wiley & Sons, 1986.

Mattox KL, Moose EE, Feliciano DV. Trauma. Norwalk, Connecticut: Appleton & Lange, 1988.

Ravitch MM, Steichen FM. Atlas of general thoracic surgery. Philadelphia: WB Saunders, 1988.

Roth JA, Ruckdeshel JC, Weisenburger TH. Thoracic oncology. Philadelphia: WB Saunders, 1989.

Sabiston DC, Spencer FC. Surgery of the chest. 5th ed. Philadelphia: WB Saunders, 1990.

Shields TW. General thoracic surgery. 3rd ed. Philadelphia: Lea & Febiger, 1989.

Stark J, deLaval M. Surgery for congenital heart defects. New York: Grune & Stratton, 1983.

Skills

1. Recognize normal pressure tracings encountered during the insertion of a Swan-Ganz catheter.
2. Accurately assess tachyarrhythmias on ECG and determine the etiology.
3. Analyze arterial blood gases as a guide for ventilatory support.
4. Adjust ventilator settings in an ICU patient to improve oxygenation or ventilation.
5. Direct initial mechanical ventilation therapy in the postoperative patient.

TUBE THORACOSTOMY

1. Preparation. Assemble proper antiseptic, instruments, gloves, and receptacles. Apply antiseptic to area to be aspirated, as judged by chest x-ray, CT scan, ultrasound, or percussion.
2. Local Anesthetic. Infiltrate with 1/2% or 1% Xylocaine. Take care to anesthetize a sizable skin wheal, subcutaneous tissues, periosteum of rib, and especially the pleura. At least 20–30 mL of anesthetic will be required. Area chosen must enable aspiration of substance (blood, pus, air), or location must be changed.
3. Incision. In the appropriate location, make an incision slightly larger than the tube. Carry blunt dissection down to the intercostal muscle after having tunneled up one rib to provide a subcutaneous tunnel to seal the tract after the tube is removed. With an instrument, perform blunt penetration into the pleura over the top of the rib. Enlarge the opening and insert a finger into the pleura to confirm intrapleural location and absence of adhesions.
4. Insertion. Insert the appropriate tube (#24 or #28 for air, #32 or #36 for fluid) using the instrument to guide the tube into an intrapleural location.

   Note: Tubes expected to evacuate apical pneumothoraces should be placed through the second intercostal space anteriorly and directed to the apex. Tubes expected to drain blood or fluid should enter via the 4–5 intercostal space in the anterior axillary line and should be directed dorsally for optimal drainage.

   Correct underwater seal and suction. Suture the tube to the skin with a heavy material (2-0 or 0 silk) and apply a dressing. Obtain a chest x-ray to confirm tube position and evacuation of pleural space.

   Upon tube removal, cover the wound with an impervious dressing (petrolatum gauze) to prevent air entry into the pleural space.

THORACENTESIS

1. Preparation. Assemble proper antiseptic, instruments, gloves, and receptacles. Apply antiseptic to area to be aspirated, as judged by chest x-ray, CT scan, ultrasound, or percussion.
2. Local Anesthetic. Infiltrate with 1/2% or 1% Xylocaine. Take care to anesthetize skin, subcutaneous tissues, periosteum of rib, and especially the pleura. At least 10–20 mL of anesthetic will be required.
3. Aspiration. Using either an Angiocath R or similar plastic catheter, advance the needle just over the top of the rib in question so as to avoid the neurovascular bundle that courses along the lower border of the rib.

   Begin aspiration after the needle is removed, taking care not to allow air into the chest during needle removal. Cessation of respiration is helpful in this regard. A three-way stop-lock or commercial one-way valve facilitates fluid removal.

   Culture, cell count, and chemical studies may be performed on an aliquot of the fluid.

   Postprocedure precautions. A chest x-ray (PA in maximal expiration) should be obtained to ensure absence of pneumothorax. Vagotonia or syncope may occur; patients may need to rest supine.

Study Questions

1. Describe the principles involved with the use of a pulmonary artery catheter to investigate and delineate circulatory status. What are the implications of volume versus pressure measurements?
2. What are the clinical and measurable hallmarks of cardiac tamponade?
3. Describe the sequential workup of a patient with suspected ischemic heart disease. What is the most definitive study?
4. Discuss the indications for coronary revascularization, including symptoms, anatomy, and clinical syndromes.
5. What are the advantages and disadvantages of mechanical and bioprosthetic heart valves?
6. What are the most common acyanotic congenital heart defects? Which have increased pulmonary blood flow and which do not?
7. What are the indications for an artificial pacemaker? Discuss the merits of atrioventricular sequential pacing.
8. How can a diagnosis be made of a mass in the lung? What diagnostic studies are used first?
9. A 24-year-old patient with shortness of breath and evidence of a pneumothorax is presented to you. How would you manage the patient? What would influence you to operate upon him? What procedure would you perform? What is the natural history of this lesion?
10. A patient presents with a painful mass in his sixth rib. How would you proceed to work the patient up? What lesions are in the differential? Describe the definitive procedure.
11. Urgent workup of hemoptysis entails which studies and/or procedures? What are the usual causes? Describe the treatment options for recalcitrant or massive hemoptysis.

7 Orthopedic Surgery: Diseases of the Musculoskeletal System

Eugene E. Berg, M.D.
Larry B. Conochie, M.D.

ASSUMPTIONS

The student has knowledge of the anatomy, physiology, biochemistry, and pathology of the musculoskeletal system (bone, hyaline, and growth plate cartilage; tendon; muscle; and collagen).

The student understands principles of bone and soft tissue repair.

OBJECTIVES

1. Define open and closed fractures, dislocations, and subluxations.
2. Describe the clinical and radiological features of fractures.
3. Outline the management priorities in treating fractures.
4. List the complications of cast immobilization of acute extremity injuries.
5. List and discuss principles of physical rehabilitation of an extremity following immobilization for fracture healing.
6. List vascular, neurological, and musculoskeletal complications commonly associated with fractures.
7. Describe the clinical and radiological features of dislocations and subluxations; outline their treatment.
8. Define and list the symptoms, signs, and diagnostic criteria of a compartment syndrome; discuss its treatment.
9. Discuss common fractures and joint injuries; identify specific problems with their diagnoses and management.
10. Describe the indications and contraindications for replantation of an amputated appendage. Discuss the proper method of transporting the amputated part.
11. Describe the pathophysiology of attritional sports-related injuries as they affect bone, muscle, and tendon.
12. Define the term *sprain* and its three gradations. Explain the methods of diagnosing the common sprains at the knee and ankle.
13. Demonstrate recognition of pediatric musculoskeletal problems such as limb torsion and deformity, flat feet, developmental dysplasia of the hip, slipped femoral capital epiphysis, club foot, Legg-Calvé-Perthes disease, and scoliosis.
14. Describe the symptoms and signs of infectious processes of bone and joints (osteomyelitis and septic arthritis).
15. List and discuss the diagnostic workup used in making a definitive diagnosis of bone or joint infection.
16. Describe the symptoms and signs of inflammatory (noninfectious) joint disease.
17. List and discuss the laboratory and radiological techniques used in making the diagnosis of rheumatoid arthritis and osteoarthritis.
18. List and discuss the nonsurgical and surgical treatment options of degenerative joint disease of the hip, knee, and spine.
19. Describe the pathophysiology of osteonecrosis.
20. List and discuss common causes of low back pain and cervical pain.

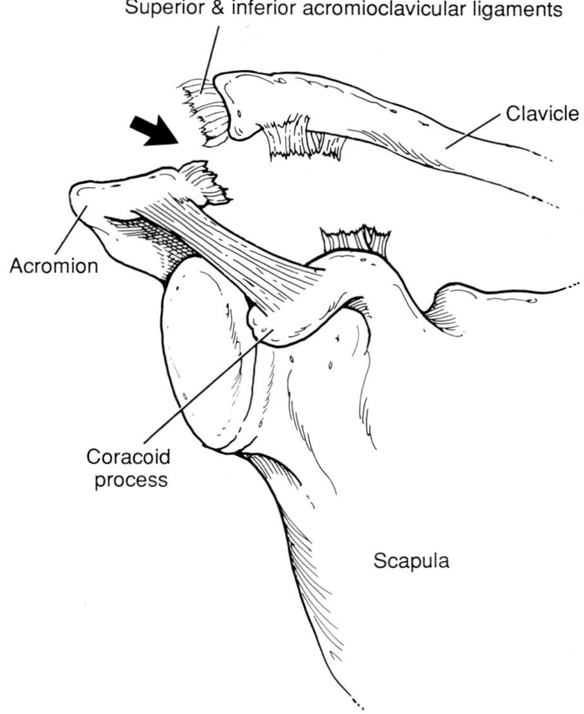

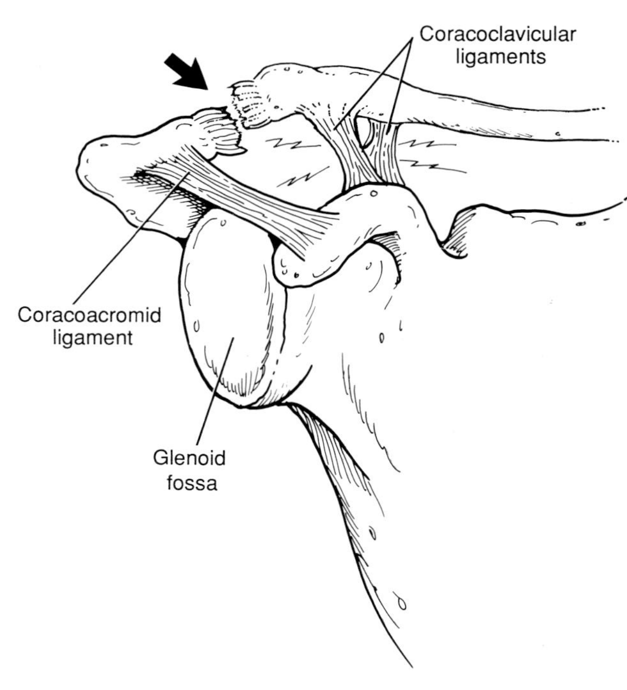

Figure 7.1. **A**, Fracture: a break in continuity of a bone. **B**, Dislocation: complete displacement of apposing joint surfaces. A reduction maneuver is often needed to restore joint alignment. **C**, Subluxation: partial displacement of apposing joint surfaces. This phenomenon may be transient and reduce itself.

21. Describe the symptoms and signs and outline the diagnostic workup for a patient with lumbar or cervical disc herniation.
22. Define osteoporosis and osteomalacia and list common etiologies of each.
23. Discuss the pathophysiology, symptoms, and laboratory and radiographic findings of hyperparathyroidism and Paget's disease.
24. List common primary and secondary malignant neoplasms of bone.
25. Outline the diagnostic workup for a patient with a suspected primary and secondary malignant neoplasm of bone.
26. Describe the basic components of gait and discuss common gait abnormalities in relation to mechanical or neurological disorders.

The musculoskeletal system is composed of connective tissue of mesodermal origin. Bones, joints, muscles, tendons, ligaments, and aponeurotic fascia constitute 70% of total body mass. While afflictions of the musculoskeletal system do not usually affect longevity, they frequently interfere with the quality of life. Musculoskeletal problems are the second most frequent cause of visits to a physician and are second in the consumption of health care dollars. Forty percent of emergency room visits are related to musculoskeletal problems. It is estimated that osteoporosis affects over 20 million premenopausal women and that associated hip fractures occupy almost 20% of surgical hospital beds. Back pain is the most common cause of time lost from work and disability in patients under 45 years of age. The annual cost of treatment and compensation for back conditions is greater than 14 billion dollars. From these impressive statistics, it is clear that a working understanding of the musculoskeletal system is necessary to all physicians, especially those who render primary care.

Fractures, Dislocations, and Subluxations

A fracture is defined as a break or loss of structural continuity in a bone. A dislocation or subluxation alters the normal relationship between joint surfaces. In a dislocation the normally apposing joint surfaces are completely displaced (Fig. 7.18**A**), while in a subluxation those surfaces are partially displaced (Fig. 7.1). Joint subluxation may be a transient phenomenon in which the joint becomes displaced to the verge of dislocation but reduces itself.

Fractures

Description. Knowledge of accepted fracture nomenclature allows for communication between medical

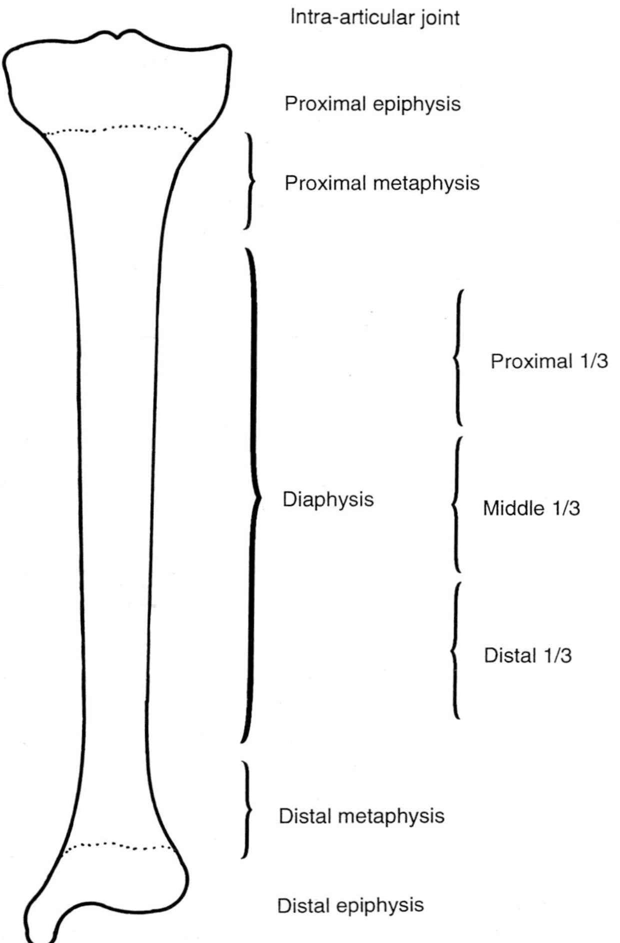

Figure 7.2. Anatomical regions of a long tubular bone.

colleagues and can affect decision making. It is essential that fractures be described in a precise and detailed manner. Fractures are described according to type, site, pattern, and degree of displacement.

Type. Fractures are either *open* or *closed*. A fracture is open (compound) when there is a break in the surrounding skin or mucosa that allows the fracture to communicate with the external environment. While most open fractures are obvious to cursory inspection, others, such as pelvic fractures, may communicate with the rectum or vagina and are only discovered in the course of a thorough physical examination. All open fractures are by definition contaminated and require emergency treatment to prevent infection. A fracture is closed (simple) when the skin or overlying mucosa is intact.

Fractures usually are the result of a single injury. However, repeated submaximal stress can produce microscopic fractures, which, if not allowed to heal, will coalesce into a *stress fracture* (Fig. 7.23). Such fractures are seen in Army recruits or in patients who participate in vigorous athletic training routines. A fracture produced by minimal trauma through abnormal bone is termed a *pathological fracture*. Such fractures occur in bone weakened by metabolic bone diseases such as osteoporosis, or in bone harboring primary or metastatic tumors.

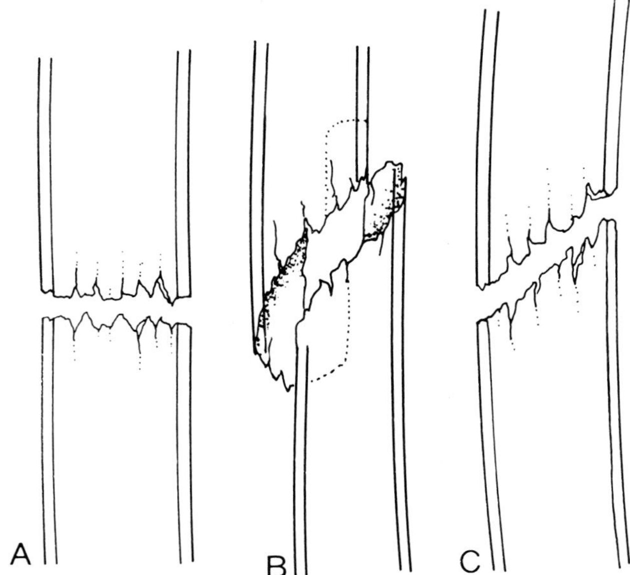

Figure 7.3. Common fracture patterns. **A**, Transverse fracture. **B**, Spiral fracture. **C**, Oblique fracture.

Site. When describing the location of a fracture, the bone affected is identified as well as the specific site involved, such as the proximal or distal epiphysis, metaphysis, or diaphysis (Fig. 7.2). A fracture in the epiphyseal region suggests intra-articular fracture extension that would violate the joint surface and could result in traumatic arthritis. By convention, the diaphysis of a long bone is described in thirds: proximal, middle, or distal (Fig. 7.2). Fracture location has implications for healing. Fractures of metaphyseal or cancellous bone with a rich blood supply and high bone turnover rates usually heal quite rapidly. In contrast, cortical, diaphyseal bone heals more slowly. Diaphyseal fractures, therefore, require lengthier periods of stress protection.

Pattern. The fracture pattern relates to fracture geometry, which suggests the type and amount of kinetic energy imparted to the bone. A *transverse fracture* (Fig. 7.3**A**) is a low-energy injury, usually the result of either a direct blow to a long bone or a ligament avulsion. A "nightstick" fracture is a transverse fracture of the ulna that occurs when the forearm is used to fend off an assault. Stress and pathologic fractures usually have a transverse pattern. *Spiral* or oblique fractures (Figs. 7.3**B** and 7.3**C**) result from a rotatory, twisting injury. These fractures have a tendency to displace after reduction and immobilization. A fracture with more than two fragments is termed *comminuted*. If the middle fragment is triangular, it is sometimes called a butterfly fragment (Fig. 7.4**A**). If cylindrical in configuration, it is described as segmental (Fig. 7.4**B**), which implies a greater degree of damage due to the interruption of the intramedullary blood supply to the bone, and thus healing at one or both fracture sites may be compromised. An *impacted*

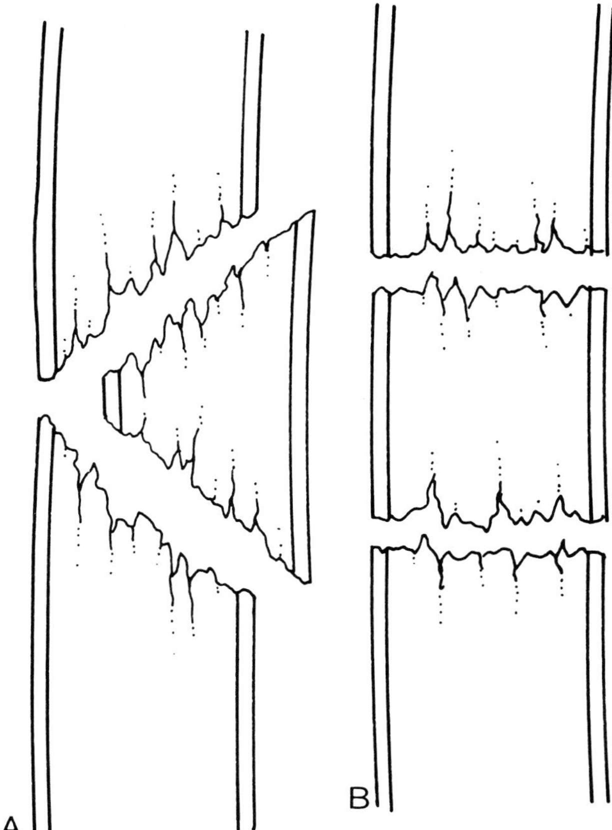

Figure 7.4. **A**, Comminuted fracture with butterfly fragment. **B**, Segmental fracture.

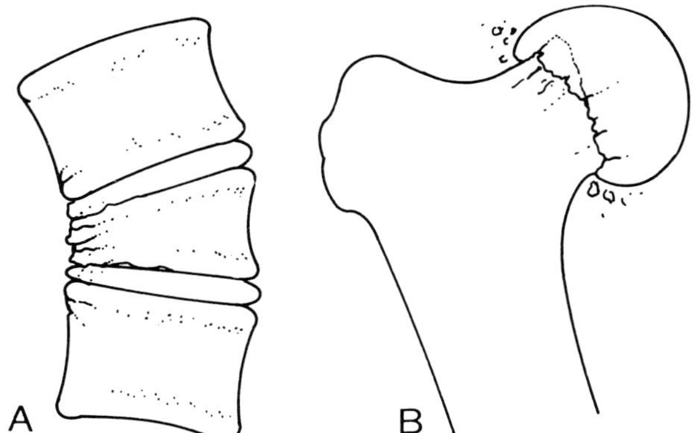

Figure 7.5. **A**, Impacted femoral neck fracture. **B**, Anterior compression fracture of vertebral body.

fracture (Figs. 7.5**A**, 7.16) is commonly seen in metaphyseal bone, such as with femoral neck, distal radius, or tibial plateau fractures. These are low energy injuries in which two bone fragments are jammed together. A *compression fracture* signifies that trabecular or cancellous bone is crushed; it often occurs in vertebral bodies (Fig. 7.5**B**). While most bone fractures are complete, an incomplete buckling of only one cortex is seen in children and is known as a *greenstick* fracture (Fig. 7.6).

Displacement. Fractured bone fragments can be displaced because of force of injury, gravity, or muscle pull. Displacement is described in terms of (*a*) apposition, (*b*) angulation, (*c*) rotation, and (*d*) length (either shortening or distraction).

Apposition and angulation are described in both the mediolateral (coronal) plane and the anteroposterior (sagittal) plane. By convention, the position of the distal fragment is always named relative to the proximal fragment. This convention is helpful because most fractures are aligned by reducing the displaced distal fragment to the proximal one. Fracture displacement is customarily quantified as a percentage (Fig. 7.7). This description can be misleading because 50% posterior (Fig. 7.7**B**) and 50% lateral displacement (Fig. 7.7**A**), may, when viewed in three dimensions, represent only 25% bone apposition (Fig. 7.7**C**). Angulation may be described by one of two conventions. In one, the direction to which the distal fragment is inclined is identified (Fig. 7.8). Alternatively, angulation can be noted by location of the fracture angle apex. Reference to either distal fragment or apical angulation should be mentioned in reports of fracture alignment. In Figure 7.8, for example, the distal fragment is angled or inclined in the posterior and lateral directions, and the fracture apex is angled anteromedially.

The terms *varus* and *valgus* are also used in the descriptions of fractures and postural deformity. They refer to the direction of an angular deformity in relation to the midline of the body. If the deformity apex is pointed away from the midline (Fig. 7.9**A**), the term *varus* is used. When the deformity apex is directed toward the midline (Fig. 7.9**B**), it is called *valgus*. Thus, bowlegs in which the deformity apex at the knee (*genu*) is away from the midline are called *genu varum*, while knock-knees are termed *genu valgum*.

Fracture apposition, angulation, and shortening are quantified in percentage, degrees, and centimeters, respectively, from their radiographic depiction. Although rotation may be discerned radiographically, it usually is more apparent clinically. Rotational deformity is expressed by identifying the position of the distal fragment as it relates to the proximal one. For example, if the foot is twisted outward, the fracture is externally rotated.

Growth Plate Fractures. In children the growth plate (physis) is a zone of cartilage situated between the epiphysis and the metaphysis of long bones. As cartilage is weaker than bone mineral, it is a common site of fracture. The Salter-Harris classification of growth plate injuries is descriptive, generally recognized, with important prognostic implications.

The Salter-Harris type I fracture is a separation of the epiphysis from the metaphysis (Fig. 7.10). If the periosteum is not torn, the fracture may not be displaced. The patient will be tender over the growth plate. The Salter-Harris type II fracture passes through the growth plate and exits through the metaphysis. This fracture is due to a bending movement that tears periosteum on the side opposite the triangular metaphyseal fragment. In a Salter-Harris type III injury the fracture extends from the growth plate through the epiphysis to enter the joint. This fracture is intra-articular and requires a per-

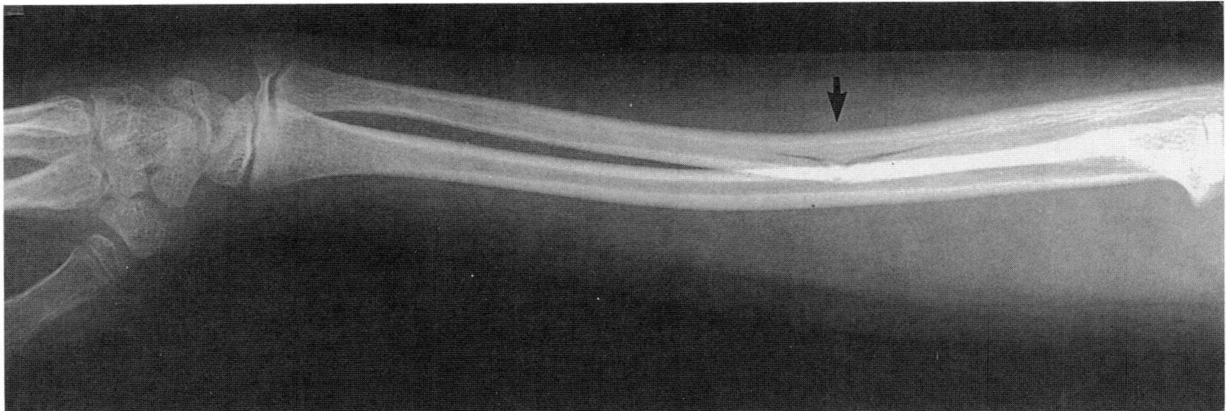

Figure 7.6. Greenstick fracture of the ulna in which only one cortex is broken (arrow) and the bone is bowed with its apex anterior. The fracture must be complete (the other cortex broken) to prevent angular deformity. Greenstick fractures typically occur in children whose bones are more plastic and less brittle than those of adults.

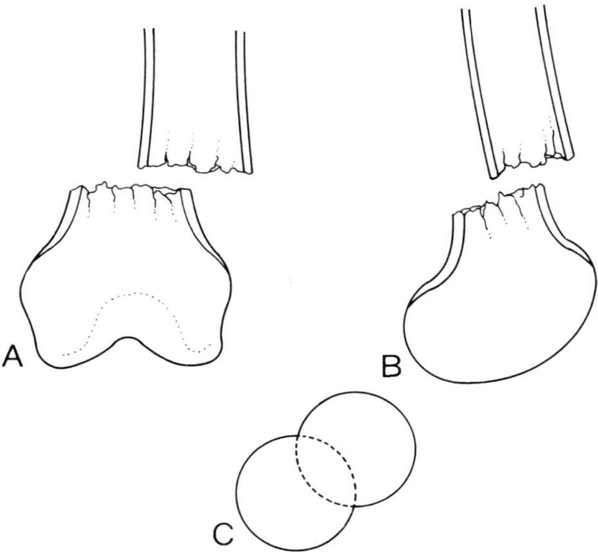

Figure 7.7. Fracture displacement. **A**, The anterior-posterior (AP) view reveals approximately 50% lateral displacement of the distal fragment. **B**, The lateral view demonstrates 50% posterior displacement of the distal femur. **C**, Additively in three dimensions, the amount of bone apposition is approximately 25%, an amount that is underestimated by either **A** or **B** in isolation.

fect reduction. The Salter-Harris type IV fracture line extends from the metaphysis through the growth plate cartilage into the epiphysis. This fracture pattern is also intra-articular. These fractures must be operatively fixed to prevent nonunion and joint surface incongruity. These fractures have the highest incidence of growth disturbance if not properly managed. A Salter-Harris type V fracture involves a crushing of the epiphyseal growth plate. These fractures may appear innocuous on radiographs and therefore are difficult to identify prospectively. The type V injury causes a bony bar to replace the growth plate, which will result in asymmetric, angular growth.

Growth plate injuries, no matter how trivial, have the potential to cause growth disturbance of the involved long bone. The larger Salter-Harris numbers represent greater degrees of violence to the growth plate. Consequently, the type IV fracture has a poorer prognosis and higher incidence of growth disturbance than the type I injury. The possibility of a growth disturbance requires that all growth plate fractures be followed radiographically for at least 1 year after injury.

Evaluation of Patients with Musculoskeletal Trauma. The patient usually presents with a history of injury, although in pathological fractures, as mentioned, the injury might be minimal. In children, either a limp or the refusal to use an extremity should lead the physician to suspect a possible fracture. Symptoms of musculoskeletal injury include pain, swelling, and deformity. Bony tenderness, crepitus, or deformity strongly suggest a fracture. The examiner should inspect the extremity circumferentially for small puncture wounds. Vascular integrity (pulses, capillary return) and neurological status (sensory, motor, and reflex functions) must be assessed and documented. Motion of articulations distal to the fracture site implies an element of soft tissue integrity and neurological function.

A complete radiological evaluation must include the following.

1. Two views at right angles to each other must be taken. Since fractures occur in three dimensions, a solitary x-ray view will not demonstrate enough of the fracture to permit an accurate description (i.e., displacement and angulation) of the injury (Fig. 7.7). Two views taken perpendicular to each other, usually an anterior-posterior (AP) and a lateral view meet these requirements.
2. The joint above and the one below the injured area must be depicted. It is not uncommon for a knee injury or hip fracture to be associated with a fracture of the femoral shaft.

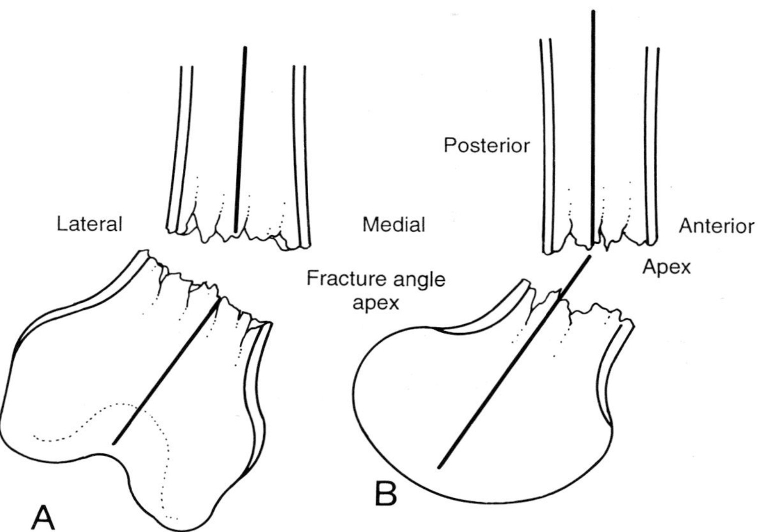

Figure 7.8. **A**, On the anterior-posterior view (coronal plane), the distal fragment is angulated laterally and the fracture angle apex is medial. **B**, On the lateral view (sagittal plane), the distal fragment is angulated posteriorly and the angle apex is anterior.

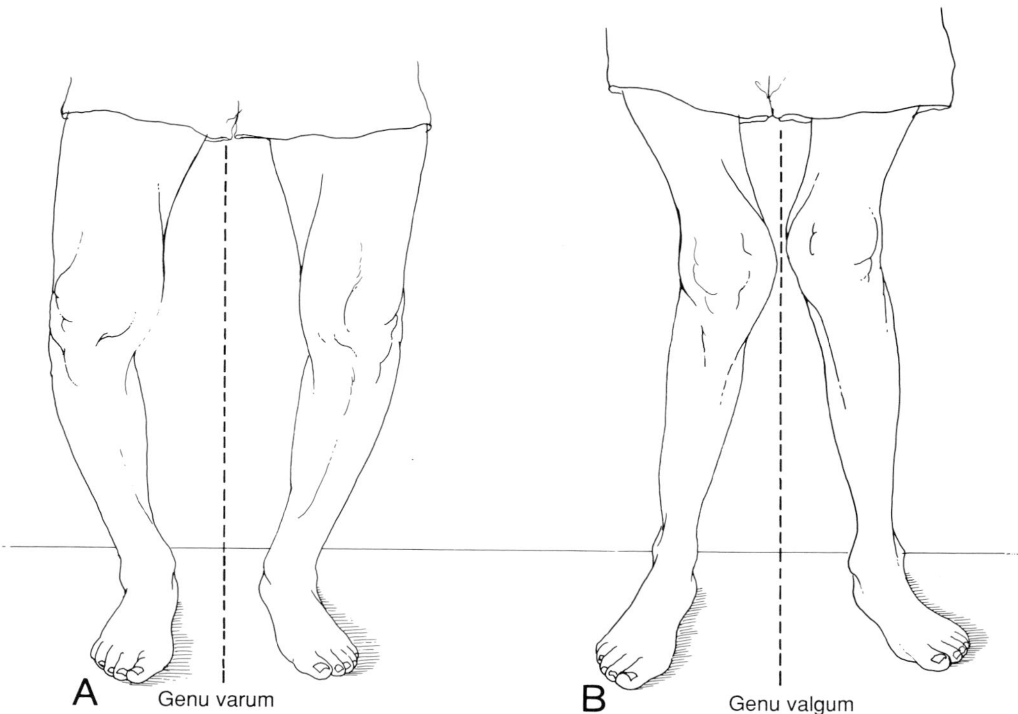

Figure 7.9. The terms "varus" and "valgus" refer to the relation of a deformity to the midline of the body. When the deformity apex is pointing away from the midline, the term "varus" is used: **A**, genu varum or bow legs. When the deformity apex is directed toward the midline, it is called "valgus": **B**, genu valgum or knocked knees. In knocked knees the knee resembles the letter L, which is a helpful mnemonic in distinguishing between these confusing terms.

3. Known injury associations warrant special radiographic examination. For instance, cervical spine x-rays are mandatory in all patients with facial and head injuries. Hip dislocations are associated with dashboard injuries to the knee. Fractures of the axial skeleton (spine and pelvis) should be assessed for concomitant injuries to the thoracic, abdominal, or pelvic viscera as well as neural structures.
4. If a fracture is not evident radiographically but is suspected clinically (such as a scaphoid fracture), the patient will not be harmed if the extremity is treated presumptively as though it were fractured. Repeated x-rays, stress views, or other imaging techniques

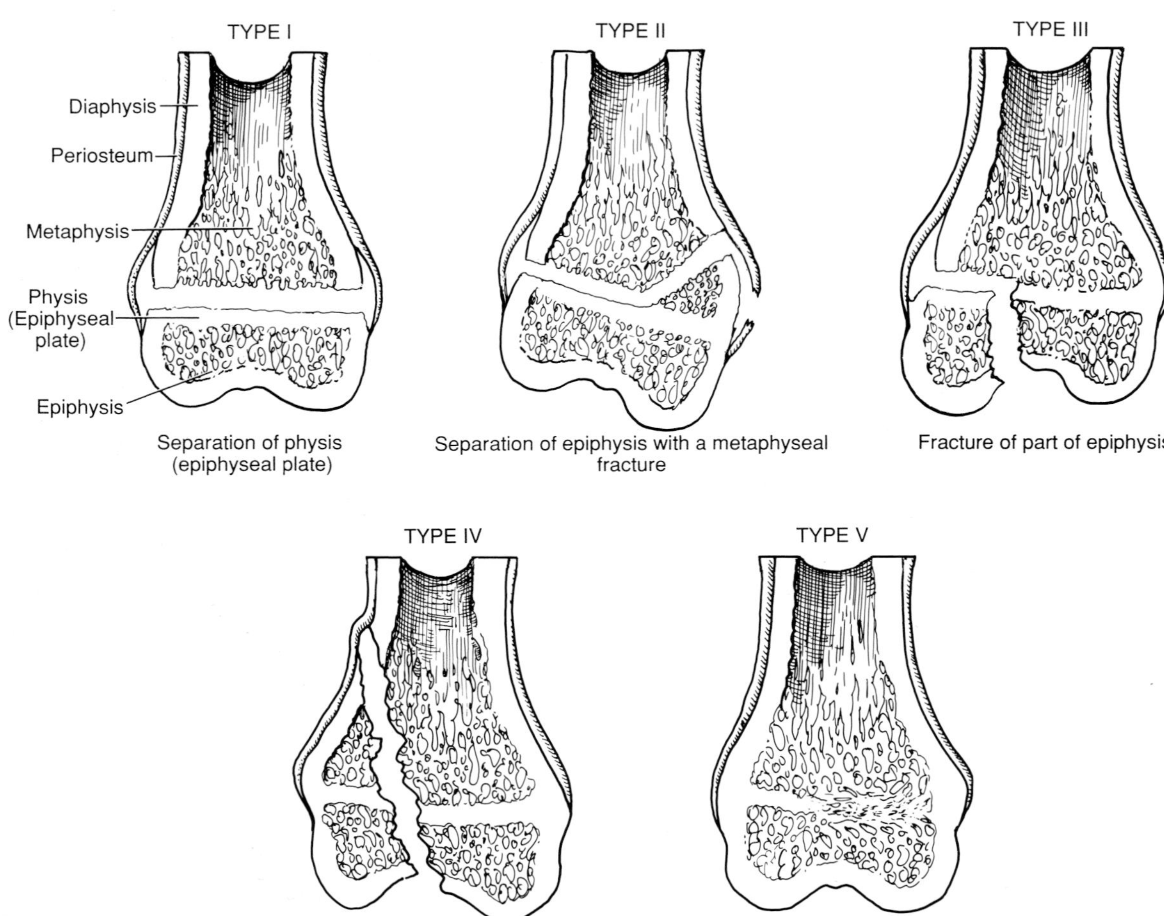

Figure 7.10. Salter-Harris classification of pediatric growth plate fractures. The greater the classification number, the more violent the injury to the epiphyseal plate and the greater the risk of long bone growth and healing problems.

such as polytomography, bone scan, computed tomography (CT), or magnetic resonance imaging (MRI) may be needed to establish the diagnosis.

Principles of Fracture Management. A patient with a fracture should be managed as a traumatized patient (see EGS2, Chapter 14). Life-threatening conditions always receive first treatment priority. It is essential to check the integrity of neural and vascular structures distal to the fracture site. All musculoskeletal injuries must be splinted in the field. Splints are to remain in place whenever the patient is transported. Splinting prevents fracture motion, thus minimizing further damage to the surrounding soft tissues (nerves, blood vessels, and muscle—Fig. 7.17), limits blood loss, and decreases the pain of injury. Proper splinting requires that the joint above and the one below the fracture site be immobilized. Similarly, with a dislocation, the bone above and the one below the joint should be splinted.

All open fractures are considered contaminated and treatment is aimed at preventing subsequent infection. After the extremity has been splinted, a culture is taken from the wound and the wound is covered with a sterile dressing. Tetanus prophylaxis is administered if necessary (see Chapter 4, Diseases of the Skin and Soft Tissue), and antibiotic treatment initiated. The patient is prepared for surgery, preferably under general anesthesia. A 1-mm margin of devitalized skin is excised, with care being taken not to sacrifice viable skin. The wound is extended as needed to expose the bone ends and debride all foreign material and necrotic tissue. Pulsatile irrigation with copious (10 or more liters) amounts of normal saline mechanically flushes the wound which is then left open and a sterile dressing is applied. Only after a thorough irrigation and surgical debridement is an open fracture reduced and immobilized. The wound is reexplored 48–72 hours later for debridement of tissue that was marginally viable at first surgery and has subsequently necrosed. Delayed wound closure or the need for special soft tissue coverage techniques (a myocutaneous or a free microvascular flap) are planned at the "second look" procedure (see Chapter 4, Diseases of Skin and Soft Tissue).

Fracture management requires a knowledge of the stages of fracture healing (Table 7.1). The three principles of fracture care are (*a*) reduction of deformity, (*b*) maintenance of reduction, and (*c*) rehabilitation of function.

Table 7.1.
Stages of Fracture Healing

1. Hematoma formation
2. Inflammation and cellular proliferation
3. Soft callus formation
   Chondrogenic and osteogenic cell proliferation, formation of woven or fiber bone
4. Consolidation (1 to 3 months)
   Transformation of woven bone to lamellar bone
5. Bone resorption (4 to 8 months)
   Callus remodeling, reconstitution of the medullary cavity

Reduction. Fracture deformity is reduced to restore bone apposition and alignment. Reduction can be achieved by closed or open methods. Closed reduction involves the manual manipulation of the fracture into a functional position. Generally, in a closed reduction traction is applied to separate impacted fractures. The deforming forces are then reversed to realign the bone fragments. In an open reduction the fracture is surgically exposed and bone fragments are manipulated directly. Open reduction is indicated when closed reduction methods fail or with intra-articular fractures in which the joint surface must be perfectly restored to prevent the development of traumatic arthritis.

Maintenance of Reduction. Once the fracture has been reduced, alignment must be maintained until the process of bone healing has been completed. Maintaining alignment requires some form of fracture immobilization, which can include casting, traction, functional bracing, and internal or external fixation. The type of immobilization employed depends upon fracture stability or its propensity for displacement. A circumferential plaster or fiberglass cast is the traditional method of immobilization. A cast is not indestructible nor does it confer strength to the fractured bone. A cast merely protects and maintains fracture alignment until healing occurs.

Continuous traction applied through the skin, the skeleton, or by gravity is a technique that can both effect and maintain reduction. With skin traction, a foam rubber appliance is wrapped directly against the skin and traction is applied via friction of the foam-skin interface. The risk of skin breakdown limits the amount of traction that can be used to no more than 7 pounds. Thus skin traction is useful in small children or to temporarily splint an adult with a hip fracture before surgery. Skeletal traction requires that a pin be inserted through bone distal to the fracture site. Large distraction forces can then be applied directly to the bone and can overcome the contractile forces of large muscles in patients with pelvic, femoral, or tibial fractures (Fig. 7.11). A common site for skeletal traction pin placement is the proximal tibia (occasionally, the distal femur or calcaneus); in the upper extremity it is through the olecranon process of the ulna. Gravity acting through a dependent extremity can also act as a traction force. In humeral fractures the weight of the distal arm will apply traction if the body is kept upright (Fig. 7.12**A**). Application of a forearm cast can augment this type of traction (Fig. 7.12**B**).

Several complications are associated with casts and traction. Circumferential bandages may cause circulatory impairment in acutely traumatized limbs in which further swelling is expected. A cast or dressing that is too tight must be completely released despite the adequacy of reduction or inconvenience to the physician. Excessive traction can cause nonunion and peripheral nerve injury. Ulcerative skin problems can occur with both skin and skeletal traction. Skeletal traction causes frictional shearing forces between the patient's sacrum and the bed, which can result in a sacral decubitus ulcer. A poorly applied cast can cause a pressure ulcer over an unsatisfactorily padded bony prominence. Joint stiffness and muscle atrophy are common problems after prolonged immobilization.

Functional braces allow for early joint motion while maintaining fracture alignment through a compressive hydraulic effect on the investing soft tissues. Conversion to a functional brace after early evidence of fracture healing hastens both healing and rehabilitation.

Internal fixation devices include screws, plates (Fig. 7.13), circumferential wires or bands, and intramedullary rods (Fig. 7.14). Indications for internal fixation are listed in Table 7.2. While metallic fracture fixation implants may appear sturdy on x-rays, they, like a cast, are intended simply to position the fracture until healing is complete. Fracture fixation hardware should be considered an internal splint that must respect the biology of fracture healing. The mere presence of an internal fixation device does not guarantee fracture healing. If the fracture does not unite, repetitive (cyclic) loading of a fracture implant will ultimately lead to its loosening or to metal fatigue and breakage. Any time internal fixation is employed, there is a race between fracture healing and implant failure. While internal fixation enhances early patient mobility, it has a host of potential complications. Internal fixation requires a surgical exposure that itself can devitalize tissue and adds to the risk of infection and nonunion. A second surgical procedure is needed if the implant is to be removed. Finally, after hardware removal, the bone can refracture through old screw holes, especially when they are in cortical diaphyseal bone.

External fixation is a minimally invasive method of securing fracture alignment. Small threaded pins are placed into the bone above and below the fracture site and are attached to a strong external frame to immobilize the fracture (Fig. 7.14). Indications for external fixation are listed in Table 7.3. Complications include pin track infection and delayed union.

Joint Dislocation: Diagnosis and Management Dislocations of appendicular joints are often visually apparent. Subluxation of a joint is usually a transient phenomenon and more subtle in presentation. When a joint is dislocated the patient is reluctant to move it. The limb may be held in a typical posture. For example, when a hip is posteriorly dislocated the thigh is held in flexion, adduction, and internal rotation. Neurovascular structures, in close proximity to joints, are frequently injured with dislocations, especially in older patients whose arteries may be thickened by atherosclerotic plaque. Not all vascular injuries are acute occlusive phenomena. Omi-

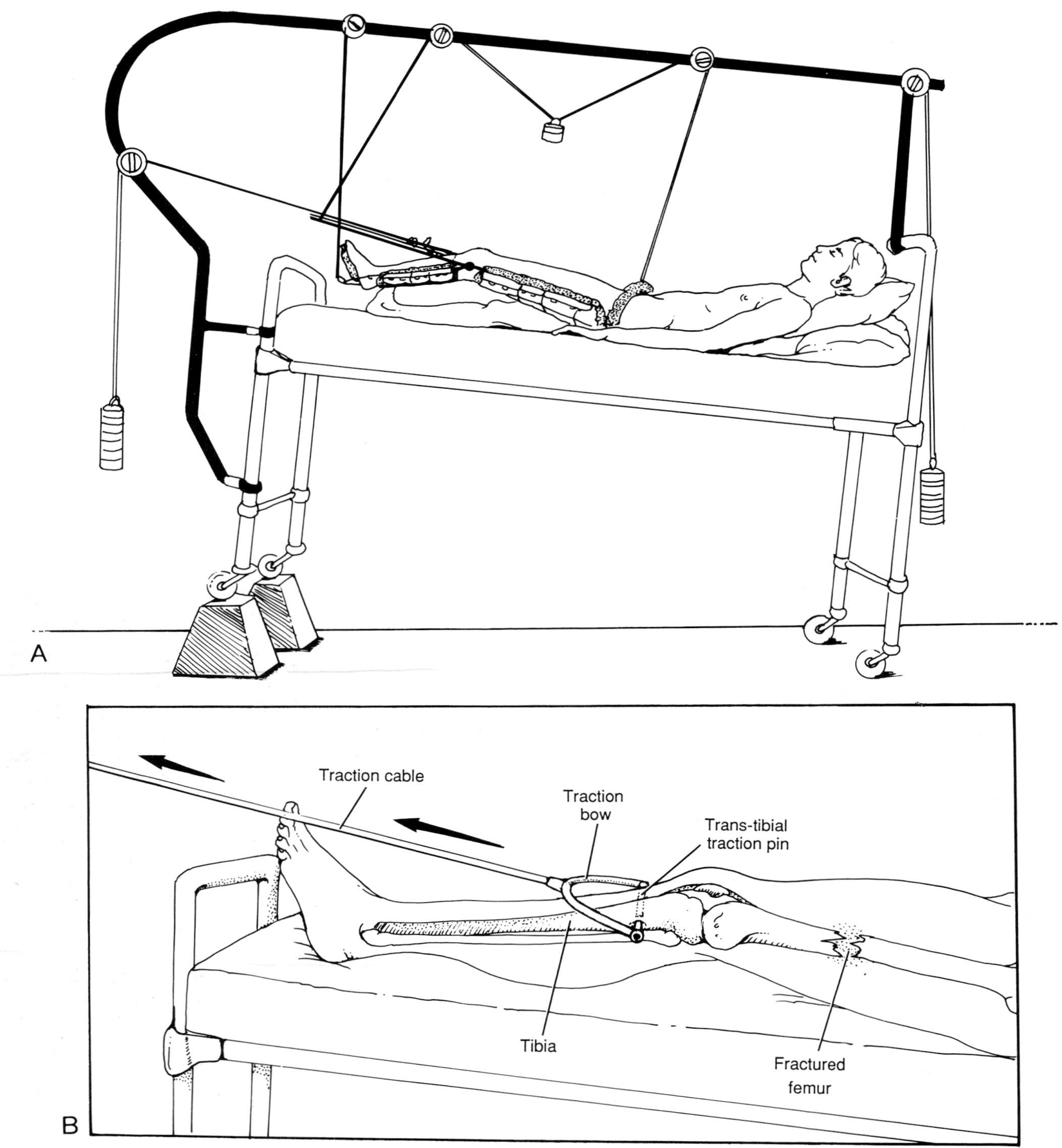

Figure 7.11. Skeletal traction applied through a pin placed in the tibia is useful for treating femur or pelvic fractures. The leg is supported in a suspension apparatus and the foot of the bed is raised to permit the body to act as countertraction.

nously, a partial arterial injury may slowly cause thrombus formation, delaying the presentation of vascular compromise. Serial neurovascular evaluations are essential before and after the reduction of a joint dislocation. Any asymmetry in pulses (detected by palpation or by Doppler ultrasonography) warrants further vascular workup, especially in young patients who have had little stimulus to develop collateral circulation.

Radiographs of the involved joint are obtained in the dislocated posture. This x-ray demonstrates the pathology and allows the treating physician to infer which specific ligamentous structures are damaged.

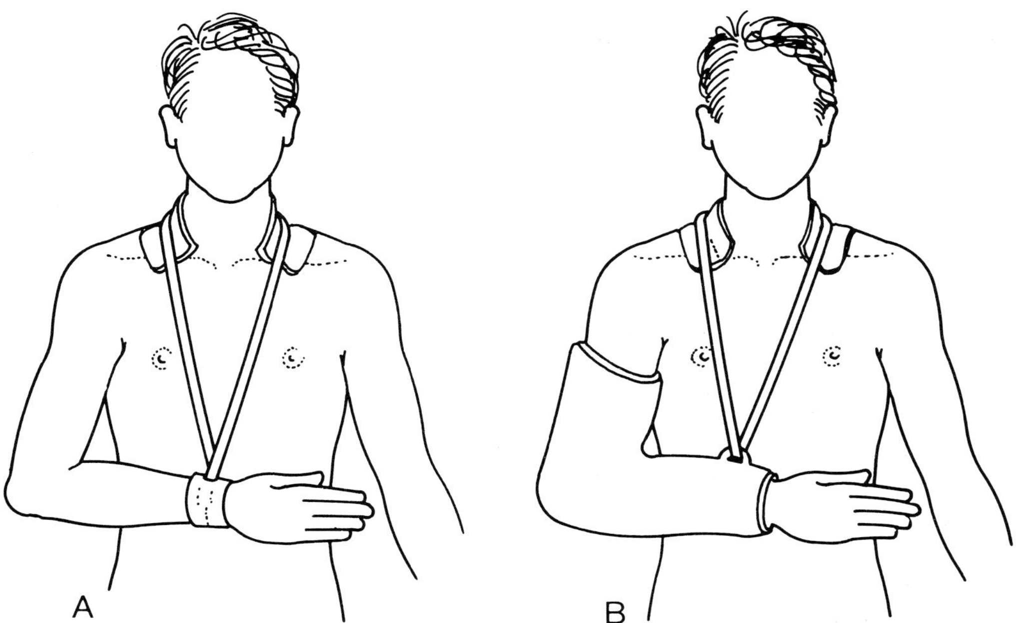

Figure 7.12. Gravity traction. **A**, With collar and cuff. **B**, With hanging cast.

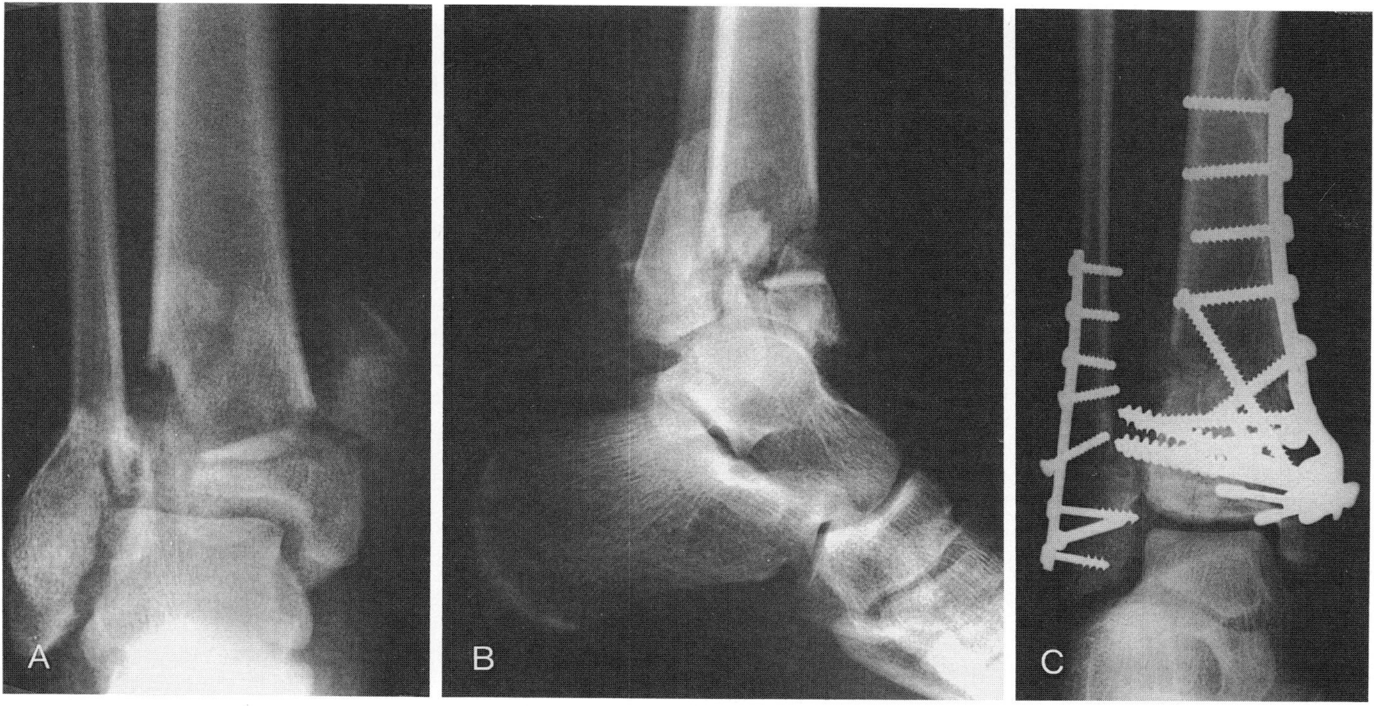

Figure 7.13. **A**, AP and **B**, lateral x-ray of a comminuted ankle fracture. This intra-articular fracture was treated with a complex array of internal fixation plates and screws (**C**).

Like a fracture, a dislocation can be described as open or closed and according to the position of the distal fragment relative to the proximal fragment. If radiographic assessment will be delayed and if skin is compromised (as in an ankle fracture-dislocation), or if neurovascular integrity is in question (as in knee dislocations), then reduction should be attempted.

Dislocations are usually reduced by closed methods. Occasionally, bone or soft tissue may be interposed between joint surfaces and will require a surgical (open) reduction. Postreduction radiographs must be taken to

Table 7.2.
Indications for Internal Fixation of a Fracture

Failure of nonoperative reduction methods
Anatomical reduction of intraarticular fractures
Fractures not amenable to traction or cast immobilization (such as femoral neck fractures or intertrochanteric fractures in the elderly)
Pathological fractures
Multiple fractures in the same extremity or same patient
Fractures in paraplegics (to assist nursing care)

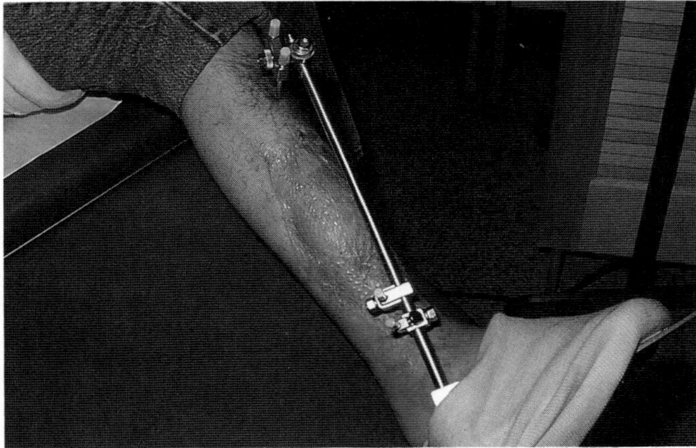

Figure 7.14. Severely comminuted open tibia fracture treated with an external fixator. This form of fixation immobilizes the fracture while permitting access to the wound for observation and care.

Table 7.3.
Indications for External Fixation of a Fracture

Open, unstable fractures to allow access and care of the wound and avoid the use of internal fixation devices in contaminated wounds
Infected fractures
Unstable pelvic fractures
Severely comminuted or unstable fractures not amenable to internal fixation
Fractures involving bone loss in which bone length must be maintained until a bone graft can be performed

assure the adequacy of reduction and rule out a concomitant fracture.

Rehabilitation of Function. Rehabilitation planning begins with the initial phases of fracture management. To avoid joint stiffness common to peri- and intra-articular fractures, the limb is immobilized in a position of maximum function. Isometric exercises of immobilized muscles are started to avoid excessive atrophy. Range of motion exercises for adjacent joints that are not immobilized are encouraged from the onset of care. After a cast or brace is removed, active range of motion and resistive muscle strengthening exercises are started.

The speed of rehabilitation depends upon the rate and quality of fracture healing. Overly exuberant rehabilitative activities or exercises can result in delayed healing, implant failure, and loss of reduction. Thus a rational rehabilitation plan acknowledges those factors that influence the speed and success of fracture healing, such as the amount of energy imparted to the bone (comminuted, open, and displaced fractures all heal slowly), the type of bone involved (cancellous or cortical), the integrity of the soft tissue envelope, and the patient's general health and age (children heal more rapidly than adults).

Bone healing is evaluated by two methods, one clinical and the other radiologic. Clinical healing is evident when the fracture is no longer tender to palpation or stress. Radiographic healing occurs when distinct bony trabeculae are seen crossing the site.

Complications

Local. Local bone complications include infection, delayed union, nonunion, malunion, avascular necrosis, and, in children, growth disturbance. Fractures that are open, either from injury or surgical intervention, have a higher incidence of infection than closed fractures. When fracture healing exceeds the usual timetable but still appears to be taking place, the bone is considered to have a delayed union. When fracture healing is incomplete and nonprogressive, the bone is considered to have a nonunion. The ununited fracture gap may be filled with fibrous tissue or, if subjected to a lot of motion, may form a synovial membrane with joint fluid called a pseudarthrosis, which acts like a "false joint." Delayed unions and nonunions are caused by fracture separation, soft tissue interposition, excessive fracture motion, inadequate vascularization of the fracture segments, or an infectious process. When a fracture heals with a deformity that causes cosmetic or functional impairment, it is called a malunion. Shortening, angulation, or rotational deformities constitute malunion and require surgical refracture (osteoclasis) or corrective osteotomy.

Avascular necrosis occurs when the blood supply to a bone is injured by the traumatic event (see Bone Necrosis later in this chapter). Bones that are extensively covered by articular cartilage and have a minimal muscular envelope are particularly vulnerable to osteonecrosis, for example, the femoral head after a femoral neck fracture or hip dislocation, and scaphoid or talus fractures.

Growth disturbance is a fracture complication specific to children. The epiphyseal plate is composed of cartilage and is the site of longitudinal growth. As cartilage is weaker than bone mineral, the growth plate is often involved in pediatric fractures. Understandably, fractures in children may damage the growth plate, especially by compressive or shearing mechanisms. When the entire growth plate is damaged, growth will cease and cause limb shortening. If only part of the epiphyseal plate is damaged, the bone will grow asymmetrically and cause an angular deformity. A growth plate injury can be detected only by serial x-rays. Most growth plate problems can be identified by x-rays taken at the 1-year anniversary of the injury, a date that parents should be made to remember. Lower limb shortening of less than 1 cm is well tolerated. Between 1 and 2 cm can be managed by a shoe lift. A leg length discrepancy of more than 2 cm can be corrected by fusion of the opposite growth plate, a procedure known as epi-

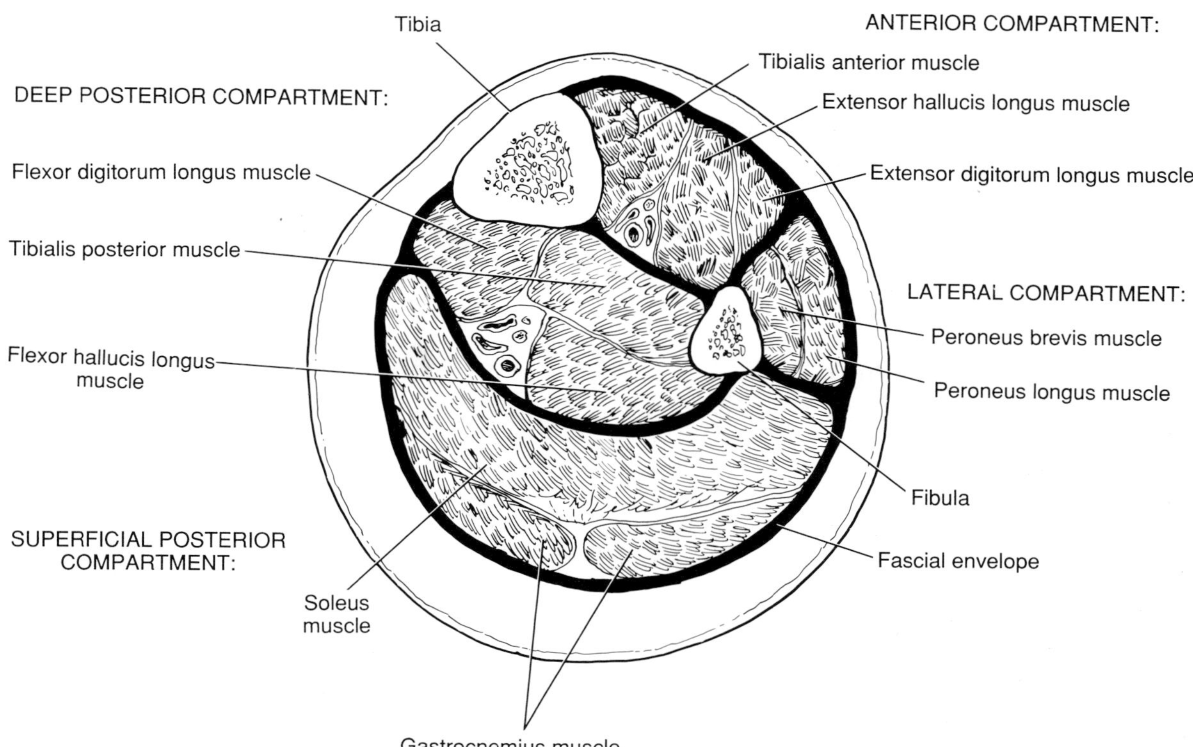

Figure 7.15. Four distinct leg compartments are separated by thick, unyielding fascial planes.

physiodesis. The timing of this procedure is calculated from growth tables. Angular deformity from a partial growth plate arrest is managed surgically and is best handled when diagnosed early.

Posttraumatic arthritis is a complication of intra-articular joint surface fractures. Articular cartilage has no blood supply and depends on synovial fluid diffusion for cellular nourishment. Therefore when injured, cartilage mounts a minimal healing response and usually suffers some permanent damage. The hyaline cartilage joint surface has a low coefficient of friction; however, if interarticular fractures are not perfectly restored, the irregular surface will cause rapid arthritic change.

Arthritis can also develop from a severe angular deformity. Weight-bearing forces will be unevenly distributed upon the joint, causing abnormal stress concentration and joint wear. Depending upon the magnitude of injury, posttraumatic arthritis can occur rapidly or slowly over a decade or more. Patients who have had a traumatic hip dislocation, for example, usually develop hip arthritis in their fifties, one decade before the usual onset of this condition in their peers.

Systemic. Systemic complications usually result from trauma in general and not from the fracture itself. They include shock, sepsis, tetanus (in open injuries), gas gangrene, venous thrombosis, pulmonary embolism, and fat embolism. The emergent stabilization of spine, pelvic, and long bone fractures is necessary to allow a patient to sit upright and receive proper pulmonary physiotherapy; this been shown to significantly decrease the incidence of respiratory insufficiency in multisystem trauma patients.

Compartment Syndrome

Muscles, nerves, and blood vessels are housed in osseo-fascial compartments (Fig. 7.15). Fascia, composed of fibrous collagen and having limited extensibility, focuses the contraction of a muscle and contributes to muscle strength. Bleeding and tissue swelling cause increased compartment pressure within the unyielding osseo-fascial envelope. Capillary blood flow to muscle and nerve is thus reduced, causing local acidosis, cell injury, and further edema. Compartment pressures can become so elevated that muscle and nerve necrosis result. Dead fibrotic muscle will cause joint contractures, and the insensate limb will be totally dysfunctional.

A compartment syndrome can be caused by fractures, severe muscle contusions, crush injuries, and even casts. Fractures associated with unyielding compartments that are likely to cause compartmental syndrome should therefore be observed closely; they include supracondylar distal humerus (Fig. 7.17), double bone (radius and ulna) forearm, and proximal third tibia fractures.

The classic signs of a compartment syndrome are described by the "4 Ps": *pain*, *paresthesia*, *paralysis*, and *pallor*. Pain is intense and usually out of proportion to the injury. It is intensified on passive stretching of the muscles within the suspected compartment. As nerve ischemia progresses, paresthesias involving the nerve within the compartment are noted and later paralysis occurs. Pallor is apparent because of decreasing blood flow. A fifth P, pulselessness, is mentioned only to con-

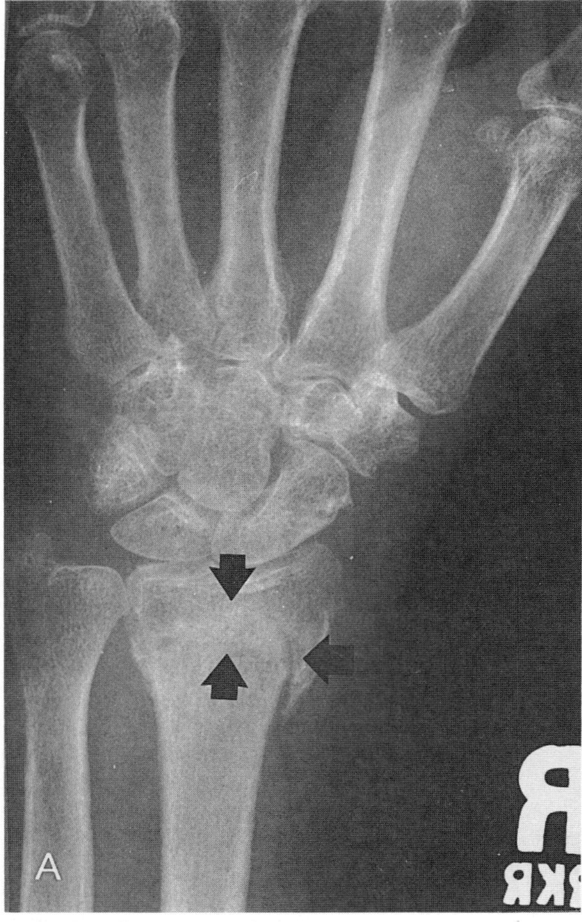

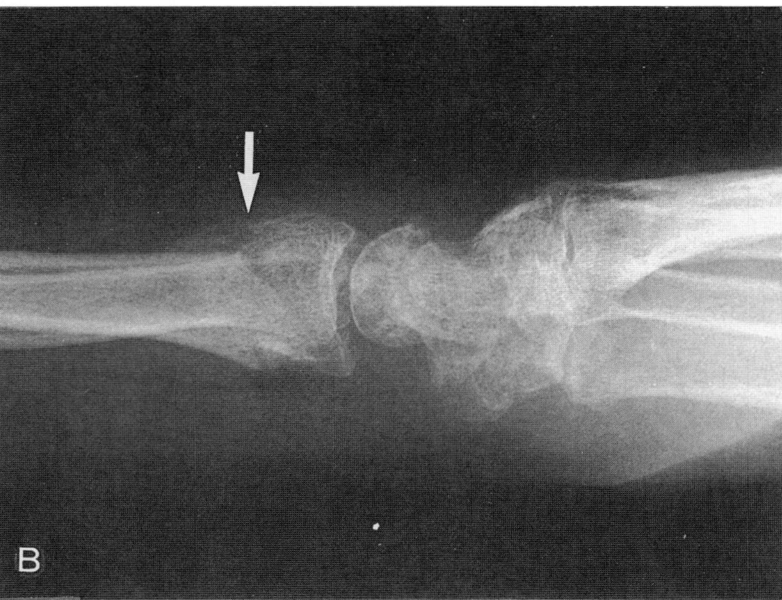

Figure 7.16. Colles' fracture of the distal radius is common to osteoporotic patients. The fracture occurs from a fall on an outstretched dorsiflexed hand. The AP view (**A**) demonstrates the impaction and shortening of the distal fragment (arrows). The lateral x-ray (**B**) shows the dorsal cortex of the radius to be comminuted and impacted, which results in apex palmar angulation.

demn it as a sign. A full-blown compartment syndrome can occur and the pulse will still be present. Systolic arterial pulse pressures are usually much higher than the 30 mm Hg interstitial compartment pressure at which myonecrosis begins to occur.

A high index of suspicion and unaccountable pain are sufficient to initiate removal of all circular bandages or casts. One need not wait for paresthesia, paralysis, or pallor. Decompression by open fasciotomy is indicated if compartment pressure is greater than 30–40 mm Hg in an unconscious or paralyzed patient. (Compartment syndrome is also discussed in Chapters 4, Skin and Soft Tissue, and 8, Neurosurgery.

Common Fractures, Dislocations, and Ligament Injuries

Upper Extremity

Carpal Scaphoid Fracture. A fracture through the waist of the scaphoid usually occurs after a fall on the outstretched hand, with the wrist positioned in dorsiflexion and radial deviation. If a fracture is suspected both from the mechanism of injury and tenderness in the anatomical snuff box, the patient should be treated as if there were a fracture, even though radiographic views do not indicate a fracture. A bone scan or follow-up radiographs at 7–14 days will prove or disprove the diagnosis. The scaphoid bone is extensively covered by hyaline cartilage and has limited soft tissue attachments and blood supply. Complications of avascular necrosis, delayed union, and nonunion are increased by failure to treat a scaphoid fracture initially. Treatment consists of a below-elbow cast with the wrist slightly dorsiflexed; the thumb, in the pinch position, is incorporated in plaster to the interphalangeal joint. This cast is known as a thumb spica cast.

Colles' Fracture. A Colles' fracture is also due to a fall on an outstretched hand. This mechanism causes a transverse fracture of the distal radius just proximal to the wrist. It is a common fracture in elderly osteoporotic patients. Radiographically, dorsal comminution can be noted and the distal fragment is impacted and shortened with apex volar angulation. The ulnar styloid is often fractured (Fig. 7.16).

The reduction maneuver recreates the hyperextension wrist deformity. Manual traction then is applied to

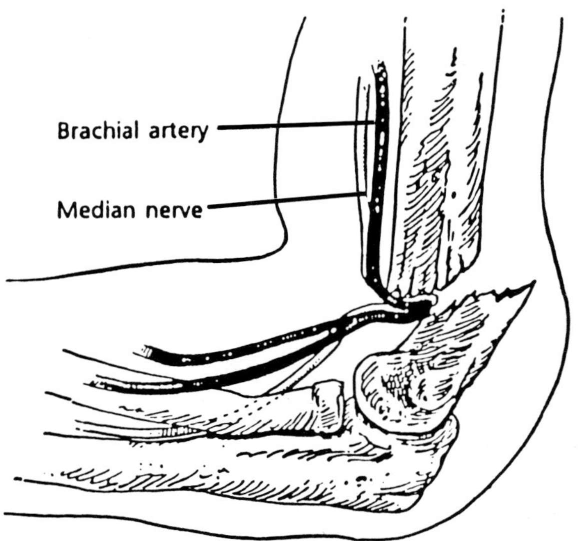

Figure 7.17. The dangerous supracondylar distal humerus fracture may entrap the brachial artery and the median and radial nerves. This fracture is associated with forearm compartment syndrome and warrants cautious and frequent neurovascular monitoring.

the hand, disimpacting the fracture. The wrist and distal fragment are manipulated into flexion and ulnar deviation to correct the dorsal and radial displacement. The deformity tends to recur because of dorsal cortical comminution. Occasionally, a Kirschner or K-wire is inserted percutaneously to prevent loss of fracture alignment.

Following reduction, a cast is applied from the elbow to the palm. A repeat radiograph should be taken at approximately 10 days to assess whether the reduction has been maintained. If it has not, a repeat manipulation or external fixation is required.

Because the median nerve is in close proximity to the fracture, it may be injured. Its function must be documented before and after fracture manipulation. A common complication of a Colles' fracture in the elderly is the "shoulder-hand syndrome," in which shoulder and finger stiffness results from disuse during the treatment period. Patients are therefore encouraged to exercise these joints while the wrist is immobilized by the cast.

Olecranon Fracture. An olecranon fracture usually occurs after a fall in which there is a direct blow to the point of the elbow. The fracture is displaced by contraction of the triceps muscle. Thus, there is loss of active elbow extension necessary for crutch use and pushing. The fracture also involves the elbow joint surface. Any displacement requires an open reduction to restore the articular surface and triceps integrity.

Supracondylar Humerus Fracture. The supracondylar humerus fracture is dangerous and is seen in children between 5 and 10 years of age. It also occurs from a fall on an outstretched hand with the elbow extended. The distal fragment is usually displaced posteriorly and can entrap the brachial artery and the median and radial nerves either at injury or upon reduction (Fig. 7.17). This fracture is at notorious risk for the development of a forearm compartment syndrome (Volkmann's ischemic contracture) and needs to be treated with great care and vigilance.

Shoulder Dislocation. The shoulder is the most frequently dislocated joint in the body. In more than 90% of cases the humeral head is dislocated anterior to the scapular glenoid fossa (Fig. 7.18**A**). The axillary nerve and artery can be endangered by this injury. The integrity of the axillary nerve should be documented before and after reduction of the shoulder dislocation. An anterior shoulder dislocation occurs with the shoulder in the position of vulnerability—abduction and external rotation—from a blow on the anterior arm. Such an injury would occur from an arm tackle in football or from blocking a basketball shot.

Reduction can be effected by gradual shoulder abduction while longitudinal traction is placed upon the arm and counter traction is placed through the axilla with a sheet (Fig. 7.18**B**). Sedation and muscle relaxation facilitate the manipulation.

Posterior shoulder dislocations, although rare, are often missed because of improper interpretation of the AP radiograph, which appears to show the humeral head aligned with the glenoid. An axillary lateral view, however, will show posterior displacement of the humeral head, demonstrating the principle that two radiographs taken in perpendicular planes are needed for proper x-ray evaluation. Clinically, the arm is held internally rotated and cannot be externally rotated beyond the neutral position. A posterior dislocation should be considered in all patients with shoulder symptoms following an epileptic seizure or an electrocution because of the overpowering strength of the shoulder internal rotators.

Lower Extremity

Hip Fractures. Low energy hip fractures are common in elderly osteoporotic patients, accounting for about one-third of admissions to large orthopedic centers. The two most common types are femoral neck (Fig. 7.5**A**) and intertrochanteric hip fractures (Fig. 7.19). In both fractures, the affected limb will be externally rotated and shortened. The patient will be unable to bear weight and slight amounts of hip motion will cause pain.

The blood supply to the femoral head comes from retinacular vessels that run along the femoral neck. These vessels can be damaged by a femoral neck fracture. When this happens, the femoral head can undergo avascular necrosis, which when subjected to weight-bearing loads will collapse and fragment. Similarly, since the femoral neck is an intracapsular bone with a thin periosteum and no muscle envelope, this fracture has a high incidence of nonunion.

An intertrochanteric hip fracture is extracapsular and will invariably heal (Fig. 7.19**A**). Intertrochanteric fractures are reduced under radiographic guidance and fixed with a sliding screw and side-plate device (Fig. 7.19**B**). Femoral neck fractures are either reduced and surgically fixed or, because of attendant complications,

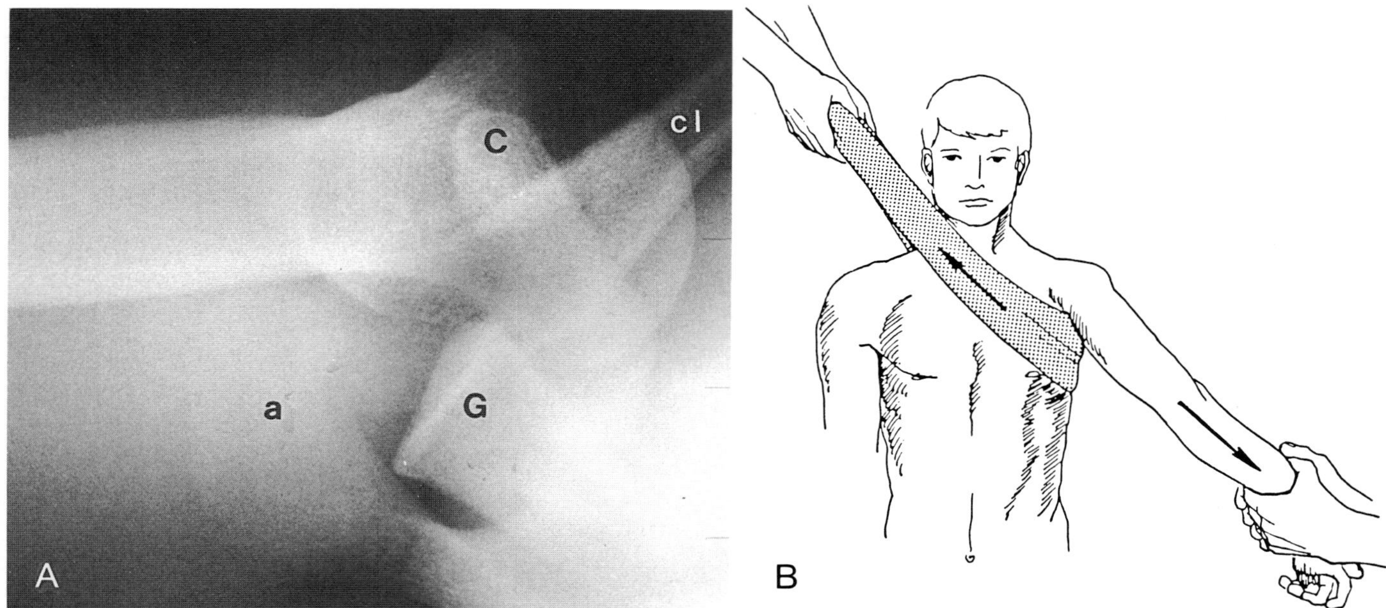

Figure 7.18. **A**, Axillary lateral x-ray of an anterior shoulder dislocation (a = acromion, cl = clavicle). The humeral head lies out of the glenoid fossa (G). The coracoid process (C) is an anterior scapular structure and orients the film. **B**, Closed reduction of an anterior shoulder dislocation via traction countertraction.

replaced with a metallic hemi-joint in patients with decreased life expectancies. Surgical treatment allows for early patient mobilization and decreases problems related to prolonged bed confinement, such as pneumonia, thrombophlebitis, and decubitus ulcers.

Femoral Shaft Fractures. The femoral shaft is the strongest bone in the body. In young patients, femur fractures require high-energy trauma and are incurred by motor vehicle accidents and falls from heights. Blood loss may be considerable. In a closed fracture, 1 to 3 units of blood may be lost into the thigh, and the patient may present in hypovolemic shock. Other sources of hypovolemia, such as intra-abdominal and intrathoracic injuries, or pelvic fractures, must be excluded. In all patients with a fractured femur, the pelvis and hip must be assessed radiologically to rule out associated fractures or dislocations. Knee ligament injuries are possible and should be assessed.

Closed fractures of the femur were traditionally treated by skeletal traction. This technique required prolonged periods (months) of bed rest immobilization, with the attendant morbidity of venous thrombosis, knee stiffness, quadriceps contracture, generalized muscle atrophy, and disuse osteoporosis. A newer technique, closed interlocked intramedullary nailing, has become the treatment of choice (Fig. 7.20). Because the rod can be locked proximally and distally, the fracture can be rendered quite stable and allow early ambulation. The prolonged bed rest required by skeletal traction with its subsequent morbidity can thus be avoided.

Hip Dislocation. Hip dislocation commonly occurs after a deceleration injury in which the knee strikes the dashboard. Seated posture places the hip in adduction and 90° of flexion. The axial load of unrestrained dashboard impact drives the hip posteriorly out of the acetabular socket. A sciatic nerve traction palsy is frequently associated with the dislocation and can cause a foot drop.

Tibia/Fibular Shaft Fracture. Shaft fractures of the tibia and fibula occur nine times more frequently than femoral shaft fractures. Almost one-third of the tibial surface is subcutaneous. For this reason, tibia fractures are often open and contaminated. The limited blood supply to the tibia causes fractures of this bone to have healing difficulties. Tibia fractures are often complicated by a compartment syndrome that requires attentive observation and early diagnosis. Complications related to tibia fracture management are the number one cause of trauma-related orthopedic malpractice suits.

Closed reduction and above-knee cast immobilization are the usual treatment for uncomplicated tibia fractures. Open reduction and internal fixation are considered only when an acceptable reduction cannot be achieved by closed means or the reduction cannot be maintained by a plaster cast. External fixation represents a significant advance in managing open fractures of the tibia: stability and alignment of the fracture fragments are maintained as is access to treat the soft tissue wound.

Ankle Injuries. Ankle injuries are common in young, athletic individuals and may involve both ligamentous and bony structures. The ankle is a mortise and tenon joint. The three-sided mortise is composed of tibial malleolus, tibial plafond (ceiling), and the fibular malleolus. The talus represents the tenon. The mechanism of injury can be inferred from the plane of the

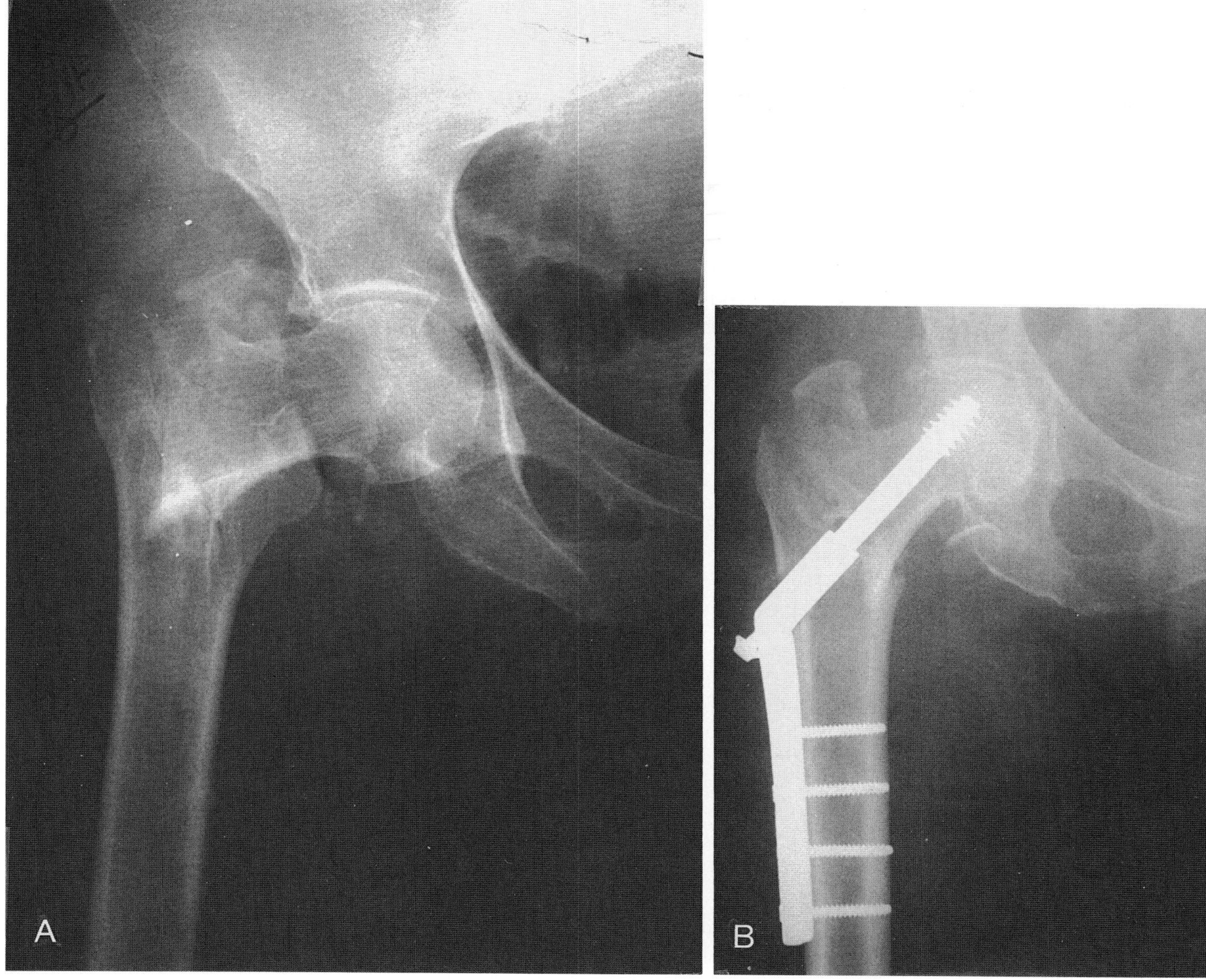

Figure 7.19. **A**, Intertrochanteric hip fracture. The bone is osteopenic and rarefied. **B**, This fracture has been reduced and internally fixed with a screw and sideplate device. This type of fixation will permit early patient mobilization.

fracture line (Fig. 7.21). A transverse fracture line occurs from a tensile or "pulling off" force. Thus, when the medial malleolus fracture is transverse, it suggests an abduction (eversion or pronation) force of the foot on the leg (Fig. 7.21**B**, **C**). If the lateral malleolus fracture is transverse, the force applied to the foot is adduction (inversion or supination—Fig. 7.21**A**). A spiral fracture configuration implies a rotatory force. A coronal plane spiral fracture is a common lateral malleolar fracture pattern and is seen when the foot is externally rotated on the leg and body (Fig. 7.21**C**). Bimalleolar ankle fractures are common. When a posterior tibial fragment is seen on the lateral x-ray, it is called a trimalleolar fracture and results from vertical loading of the plantar flexed ankle (Fig. 7.21**D**).

Since ankle fractures are intra-articular, anatomic restoration of the joint congruity is an essential treatment principle. One millimeter of ankle displacement can reduce joint surface contact by 40%. Therefore, a perfect open reduction with internal fixation is required.

Spinal and Pelvic Fractures. Spinal and pelvic fractures in young people result from high velocity trauma and are associated with intrathoracic, intra-abdominal, and extremity injuries. In the elderly, spine fractures can occur after minimal trauma in bone weakened by osteoporosis or tumor.

Spinal Fractures. Spinal stability is the critical concept in the treatment of spinal fractures. The spine is unstable if unprotected movement will cause fracture displacement that can compromise the integrity of neural structures. In all cases of suspected spinal injury, a complete and detailed baseline neurological assessment should be performed and documented as soon as the patient's condition permits. In unconscious patients or in those with any injuries above the level of the clavicle (facial), the cervical spine is presumed to be injured un-

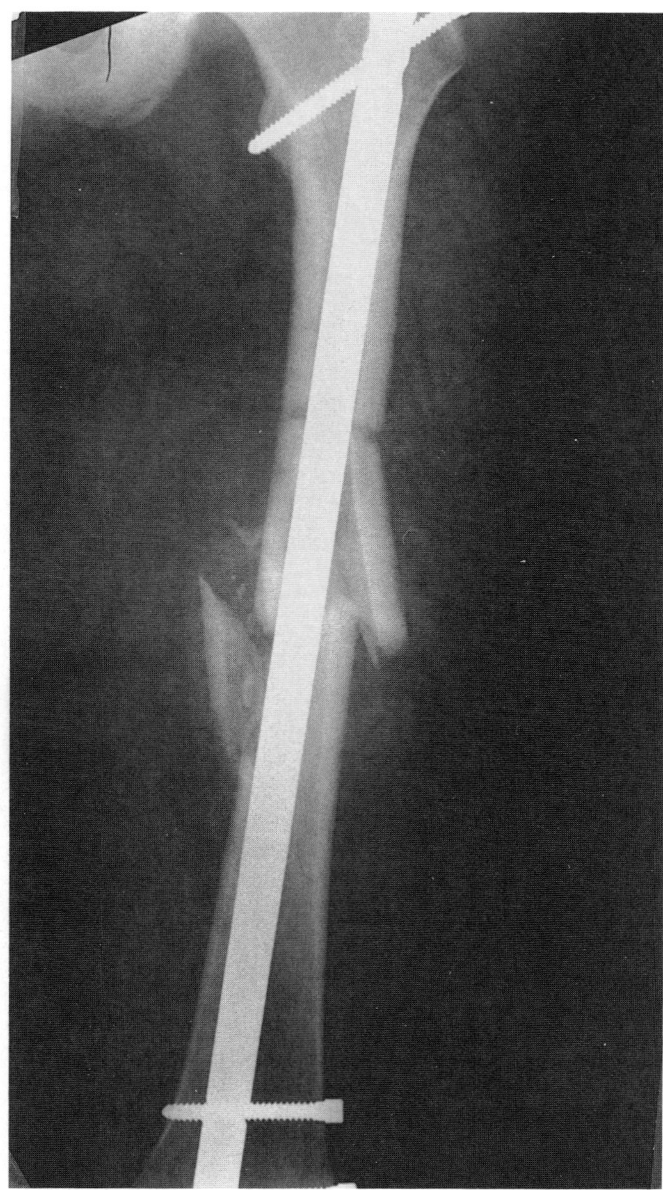

Figure 7.20. Comminuted femoral shaft fracture after internal fixation with an interlocked intramedullary nail.

til proven otherwise (see EGS2, Chapter 14). Patients with minor wedge compression fractures (Fig. 7.5**B**) of the lower thoracic or lumbar spine often develop an ileus from retroperitoneal bleeding and should not be fed enterally until the ileus has resolved. If paraplegia results from a catastrophic spinal column injury, the signs of other injuries will obviously be masked by the lack of sensation. A systematic and thorough examination of all vital structures must therefore be carried out in paraplegics. The patient with suspected spine trauma is properly splinted in a cervical collar with the head secured by taped sandbags; the thorax, abdomen, and extremities are strapped to a spine board. Consultation with a neurosurgeon or an orthopedic surgeon is indicated if the physician has any doubt about the stability of the spine injury.

Pelvic Fractures. The pelvis facilitates body weight transfer through the sacroiliac joints and acetabula in stance, and through the ischial spines in seated postures. The pelvis also confers bony protection to the lower abdominal and genitourinary tracts. The pelvis houses the extensive vascular arborizations of the iliac vessels and the lumbosacral plexus of nerves. Pelvic fractures usually occur with high velocity blunt trauma and can therefore be associated with massive blood loss and multiorgan system injuries (Fig. 7.22). Therefore, in a hemodynamically unstable patient, emergency pelvic stabilization with external fixation is considered essential to the trauma resuscitation. The two goals of acute pelvic fracture surgery are to tamponade bleeding and confer sitting stability to facilitate aggressive pulmonary physiotherapy.

Almost one in five pelvic fractures has a concomitant bladder or urethral injury. When blood is seen at the external urethral meatus, or when the patient is unable to pass urine, a retrograde urethrogram should be obtained to evaluate the integrity of the urethra before placement of an indwelling catheter. With hematuria, an IVP should also be procured to demonstrate renal function. Pelvic fractures may be open injuries if they have even a subtle rent in the rectal or vaginal mucosa. The former require a diverting colostomy after debridement and external fixation to prevent ongoing fecal soilage of the fracture.

Traumatic Amputations and Replantation

With the advent of microsurgical techniques, completely severed digits and limbs can be surgically reattached. Limb replantation is most successful if the part is amputated cleanly with a minimum of crushed tissue. Children enjoy better nerve regeneration than adults and are ideal candidates for replantation. As a general rule: because muscle tissue is sensitive to ischemic injury, the greater the amount of muscle attached to the amputated part, the poorer the prognosis for its function after replantation.

The best amputation levels for replantation in adults are the thumb, multiple digits, and the wrist or metacarpal level of the hand. In children amputations at any level have a good chance of successful replantation. Contraindications to replantation include: (*a*) amputations with large crush or avulsive components; (*b*) body parts that have been amputated at multiple levels; (*c*) individual digit amputations (other than the thumb), especially proximal to the middle phalanx; (*d*) amputation in older patients with concurrent disease or mental instability.

An amputated part may remain viable for approximately 6 hours of warm (52°C) ischemia. Cooling decreases tissue metabolism and increases the duration of viability. Amputated tissues can tolerate up to 16 hours of cold (10°C) ischemia. Thus, preparation of a severed part for transportation should include: cleansing of superficial contamination, wrapping in moist gauze, and placement in an air-tight plastic bag that is then im-

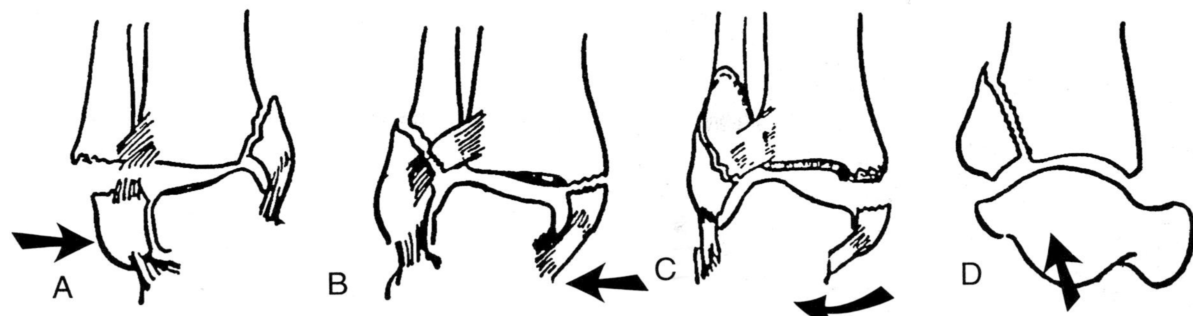

Figure 7.21. Ankle fractures. The basic mechanism of injury can be identified by the characteristic fracture patterns. A transverse fracture line implies that tensile, avulsive force was applied to the bone and is usually the first fracture to occur in the injury pattern. **A**, Adduction (inversion): the lateral malleolus is pulled off transversely and the medial malleolus is pushed off obliquely by the talus. **B**, Pure abduction (eversion): the medial malleolus is pulled off transversely, the fibula pushed off obliquely by the talus. The lateral malleolus is fractured in the sagittal plane. In some cases, the fibula is fractured above the joint line, indicating a tear in the interosseous membrane. **C**, Abduction (eversion) and external rotation (common): the medial malleolus is pulled off transversely while the lateral malleolus is obliquely fractured by the talus as it externally rotates and abuts the fibula. The fibular fracture is in the coronal plane. **D**, Vertical load: the "posterior malleolus," seen best on lateral x-ray, can be fractured by a vertical compression load, as the talus impacts the posterior tibia. The addition of this fracture fragment to any of the above constitutes a trimalleolar fracture.

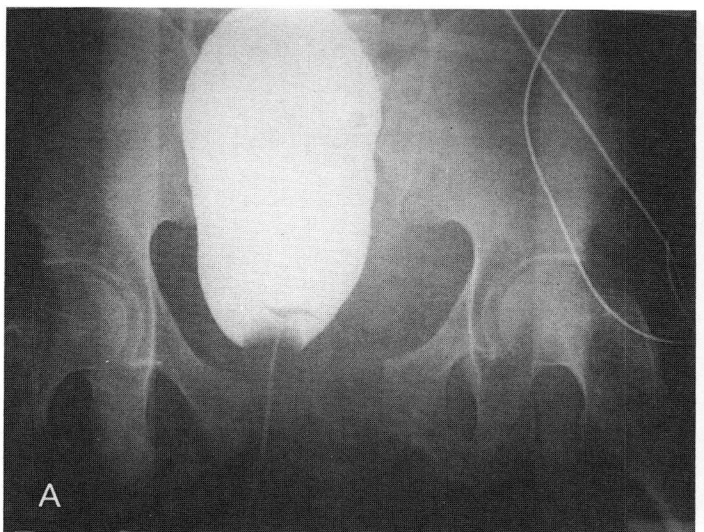

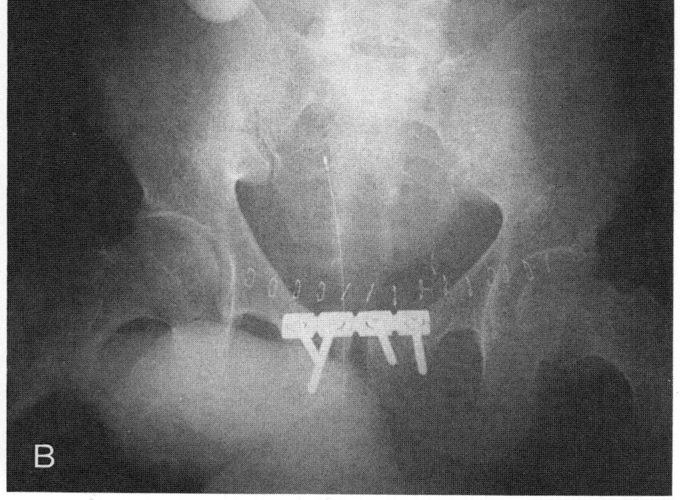

Figure 7.22. **A**, AP pelvis x-ray depicting diastasis of the symphysis pubis. The retrograde cystogram demonstrates bladder compression from a large pelvic hematoma. This type of pelvic injury can cause massive amounts of internal hemorrhage. **B**, AP pelvis x-ray after internal fixation with a plate and screws. Fracture reduction decreases pelvic volume, which both stabilizes and facilitates tamponade of bleeding fracture surfaces.

mersed in ice water. Dry ice is *never* used, because it causes frostbite and further tissue damage.

Of digital replants, 85% remain viable. Joint motion is usually about 50% of normal, and two-point sensory discrimination is protective (>10 mm) in half of adults while being almost normal (>5 mm) in children. All digits are cold intolerant for a period of at least 2 years, and 80% of epiphyses will continue to grow after replantation.

Sports Medicine

The recent emphasis on physical fitness has led to an increase in sports-related injuries. These injuries can be classified into those caused by acute trauma and those caused by repetitive stress. All musculoskeletal tissues are composed of living cells that are stimulated by physical stress to self-fortify and become stronger. When these tissues are not stressed, bones, ligaments, muscles, and tendons will atrophy. The goal of exercise, therefore, is to produce beneficial increases in physical strength and endurance through the controlled application of stress. Tissues gain strength following stress-induced microscopic breakdown by a process of hypertrophic repair. When the stresses of exercise overwhelm normal reparative process, tissues become chronically injured, inflamed, and ultimately fail. Unfortunately, much is unknown about proper training techniques. The proper duration, frequency, and inten-

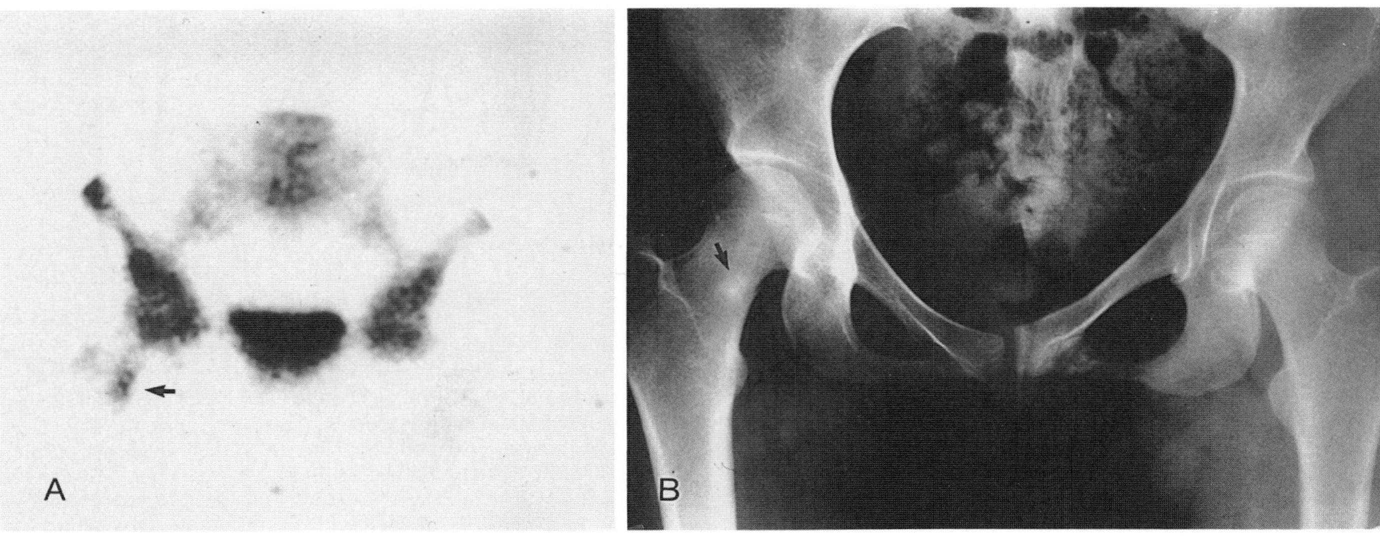

Figure 7.23. **A**, Femoral neck stress fracture detected by increased radioisotopic uptake on bone scan (arrow) 2 weeks before **B**, radiographic evidence of the fracture (arrow).

sity of exercise are therefore surrounded by myth and superstition. The "no pain, no gain" attitude toward exercise, for example, often exacerbates many injuries. While pain may be an annoyance, it is also appropriate biofeedback signifying injury and the need for rest.

It has been calculated that in running the foot strikes the ground between 800 and 2000 times per mile at a force of 2 to 4 times body weight. An average, 140-pound man will generate between 110 and 560 tons of ground reaction force per mile. This tremendous amount of force is dissipated by the shoe, the many small joints of the foot, and the bones and muscles of the leg. Any of these tissues can and do fail with injudicious exercise.

This section describes the more common injuries related both to acute trauma and to chronic, repetitive overuse. Many of the syndromes described below often occur as occupational injuries in which a given task is repeated with great frequency and without adequate periods of restorative rest.

Stress Fractures

Stress fractures are the archetypical overuse disorder. They occur when individuals are subjected to increased activity levels or changes in habits and training methods. Historically, stress fractures were first identified in the metatarsals of Prussian military recruits who were expected to endure arduous marches. Stress fractures have been identified in most bones of the body, including femur, tibia, calcaneus, and metatarsals in runners; humerus in throwers; ribs in oarsmen; and wrists and L5 vertebrae in gymnasts.

Stress fractures are postulated to be a consequence of muscle fatigue. Not only do muscles cause locomotion, they also absorb shock. Eccentric muscle contraction, or controlled muscle lengthening, decelerates the body, absorbs shock, and diffuses stress away from bone. When muscles tire, this stress-shielding effect is negated and stress is transferred directly to bone. Repeated submaximal stress will cause bone as a material to fatigue. Microfractures result and may cause an achy discomfort. The traditional treatment of rest and stress protection permits these microscopic fractures to heal. Normal cellular bone healing mechanisms permit the bone to strengthen in response to increasing demands. If the bone's ability to heal itself is overwhelmed by repeated, unremitting stress, these microfractures will coalesce, resulting in a gross, macroscopic fracture. Since stress fractures are initiated on a microscopic level, x-rays lack diagnostic sensitivity and have high false-negative rates, missing as many as 70% of these injuries. Radioisotope-labeled technetium pyrophosphate bone scans, which detect cellular bone formation, can identify a stress fracture at an earlier stage of its pathogenesis (Fig. 7.23).

Lateral Epicondylitis (Tennis Elbow)

Lateral epicondylitis, popularly known as tennis elbow, is an overuse injury of the wrist extensor muscle origin. This condition affects players of racquet sports, as well as laborers who use their hand in repetitive forceful gripping. Wrist extension is necessary for power grip (try to grip with your wrist flexed!).

The wrist extensor muscles also dissipate force when a hand-held object is used in striking. In tennis elbow, the common wrist extensors are damaged and inflamed at their lateral epicondylar origin. The majority of these injuries respond to nonoperative methods that include rest, heat, anti-inflammatory agents, wrist extensor muscle stretching, and antagonist (wrist flexor) strengthening exercises. In the few cases that are managed operatively, chronic granulation tissue is found in the origin of the extensor carpi radialis brevis and is resected.

Rotator Cuff Tendinitis (Shoulder Bursitis)

The glenohumeral joint of the shoulder is the most mobile joint in the body. The four rotator cuff muscles, supra- and infraspinatus, subscapularis, and teres minor all take broad origin from the scapular body and insert just lateral to the articular surface of the humeral head. These muscles act to stabilize the joint by pulling the humeral head into the shallow scapular glenoid fossa. The combined cross-sectional area of the rotator cuff musculature is equal to that of the imposing deltoid muscle. As cross-sectional area is directly related to muscle strength, it is interesting that the amount of shoulder muscle strength expended on joint stability—through the rotator cuff—is equal to that of the deltoid, which is responsible for joint mobility.

Rotator cuff tendinitis or subacromial bursitis is common to sports or jobs in which the arm is used overhead (e.g., throwers, swimmers, mechanics). As the shoulder abducts away from the body, the rotator cuff muscles (especially supraspinatus) contact and are positioned under the coracoacromial arch. As the arm is raised, this arch becomes narrower, impinging upon and mechanically irritating the tendon. A bursa, which is a fluid-filled synovial sac, develops under these conditions of friction and acts as an interposed subacromial cushion. Yet, pathologic changes can also affect the tendon and run the gamut from edematous inflammation to calcific degeneration to tendon attrition with tearing (Fig. 7.24). Painful inflammatory changes can also affect the subacromial bursa. It is difficult to distinguish which structure is painful, the bursa or the tendon proper. A rotator cuff tear may demonstrate weakness of shoulder external rotation strength. Pain, however, also inhibits the reliability of strength testing. A shoulder arthrogram, ultrasound, or MRI scan can diagnose the presence of a rotator cuff tear with good dependability.

Factors that contribute to rotator cuff pain include overuse, muscle weakness, improper throwing technique, strenuous training techniques, and an unstable glenohumeral joint. Treatment consists of rest, eccentric rotator cuff strengthening exercises, and anti-inflammatory medication. Surgical decompression of the coracoacromial arch is indicated if the condition becomes chronic or if it is necessary to repair a torn rotator cuff tendon.

Plantar Fasciitis (Heel Spur)

Plantar fasciitis, commonly known as heel spur, is a problem common to runners. The plantar fascia is a thick, fibrous structure attached to the calcaneus that fans distally to envelop the metatarsal heads. It increases and stiffens the longitudinal arch of the foot during the propulsive toe-off phase of gait. When the inflexible plantar fascia is repeatedly impacted and stretched by running, it is injured at its calcaneal origin, becoming inflamed and painful. The inflammatory reaction can produce a traction spike of new bone, which when seen on x-rays is called the heel spur.

Classically, plantar heel pain is worse whenever gait is initiated in the morning, after sitting, or at the start of jogging. Contributory factors include both flat (planus) and high, arched (cavus) feet, toe or sand running, obesity, and improper shoe (such as slippers) wear. Nonoperative treatment includes rest, medication, weight loss, proper shoe wear, heel padding, or cushioned shoe orthoses. If the condition has been of longstanding duration, recovery may be slow. Surgical release of the plantar fascia from its calcaneal origin is reserved for the most recalcitrant cases.

Patellar Overload Syndrome (Chondromalacia Patella)

Anterior knee pain is common to sports participants. The patella is embedded in the quadriceps muscle and glides through the femoral groove. The patella functions much like a pulley to increase the mechanical efficiency of the quadriceps in extending the knee joint. When the patella is abnormally loaded or malaligned, abnormal patellar wear and irritation produce *chondromalacia*, a term meaning cartilage (*chondro-*) softening (*malakia*).

The knee discomfort is located anteriorly and is aggravated by climbing or descending stairs and hills, squatting, kneeling, arising from a chair, or after prolonged sitting. These activities all stress the quadriceps mechanism. As the quadriceps muscle is inhibited by the discomfort, it begins to atrophy. Nonoperative treatment is often effective. Rest, anti-inflammatory medications, and patellar knee sleeves are effective treatment adjuncts. Straight leg raising, quadriceps strengthening exercises, are important to successful rehabilitation. Quadriceps exercises over a full arc of motion are to be avoided, since they place excessive load on the patella and exacerbate the condition.

Exercise Compartment Syndrome (Shin Splints)

Shin splints describes leg pain that is intensified during exercise. In recreational runners the pain is usually localized to the anterior leg compartment (Fig. 7.15) containing the anterior tibialis, extensor digitorum, and extensor hallucis longus muscles. In competitive runners the pain often emanates from the distal medial leg in the deep posterior compartment musculature (posterior tibialis, flexor digitorum, and flexor hallucis longus). Intramuscular pressures increase during contraction, which decreases blood flow. Muscle perfusion therefore occurs primarily during muscle relaxation. Sustained increases in compartment pressure decrease muscle perfusion, producing pain and the cessation of exercise. This phenomenon is known as an exercise compartment syndrome. When measured, compartment pressures can rise to well over 100 mm Hg with exercise. In the asymptomatic individual, pressures return to normal levels very rapidly during periods of rest. In patients with exercise compartment syndromes, interstitial tissue pressures fall off slowly and have a delayed return to normal values. Tibia stress fractures,

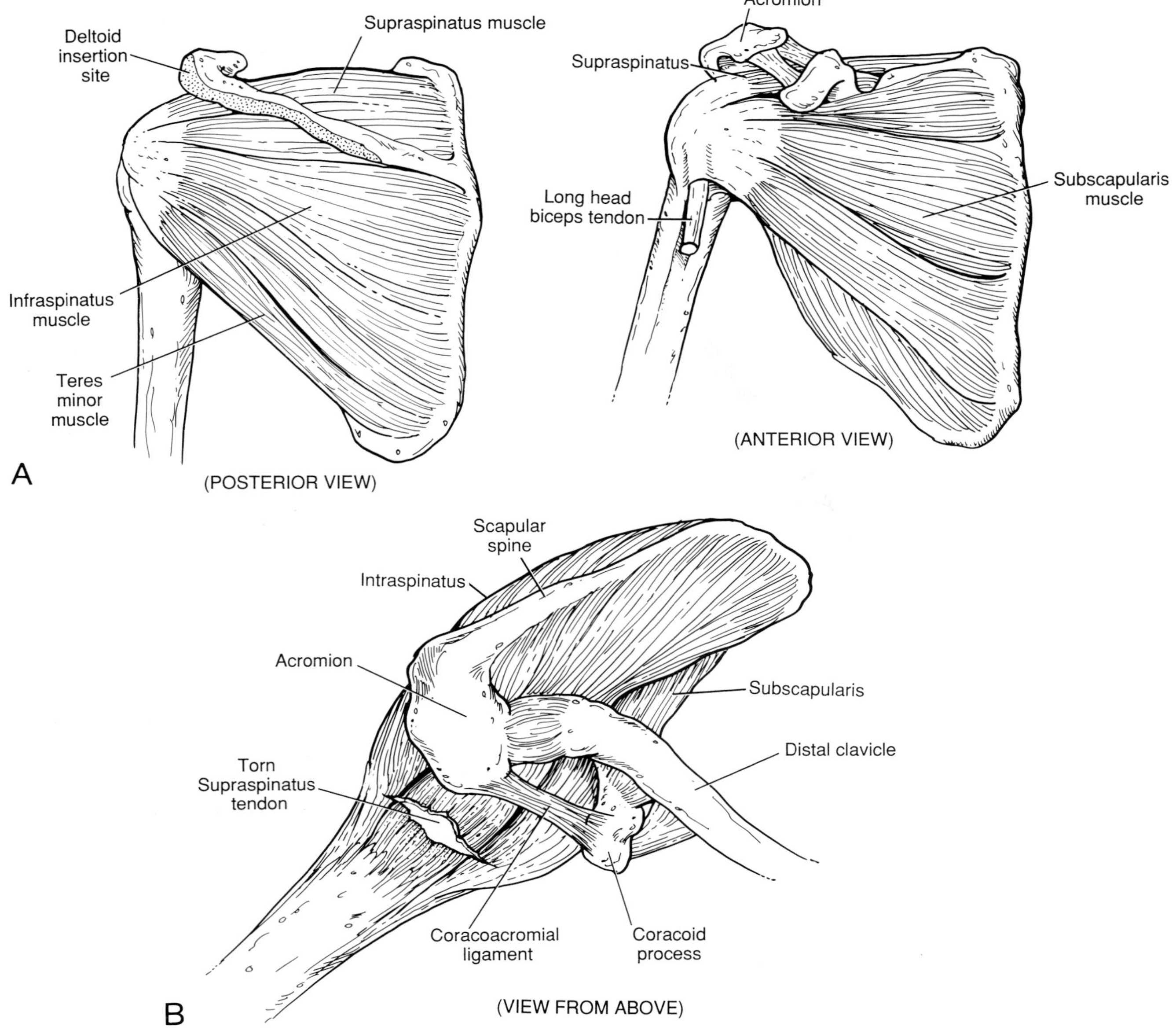

Figure 7.24. Viewed from the anterior and posterior perspectives, the cowl of rotator cuff muscles takes broad origin from the scapula and inserts close to the articular margin of the humeral head. The rotator cuff acts to pull the humeral head into the glenoid fossa as the arm is abducted away from the body. Viewed from its superior surface, the supraspinatus tendon is torn near its humeral insertion. The tear results from acromion and coracoacromial ligament attrition, when the shoulder is abducted and forward flexed.

periostitis, nerve entrapment, and fascial muscle hernias have a similar clinical presentation. The diagnosis of exercise-related compartment syndrome is based on objective pressure measurements. When conservative treatment measures fail (such as rest, cushioned shoe orthotics, and changes in training patterns and running surfaces), the condition can be successfully treated with a complete surgical fasciotomy of the involved leg compartment.

Sprains

A sprain is a ligament injury. Ligaments are collagenous structures that originate and insert on bone and act to stabilize joints. They are injured under tensile or stretching loads. Sprains are classified according to the three grades of damage. A grade I sprain exhibits microscopic ligament damage, which produces ligament tenderness but no change in joint laxity when the joint is subjected to stress. Grade II sprains demonstrate a greater degree of damage, with rupture of entire fascicles of ligament collagen. The ligament is in macroscopic continuity but is stretched or partially torn and therefore demonstrates joint laxity when stressed. When grossly disrupted with total loss of joint stability, the ligament injury is classified as a grade III sprain.

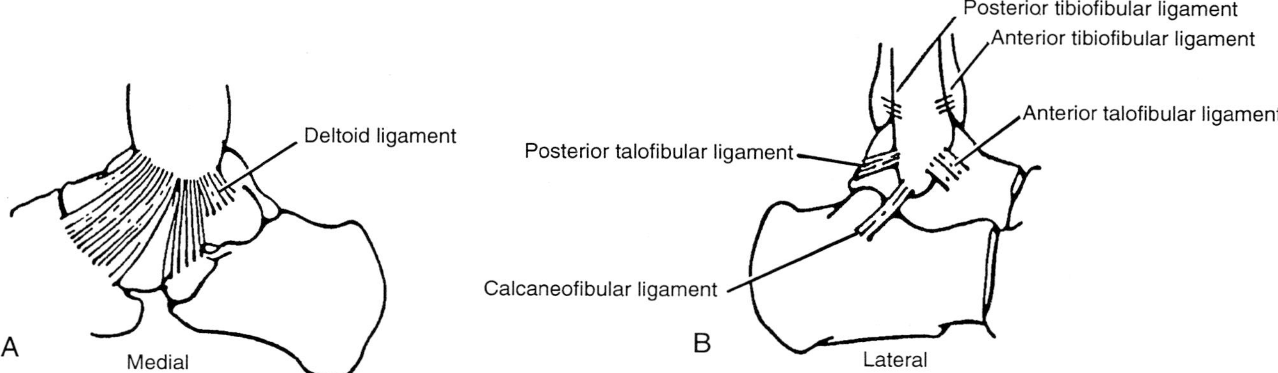

Figure 7.25. **A**, Extensive medial deltoid ligament of the ankle. **B**, The lateral ankle is supported by three discrete ankle ligaments. The most commonly sprained anterior talofibular ligament, the calcaneofibular, and the posterior talofibular ligaments. The anterior talofibular ligament resists anterior translation of the ankle (anterior drawer test); the calcaneofibular resists inversion stress (talar tilt).

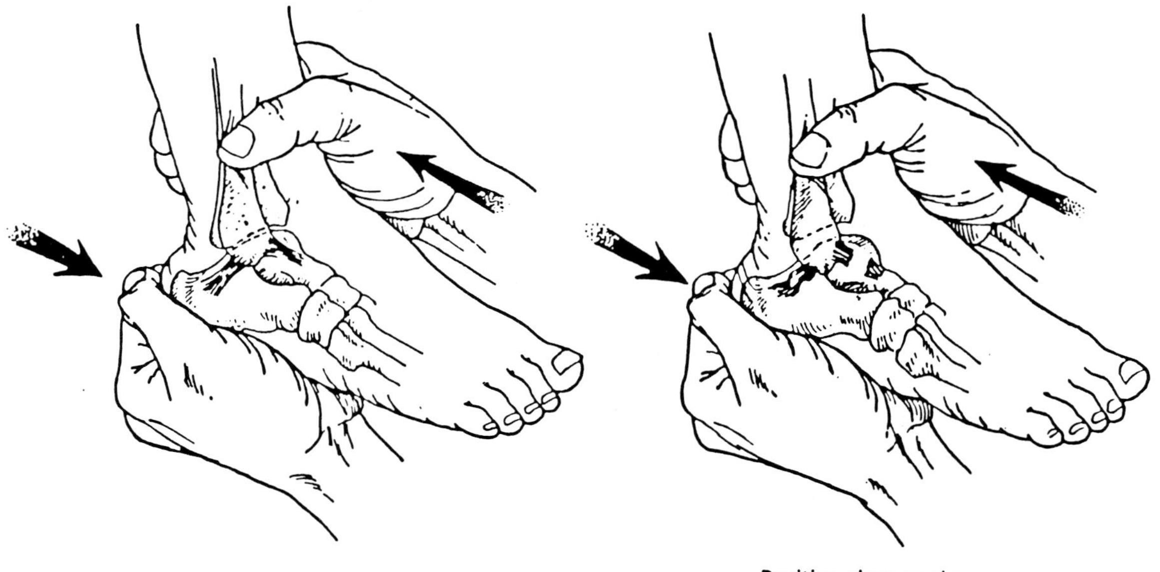

Figure 7.26. Anterior drawer test. The anterior talofibular ligament resists anterior ankle stress. The anterior drawer test is positive when this ligament is disrupted and will detect excessive anterior translation of the foot on the leg.

Ankle Sprains

The lateral ankle ligaments are the most commonly sprained ligaments in the body. The lateral ankle is supported by 3 discrete ligaments: the anterior talofibular, calcaneal-fibular, and posterior talofibular ligaments (Fig. 7.25). Because the longer fibular malleolus buttresses the ankle from abduction or eversion stress, the broad deltoid ligament that connects the medial tibial malleolus to the talus is not commonly injured.

When the ankle is subjected to an inversion stress, the anterior talofibular ligament is the first lateral ligament to be torn. With more severe injury, the calcaneal-fibular ligament will also be disrupted. These two ligaments resist anterior talar displacement on the tibia (anterior drawer, Fig. 7.26) and abnormal inversion talar tilt, respectively.

The diagnosis of a lateral ankle ligament sprain and its severity is ascertained by the extent of ligament tenderness and by manual and radiographic stress tests. Treatment consists of ice, elevation, compressive wraps, and early weightbearing. Primary surgical ankle ligament repair is rarely indicated, since most ankle sprains have no residual joint instability and the outcomes of early versus late ankle reconstruction are similar. Ligaments contain proprioceptive nerve endings that are also injured by a sprain. Recurrent ankle sprains may be the result of inadequate proprioceptive feedback. Balance board proprioceptor retraining is an effective component of ankle rehabilitation.

Knee Ligament Sprains

Since the knee is situated between the two largest bones (femur and tibia) and is spanned by the body's

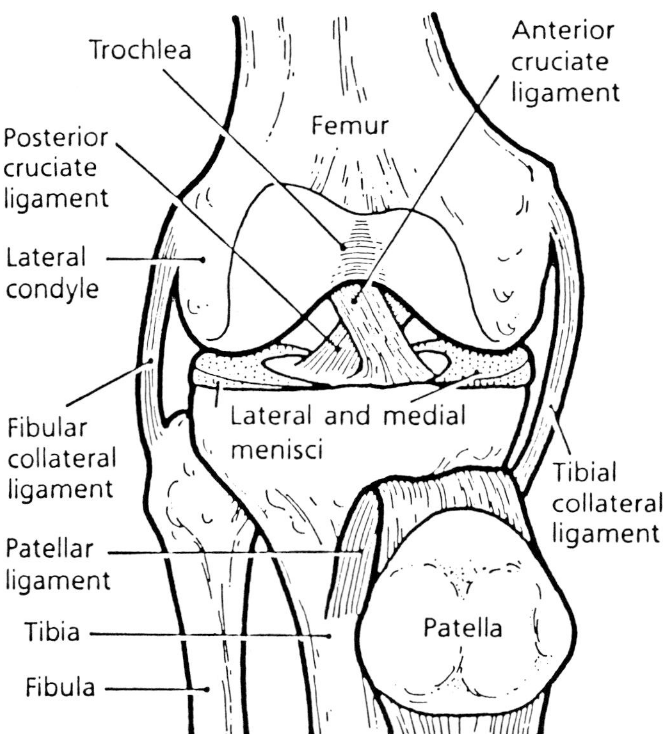

Figure 7.27. Knee joint stability depends on the two collateral and cruciate ligaments. The medial collateral ligament is broad and large and resists varus or abduction stress. The anterior cruciate ligament resists anterior tibial translation, while the posterior cruciate prevents posterior tibial shear.

strongest muscles (quadriceps and hamstrings), it is not surprising that this joint is often injured. In general terms, the knee is stabilized by four ligaments: the two collateral ligaments that resist varus and valgus (abduction-adduction or medial-lateral) stress and the two cruciate ligaments that primarily resist anterior-posterior motion (Fig. 7.27).

The collateral ligaments are usually damaged by direct traumatic violence. The anterior cruciate ligament (ACL) can be injured in isolation in twisting, hyperflexion, and hyperextension noncontact modes. The ACL is the only one of the four ligaments that is intrasynovial. Of patients with bloody knee joint effusions, 70% have an anterior cruciate ligament injury. Of those with an acute ACL tear, 50% have a concomitant meniscus tear. The medial collateral and anterior cruciate ligaments are frequently injured in combination from a valgus stress, such as occurs from a direct blow to the lateral thigh. When a collateral ligament is severely injured, the knee joint capsule and lining synovium are disrupted. The knee will not contain an effusion, and hemorrhage will diffuse into the soft tissues. The posterior cruciate ligament is injured 10 times less commonly than the anterior cruciate ligament, but when torn it is often associated with a popliteal artery injury. Lateral collateral ligament and peroneal nerve injuries frequently occur in combination.

Collateral ligament damage can be detected by local tenderness, pain, and laxity when the knee is manually stressed in a mediolateral (varus/valgus plane). Laxity tests of an injured knee should always be judged in comparison to the normal side. Abduction (valgus) of the tibia on the femur will stress the medial collateral ligament, whereas adduction (varus) will test the integrity of the lateral collateral ligament. Full knee extension places the joint in a position of maximal geometric stability. Joint laxity in knee extension therefore implies a greater degree of collateral ligament damage. Subtle differences between the laxity on the normal versus the injured side can best be detected with the knee in the less stable, 20° knee flexion position.

The drawer test is used to evaluate cruciate ligament integrity. With the knee flexed 90°, the tibia is pulled forward like a bureau drawer against a fixed femur (Fig. 7.28). If there is abnormal anterior tibial translation, the anterior drawer test suggests that the anterior cruciate ligament is incompetent. Conversely, abnormal posterior tibial translation to a posteriorly directed tibial force indicates a posterior cruciate ligament injury. Anterior knee laxity may be better appreciated in the 20° knee flexed position, which is called the Lachman test.

Isolated medial collateral ligament injuries heal well with immobilization in a hinged cast-brace, which protects the knee from abduction (valgus) stress. An anterior cruciate ligament injury is disabling to most athletes. With cutting and twisting movements, the knee will transiently subluxate and give way. Posterior cruciate ligament deficient knees are associated with patellar overload and arthritis as the quadriceps muscle attempts to compensate for increased posterior tibial displacement. The less stout lateral collateral ligament is often injured in conjunction with one of the two cruciate ligaments. Acute repairs of combination knee ligament injuries should be strong enough to tolerate early motion to prevent the common postoperative complication of joint stiffness.

The indications for surgical ligament repair and reconstruction are controversial. In general, younger patients whose activities stress the knee are candidates for surgery. The intra-articular cruciate ligaments, if torn interstitially, heal poorly and are generally reconstructed with soft tissue autografts or allografts (for example, from the patellar tendon or the fascia lata). The collateral ligaments often respond well to direct sutured repair.

Meniscal Injury

The knee joint is inherently unstable by virtue of its bony geometry. The medial and lateral meniscal fibrocartilages increase joint surface contact and aid in joint stability. In stance, the menisci transmit between 40 and 60% of the weight-bearing load placed across the joint. The menisci also assist with joint lubrication and hyaline cartilage nutrition. The menisci move anterior to posterior as the knee is flexed. In flexion, the menisci are trapped between the femoral condyle and tibial plateau. If a twisting, rotatory motion occurs when the knee is flexed, the menisci may split longitudinally (Fig. 7.29**C**, **D**). Meniscal tissue loses hydration and becomes

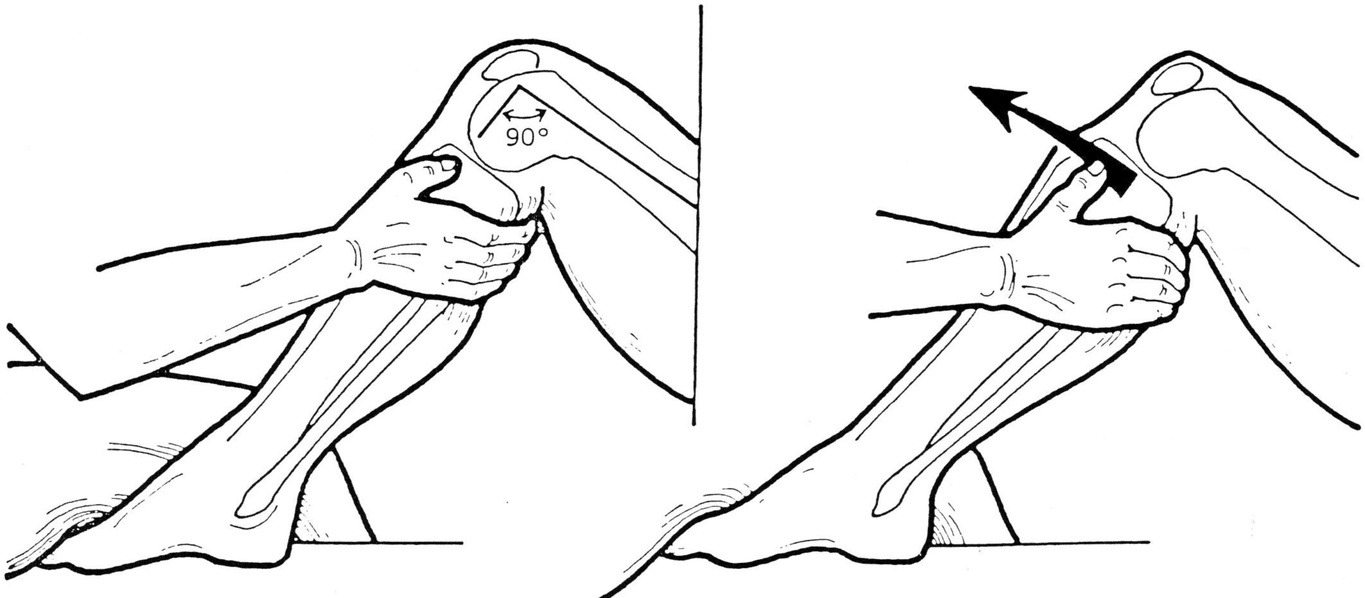

Figure 7.28. The anterior drawer test is performed with the foot stabilized and the knee flexed 90°. With the examiner's thumb placed on the joint line, the tibia is pulled anteriorly. Excessive anterior tibial shift suggests that the anterior cruciate ligament is incompetent. The contralateral side can be used as a comparative reference. A similar test performed in 20° of knee flexion is called the Lachman test and is more sensitive in the evaluation of acute injuries.

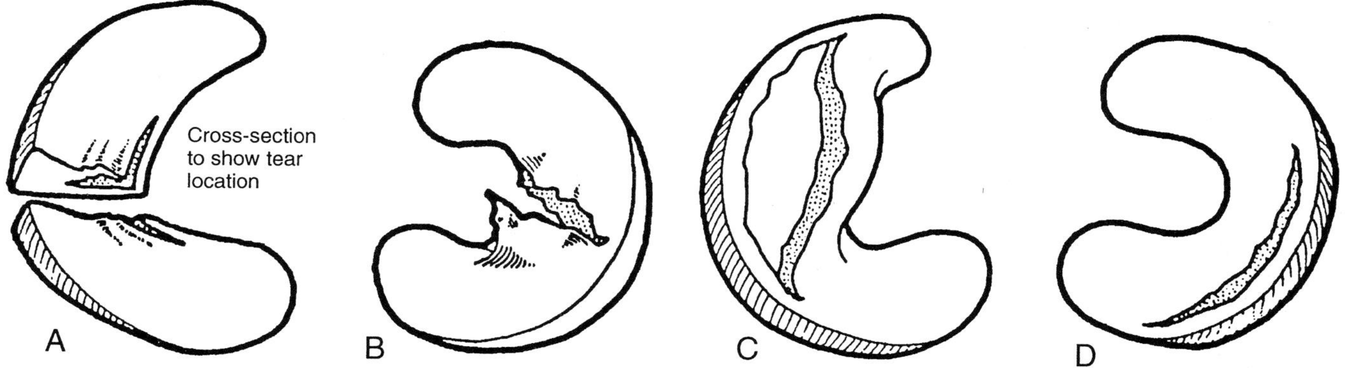

Figure 7.29. Meniscal tears. **A**, Degenerative horizontal tear. **B**, Radial tear. **C**, Displaced bucket handle tear. **D**, Longitudinal tear.

more brittle with age. Shearing, horizontal cleavage tears, not seen on the meniscal surface, are frequently found in older patients (Fig. 7.29**A**).

Patients with meniscal pathology present with pain and tenderness localized to the joint line. There may be recurrent swelling. A history of giving way suggests a tear located in the posterior portion of the meniscus. Symptoms of intermittent joint locking occur with bucket handle tears (Fig. 7.29**C**), when the torn component of the meniscus slides between the condyle and acts as a mechanical block to joint motion. Longitudinal tears (Fig. 7.29**D**) in the peripheral third of the meniscus will heal when repaired since this zone is well vascularized. Total meniscectomy leads to the slow development of tibiofemoral arthritis; therefore, irreparable and displaceable meniscal tears causing mechanical symptoms are best treated by partial excision, leaving the stable, untorn meniscus in situ. Meniscal surgery is performed arthroscopically because it is less traumatic, more precise, and can be performed on an outpatient basis.

Acromioclavicular (Shoulder) Separation

In addition to the glenohumeral articulation, the shoulder is composed of three other joints: the acromioclavicular, sternoclavicular, and scapulothoracic articulations. The acromioclavicular joint rotates approximately 20° with flexion and extension of the shoulder and is stabilized in this AP (horizontal) plane by the acromioclavicular ligaments (Fig. 7.1). In the craniocaudal direction (coronal plane), the joint is constrained by the stronger coracoclavicular ligaments.

The acromioclavicular joint is injured after a blow to the point of the shoulder. The scapular acromion is driven

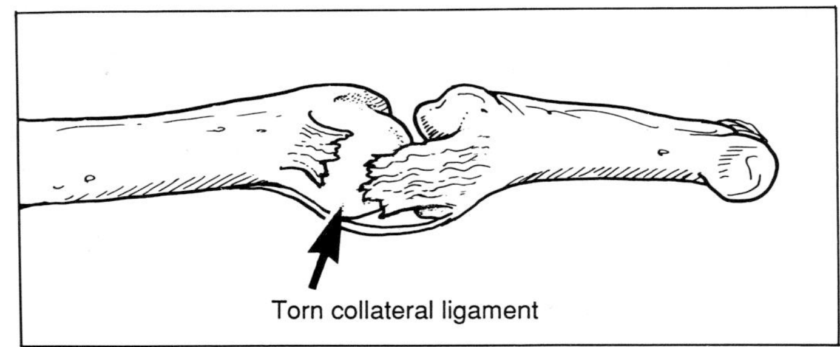

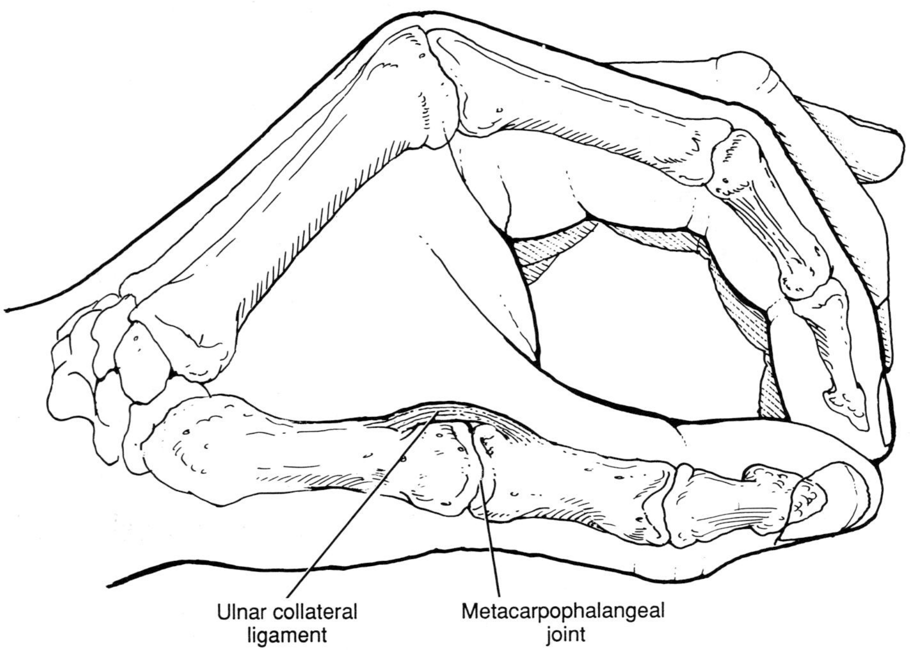

Figure 7.30. **A**, Lateral depiction of a torn collateral ligament metacarpophalangeal joint. **B**, The ulnar collateral ligament of the thumb metacarpophalangeal joint is critical to opposable thumb function. Injury to this ligament (gamekeeper's thumb) renders the thumb unstable and weakens its contribution to pinch and grip strength.

caudally, while the clavicle remains fixed to the chest. If the acromioclavicular ligaments alone are torn and the coracoclavicular ligaments stretched, the injury is classified as grade II, in which the clavicle is partially displaced (subluxated) from the acromion (Fig. 7.1**C**). This situation may not be obvious but can be determined by stress radiographs in which weights are strapped to dependent wrists. The distance between the clavicle and coracoid process will be widened. When both acromioclavicular and coracoclavicular ligaments are disrupted (grade III), the joint will be dislocated. The distal clavicle will be dislocated and elevated above the acromion, which is obvious to inspection (Fig. 7.1**B**). Treatment of a grade III shoulder separation is controversial. Both surgical and nonsurgical methods yield functional results.

Gamekeeper's Thumb

The ulnar collateral ligament of the thumb metacarpophalangeal (MCP) joint is a critical structure. It resists the forces of opposable thumb-index finger pinch. As the thumb is out of the plane of the hand, this ligament is vulnerable to thumb abduction stress. It is injured in skiers who fall while still gripping their pole or ball handling sports (Fig. 7.30). Loss of the stabilizing effect of the thumb MCP ulnar collateral ligament renders pinch weak and painful. To test the ligament it is stressed in 35° of flexion to relax the volar plate and the short thumb flexor. The adductor pollicis aponeurosis is often interposed between the ligament and the proximal phalanx, which can prevent ligament healing. Thus, ligament exploration with repair or reattachment is the preferred treatment of this small but important ligament.

Mallet (Baseball) Finger

A sudden jamming blow to the tip of the extended finger can cause rupture of the digital extensor tendon. The finger distal interphalangeal (DIP) joint will be in a flexed habitus, and there will be loss of active DIP extension (Fig. 7.31). This injury heals well if immobilized in full DIP extension.

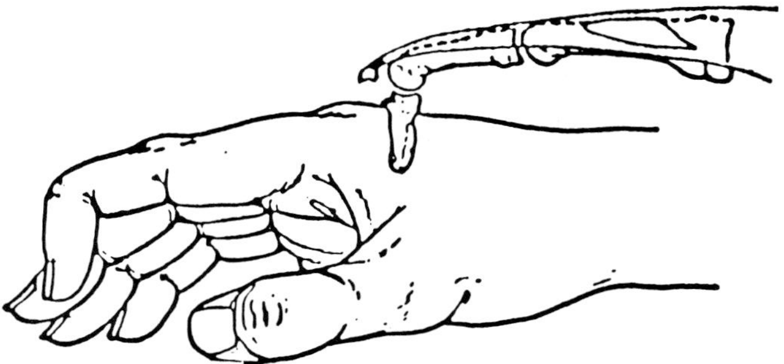

Figure 7.31. A mallet or baseball finger, which results from rupture of the extensor tendon.

Boxer's Fracture

The index and long finger metacarpals have limited mobility and act as rigid posts for the fine precision work of the hand. The ring and little finger metacarpals are more mobile and are important to power grip as motion is needed for these fingers to surround an object. For a fist to impart maximal kinetic energy, the more rigid radial side of the fist should strike the object. When the ulnar fist strikes an object the little finger metacarpal neck often fractures. This is known as a boxer's fracture and results from poor pugilistic technique. Closed reduction and plaster immobilization is the preferred and usually successful treatment.

Achilles Tendon Rupture

Achilles tendon ruptures occur in the middle-aged, out-of-shape, weekend athlete who enthusiastically stresses the tendon beyond its customary demands. Systemic and local steroid injections weaken tendinous tissue and also predispose it to rupture. With an Achilles tendon rupture, the athlete feels a severe pain in the calf. There may be swelling, ecchymosis, and sometimes a palpable gap between tendon ends. Active plantar flexion of the ankle will be weak but present because the tibialis posterior and long toe flexors are still functional.

The Thompson test (Fig. 7.32) verifies whether the gastrocnemius-soleus complex is intact: with the patient kneeling and the foot hanging free, the examiner squeezes the calf muscle belly. Normally, the foot responds with plantar flexion. Lack of plantar flexion indicates that the Achilles tendon is torn.

Nonoperative treatment in a long leg cast with the foot in plantar flexion will permit excellent tendon healing but is quite cumbersome. Surgical treatment may be more expeditious for athletes. Both types of treatment are effective.

Turf Toe

Turf toe is a hyperextension injury to the great toe metatarsophalangeal (MTP) joint (Fig. 7.33). The flexor hallucis brevis tendon is ruptured either at its proximal phalangeal insertion or by a fracture of its sesamoid bones. The plantar plate may also be torn. The injury occurs during football pile-ups, in which an opposing player falls on the posterior aspect of a prone player's foot, hyperextending the great toe. The injured player experiences exquisite plantar great toe pain exacerbated by passive extension of the MTP joint. The toe-off, propulsive phase of gait is painful. Treatment consists of rest, taping of the toe in plantar flexion, and the wearing of stiff forefoot, in-shoe orthosis. Untreated turf toe has been implicated as the cause of great toe MTP arthritis and loss of extension known as hallux rigidus.

Myositis Ossificans

Bone deposited in a muscle after a blunt injury is known as traumatic myositis ossificans (Fig. 7.34). When a deep muscle (frequently the quadriceps) is contused, the muscle closest to bone will suffer the greatest amount of direct damage. Either a metaplasia of muscle cells or a release of osteogenic material from the underlying bone causes bone to form within the injured muscle. Early symptoms are deep muscle tenderness and loss of joint motion. The condition is self-limited, but may be retarded by nonsteroidal anti-inflammatory agents. If the lesion is large or causes mechanical problems, surgical excision is indicated. When a lesion is resected early (before 18 months), there is a high rate of recurrence. A systemic form of myositis ossificans occurs in patients with paralysis or extensive burns.

Pediatric Musculoskeletal Problems

The term *orthopedic* derives from the Greek word for straight, *orthos*, and the word for child, *pais*, (combining form *paid-*). The diagnosis and treatment of pediatric deformities thus represent the origin of the specialty of orthopedics. This section deals with common pediatric musculoskeletal disorders.

Lower Limb Torsion (In- and Outtoeing)

The most common group of childhood "deformities" are actually normal variations of musculoskeletal form. Flat feet, bow legs, knock-knees, and in-and outtoeing are commonly seen in young children but are unusual in adolescence. Because these conditions seem to resolve spontaneously, they must be considered part of the natural process of skeletal development. The first two years of life are a remarkable period of physical growth. The average child attains almost half of its adult size and stature during these first two years. Body structure also changes radically as the skeletal frame is subjected to the demands of locomotion and bipedal gait.

The common rotational deformities of in- and outtoeing can be ascribed to one of three lower limb sites: the femur (ante- or retroversion), the tibia (internal or external torsion), or the forefoot (metatarsus adductus). Although rotational variations may run in families, the most common cause is the restricted confines of intrauterine positioning (Fig. 7.35). Certain sleeping or

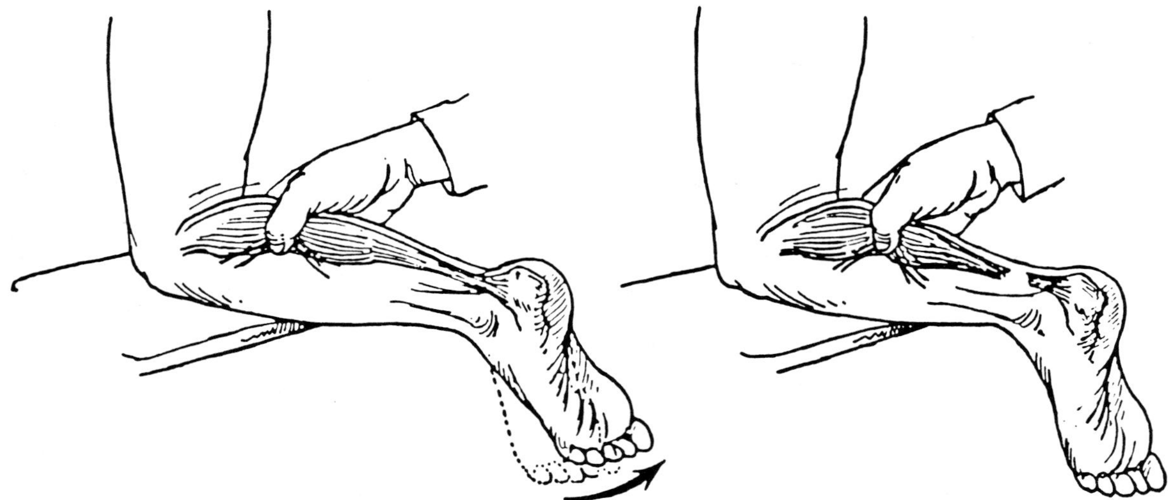

Figure 7.32. The Thompson test will provoke a plantar flexion response when the gastrocnemius-soleus Achilles tendon complex is intact. Absence of this response indicates a tear of the Achilles tendon.

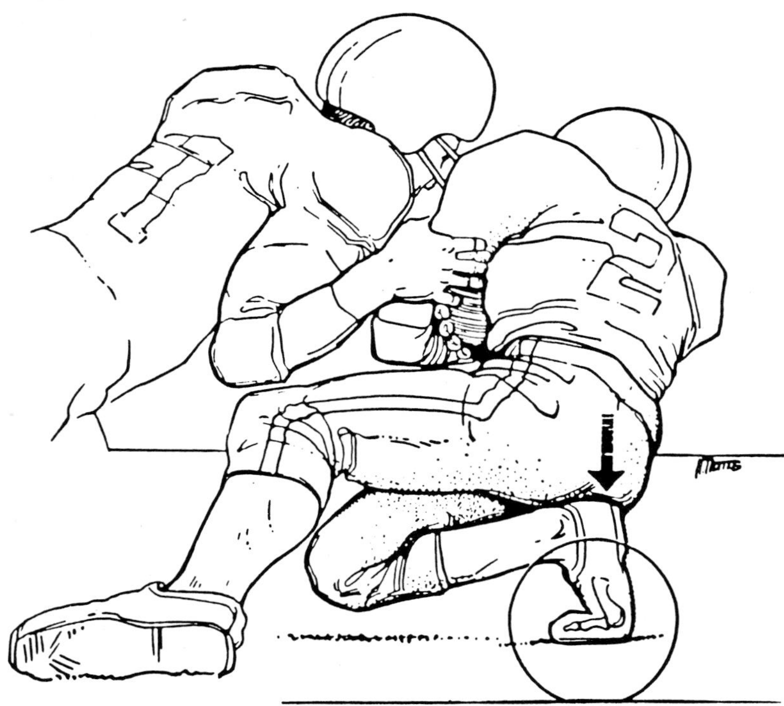

Figure 7.33. A turf toe injury occurs from hyperdorsiflexion of the great toe metatarsophalangeal joint and ruptures the flexor hallucis brevis mechanism through the tendon or the sesamoid.

sitting postures may accentuate these conditions and delay their resolution. Femoral version describes the anatomic relationship of the femoral head and neck that are not coplanar with the femoral shaft. The femoral neck is offset from the shaft in the coronal plane. This relationship, called femoral anteversion, can be seen if one sites down the shaft of the femur as one would a gun barrel: the femoral neck is canted an average of 10–15° anterior (Fig. 7.36). At birth, femoral anteversion averages about 40°. It decreases to 10° by adulthood, with most of the change occurring in the first 3 years of life (Fig. 7.37).

All rotational deformities are best evaluated with the child placed prone. Femoral anteversion (intoeing) is present when medial or inward rotation of the femur is in excess of 30° more than external femoral rotation (Fig. 7.38). When external (outward) femoral rotation is excessive, femoral retroversion is present as a cause of outtoeing, and the person is colloquially called *slew-footed*.

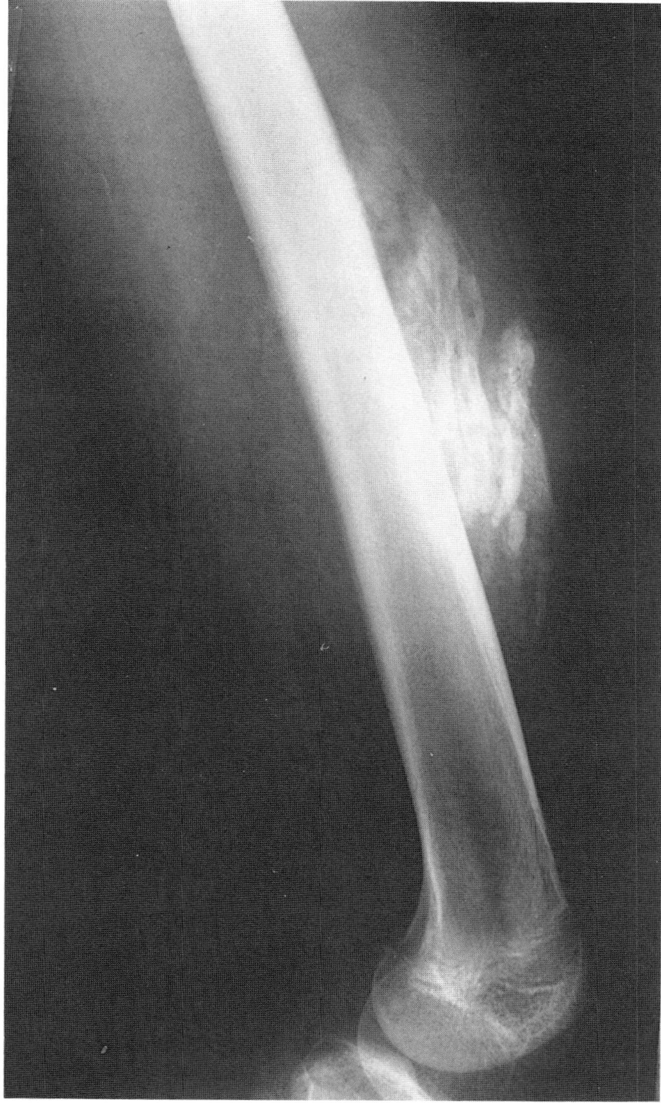

Figure 7.34. Myositis ossificans. Bone deposition in the quadriceps muscle after an anterior thigh contusion.

When the child is viewed from above with its knee flexed, the angle the sole of the foot makes with the thigh (thigh-foot angle) allows for assessment of internal versus external tibial torsion (Fig. 7.39**A**). The normal lateral border of the foot is straight. If it is curved inward or its lateral border is convex, metatarsus adductus is present (Fig. 7.39**B**). If the foot is flexible and can be passively corrected to neutral alignment, treatment is probably unnecessary. When the deformity is rigid, corrective serial casting is beneficial. Metatarsus adductus is often associated with internal tibial torsion. Both result from fetal in utero positioning, the latter being the most common cause of rotational lower extremity problems (Fig. 7.35).

As the skeleton adapts to growth and bipedal posture, these torsional "deformities" regress. A slight amount of intoeing has been noted in the better athletes. Intoeing is advantageous during cutting maneuvers, since a limb that is internally rotated will be aligned with the intended change of direction and is more effective in push-off acceleration. A variety of orthotic devices are available to treat these rotatory conditions. However, their true efficacy in altering the natural history of these developmental variations is uncertain. Orthotic appliances can be used to prevent certain sleeping postures that may aggravate these conditions.

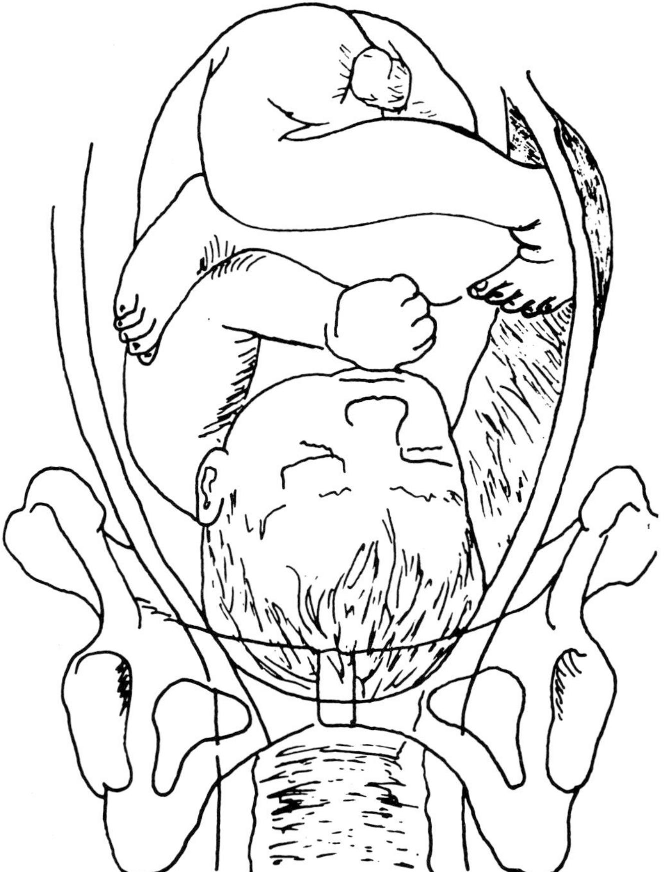

Figure 7.35. Cramped intrauterine confines often mold the child's plastic bone structure. Note that in utero fetal posture forces the tibias to be internally rotated and the forefoot adducted.

Angular Limb Deformities (Bowlegs, Knock Knees)

Angular lower limb alignment, bowlegs and knock knees (genu varum and valgum—Fig. 7.9), are another common cause for an orthopedic consultation. For most children, these conditions represent the spectrum of normal development. It is rare for limb malalignment to persist and cause functional or cosmetic impairment sufficient to require surgical intervention. Normal, nonambulatory infants have physiologic bowlegs with tibiofemoral angles of 20° or more of varus (bow). At approximately a year-and-a-half of age, the angle corrects as the femur and tibia become colinear. After the

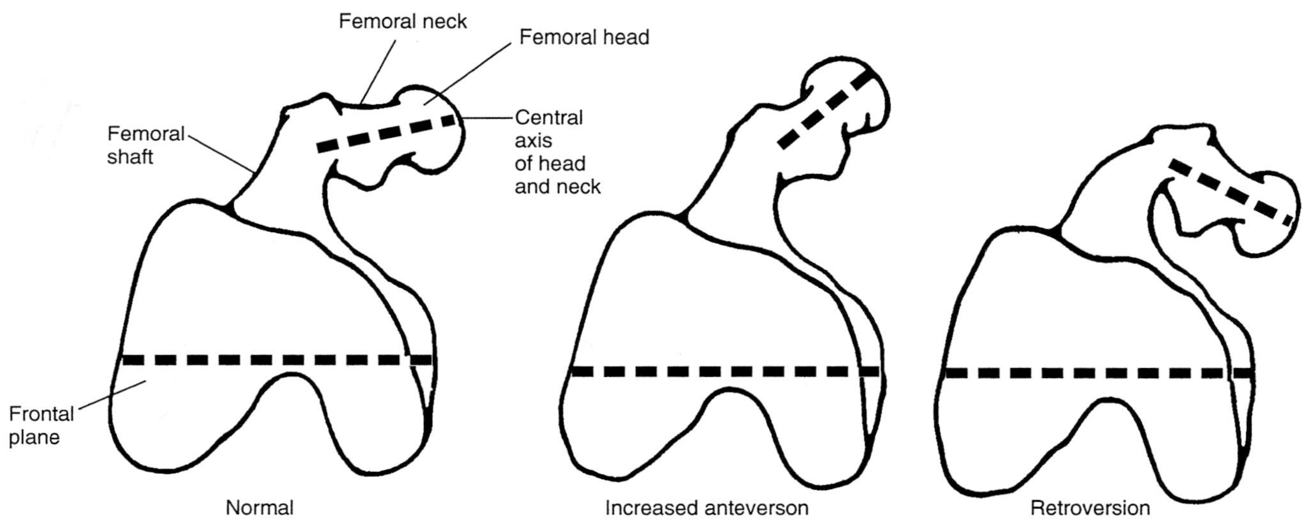

Figure 7.36. Femoral neck version or torsion as seen from the distal femoral condyles.

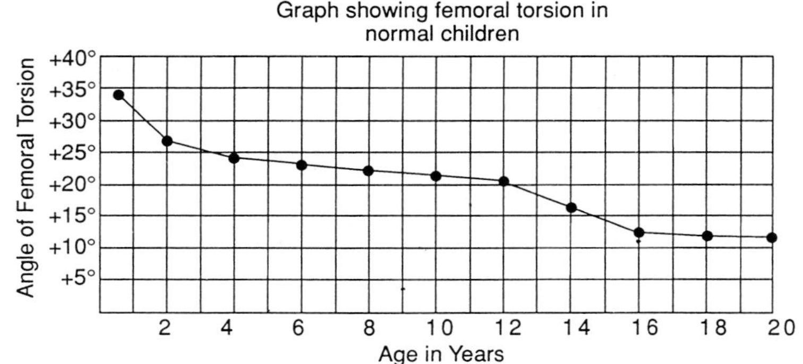

Figure 7.37. The average amount of femoral anteversion decreases from about 40° at birth to the normal 10° in adulthood. The most dramatic change occurs within the first 2 years of life.

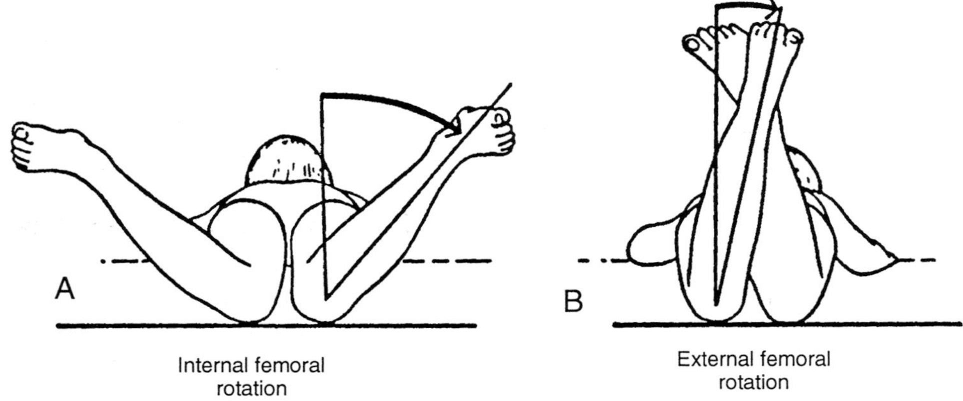

Figure 7.38. Clinical evaluation of a patient with intoeing due to femoral anteversion will demonstrate internal femoral rotation (**A**) in greater excess than external femoral rotation (**B**).

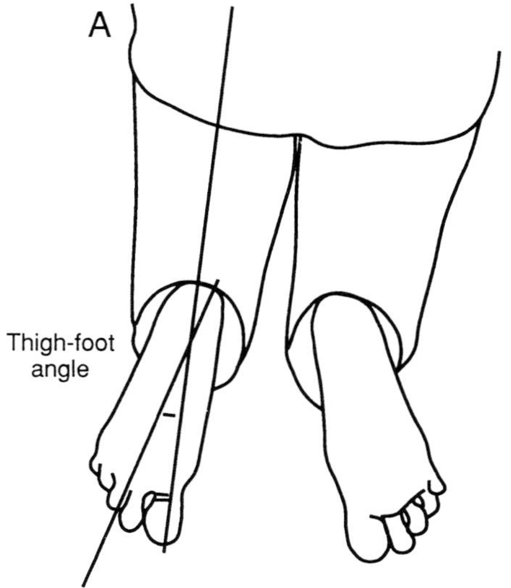

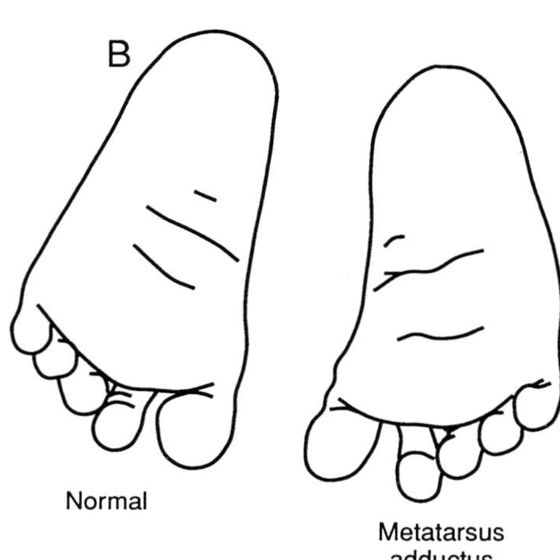

Figure 7.39. **A**, External tibial torsion is detected by a thigh-foot angle pointed away from the midline. **B**, Metatarsus adductus as a cause of intoeing is noted by a convex lateral foot border. If the foot cannot be passively corrected to neutral, the deformity is rigid and may require serial casts for correction.

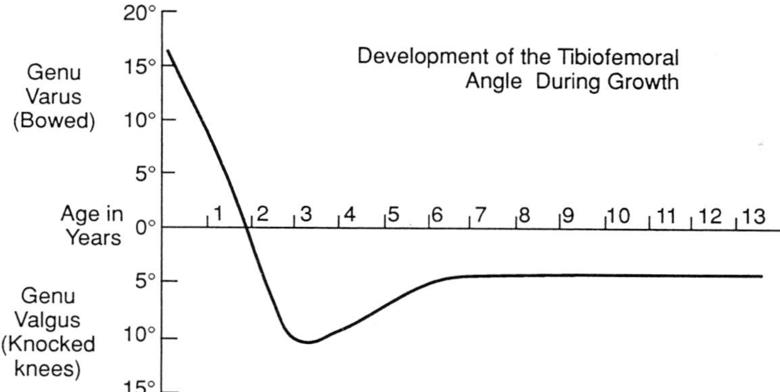

Figure 7.40. Changes in tibiofemoral alignment with growth shows that there is a natural progression from bowlegs at birth to physiologic knocked knees by the age of 3.

third year of life, the limbs assume the normal adult, "knock-knee" habitus of 7° of valgus (Fig. 7.40).

Pathologic conditions can cause knee bowing, including chondrodysplastic dwarfism and Vitamin-D-resistant (hypophosphatemic) rickets. These systemic conditions also deform other bones and joints. If bowlegs persist beyond the second year of life, radiographic evaluation may be warranted.

Flat Feet

Flat feet are another common skeletal variation. The most common type is the hypermobile or flexible flat foot. The longitudinal arch of the foot is absent or flat in stance, but reconstitutes when the foot is non-weight-bearing. Most flexible flat feet are asymptomatic and result from ligamentous laxity affecting the many small joints of the midfoot. A flat foot that is rigid and has little passive motion may be caused by a congenital coalition of the tarsal bones. A flat foot associated with a tight heel cord may be caused by muscular dystrophy or cerebral palsy. High arched feet (pes cavus) with clawed toes are the sequelae of peripheral neuropathies such as Charcot-Marie-Tooth disease.

Developmental Dysplasia of the Hip

The incidence of developmental dysplasia or instability of the hip (DDH)—formerly called congenital dislocation of the hip (CDH)— is 1.5 per 1000 newborns. One-third of cases are bilateral. The condition shows a familial predisposition and is associated with intrauterine breech presentations. Females are affected much more frequently than males, since their ligaments are more sensitive to the relaxing effects of maternal estrogen released in preparation for birth.

The early diagnosis of congenital hip instability renders treatment more effective. All newborns and infants

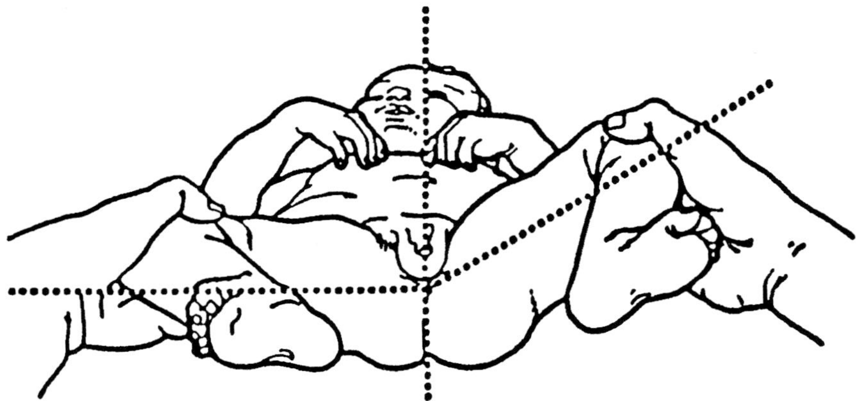

Figure 7.41. Limited hip abduction in congenital hip dislocation. The perineum should be perpendicular to the table. The limit of true hip joint motion is evidenced by concomitant movement of the perineum.

must therefore be examined for hip instability. The diagnosis is never obvious but must be sought by careful examination. Limited or asymmetric thigh abduction should raise the suspicion of a hip abnormality (Fig. 7.41). The infant's thigh is gently grasped by the long finger and thumb. With the hip and knee flexed 90°, the thigh is abducted while the greater trochanter is gently pressed forward in an anterior direction. A palpable jump or click during this maneuver (Ortolani's sign) signifies that the femoral head has been reduced into the acetabulum and that the hip was dislocated. An opposite, provocation maneuver in which adduction and posterior pressure is applied by the thumbs over the femoral head will lever the hip out of the acetabulum (Barlow's sign) if the hip is unstable. These two tests are useful in the first 2 weeks of life when the child's ligaments are under the relaxing influence of maternal hormones. Treatment is most successful early in life and is accomplished by manipulative reduction (Ortolani's maneuver) and immobilization with the hips in a stable position of flexion and abduction. If the hip remains dislocated, the acetabular socket does not develop and remains shallow. Reduction is therefore critical to acetabular development.

After 1 month of age, limited hip abduction is the most reliable sign of congenital hip dislocation (Fig. 7.41). Asymmetry of thigh and buttock folds or telescoping of the flexed femur are other signs of late hip dislocation. When the condition is bilateral, all physical signs that depend on noting asymmetry will be absent, making diagnosis more difficult. When the child begins walking, a short leg limp is evident when the hip dislocation is unilateral. A waddling, hyperlordotic gait will be apparent if the condition is bilateral. Treatment after walking age is more difficult. Contracted hip muscles must be gradually stretched with traction, or an adductor muscle release. Operative hip reduction is likely to be needed and must be maintained in a cast.

The head of the femur is cartilaginous until almost 9 months of age and is not visible on x-rays. Radiographs are therefore of limited early diagnostic value. Ultrasonography images cartilage well and is useful in early infancy. Hip joint ultrasound can dynamically evaluate the hip under positional stress. Once the femoral head has ossified, an x-ray will show a dislocated hip to be displaced lateral and superior to a shallow acetabulum.

The management of congenital hip instability requires the prompt attention by an orthopedic specialist. When treatment is begun early and followed closely, the prognosis for normal hip function is good.

Legg-Calvé-Perthes Disease

Legg-Calvé-Perthes disease is a condition of unknown etiology that causes osteonecrosis of the femoral head in children between the ages of 4 to 8 years. Males are affected eight times more commonly than females. Hip discomfort may be referred to the medial knee in the distribution of the obturator nerve. Therefore, every knee exam should mandate an examination of the hip. The hip will display a subtle decrease in all ranges of motion, especially abduction and internal rotation. Hip abduction strength is also decreased and will cause a Trendelenburg limp in which the torso lurches over the affected side.

Legg-Calvé-Perthes disease is self-limited and runs a 2- to 4-year course. Initial x-rays have minimal findings and may show disuse osteoporosis and hip joint space widening. Later, when the dead bone is being resorbed and revascularized, new bone is laid down on dead bone, causing the femoral head to appear dense (sclerotic). During this revascularization stage, radiographic changes are most dramatic. Pathologic fractures of dead trabeculae can occur with weight-bearing loads, causing a flattening of the femoral head. The femoral head can appear fragmented and laterally displaced; the metaphysis may be rarefied and broadened. The child with Legg-Calvé-Perthes disease should be referred to an orthopedic surgeon. Treatment consists of traction to regain motion followed by bracing or surgical osteotomy to protect the hip from localized stress concentration and bony collapse.

Slipped Capital Femoral Epiphysis

Another cause of childhood limping is a fracture of the proximal femoral growth plate, also called a slipped

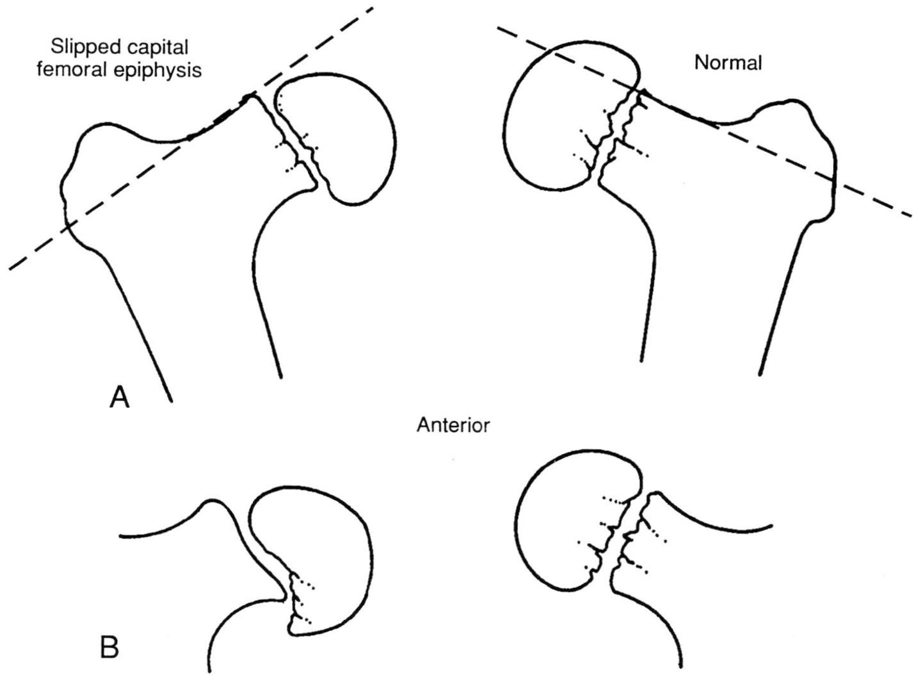

Figure 7.42. Slipped capital femoral epiphysis. The slipped capital femoral epiphysis on the left is compared to the normal hip on the right. **A**, On AP x-rays a line drawn tangential to the top of the femoral neck should pass through the normal femoral head (right). In a slipped femoral epiphysis the line does not intersect the head but passes above it (left). **B**, On a lateral radiograph the head of the femur has slipped posterior to the femoral neck (left).

capital femoral epiphysis (SCFE). SCFE is more common in males than females, is bilateral in approximately one-third of cases, and usually occurs during the prepubescent growth spurt, that is, between 10 to 14 years of age. Two distinctly different body types are susceptible to the condition. One group consists of fat children with delayed gonadal development, and the other includes very tall children who have grown rapidly.

In addition to a limp, patients may have pain localized to the knee or, less frequently, to the groin. The affected leg is held externally rotated. Internal hip rotation is limited and painful. On AP radiographs, a line drawn tangential to the superior neck does not intersect the femoral head epiphysis as it does in a normal hip (Fig. 7.42**A**). Displacement is more apparent on the lateral radiograph in which the femoral head appears posteriorly on the femoral neck (Fig. 42**B**). Untreated, this femoral head/neck slippage can continue until growth ceases. To prevent further displacement, the femoral head is fixed with multiple pins.

Congenital Club Foot

The etiology of congenital club foot (talipes equinovarus) is unknown. It occurs in approximately 1:1000 births, is twice as common in males as in females, and is bilateral in one-third of cases. The condition is characterized by three deformities: (*a*) the ankle or talus is plantar flexed (equinus), (*b*) the hindfoot or calcaneus is inverted into varus, and (*c*) the navicular bone and forefoot is shifted medially and supinated (metatarsus adductus, Fig. 7.39**B**). Untreated, this deformity would cause the patient to walk on the lateral border of the foot, not upon the sole. The posterior muscles of the leg are atrophic and contracted; therefore, neuromuscular abnormalities must be excluded in children with a club foot. Corrective casts are applied immediately with the gradual application of force directed to correct each of the three deformities. When a club foot is refractory to serial cast correction, surgical release of the tight, soft tissue structures of the posteromedial foot and ankle is indicated.

Scoliosis

Scoliosis is a lateral curvature of the spine that is either flexible (correctable) or fixed (structural). A mobile form of scoliosis may be due to poor posture, the muscle spasm secondary to a prolapsed disc, or as compensation for a shortened leg. A fixed, structural scoliosis is accompanied by a rotational vertebral deformity that is not correctable by a change in posture. Scoliosis causes an asymmetry of the rib cage that is most noticeable when the patient bends forward. In stance if the trunk is laterally shifted and not centered over the pelvis, the scoliotic curve is said to be decompensated. Decompensated scoliosis may be associated with a higher incidence of back pain.

Structural scoliosis has many etiologies, including congenital, idiopathic, neuromuscular, or neurofibromatosis. Congenital scoliosis is due to developmental abnormalities of vertebral formation and is rapidly progressive. Because the abnormality of vertebrae formation occurs during the first trimester of embryologic organogenesis, congenital scoliosis is associated with congenital anomalies of the neural tube, the genitourinary, and cardiovascular systems, which are developing concurrently. When a congenital scoliosis is identified, cardiovascular and genitourinary system evaluations should be performed. Idiopathic scoliosis, the most common variety, is seen in adolescence. Girls are affected nine times more frequently than boys. Neuromuscular scoliotic curves are usually long and involve the entire thoracolumbar spine. These curves result from paraspinal muscle imbalance produced by diseases such as polio, spinal muscle atrophy, cerebral palsy, and the muscular dystrophies. The scoliosis of neurofibromatosis is characterized by a short, severe curve.

Scoliotic deformity progresses most rapidly during periods of skeletal growth. As curvature and vertebral rotation increase, the vertebrae themselves become wedge shaped and the ribs are prominent on the convex side of the curve. These changes of vertebral structure explain the inflexibility of the curve. Aside from its cosmetic implications, severe thoracic spinal curves can compromise cardiopulmonary function. Some patients with large curves also develop degenerative spinal joint pain. Curve progression is more likely in young patients with larger curves.

Treatment is intended to prevent the curve from increasing in magnitude. Spinal braces work well in smaller curves but must be worn until the cessation of growth. Larger curves or ones that progress in severity despite bracing are managed with surgical spine fusion.

Musculoskeletal Infection

Musculoskeletal infection involves either bone (osteomyelitis), or joints (septic arthritis). Gram-positive organisms, primarily staphylococci, are usually the causative microbes. Gram-negative organisms have been increasing as a cause, especially in compromised hosts and in the nosocomial environment.

Osteomyelitis

Bacteria may infect bone by one of four mechanisms.

Hematogenous spread from a distant site
Contamination from an open fracture
After an operative procedure on bone
Extension from a contiguous infected foci

Acute Hematogenous Osteomyelitis. Acute osteomyelitis occurs most commonly in children and is due to hematogenous spread from a distant site of infection. In the 0 to 3 month age group the common causative organisms are coliforms from the maternal birth canal to which the infant is exposed during delivery. *Haemophilus influenzae* from otitis media and pharyngeal sources is common until age 3. *Staphylococcus aureus*, which predominates in skin infections, is common in all age groups. In adults, hematogenous osteomyelitis occurs in the immunocompromised patient.

Pathology. In children, metaphyseal capillaries turn back toward the diaphysis at the level of the growth plate, forming a turbulent area where organisms can be entrapped. Due to this peculiarity of interosseous vascular anatomy, the metaphyses of long bones are the most common foci of acute hematogenous osteomyelitis. Metaphyseal vessels cross the epiphyseal plate during a brief period of neonatal development, which permits epiphyseal infection to occur in infancy.

As trapped bacteria multiply and suppuration occurs in metaphyseal tissue, the pressure within the unyielding bone causes intense pain, forcing the infection through the thin metaphyseal cortex to elevate and spread beneath the periosteum as a subperiosteal abscess (Fig. 7.43). Periosteal stripping will stimulate new bone formation, which can be seen on radiographs. The infection may envelop the bone or burst through the periosteum into the soft tissues.

Clinical Presentation. Onset is acute and progression can be rapid, even life threatening. The child experiences severe pain near the end of a long bone and guards the limb, unwilling to move it. With septicemia there may be fever, increased irritability, or malaise. Soft tissue swelling occurs late and indicates that the infection has spread beyond the bone. The white blood cell count and erythrocyte sedimentation rate are usually elevated. Radiographic changes occur slowly and may not provide evidence of infection for a week or more. A three-phase technetium pyrophosphate bone scan can distinguish among soft tissue cellulitis, rheumatic fever, and acute hematogenous osteomyelitis earlier in its clinical course.

Evaluation and Treatment. Blood cultures should be obtained along with a bone marrow aspirate for cultures and Gram's stain. Parenteral antibiotic treatment should be initiated to cover organisms common to the child's age group. Final antibiotic selection will depend on the results of bacteriologic cultures and sensitivities. If local and systemic manifestations of the infection have not improved within 24 hours, open surgical drainage of subperiosteal pus is indicated as is bone drilling. Antibiotic therapy should be continued for at least 3 weeks to fully eradicate the organism. Serial sedimentation rates are useful in monitoring the therapeutic response: elevated rates should return to normal values as the infection resolves. Late complications of hematogenous osteomyelitis include the development of persistent or recurrent chronic osteomyelitis, pathologic fractures, and growth disturbances from epiphyseal plate injury.

Adult osteomyelitis typically occurs after an open fracture or as a postoperative complication. Proper management of open fractures with aggressive and repeated debridement of devitalized tissue, wound irriga-

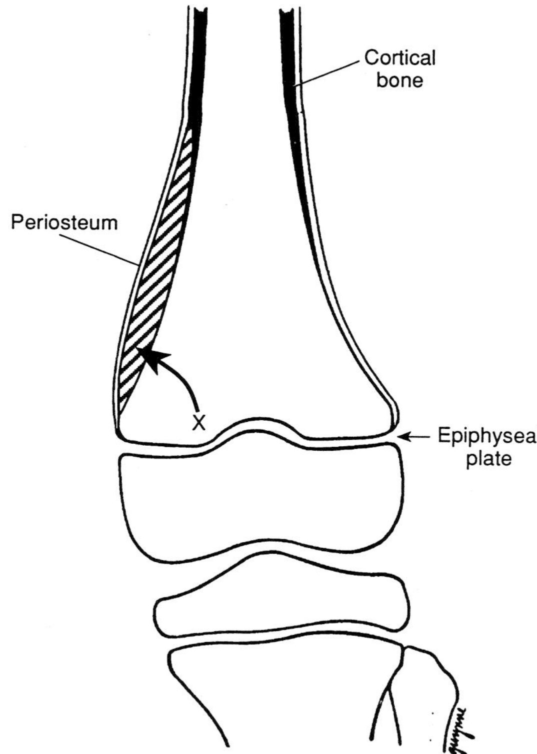

Figure 7.43. Osteomyelitis begins in the bony metaphysis where hematogenous spread leaves bacteria entrapped in the end arteriolar system of interosseous blood vessels. With exponential bacterial reproduction, pressure within the unyielding bone causes pain and forces the infection through the thin metaphyseal cortex to form a subperiosteal abscess. The epiphyseal plate and periosteum provide a temporary barrier to the infection. X = infected foci; arrow shows path of infection; shaded area = periosteum stripped from bone.

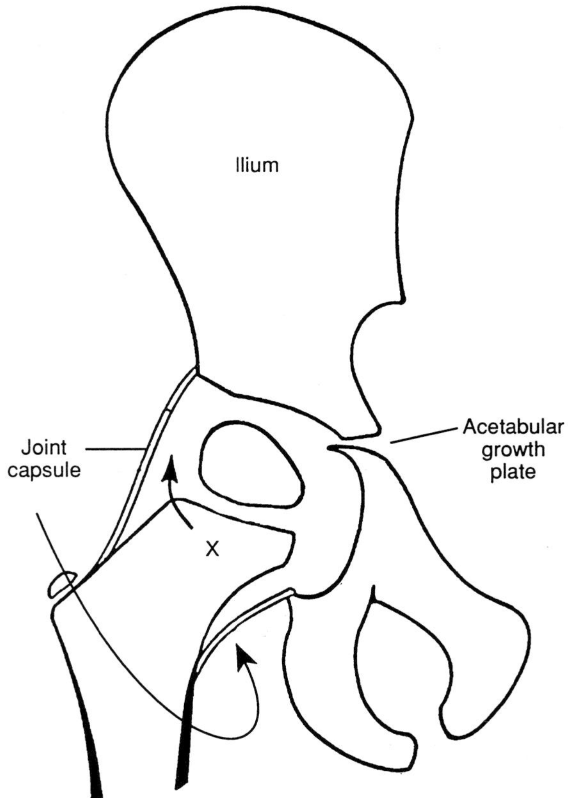

Figure 7.44. In children, septic arthritis occurs as a consequence of hematogenous osteomyelitis. The joints involved are those in which the bony metaphysis resides within a joint capsule such as the hip. When osteomyelitis erupts through the metaphyseal cortex, it will infect the joint space. X = infected foci; arrow shows path of infection.

tion, appropriate antibiotic coverage, fracture stabilization, and dressing the wound open serve to decrease the incidence of posttraumatic infection. A clean operative environment (room, air, personnel), atraumatic tissue handling, adequate hemostasis, suction drainage, and prophylactic antibiotic administration—especially in implant surgery—are surgical methods that have been shown to prevent postoperative infections. Effective treatment of an infected implant requires its surgical removal, host tissue debridement, and parenteral antibiotics. Many less virulent organisms such as *Staphylococcus epidermidis* are responsible for infected total joint replacements.

Chronic Osteomyelitis. The incomplete eradication of a previous bone infection results in chronic osteomyelitis. Bacteria that have been protected from leukocytes and antibiotics by a surrounding wall of avascular dead bone (known as a sequestrum) remain dormant in the canaliculi of dead bone. Many years after the initial infection, the bacteria can suddenly multiply, form a sinus, and drain, or they can cause an acute recurrence of the osteomyelitis. Infected, sequestered bone needs to be surgically debrided (saucerized). Soft tissue coverage may be required to enhance local blood supply and antibiotic delivery. A bone graft may be necessary if radical amounts of infected bone have been resected.

Septic Arthritis

Pathology. While bacteria can gain entrance to the joint through hematogenous spread, joint infections in adults more commonly appear following a penetrating wound or an operative procedure. When bacteria invade a synovial joint the inflammatory process can result in rapid and severe destruction of the fragile joint surface cartilage. In children septic arthritis occurs as a consequence of acute hematogenous osteomyelitis. The joints commonly involved are those in which the metaphysis resides within the joint capsule, such as the hip, elbow, and shoulder. Because the metaphysis is enclosed in the joint capsule, what begins as osteomyelitis will erupt through the cortex to involve the joint in the septic process (Fig. 7.44). Thus in children the causative organisms of septic arthritis are the same as those involved with osteomyelitis. (Staphylococcus predominates in all age groups. Gram-negative organisms have a special propensity for neonates, as do *Haemophilus influenzae* bacteria for children under the age of 3.)

Evaluation. If a newborn is profoundly ill and unresponsive, the diagnosis of septic arthritis can be difficult to make. The major finding on physical examination is restricted, painful joint motion. The joint will also be tender to palpation. Early radiographs and peripheral white blood cell counts are usually nonspecific. Since the consequences of treatment delay are so dire, the clinical suspicion of a septic joint is enough to warrant emergency joint fluid aspiration for culture and Gram's stain. To document that the joint has been entered, an arthrogram should be performed after aspiration. Joint aspiration through an area of cellulitis is contraindicated, since it may introduce organisms into the joint.

In the patient with active rheumatoid arthritis on suppressive medications, acute septic arthritis must not be mistaken for an acute flare of rheumatoid arthritis. The two can be distinguished only by joint aspiration with culture of the synovial fluid.

Treatment. To prevent the rapid degradation of articular cartilage by pyogenic toxins, treatment of a septic joint is an emergency. The most effective treatment is surgical incision of the joint capsule (arthrotomy), abscess drainage, debridement of infected loculated tissue, and joint irrigation. Intravenous antibiotic therapy is started and the wound is packed open or loosely closed over a drain. In the knee, arthroscopic drainage, irrigation, and synovectomy has been successful in eradicating joint sepsis. The potential complications from septic arthritis include: painful arthritis, epiphyseal necrosis, pathologic joint dislocation, growth disturbances, leg length discrepancies, and limb deformity.

Infected Hand Flexor Tenosynovitis

Improperly treated hand infections can result in severe disability. A flexor tendon sheath infection is especially serious as it can rapidly destroy the tendon's gliding mechanisms, create adhesions, and cause severe loss of joint motion. Tendon sheath infection can even result in tendon necrosis.

The prevailing infecting organism is *S. aureus*. Pyogenic flexor tenosynovitis is commonly caused by a penetrating palmar injury but can also occur by means of hematogenous seeding.

Kanavel described the four classic physical signs of infected flexor tendon sheaths:

The entire digit is enlarged and swollen
The finger is held in a flexed posture
The patient experiences tenderness over and limited to the course of the tendon sheath
The patient feels exquisite pain with passive digital extension

Pyogenic hand infections are limb threatening and require emergency care. If treated early with parenteral high-dose antibiotic therapy, the infectious process may be halted. Delayed resolution of symptoms and signs warrants surgical drainage with antibiotic irrigation.

Arthritis

Arthritis means joint inflammation. The two common forms are osteoarthritis and rheumatoid arthritis. The management of arthritis as it affects specific joints is the province of a more specialized text; treatment in this section will be discussed in general terms.

Osteoarthritis

Osteoarthritis is the prevalent form of arthritis affecting adults. In the adult population over age 65, there will be radiographic evidence of osteoarthritis affecting one or more joints. Osteoarthritis, also called degenerative joint disease, is characterized by the progressive deterioration of joint surface cartilage and a hypertrophic response of misdirected bone and cartilage growth. Its incidence increases with age and has no sex predilection. The etiology of osteoarthritis is not clearly understood, yet mechanical joint stresses are related to its development. Arthritis will result from joint surface incongruity, malalignment, and joint instability. Overuse related to handedness, obesity, and certain occupational tasks often affects the distribution of involved joints.

Pathology. Joint cartilage has physical properties that tolerate a limited amount of stress per unit surface area. When these forces are exceeded, the cartilage will show signs of wear. Pathologically, articular cartilage becomes softened, frayed, and fibrillated. Focal cartilage erosions become widespread and expose the underlying subchondral bone. This bone becomes sclerotic and stiff as the trabeculae thicken and cysts form. At the periphery of the joint, spurlike bony outgrowths covered by hyaline cartilage called osteophytes develop. Osteophytes are a biological attempt to decrease joint stress by increasing joint surface area and decreasing motion. The radiological hallmarks of osteoarthritis are (Fig. 7.45):

Joint space narrowing
Subchondral bone sclerosis and cyst formation
Osteophytic bone hypertrophy

Symptoms begin insidiously with local pain brought on by activity and relieved by rest. The patient will report a history of joint stiffness and the slow, progressive loss of joint motion. Since cartilage has no nerve supply, the pain arises from periarticular structures. In superficial joints, swelling may be apparent. Pain and crepitus (a crackling sensation) occur with joint motion. As the disease progresses, deformities from proliferative bone and cartilage changes become evident. Signs and symptoms often correlate with the degree and extent of radiographic abnormalities. It must be emphasized that osteoarthritis is generally a local disease. Multiple joint involvement suggests a systemic process such as collagen vascular disease.

In the hands, osteophytes form over the dorsolateral distal interphalangeal joints of the fingers and are called Heberden's nodes. The disease commonly affects the thumb trapeziometacarpal joint, causing pain at the

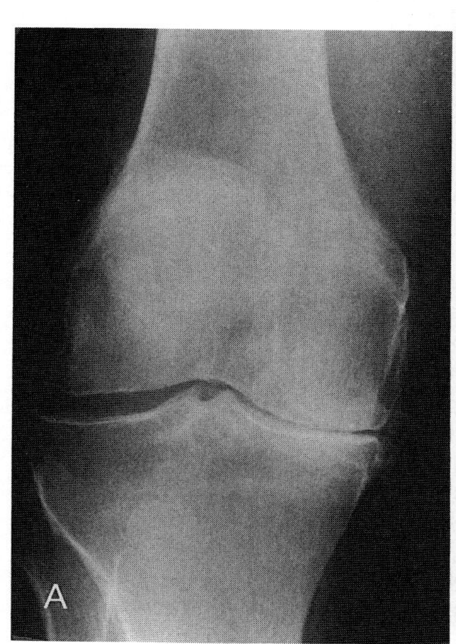

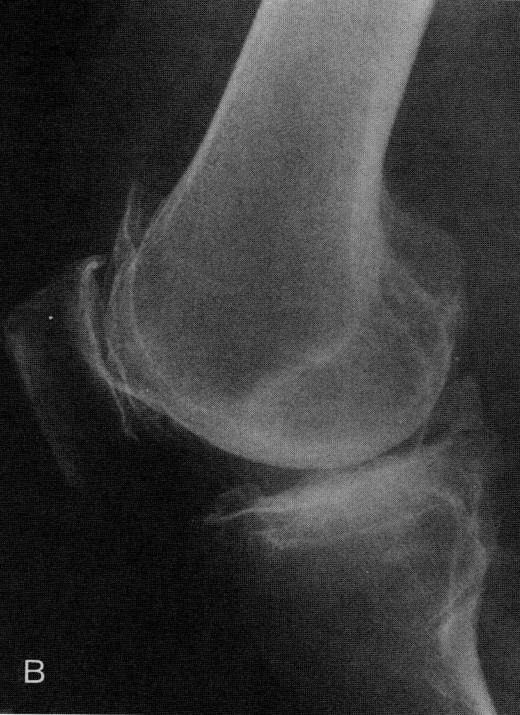

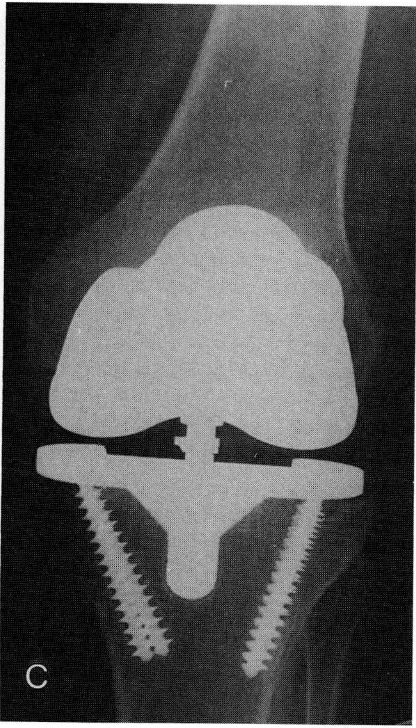

Figure 7.45. Osteoarthritis affecting the knee joint. **A**, The AP x-ray shows joint space narrowing, subchondral sclerosis, and a hypertrophic osteophytic response of the bone at the joint margins. **B**, Osteophytes (seen better on this lateral x-ray) decrease joint motion and increase joint surface area, in a biological attempt to decrease excessive joint surface stresses. **C**, The knee ultimately required total joint replacement.

base of the thumb with pinching. Weight-bearing joints such as the lumbar spine, hip, and especially the knee are frequently involved. Osteoarthritis often affects the great toe metatarsophalangeal joint of women. The hypertrophic bunion deformity (hallux valgus) of this joint is due to the abnormal stress placed upon it by pointed toe, high-heel shoe wear. Bunions are rarely seen in societies in which shoes are not worn.

Treatment

Nonsurgical Treatment. The goal of nonsurgical treatment of osteoarthritis is to relieve pain and to maintain strength and motion. Reduction of joint load by means of activity modifications, weight loss, or appliances such as a cane are attempts to protect the joint from excessive wear. Physical therapy alleviates pain with the use of heat while attempting to maintain joint motion and muscle strength through exercise. Nonsteroidal anti-inflammatory drugs that interfere with the pain-producing products of inflammation (prostaglandins, lymphokines, kinins) are palliative. Most of these drugs share toxic side effects that include rashes, peptic ulceration, and tinnitus. Analgesics should be prescribed only for acute arthritic flares. The chronic use of narcotics is to be avoided. Intra-articular steroid injections provide dramatic relief of acute symptoms. However, the repeated use of steroids may accelerate joint deterioration by direct cartilage effects as well as by masking painful joint biofeedback.

Surgical Treatment. The selection of surgical procedures depends upon the stage, site, and debility caused by the arthritis. Bony procedures fall under three categories: angular osteotomy for joint realignment, total joint replacement, and joint fusion or arthrodesis. An osteotomy realigns the extremity, corrects deformity, and shifts weight-bearing forces from worn joint surfaces to healthier cartilage. An osteotomy is analogous to rotating worn tires on a car and should be considered in younger patients with focal arthritis. An example would be a valgus producing tibial osteotomy to decompress medial compartment knee osteoarthritis from the varus deformity caused by a prior medial meniscectomy.

Total joint arthroplasty (Fig. 7.45**C**) involves the replacement of articulating biological surfaces with low friction, artificial metal and high-molecular-weight polyethylene surfaces. Total joint arthroplasty is an extremely successful procedure that profoundly relieves pain in over 90% of cases. Joint replacement is not without complications: prosthetic components wear out, loosen, become infected, and cause local osteoporosis and periprosthetic fractures. Joint replacement is thus reserved for older patients with advanced arthritis.

Joint arthrodesis is an effective procedure that converts painful arthritic joint motion into a painless, stable, fused joint. Arthrodesis is a durable procedure that is indicated in young, very active patients with isolated

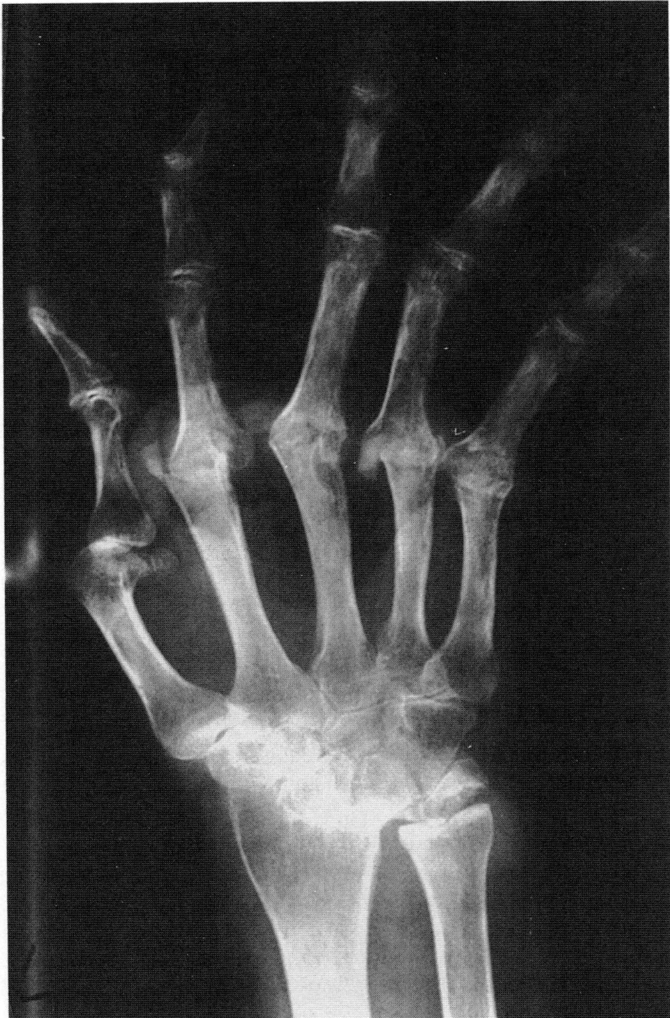

Figure 7.46. Radiographic evidence of rheumatoid arthritic joint involvement, with soft tissue swelling and multiple metacarpophalangeal joint palmar dislocations. Disuse osteoporosis is evident. Actual cartilage destruction causes joint space narrowing as exemplified at the proximal interphalangeal and wrist joints. Bone erosions occur at the site of synovial attachments. Osteophytic changes of bone hypertrophy typical of osteoarthritis are unusual with rheumatic diseases.

joint involvement. Large joint arthrodesis is contraindicated in patients with systemic multiple joint inflammatory arthritis.

Rheumatoid Arthritis

Rheumatoid arthritis is an inflammatory disorder of unknown etiology. It is a chronic polyarthritis with a relapsing, remitting course that ultimately leads to progressive joint destruction, deformity, and incapacitation.

Rheumatoid arthritis is a common illness with a female predominance of 3 to 1. The disease has a genetic basis in that individuals with the HLA-DR4 haplotype are at high risk for developing rheumatoid arthritis. Whatever the inciting factor, the immune system is involved in the disease process. Of rheumatoid patients, 80% have autoantibodies to the Fc region of the IgG immunoglobulin. The IgM autoantibody is called the rheumatoid factor. While the presence of the rheumatoid factor is not diagnostic of the disorder (1–5% of normal subjects have it) high titers are associated with severe joint disease, multisystem involvement, and a poor prognosis.

Pathology. The pathology of rheumatoid arthritis results from synovial inflammation of joints and tendon sheaths. As the delicate synovial membrane becomes infiltrated by macrophages and lymphocytes, it undergoes hypertrophy and causes joint swelling and effusions. The cytotoxic and enzymatic byproducts of the inflammatory process cause destruction of both bone and cartilage. Hypertrophic synovial cells proliferate and invade the cartilage. This synovial overgrowth of the joint surface is called pannus formation. Recurrent joint swelling stretches the capsular and supportive ligaments, which causes joint instability, deformity, and further mechanical injury. Similar inflammatory processes weaken tendons and cause muscle imbalance in the complex joint systems of the hand. Joint and tendon subluxation is common in rheumatoid hands that become weak and deformed (Fig. 7.46). The systemic nature of the disease is made evident by its extra-articular manifestations: vasculitis, neuropathy, iritis, lymphadenopathy, splenomegaly, and polyserositis. Just as the pathophysiology of rheumatoid arthritis differs from that of osteoarthritis, so the radiologic pictures differ. Soft tissue swelling and periarticular osteoporosis are the early signs of rheumatoid arthritis. Diffuse cartilage destruction leads to joint space narrowing and bone erosions at the site of synovial attachments (Fig. 7.46). Joint deformity, cystic bone destruction, and joint ankylosis mark end-stage disease. Hypertrophic osteophytic radiographs are much less common to rheumatologic conditions.

Treatment. The treatment of rheumatoid arthritis is directed toward pain relief, suppression of the inflammatory synovitis, prevention of joint deformities, and early joint reconstruction to maximize patient function and productivity. In its early stages the synovitis is managed either by drug inhibition or by surgical removal of the diseased synovium (synovectomy). Splinting the involved joints in functional positions during acute flare-ups rests the joint, prevents contractures, and minimizes deformity. Exercises to maintain range of motion and muscle strength, while painful and frustrating to the patient, are encouraged. With advanced joint destruction, tendon ruptures are repaired, and either excisional or replacement arthroplasty helps to restore mobility and function.

To optimize the patient's function, it is often necessary to employ mechanical aids and adaptive apparatus and to modify the physical layout of both the home and work place. The proper management of rheumatoid arthritis requires the multidisciplinary teamwork of a social worker, rheumatologist, surgeon, physiotherapist, and occupational therapist.

Other Arthritides

While rheumatoid and osteoarthritis are the most common arthritic conditions, there are a myriad of other arthritic diseases, including juvenile arthritis, the spondyloarthropathies of ankylosing spondylitis, Reiter's disease, and psoriatic arthritis. In the arthropathies of gout and pseudogout, insoluble crystals are deposited in joints. With gouty arthritis, microscopic analysis of joint fluid under polarized light reveals splinterlike, monoclinic, negatively birefringent uric acid crystals. Whereas in pseudogout, positively birefringent, rhomboid-shaped, calcium pyrophosphate dihydrate crystals are apparent. Radiographs of the latter may reveal typical articular cartilage or meniscal calcification. Some arthritides are caused by infectious agents such as gonococcal arthritis and Lyme disease (*Borrelia burgdorferi*). Neuropathies, hemophilia, and a host of other diseases also have arthritic manifestations.

Bone Necrosis

Interruption of the blood supply to bone results in bone cell death termed *osteonecrosis* or *avascular necrosis*. Traumatic causes of osteonecrosis have been discussed and involve interruption of the macrovascular blood supply to bones. The femoral head, talus, carpal lunate, and scaphoid are prone to avascular necrosis, as these bones all are extensively covered by articular cartilage and have limited soft tissue attachments. Legg-Calvé-Perthes disease of the femoral head represents a pediatric form of avascular necrosis. Atraumatic causes of osteonecrosis involve interosseous microvascular disturbances that result from either embolic arterial interference or impairment of venous outflow, which increase interosseous pressures that compromise bone perfusion.

Patients on glucocorticoid therapy (especially systemic lupus erythematosus and renal transplants) constitute the largest group developing nontraumatic osteonecrosis. The thrombi of hemoglobinopathies (e.g., sickle cell disease), the nitrogen bubbles of decompression sickness (dysbarism), the glucocerebroside deposits of Gaucher's disease, hyperuricemic crystals, fat emboli of alcoholism, and pancreatitis all cause an occlusive form of bone infarction. Affected bones have a paucity of arterial anastomoses, with the femoral head of the hip being the most frequently symptomatic and debilitated by avascular necrosis.

Pathology

Bone is a dynamic, cellular, living tissue that undergoes homeostatic resorption, replacement, and remodeling, albeit slowly. Following a loss of blood supply, bone cell and marrow necrosis occur within 24 hours. While these changes can be detected microscopically by the absence of osteocytes from their lacunae, there is often a delay of as much as 5 years between the onset of symptoms and the appearance of radiological abnormalities. Magnetic resonance imaging is the most sensitive method of detecting early osteonecrosis.

The revascularization process is slow. The living bone surrounding the infarction becomes hypervascular. The hyperemia of the surrounding bone causes osteoporosis, while the dead tissue retains its density and appears white (sclerotic) on x-rays. As new vessels invade the necrotic zone, new bone is laid down on the old trabeculae and dead bone is removed by osteoclasts. This reparative bone resorption weakens the femoral head at the periphery of the infarct. With persistent weight-bearing stress, the necrotic subchondral bone may collapse, resulting in painful joint degeneration (Fig. 7.47). Initially, the articular cartilage remains intact because it is nourished by synovial fluid. When bone support is lost, however, the cartilage becomes mechanically injured and a process similar to osteoarthritis causes joint destruction.

Evaluation and Treatment

The symptoms of osteonecrosis may not become manifest for a long time following an avascular incident. Symptoms begin with painful limited active motion. Two-thirds of patients complain of pain at rest. In the elderly, a condition known as *spontaneous osteonecrosis* of the femoral condyle occurs with the sudden onset of severe knee pain not associated with trauma. Many cases will demonstrate increased bone scan activity over the femoral condyle that will resolve with symptomatic care.

The prevention of joint loading until natural healing processes are completed is the basis of conservative treatment. Core decompression, in which dead cancellous bone is trephined from the ischemic segment, is best employed early in the disease process. Interosseous pressure is decompressed as the biopsy track creates an avenue for revascularization.

Although the inciting agent is vascular, the joint deterioration results from mechanical factors similar to osteoarthritis. The management principles for advanced disease are similar to those employed in the treatment of osteoarthritis. However, if the volume of dead bone is large, realignment osteotomy or arthrodesis may further compromise bone healing, and consequently joint replacement with a prosthesis is a reasonable treatment option. Unfortunately, avascular necrosis occurs in younger patients whose high activity levels place potentially dangerous stresses upon prosthetic joints.

The Spine

Lumbar Spine

Low back pain is a common musculoskeletal problem for the 30- to 65-year age group. At some time in their lives, 80% of the population will experience an episode of low back pain severe enough to interfere with normal daily activities. In the United States, the annual cost of back-related medical payments has been estimated at $16 billion. An additional $50 billion is attributed each year to lost worker productivity.

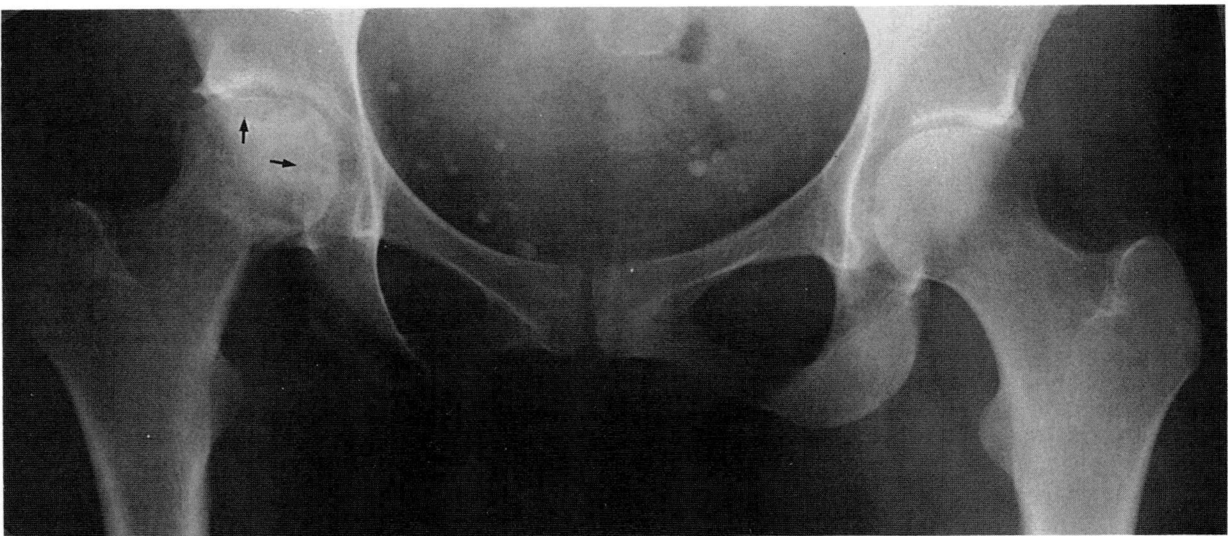

Figure 7.47. Advanced avascular necrosis of the femoral head in a patient with sarcoidosis who had been treated with systemic steroids. The femoral head is dense (sclerotic). There is evidence of a subchondral lucency (arrows) with joint surface flattening, collapse, and marginal osteophyte formation.

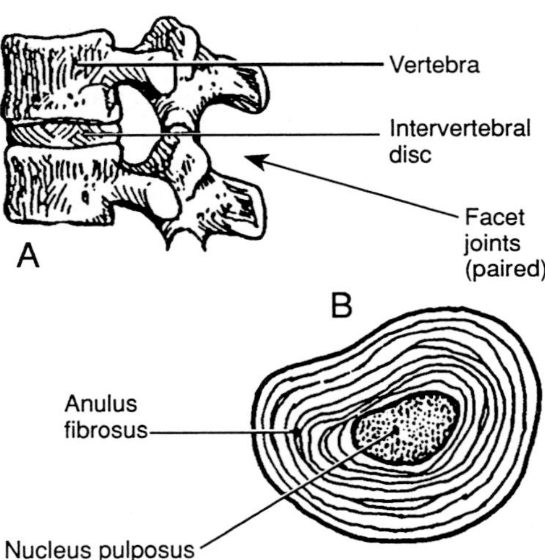

Figure 7.48. **A**, The spinal motion segment consists of two vertebral bodies and the intervening disc. Motion occurs through two paired facet joints and the disc. The vertebrae rock or pivot over the disc in flexion and lateral bending. **B**, The disc is comprised of a central gelatinous nucleus pulposus and its peripheral fibrous encasement, the annulus fibrosus.

Etiology of Low Back Pain. Degenerative joint disease is far more common to the joints of the spine than to the joints to the limbs. The spine is an articulated column of vertebrae that protects the spinal cord and nerve roots. These neural elements can also be affected by degenerative spinal pathology. The motion segment of the spine is composed of two bony vertebrae covered with cartilage end plates and the interposed disc. Vertebral motion takes place through a three-joint complex: the symphyseal disc and two posterior synovial facet joints (Fig. 7.48**A**). The disc is composed of a central gelatinous nucleus pulposus and an elastic peripheral incasement, the annulus fibrosus (Fig. 7.48**B**). In flexion-extension and lateral binding, the vertebrae rock over the disc, which acts as a pivot. The spatial orientation of the paired facet joints directs spinal motion: the lumbar vertebral facets are in the sagittal plane and permit flexion and extension, while the thoracic facets are oriented in more of a horizontal plane, allowing lateral bending and rotatory motion. Degenerative spine disease anatomically affects the two sites of spinal motion; the disc and/or the facet joints. The ligaments that tether the vertebrae together include the anterior and posterior longitudinal ligaments attached to the vertebral bodies. The ligamentum flavum connects the laminae with the inter- and supraspinous ligaments between the spinous processes (Fig. 7.49). The paraspinal muscles are complex and span between two and five segments. These muscles confer spinal motion and absorb the stresses of erect bipedal posture.

Contrary to popular opinion, the vast majority of low back pain is not due to a "slipped disc." In 80 to 90% of patients with low back pain, the pain is of unknown etiology and unidentifiable pathology. Less than 10% of patients experience pain in the sciatic nerve (L5–S3) distribution—sciatica. Only 1 to 2% of patients require surgical treatment for a disc herniation. With symptomatic care, 50% improve over 2 weeks and 90% in 3 months.

Lumbar Strain (Mechanical Back Pain). Most cases of back pain result from minor events, not from significant trauma. Many injuries involve myofascial strains, minor ligament injury, or overuse arthritis. Lack of exercise, poor muscle tone, and obesity contribute to minor postural injuries of the spine. This type of mechanical back pain is common to women during or after pregnancy. The pain of mechanical strain rarely radiates beyond the knee and remains localized to the spine

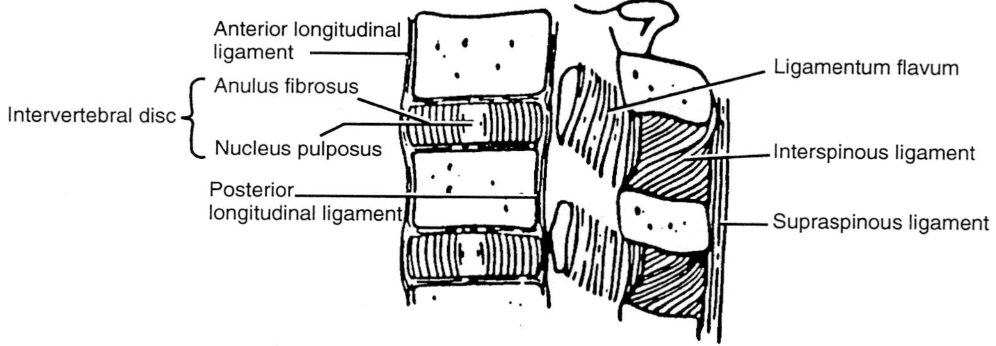

Figure 7.49. The ligaments of the spinal column.

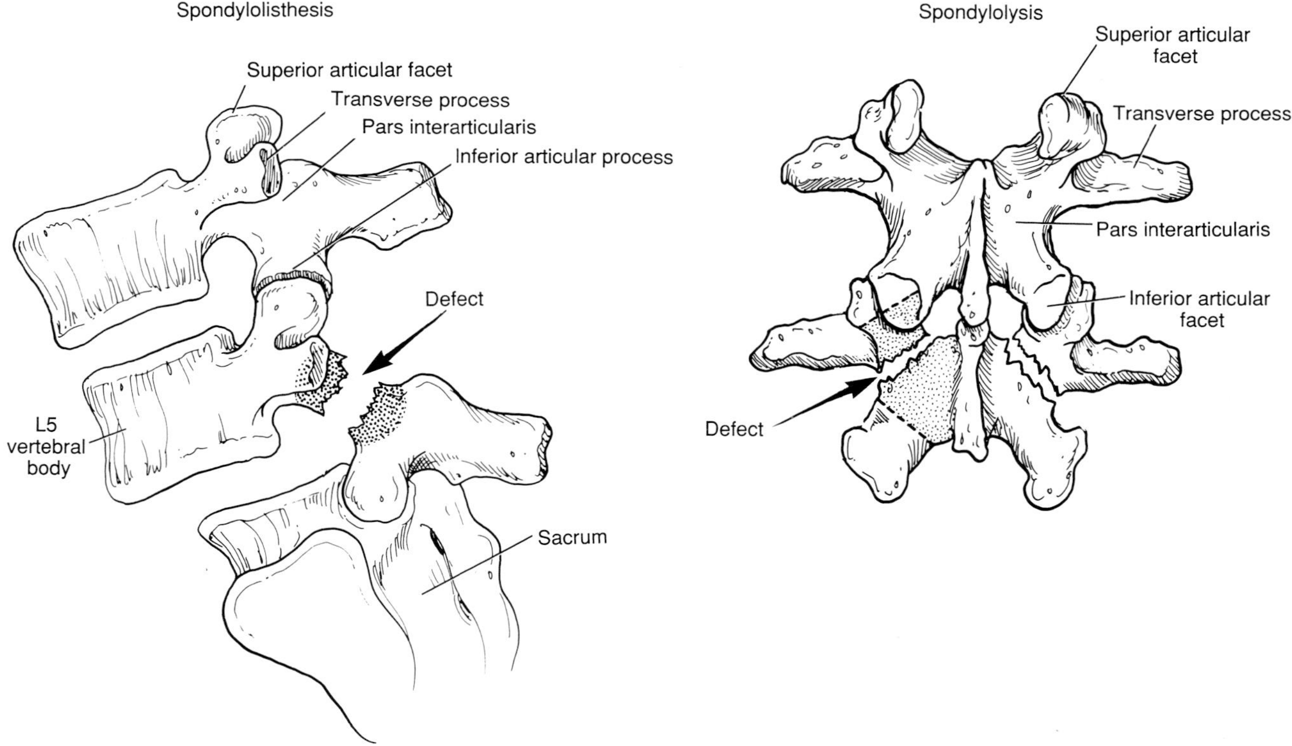

Figure 7.50. The lumbar facet joints are oriented in the sagittal plane and allow flexion and extension. With lumbar extension the facet joints engage; when a significant rotatory force is added, the lamina just inferior to the facet may fracture. This fracture is called spondylolysis, which literally means spine lysis (right). If spondylolytic fractures occur bilaterally, the unsupported superior vertebrae may translate anteriorly, producing spondylolisthesis (left).

and buttocks. Over 80% of these back problems resolve within 6 weeks of onset.

Spondylolysis. The facet joints of the lumbar spine are oriented in a sagittal plane, which permits flexion and extension while resisting rotational and lateral bending motion. When the spine is hyperextended the facet joints are engaged. If a rotational twisting force is added, the lamina may fracture, either following an acute injury or from the stress of repetitive microtrauma. The fracture occurs immediately caudal to the superior facet in a region called the pars interarticularis (Fig. 7.50**A**). This injury, spondylolysis, occurs 10 times more frequently in gymnasts than in age-matched controls and results from back extension during dismount landings. If the fracture is bilateral, the superior vertebral body lacking facet support can slide forward on the inferior vertebra. This anterior shift of one vertebrae on another is called spondylolisthesis (Fig. 7.50**B**). In young patients the condition may be painful and the amount of slippage can progress in magnitude. Spinal fusion is the standard treatment for a progressive, painful spondylolisthesis.

Disc Herniation. Disc herniation is the result of disc degeneration and is prevalent in adults between the

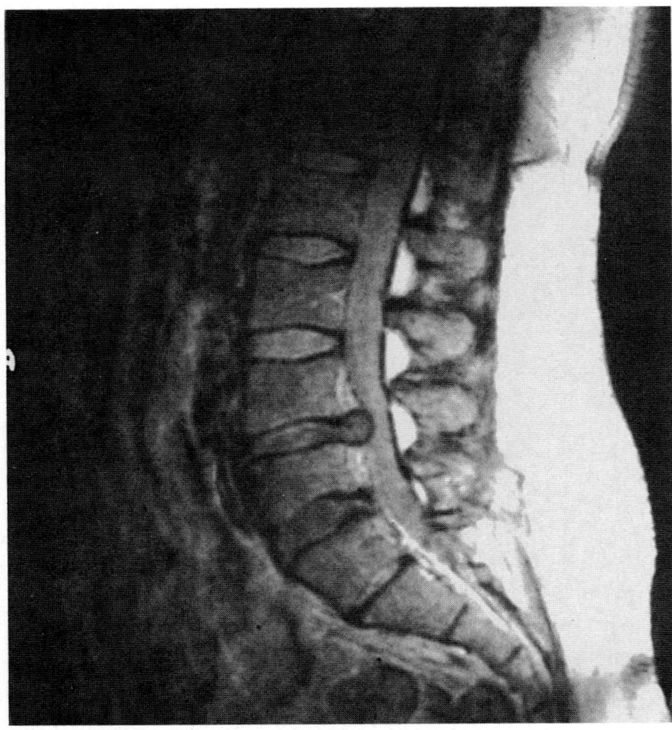

Figure 7.51. Magnetic resonance scan of a large L4-5 herniated disc. The epidural fat plane is obliterated as the disc exerts extradural pressure on the thecal space.

ages of 30 and 50, the prime of working life. The most frequently involved discs are at L4-5 and L5-S1, the most mobile lumbar spinal segments. A ruptured L4-5 disc will affect the L5 nerve root, and an L5-S1 disc the S1 root. In adult life the nucleus pulposus loses proteoglycans and water content, making it less resilient. In the aging process, the annulus fibrosus loses its elasticity, especially posteriorly where it is thinnest. The combination of age-related changes and repeated minor trauma can cause tears in the annulus. If an annular rent is large, it will permit the extrusion of the nucleus pulposus. In some cases the herniated disc material will be resorbed. In others, it will exert direct pressure on the nerve root (Fig. 7.51).

Clinically, patients complain of severe low back pain often after bending to lift or while twisting with a heavy object. The pain emanates from the back or buttock and radiates into the leg and foot in a radicular (nerve root), dermatomal distribution. The pain is accentuated by bending, sitting, and coughing. The supine straight-leg raising test places traction on the S1 nerve root and to a lesser degree the L5 root. This test will reproduce the pain. Ankle dorsiflexion will accentuate the pain (Lasègue maneuver), while ankle plantar flexion should not affect it. The latter test is helpful to determine the true organicity of the pain and to rule out malingerers. Radicular motor weakness, numbness, and reflex diminution provide objective evidence of nerve root entrapment (Table 7.4). When a large amount of disc has been extruded into the spinal canal, it may compress more

Table 7.4.
Lumbar Lesions and Associated Radicular Abnormalities

Location	Abnormality
L4 Nerve Root	
Pain/Numbness	Medial leg and ankle
Sensory	Hypesthesia, medial leg and ankle
Motor	Weak ankle dorsiflexion or weak quadriceps (knee extension)
Reflex	Decreased knee jerk
L5 Nerve Root	
Pain/Numbness	Lateral calf and dorsal foot
Sensory	Hypesthesia, dorsal foot
Motor	Weak extensor hallux longus
Reflex	Usually none; decreased posterior tibial tendon reflex possible (but that reflex present only in 20% of normal patients)
S1 Nerve Root	
Pain/Numbness	Posterior calf, lateral and plantar foot
Sensory	Hypesthesia, lateral foot
Motor	Weak toe and ankle flexors, foot evertors
Reflex	Decreased ankle jerk

than one nerve root. When multiple nerve roots are involved, the clinical picture may be confusing because of overlapping patterns of pain and functional losses. When bowel and bladder continence is lost, there is a massive disc herniation compressing multiple S1–4 roots. Called the *cauda equina syndrome*, this condition is a surgical emergency demanding decompression to prevent permanent incontinence. Myelography, CT, and MR scans effectively define pathologic anatomy (the extent of the neural canal compromise) and are helpful diagnostic modalities when surgery is anticipated.

Spinal Stenosis. The paired spinal facets are synovial joints, and likewise are subject to degenerative arthritic processes. Spondylosis is the term used for osteoarthritis as it affects the spine. Recurrent compressive and rotational spinal stresses cause disc and facet joint surface wear. The disc space may narrow, causing settling facet subluxation and infolding of the ligamentum flavum. The development of hypertrophic facet joint osteophytes may restrict spinal mobility and also narrow the spinal canal and neural foramina. These bony facet spurs can irritate and entrap the exiting nerve roots. The encroachment of spinal canal or foraminal contents by degenerative hypertrophic spondyloarthritic changes is called *spinal stenosis*.

Spinal stenosis affects the elderly and usually involves multiple spinal levels. Patients complain of back and leg pain and of weakness brought on by walking and extension of the lumbar spine (sometimes called neurogenic claudication). Spinal flexion disengages the facet joints and produces pain relief.

Surgery for spinal stenosis involves extensive multiple level cord and nerve root decompressions. Careful preoperative evaluation is necessary to properly identify the multiplicity of pathology. Myelography with CT and MR images of several spinal levels are needed to define the pathology and extent of neural canal and foraminal compromise. Each disc space is evaluated for herniation and each facet joint for stenosis of the lateral recess of the spinal canal.

Other Causes of Back Pain. There are many other causes of back pain. The medical history is extremely helpful in identifying the etiology of low back disorders. The differential diagnosis includes:

1. Disc herniation with nerve root irritation or neurological deficit
2. Spinal stenosis
3. Vertebral infection
4. Primary or metastatic (especially breast and prostate) neoplasms
5. Trauma (see Chapter 8, Neurosurgery)
6. Rheumatological conditions (e.g., ankylosing spondylitis, rheumatoid arthritis, Reiter's disease)
7. Vascular disorders (e.g., aortic aneurysm or aortic dissection)
8. Psychogenic or malingering pain (a vague history and bizarre gait with inconsistent physical findings suggest psychogenic causes)

Treatment. Nonsurgical measures are effective in most cases of back pain and should be tried before surgery is contemplated. Patient education about the causes and nature of back pain is important. Instruction in proper postural mechanics and lifting techniques will prevent reinjury. Patients should be encouraged to take an active interest in and be responsible for their own back care. Patients with back and referred leg pain may benefit from a short period of bed rest and heat followed by an active back exercise program. A brace can confer mechanical support to the lumbar spine by a hydraulic effect on abdominal contents that increases intra-abdominal pressure. The brace also acts as a proprioceptive device, reminding the patient to lift and bend properly. The excessive use of bed rest and back braces is to be condemned as both can cause paraspinal muscle atrophy.

Nonsteroidal anti-inflammatory medications are useful for their antiarthritic effects. Narcotic analgesics and antispasmodic agents are to be used with caution, however, especially with chronic back pain, since both mask symptoms and may cause chemical dependency. Since herniated disc material may atrophy or be resorbed, a conservative approach is also indicated for patients with acute lumbar disc protrusion. The two absolute indications for surgical decompression are: (*a*) when disc herniation causes a progressive neurologic deficit or (*b*) when a cauda equina syndrome is suspected and there is loss of bowel and/or bladder continence.

Approximately 10% of patients with back pain do not respond to nonoperative treatment. If sciatica persists for more than 2 months of conservative care, surgery may be considered. The results are better if surgery is performed within 6 months of the onset of symptoms. After 6 months the patient becomes physically deconditioned and psychologically dependent. The candidate for surgery should have consistent physical and radiographic findings. Spine surgery treats symptoms and does not reverse the degenerative processes of spinal aging and arthritis. Therefore, operations for disc herniations should be precisely defined so that the surgery can be effected through a small incision with maximal preservation of noninvolved tissue. In patients with spinal stenosis, decompression is more radical. All structures causing nerve root pressure, herniated discs, osteophytic spurs, and calcified ligaments are surgically removed from each involved spinal level. The indications for spinal fusion are controversial. In patients with spinal instability from progressive spondylolisthesis or after anatomically extensive decompression, spinal fusion can be an effective stabilizing and palliative procedure.

Table 7.5.
Cervical Lesions and Associated Radicular Abnormalities

Location	Abnormality
C5 Nerve Root	
Sensory	Hypesthesia lateral arm
Motor	Weak deltoid, biceps
Reflex	Decreased biceps reflex
C6 Nerve Root	
Sensory	Hypesthesia lateral forearm and palmar thumb
Motor	Weak wrist extension
Reflex	Decreased brachioradialis reflex
C7 Nerve Root	
Sensory	Hypesthesia long finger
Motor	Weak finger extension, triceps
Reflex	Decreased triceps reflex
C8 Nerve Root	
Sensory	Hypesthesiamedial froearm and little finger
Motor	Weak finger flexion
Reflex	None
Myelopathy	
Sensory	Diffuse hypesthesias
Motor	Diffuse weakness, increased muscle tone, rigidity
Reflex	Hyperreflexia with clonus
	Positive Hoffman's or Babinski's sign

Cervical Spine

Disc protrusion and hypertrophic osteoarthritic spondylosis also occur in the cervical spine. The erosive destabilizing synovitis of rheumatoid arthritis has a special propensity for the mobile cervical spine.

Cervical Disc Protrusion. The combined effects of age-related disc degeneration and abnormal stresses cause cervical disc herniations. When disc material presses upon the posterior longitudinal ligament, symptoms of stiffness and neck pain may be referred to the scapular region. When the herniated disc material occurs posterior and lateral to the posterior longitudinal ligament, it may impinge upon a cervical nerve root causing radicular pain, numbness, focal motor weakness, and diminution or loss of upper extremity deep tendon reflexes (Table 7.5). The most commonly ruptured discs are at the C5-6 and C6-7 interspaces, where cervical flexion-extension motion is the greatest. Likewise, the respective C6 and C7 nerve roots are most often affected by cervical disc pathology.

Nonoperative treatment involves rest, immobilization with a soft cervical collar, heat, and anti-inflamma-

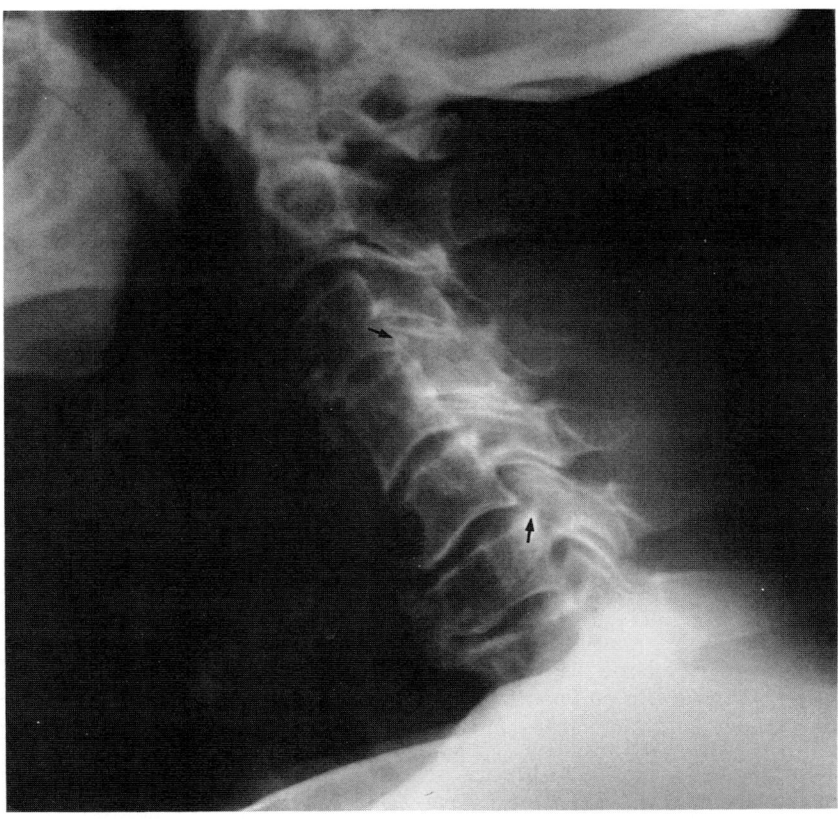

Figure 7.52. Osteoarthritic cervical spondylosis with anterior vertebral body osteophyte formation and disc space narrowing. Posterior vertebral body osteophytes also called Luschka (or uncovertebral) joints (arrows) can cause encroachment on the spinal cord. This is known as a hard disc.

tory medication. Traction may help to alleviate nerve root pressure. Indications for surgical intervention are similar to those in the lumbar spine. Emergency decompressive surgery is indicated if there is spinal cord involvement (myelopathy) with hyperreflexia, ipsilateral weakness, contralateral numbness, or the presence of pathological long tract reflexes such as the Babinski or Hoffmann signs.

Cervical Spondylosis. Degenerative changes cause disc space narrowing. Osteophytes form at the posterior disc margin, creating a "hard disc." These bone spurs, called Luschka's joints, can encroach centrally upon the spinal cord or peripherally on an individual nerve root (Fig. 7.52). The clinical picture is similar to the herniation of the nucleus pulposus (soft disc), except that the onset of symptoms is more gradual. Treatment for degenerative cervical spondyloarthrosis is similar to that for cervical disc protrusion. When refractory to conservative treatment modalities, both conditions respond to anterior cervical discectomy with a fusion.

Rheumatoid Arthritis of the Cervical Spine. Rheumatoid arthritis frequently involves the synovial joints of the cervical spine. Progressive inflammatory destruction of bone, ligaments, and articular cartilage may result in cervical spine instability, which may also cause neural compression.

Rheumatic cervical spine involvement usually takes one of three patterns:

1. Rheumatoid inflammation and swelling of the small synovial joint between the atlas and the odontoid process can stretch the stabilizing transverse ligament and cause the atlantoaxial joint to subluxate with flexion. The two vertebrae no longer move in tethered synchrony, which causes spinal canal narrowing and potential cord compromise by the posteriorly displaced dens.
2. Erosive synovitis between the atlas (C1 vertebra) and the occipital condyles causes cranial settling that may cause the odontoid process of the axis (C2) to protrude into the foramen magnum. This phenomenon is called occipitoatlantoaxial impaction.
3. Finally, facet joint synovitis affecting any cervical vertebrae below the axis can cause segmental instability known as subaxial subluxation. This instability is demonstrated on x-rays by abnormal vertebral body tilt or displacement in an anterior-posterior direction.

The prevalence of cervical instability in patients with polyarticular rheumatoid arthritis is such that flexion-extension lateral cervical spine x-rays must be obtained in any rheumatoid patient undergoing intubation for a general anesthetic. Neurological involvement does not necessarily correlate with the degree of cervical vertebral subluxation. However, when neurologic impairment does result from cervical instability, the treatment of choice is stabilization by surgical spine fusion. Most

Table 7.6.
Causes of Osteoporosis

Involutional	Postmenopausal age
Nutritional deficiencies	Scurvy
Endocrine disorders	Hypogonadism Hyperparathyroidism Cushing's disease Hyperthyroidism
Drug use	Corticosteroids Methotrexate
Disuse	Prolonged bed rest Weightlessness
Inflammatory arthritis	Rheumatoid arthritis Ankylosing spondylitis Chronic infection (tuberculosis)
Malignant disease	Multiple myeloma Leukemia
Idiopathic	

cases of rheumatoid neck pain, however are successfully managed by nonoperative treatment modalities.

Metabolic Endocrine Disorders

Bone is a biphasic material consisting of an inert mineral and an organic matrix. The mineral is composed of calcium and phosphorous in a hydroxyapatite crystal $Ca_{10}(PO_4)_6(OH)_2$. The organic matrix (osteoid) is primarily composed of type I collagen, which has high tensile strength. The mineral phase of bone resists compressive forces, while the organic collagen fiber phase provides reinforcement and resistance to bending and twisting stress (like the meshed wire in cement). Normal bone is 70% mineral and 30% organic matrix.

Osteoporosis

Bone strength depends upon the amount of bone per unit volume and its mineralization density or calcium content. In osteoporosis the chemical composition of the bone is normal, but total bone per unit volume is less than would be expected in a person of a given age and sex. Another way of stating this is that in osteoporosis, while the ratio of bone mineral to organic matrix is normal, the absolute value of each is decreased. The bone is therefore weak, less dense, and predisposed to fractures with minimal trauma. The most common type of osteoporosis is called the involutional senile type and is seen in postmenopausal, white females. Its cause is not known. Other conditions also result in osteoporosis (Table 7.6). Osteoporosis is second to arthritis in being the leading cause of musculoskeletal morbidity in the elderly. The first symptoms occur when bone mass is so compromised that the skeleton cannot withstand the mechanical stresses of everyday life. Compression fractures of vertebral bodies, fractures of the proximal femur (hip, Fig. 7.18), humerus and distal radius (Colles', Fig. 7.15) are often the first morbid manifestations of osteoporosis. These patients should be screened for the medically treatable causes of osteoporosis.

Table 7.7.
Causes of Osteomalacia

Dietary	Vitamin D deficiency (rickets)
Hereditary	Hypophosphatemic rickets
Gastrointestinal	Biliary disease Pancreatitis Celiac sprue Milk alkali syndrome Cirrhosis
Drugs	Phenytoin Barbiturates
Chronic renal disease	

Osteomalacia

Osteomalacia is the result of a deficiency in the mineral content of bone. In contrast to osteoporosis, in osteomalacia the amount of bone substance per unit volume is normal, yet because the matrix is incompletely calcified the bone quality is abnormal. Clinically and radiographically, osteoporosis and osteomalacia are similar. Often the distinction is made by histomorphometry, an analytic technique that requires ultrathin, nondecalcified, tetracycline-labeled bone biopsy specimens. In osteomalacia, wide osteoid seams of unmineralized bone are detected. The ratio of bone mineral to organic bone matrix is decreased because there is a mineral deficiency. In osteoporosis the ratio of bone mineral to matrix is normal but the quantity of each is deficient.

Inadequate bone mineralization can result from a variety of factors that affect calcium metabolism: inadequate dietary vitamin D or calcium intake, gastrointestinal malabsorption of calcium, problems with the enzymatic conversion of vitamin D, or defective renal calcium and phosphorous handling (Table 7.7). Correctable defects in the calcium pathway can be screened with serum calcium and phosphorous, blood urea nitrogen (BUN) and creatinine levels, which should help to direct appropriate gastrointestinal, endocrine, and renal workups. In addition to the generalized decrease in bone density seen radiologically, a band of bone rarefaction called a Looser zone is typical of osteomalacia (Fig. 7.53). The Looser zone represents a healing stress fracture and is most often noted in the femoral neck or pubic rami.

The pediatric form of osteomalacia is called *rickets* and is caused by dietary vitamin D deficiency and lack of exposure to sunlight. This disease was common during the industrial revolution before the advent of child

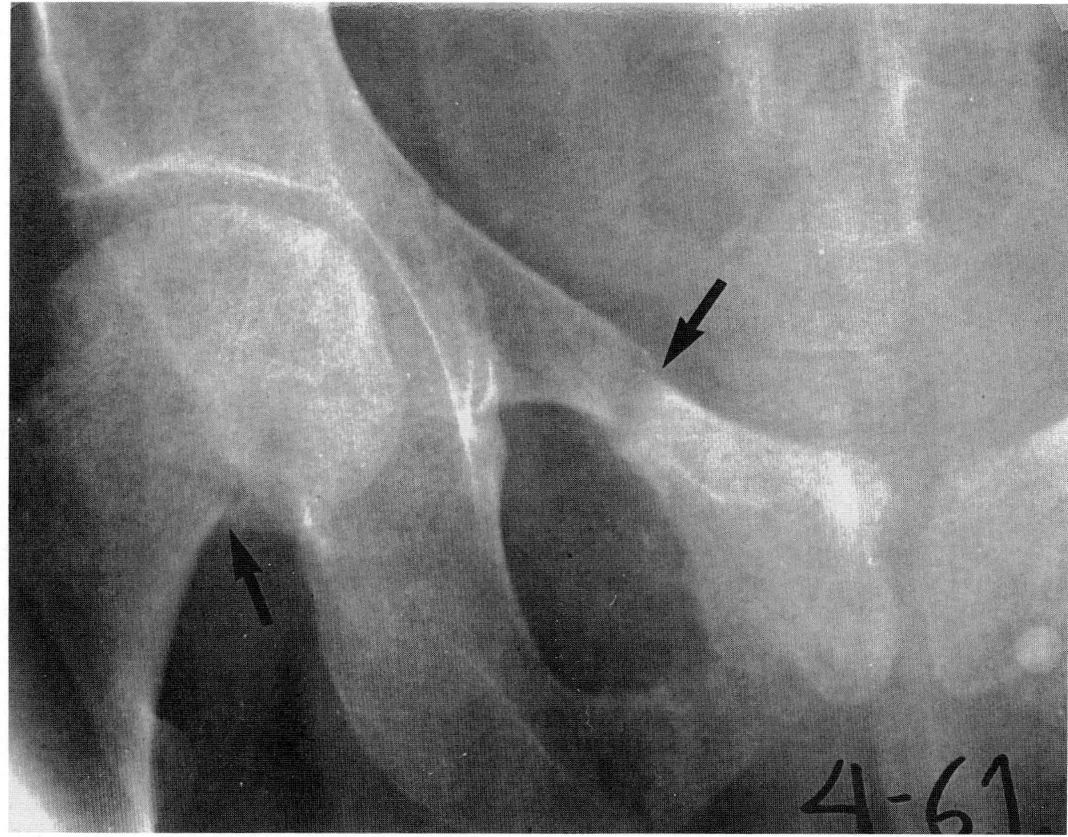

Figure 7.53. Looser line seen with osteomalacia. The band of rarefaction in the superior pubic ramus and in the femoral neck (as shown by the arrows) represents a stress fracture and is due to inadequate bone mineralization.

labor laws. Today rickets is seen primarily in a genetic disease called vitamin-D-resistant (hypophosphatemic) rickets, which is transmitted in an autosomal dominant pattern. In growing children, x-rays of osteomalacia (rickets) demonstrate widened growth plates and cupped metaphyses (Fig. 7.54). Soft, undermineralized long bones may be abnormally bowed.

Hyperparathyroidism

Hyperparathyroidism also produces diffuse bony osteopenia. Parathyroid hormone is involved with the homeostasis of ionized calcium levels in the blood. In response to low serum calcium or high serum phosphorous concentrations, parathyroid hormone acts to increase (*a*) calcium release from bone, (*b*) calcium absorption by the intestines, and (*c*) calcium reabsorption by the kidney (while decreasing renal absorption of phosphate). These changes cause a net increase in plasma calcium and a decrease in plasma phosphate levels. Primary hyperparathyroidism is due to an adenoma or hyperplasia of the parathyroid gland, which causes excess parathyroid hormone production. Secondary hyperparathyroidism is due to chronic renal insufficiency with decreased phosphate excretion. Radiographs of hyperparathyroidism show diffuse bony rarefaction but also include disseminated focal osteolytic lesions of cortical bone called *osteitis fibrosis cystica* (Fig. 7.55).

Paget's Disease

Paget's disease (osteitis deformans) is a disorder of unknown etiology characterized by excessive bone resorption and unregulated abundant bone formation. The involved areas of bone are highly vascular and can cause massive arteriovenous shunting with high output cardiac failure. In the early (osteolytic) phase of the disease, bone resorption exceeds deposition. The bone is weak and may fracture and bend. Later, bone formation predominates (osteosclerotic phase), causing the bones to become enlarged and thickened.

Pagetic patients complain of bone pain, progressive lower limb bowing, or head enlargement. Fractures prone to nonunion can occur through this pathologic bone. Serum alkaline phosphatase levels secreted by bone-forming osteoblasts can be markedly elevated with Paget's disease. Microscopically, the bone displays a wild, irregular, mosaic pattern of mature and immature bone. Radiographs show dense and irregular sclerotic bony trabeculae (Fig. 7.56). Long bone fractures are characteristically transverse and begin as a crack on the convex or tension side of the deformed bone. These wild, bone-forming cells undergo malignant degenera-

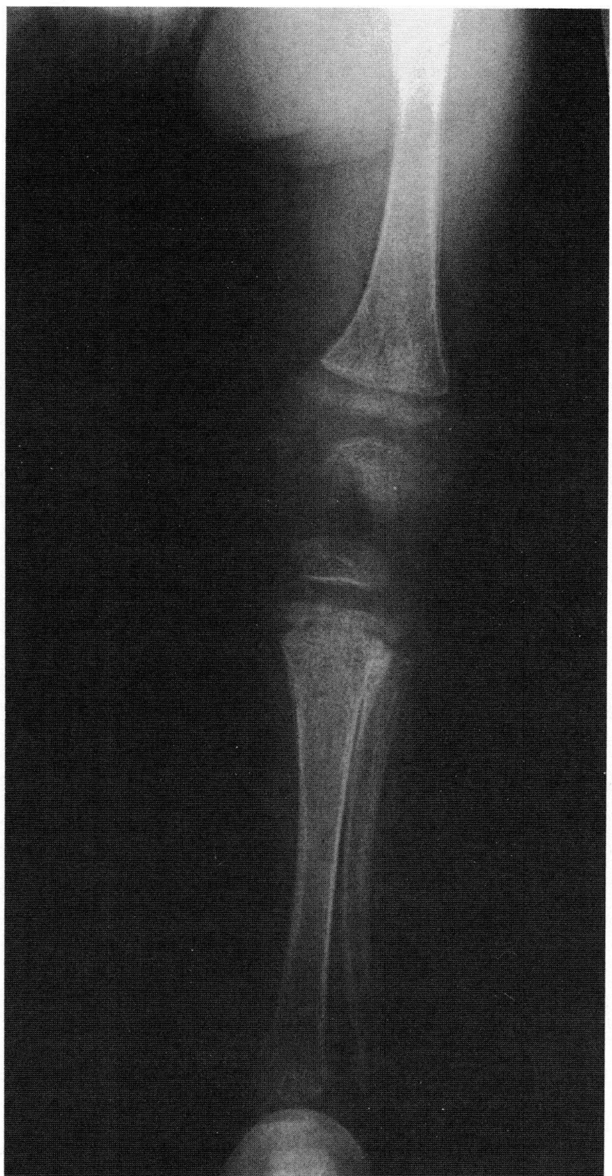

Figure 7.54. Rickets, the pediatric form of osteomalacia, is noted by diffuse osteopenia and abnormally wide growth plates. The soft bones may be bowed.

tion into osteosarcomas in less than 1% of all cases of Paget's disease. The majority of cases are asymptomatic and are discovered incidentally on pelvic x-rays, a frequent site of Pagetic involvement. The medical treatment of Paget's disease with calcitonin or diphosphonates is reserved for intractable bone pain, malignant hypercalcemia, cardiac failure, or neural involvement from bony foraminal hypertrophy.

Bone Tumors

Tumors arising from musculoskeletal tissues are rare. However, bone involvement with metastatic tumor is common in patients over the age of 50. Primary tumors of breast, prostate, lung, kidney, and thyroid frequently metastasize to bone. The sites of tumor metastasis are typically those bones involved with hematopoiesis and those with a rich blood supply, such as the spine, ribs, skull, pelvis, and long bone metaphyses. Metastases from breast and prostate may be either osteoblastic (inducing bone formation) or osteolytic (inducing bone resorption), while those from lung, kidney, thyroid, or gastrointestinal tract are usually osteolytic.

The most frequent primary bone tumors and their tissue of origin are listed in Table 7.8. Table 7.9 describes their salient features. The evaluation of primary or secondary bone tumors should be systematic and multidisciplinary. Before treatment is initiated, the physician must define the tumor according to its histology, its anatomic relationships to neuromuscular compartments and perivascular spaces, and the likelihood and mode of its metastatic spread.

Evaluation

The history is of great importance and should include: patient age, medical conditions associated with bone tumors (Paget's disease, dermatomyositis, prior radiation exposure), systemic symptoms (weight loss, bleeding diathesis, fever), and occupation (unusual environmental exposure). Lifestyle and personal expectations are also important in selecting therapy. The physical examination should note the color and temperature of overlying tissues, and the size, degree of tenderness, and mobility of the tumor if it is palpable. A tumor that is confined to bone may have no abnormal physical findings.

A complete blood count and differential help to exclude infection and hematologic malignancies. Usually, laboratory studies can detect other organ system involvement and determine the patient's overall medical condition. Liver function studies and measurements of uric acid (deoxyribonucleic acid (DNA) turnover), alkaline phosphatase, calcium, and phosphorus are helpful in the evaluation of processes that form or destroy bone. With carcinoma of the prostate, a prostatic specific antigen (PSA) level is measured before a rectal examination is undertaken. If myeloma is suspected, serum protein electrophoresis should be undertaken.

The plain film radiograph provides many clues about the behavior of the tumor, whether it is benign and slow-growing (well-demarcated with a reactive zone of bone formation) or whether it is malignant (undemarcated, destructive, with little surrounding bone formation—Fig. 7.57). Defining the specific bone and region of involvement (epiphysis, metaphysis, or diaphysis) aids in both diagnosis (Table 7.9) and staging. Subsequent radiographic investigation, be it with radioisotope scan, computed tomography, magnetic resonance imaging, or other specialized techniques is directed by suspicions generated from the plain film radiograph. A radioisotope bone scan is often an excellent screening test for metastatic disease. Radioactive, isotopically labeled technetium-99m pyrophosphate is incorporated into regions of active bone formation or increased vas-

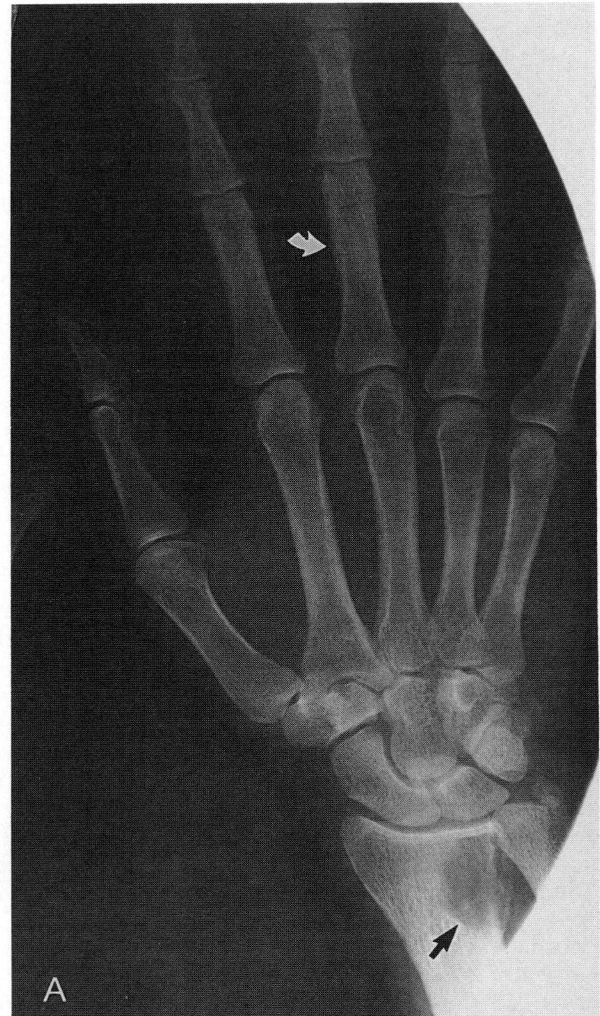

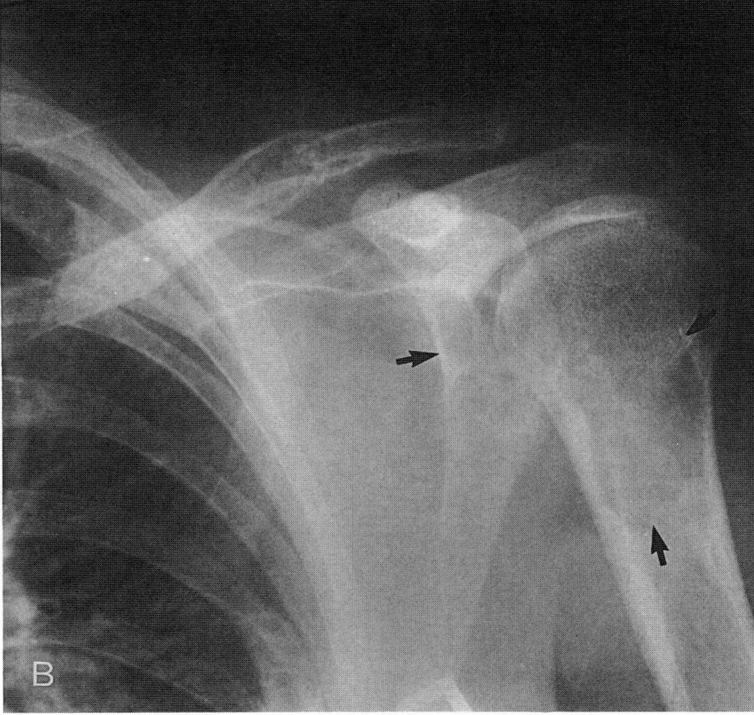

Figure 7.55. Primary hyperparathyroidism causes increased bone resorption to increase serum calcium levels. X-rays of primary hyperparathyroidism show diffuse bone rarefaction. Note the phalangeal cortices (curved arrow) and multiple focal osteolytic lesions of cortical bone (straight arrows). This explains why the radiographic picture is described as osteitis fibrosis cystica.

cularity. In multiple myeloma, however, the bone scan is characteristically negative and shows no increased uptake. Computed tomography provides the best depiction of cortical bone penetration and intraosseous detail. The CT scan is the preferred method of evaluating the lung for small pulmonary lesions. With contrast enhancement, a CT scan can define the relationship between a tumor and the surrounding neurovascular structures. Nuclear magnetic resonance imaging is used to evaluate the intramedullary (marrow) extent of a tumor. The MRI also yields the best definition of soft tissue and neurovascular tumor relationships. Angiography is used to identify vascular lesions, which can then be embolized to shrink tumor mass and decrease blood loss prior to a surgical resection. Often combinations of these special imaging techniques are obtained to study tumor and extent and behavior before biopsy.

The purpose of the surgical biopsy is to procure adequate tissue for histologic diagnosis. A biopsy may be obtained with open or closed (needle) techniques and should be performed by the surgical team responsible for definitive tumor treatment. The biopsy site should be fashioned so that the incision can be resected in total and not compromise the definitive procedure. An open biopsy incision is generally directed in the longitudinal bone axis in immediate juxtaposition to the tumor. To prevent contamination and tumor spread, extensive muscular dissection and neurovascular structures are avoided while meticulous hemostasis is maintained. When possible, an intraoperative frozen section is obtained to assure that an adequate tissue specimen has been sampled. In closed biopsies, either a fine-needle aspiration is used to remove cells for cytology or a tissue core is obtained for routine histologic preparation.

The treatment of bone tumors depends upon the tissue diagnosis, the degree of cell anaplasia, the extent of spread, the patient's medical condition, and the sensitivity of the tumor to treatment modalities. These mo-

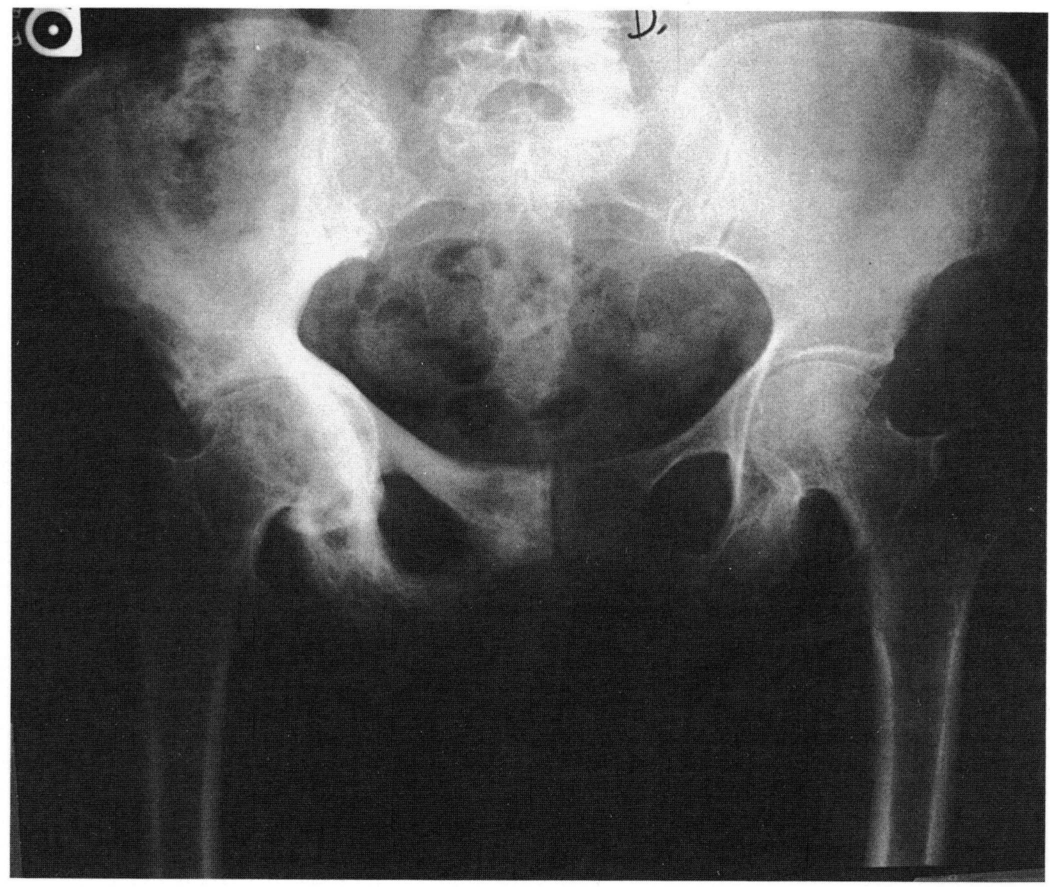

Figure 7.56. Paget's disease. The dense irregular sclerotic bony trabeculae signify the excessive, unregulated formation of bone. The bone is brittle and may fracture pathologically.

Table 7.8.
Primary Bone Tumors and their Tissue of Origin

Tissue of Origin	Bone Tumor	
	Benign	Malignant
Bone	Osteoid osteoma	Osteosarcoma
Cartilage	Osteochondroma Enchondroma	Chondrosarcoma
Fibrous tissue	Fibroma	Fibrosarcoma
Marrow elements	Eosinophilic granuloma	Myeloma Ewing's sarcoma
Uncertain	Giant cell tumor	Aggressive giant cell tumor

dalities include surgery, chemotherapy, and radiotherapy.

Benign tumors are amenable to curative local bone resection. If tumor resection will compromise the structural integrity of the bone (i.e., femoral neck), bone grafting or implant reinforcement will be necessary. Metastatic lesions may be palliated with local radiation. When a lesion occupies greater than 50% of a bone's cortical diameter, a pathologic fracture is imminent. Since fixation after pathologic fracture is more difficult technically and has a higher morbidity, prophylactic fixation is preferable with impending pathologic fractures.

Generally, malignant bone tumors are resected with wide or radical surgical margins. Adjuvant chemotherapy and ionizing radiation are employed to eradicate tumor micrometastases that are assumed to be present. In some centers innovative reconstructive techniques using bone and joint allografts alone or in combination with customized prosthetic joint replacement are used to salvage limbs and maximize patient function. Elegant limb salvage techniques should never compromise the

Table 7.9.
Salient Features of Common Bone Tumors

Tumor	Main Symptoms	Age	Common Sites	Radiographic Appearance	Other
Benign					
Osteoid osteoma	Pain, often relieved by aspirin	Under 30	Femur and tibia	Small, radiolucent area <1 cm surrounded by zone of dense sclerosis	
Osteochondroma	Palpable lump, may interfere with tendon function	Adolescence	Long bone metaphysis	Sessile or pedunculated bone excrescence, cartilage not seen unless calcified	Pain or increase in size suggests malignant change
Enchondroma (chondroma)	Swelling or pain with a pathologic fracture	Any age	Metaphysis of tubular bones of hands and feet; may be single or multiple (Ollier's disease)	Well-demarcated area of radiolucency that may contain specks of calcification	Malignant transformation is more common with multiple cartilage lesions (osteochondromas or enchondromas)
Nonossifying fibroma (fibrous cortical defect)	Asymptomatic unless pathological fracture occurs through it	Under 30	Cortical metaphysis distal femur or tibia	Well-demarcated, radiolucent, multilocular area adjacent to cortex	Ossifies with skeletal maturation
Giant cell tumor (osteoclastoma)	Pain and swelling near joint	20–40	Epiphyseal, especially distal femoral, radius, or proximal tibial epiphysis; after growth plate has closed	Epiphyseal Eccentric Expanding (EEE); expands to involve metaphysis	Frequently aggressive; should be treated as a malignant lesion
Malignant					
Osteosarcoma	Tender mass; pain worse at night	Bimodal; before 30 and after 50 due to malignant change in Paget's disease	Metaphyseal; half affect on distal femur and proximal tibia	Irregular, destructive lesion with radiodense osteoblastic and/or radiolucent osteolytic areas; periosteal new bone formation juxtaposed to a cortex that is permeated and destroyed; neoplastic bone spicules perpendicular to bone radiating in a sunburst pattern	Slightly more common in males than females
Chondrosarcoma	Increasing mass; dull, aching pain	40–60	Central sites and pelvic, shoulder girdle	Permeative radiolucent lesion with calcific densities	Malignant transformation of preexisting enchondroma or osteochondroma, especially if multiple
Fibrosarcoma	Painful, destuctive lesion	Adolescence and young adulthood	Metaphyseal regions of long bones	Poorly defined, destructive, radiolucent lesion	

Table 7.9.
(continued)

Tumor	Main Symptoms	Age	Common Sites	Radiographic Appearance	Other
Myeloma		45–65	Red marrow areas of the skeleton	Osteopenia, spinal compression fractures with minimal trauma	Most common primary malignant bone tumor of plasma cell origin; Bence Jones proteinuria, serum and urine protein electrophoresis
Ewing's Sarcoma	Enlarging, painful, soft tissue mass	10–15	Diaphysis of femur; ilium, tibia, humerus, fibula, ribs	Destructive bony lesion; onion skin layers of periosteal new bone formation	May be mistaken for osteomyelitis clinically and histologically

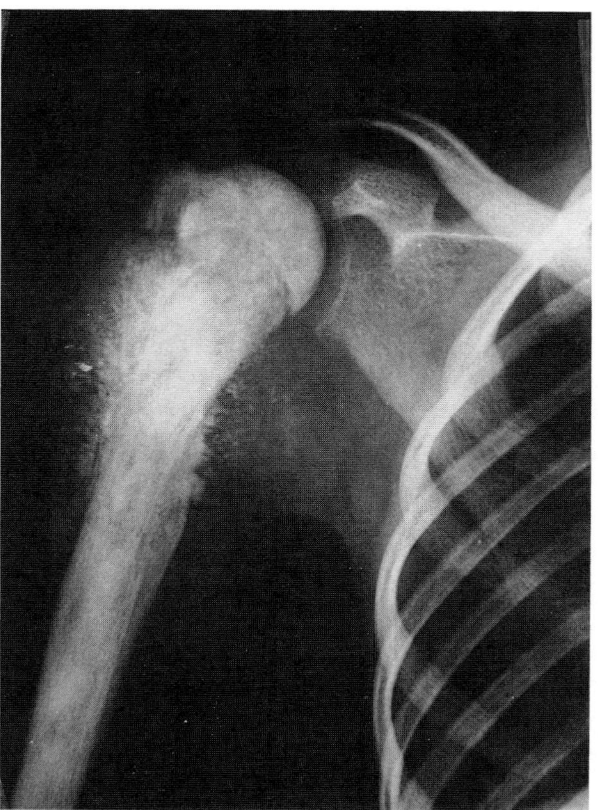

Figure 7.57. Osteogenic sarcoma of the proximal humerus metaphysis showing an aggressive, expanding, poorly demarcated, bone-forming lesion.

primary goal of tumor surgery, which is the eradication of the neoplasm.

Gait

Normal ambulation is efficient and conserves energy; abnormal ambulation is inefficient, requires increased energy expenditure, and usually is a manifestation of neuromuscular pathology. Gait observation and analysis is thus an essential part of the musculoskeletal examination. (A detailed analysis of normal and abnormal gait patterns are reviewed on video tape Program 9 in the series Physical examination of the musculoskeletal system—see Suggested Reading.)

A normal gait cycle (Fig. 7.58) extends from the heel strike of one foot to the next heel strike of the same foot. The normal cycle is divided into the *stance phase* (60% of the cycle), when the foot is in contact with the ground, and the *swing phase* (40% of the cycle), when the foot is off the ground. The stance phase begins at *heel strike*, is followed by *foot flat*, and ends with *toe off*. The swing phase is marked by advancement of the limb to the next heel strike. The *stride length* is the distance covered during one gait cycle (heel strike to ipsilateral heel strike), whereas the *step length* is the distance between the heel strike of one foot to the heel strike of the contralateral foot. Because the pelvis and trunk as well as the muscles and joints of the lower limb are involved in gait, abnormalities in these regions can also be evidenced in the gait pattern.

An abnormal gait often is called a *limp*. Most gait abnormalities are detectable during the stance phase, when body weight is supported by one lower extremity. During this phase of weight transference, pain, muscle weakness, and joint abnormalities produce their maximal effect. The typical reaction to pain is to quickly unload the affected leg. Thus, an *antalgic* (pain-relieving) gait is manifest by a decreased stance phase of the affected limb. The swing phase of the limb opposite is also decreased, which results in a shortened step length.

Muscle weakness has significant effects on gait. Quadriceps weakness interferes with the ability to lock the knee in full extension prior to heel strike. To compensate, the patient will push the thigh backwards with the hand. Weakness of the foot and ankle dorsiflexors will not allow the controlled placement of the foot following heel strike to the foot flat position; this results in a *foot slap gait* as the foot slaps to the ground following heel strike. Likewise, paralysis of the foot and ankle

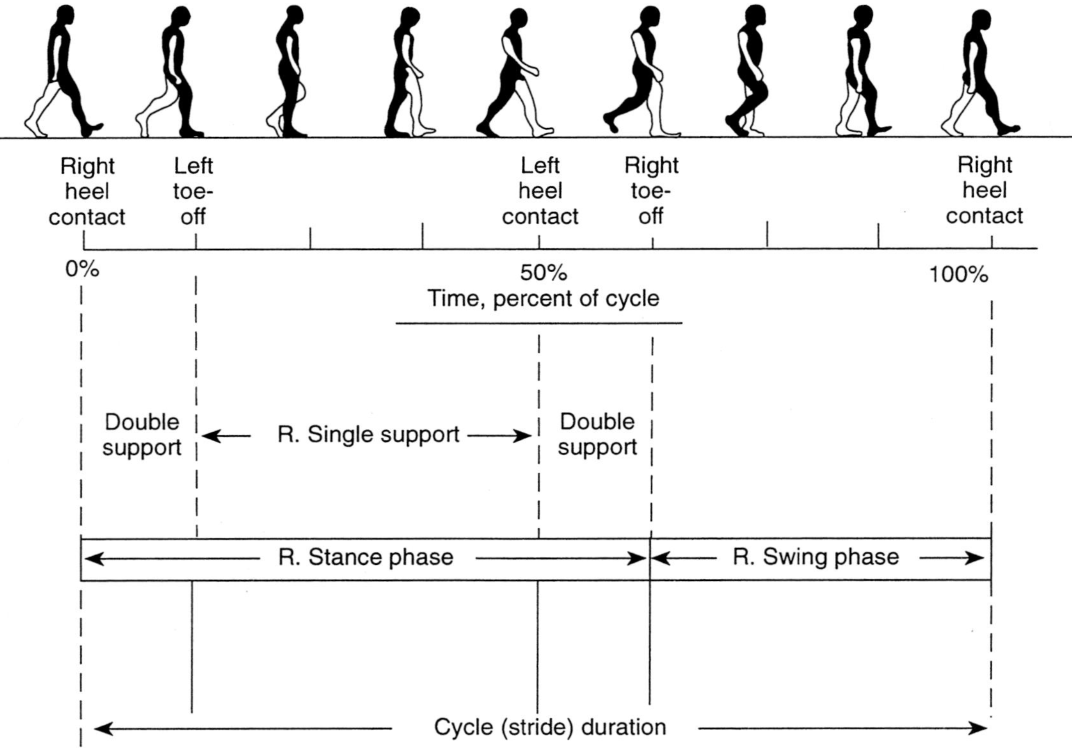

Figure 7.58. The gait cycle.

dorsiflexors due to peroneal nerve palsy will cause the patient to bring the leg up higher than normal during the swing phase in order for the toes to clear the ground . This motion may result in a *steppage gate*. Other compensatory mechanisms for clearing a dropped foot include elevating the ipsilateral pelvis (*hip-hike gait*) or swinging the leg out to the side (*circumduction gait*). A weak gluteus maximus, which serves as a hip extensor, causes the trunk to collapse forward during midstance. The patient will compensate by thrusting the trunk posteriorly in what is called an *extensor lurch* or *gluteus maximus gait*. Weakness of the hip abductor muscles (gluteus medius and minimus) allows the contralateral pelvis to sink downward during stance. To compensate, the patient's torso will lurch laterally over the weak hip in what is known as *Trendelenburg* or *gluteus medius gait*. Weakness of the calf muscles (gastrocnemius and soleus) prevents the normal propulsive toe-off push and is manifest as a *flat-footed* or *calcaneal* gait.

Joint abnormalities that interfere with the normal range of toe, metatarsophalangeal, ankle, knee, or hip joint motion will also adversely affect gait. For example, an equinus (plantar flexion) ankle contracture will cause knee hyperextension during the stance phase of ambulation.

Armed with a knowledge of gait mechanics and a critical eye, one can distinguish many of these gait patterns when observing a group of people. An abnormal gait pattern may provide the first clue in the diagnosis of a neuromuscular disease process.

SUGGESTED READINGS

American Academy of Orthopaedic Surgeons: Athletic training and sports medicine. 2nd ed. Park Ridge, Illinois: Amer Acad Ortho Surg, 1991.

American Academy of Orthopaedic Surgeons: Orthopaedic knowledge Update 3. Park Ridge, Illinois: Amer Acad Ortho Surg, 1990.

American Orthopaedic Association: Manual of orthopaedic surgery. 6th ed. Park Ridge, Illinois: Amer Acad Ortho Surg, 1985.

Apley AG, Solomon L. Concise system of orthopaedics and fractures. London: Butler Worth, 1988.

Ellison, AE. Skiing injuries. Clin Symp 1977;29:1.

Enneking WF. A system of staging musculoskeletal neoplasms. Clin Orthop Relat Res 1986;204:9.

Enneking WF, Conrad EU. Clinical symposium, common bone tumors. Clin Symp 1989;41:3.

Heckman JD. Fractures: emergency care and complications. Clin Symp 1991;43:3.

Hennsinger RN. Congenital dislocation of the hip. Clin Symp 1979;31: 1.

Kaplan FX. Osteoporosis. Clin Symp 1987;39:1.

Keim HA, Kirkaldy-Willis WH. Low back pain. Clin Symp 1987;39:6.

Kleinert HE, Kleinert JM, McCabe SJ, Berger AC. Replantation. Clin Symp 1991;43:2.

Kozinn F, Stewart C, Wilson PD Jr. Adult hip disease and total hip replacement. Clin Symp 1987;39:5.

Netter FH. Musculoskeletal system, Part I: Anatomy, physiology and metabolic disorders. The CIBA collection of medical illustrations. Vol 8. Summit, New Jersey: CIBA Pharmaceuticals, 1987.

Netter FH. Musculoskeletal system, Part II: Developmental disorders and joint replacement. The CIBA collection of medical illustrations. Vol 8. Summit, New Jersey: CIBA Pharmaceuticals, 1990.

Salter RB. Textbook of disorders and injuries of the musculoskeletal system. 2nd ed. Baltimore: Williams & Wilkins, 1983.

Schumaker HR, ed. Primer on the rheumatic diseases. 9th ed. Atlanta: Arthritis Foundation, 1988.

Thompson GH, Salter RB. Legg-Calvé-Perthes disease. Clin Symp 1986;35:1.

Wilson FC, ed. The musculoskeletal system: basic processes and disorders. 2nd ed. Philadelphia: JB Lippincott, 1983.

Video Tapes

American Academy of Orthopaedic Surgeons, Association of Orthopaedic Chairmen, and McGill University. Physical examination of the musculoskeletal system. A series of nine video programs. Park Ridge, Illinois: American Academy of Orthopaedic Surgeons, 1987.

Carette S. Intra-articular and soft tissue injection sites. Montreal, Quebec, Canada: Roussel Canada, 1990.

Skills

HISTORY

Obtain an appropriate and relevant history related to disorders of the musculoskeletal system. Patients must be allowed to state their chief complaint in their own words.

If pain is a feature of the presenting complaint, the following information must be sought:

1. Exact location of the pain.
2. Does pain remain localized or does it radiate?
3. Characteristics of the pain.
4. Factors aggravating pain (e.g., activity, position).
5. Factors alleviating pain (e.g., position).
6. Frequency of episodes.
7. Any associated factors (e.g., swelling, discoloration, deformity).

If there has been an injury, specific related information must be sought:

1. Mechanism of injury.
2. Length of time since injury.
3. Environmental factors associated with injury (e.g., heat, cold, sun, water).
4. Location (farm injuries).
5. Treatment, if any, administered since injury.

PHYSICAL EXAMINATION

Preparation

Assemble the appropriate equipment to conduct a full clinical examination of the musculoskeletal system: a marking pencil, measuring tape, goniometer to measure angles and range of motion, wooden blocks of various thicknesses from 0.5–3.0 cm, and a stethoscope. Also required is equipment to do a detailed neurological examination, including a reflex hammer, pin, cotton, tuning fork, containers to test hot and cold sensation, and a paper clip to test two-point discrimination.

Procedure

A complete physical examination of the musculoskeletal system must include the following elements: inspection, palpation, joint range of motion testing, neurological examination, vascular examination, special tests, and examination of related areas.

Inspection. The inspection must include observation for deformity, atrophy, discoloration, swelling, scars, cutaneous lesions, as well as of gait, posture, and movement.

Palpation. Anatomical landmarks must be identified and localized. Tenderness, deformity, temperature change, swelling, and crepitus must be sought on palpation.

Range of Motion. The patient's ability to perform functional movements of the joint being examined is assessed. If the shoulder is being examined, for example, the patient should be observed while combing the hair or getting a wallet out of the back pocket. The active range of motion for each joint being examined is also measured and documented. If the active range of motion is not full, then the passive range of motion must be measured in order to ascertain the cause of the deficit; e.g., is the cause due to factors such as contracture, bony block, muscle weakness, or pain inhibition?

Neurological Examination. A complete sensory, motor, and reflex examination must be carried out, including deep tendon, superficial, and pathological reflexes.

Vascular Examination. The following must be assessed during the vascular examination: skin condition, hair distribution, capillary return, status of peripheral pulses (including the effect of exercise), and venous status.

Special Tests. Special tests must be conducted as necessary; for example, the integrity of the anterior cruciate ligament should be ascertained when examining the knee.

Related Areas. Related areas must be examined; for example, the child complaining of knee pain should have the hip examined.

Joint Aspiration

Preparation. Assemble proper sterile instruments, drapes, gloves, antiseptic, and receptacles for fluid. Prep and drape the joint region to be aspirated. The patient should be in a position with the joint supported and completely relaxed.

Local Anesthetic. If the patient is not allergic to local anesthetic, the skin and subcutaneous tissues overlying the entry point into the joint may be infiltrated with 1% Xylocaine. If the joint is being aspirated for culture, a separate needle and syringe must be used, because the local anesthetic may inhibit bacterial growth on culture. The site of entry into each joint is specific and usually involves the most direct route from the skin surface that also avoids neurovascular bundles and tendons.

Insertion. The depth of the joint from the skin surface determines the length of the needle required. If frank pus is likely to be encountered, a 16- or 18-gauge needle is used. If thinner fluid is anticipated, a 20- or 22-gauge needle may be used. The needle is attached to the syringe and the joint is entered. As the plunger is drawn back, fluid will flow into the syringe.

After an adequate amount of fluid is obtained, the syringe and the needle are withdrawn and the site is covered with a small sterile dressing. Fluid should be placed in appropriate containers and sent for culture, Gram's stain, cell count, and chemical and crystal studies.

Requisition and Interpretations of Radiographs of the Musculoskeletal System

Requisition. The radiologic exam of an anatomic region should include:

1. Two views at 90° to each other, usually an anteroposterior and a lateral view.
2. When long bones are radiographed, the joint above and the joint below must be included.
3. Special views or oblique views are usually required when a joint is traumatized.
4. Occasionally, and especially in children, corresponding views of the contralateral region may be indicated for comparison.
5. In addition to plain radiographs, other imaging techniques may be required. These include plain tomography, computerized axial tomography, magnetic resonance, arthrography, angiography, and nuclear medicine scans.

Interpretation. The interpretation of radiographs must include:

1. An assessment of soft tissues as well as of bony tissues.
2. An inspection of the cortical outline of the bones for integrity.
3. An assessment of the alignment of articular surfaces with respect to each other.
4. An assessment of each bone for focal abnormalities, usually radiolucency or areas of increased density.

Study Questions

1. Describe the symptoms and signs of a patient presenting with a fracture of a long bone in the lower extremity.
2. Describe the essential features of the radiological evaluation of suspected musculoskeletal injuries.
3. Discuss the accepted conventions used for describing fracture displacement, angulation, and rotation.
4. List conditions both local and systemic that assist fracture healing and those that tend to retard it.
5. Describe the management principles of a patient with a closed fracture or dislocation.
6. Describe the management of a patient with an open fracture of a long bone but with no neurovascular compromise or deficit.
7. List the methods and devices used in maintaining a reduction of a fracture.
8. Describe the stages of fracture healing.
9. List the indications for internal fixation of a fracture.
10. List the indications for external fixation of a fracture.
11. List the local and systemic complications related to fractures.

COMPARTMENT SYNDROME

1. List the symptoms and signs of a compartment syndrome.
2. Describe the management of an adult patient with a fracture of the tibia and fibula, treated by closed reduction and an above-knee cast, in whom you suspect an anterior compartment syndrome of the lower leg.

SPORTS MEDICINE

1. Describe the pathologies seen in various degrees of ligament sprains.
2. Describe the tests used in the physical examination to assess the integrity of: (*a*) ankle ligaments and (*b*) knee ligaments.
3. Describe the symptoms and signs of meniscal injuries of the knee.

PEDIATRICS

1. Describe the physical signs and tests used in assessing the newborn for developmental dysplasia of the hip.
2. Describe the radiological features that may be seen in (*a*) Legg-CalvéPerthes disease and (*b*) slipped femoral capital epiphysis.
3. Describe the deformities found in congenital club foot.
4. Define *scoliosis* and classify the etiologies of structural scoliosis.

INFECTION

1. Describe the mechanisms by which bacteria may reach bone in order to cause an infection.
2. Describe the anatomical reasons that, in children, make the metaphysis of a long bone prone to infection.
3. In what joints can a metaphyseal osteomyelitis lead to a contiguous septic arthritis? Describe why.
4. Describe the clinical features and the laboratory investigations in:
   a. A child with osteomyelitis of the proximal tibia.
   b. An adult with septic arthritis of the knee.

ARTHRITIS

1. Describe the radiologic features of:
   a. Osteoarthritis
   b. Rheumatoid arthritis
   c. Pseudogout

2. List the nonsurgical and surgical options for the management of a 60-year-old patient with unilateral osteoarthritis of the hip.

SPINE

1. Classify the possible causes of low back pain.
2. Describe the neurological deficit that may be noted in a patient with:
   a. L4-5 disc protrusion
   b. L5-S1 disc protrusion
   c. Cauda equina syndrome
3. Describe the neurological deficits noted with:
   a. Nerve root lesions affecting C-5; C-6; C-7; C-8
   b. Cervical cord lesion
4. List the radiographic abnormalities that may be noted in the cervical spine roentgenograms of a patient with rheumatoid arthritis.

METABOLIC-ENDOCRINE

1. Define the terms:
   a. Osteoporosis
   b. Osteomalacia
2. List the causes of:
   a. Osteoporosis
   b. Osteomalacia

BONE TUMORS

1. List:
   a. The most common tumors that metastasize to bone
   b. The most common bony sites to which the above tumors metastasize
2. List the benign and malignant tumors associated with the common tissues that comprise the musculoskeletal system.
3. Describe the clinical features of:
   a. Osteochondroma
   b. Osteosarcoma
   c. Chondrosarcoma
   d. Multiple myeloma
4. Describe the systematic evaluation of a patient with a suspected neoplasm of the musculoskeletal system, emphasizing pertinent features on:
   a. History
   b. Physical exam
   c. Laboratory investigations
   d. Imaging studies

GAIT

1. Describe the components of the normal gait cycle.
2. List common gait abnormalities or limps, noting the specific pathology or pathologies associated with each.

8 Neurosurgery: Diseases of the Nervous System

Ralph A.W. Lehman, M.D.
Robert B. Page, M.D.

ASSUMPTIONS

The student has successfully completed a basic course in neuroanatomy.

The student can perform a complete neurological examination.

The student knows the organization of the cerebrospinal fluid pathways.

The student knows the organization of the brain, including its sensory input and motor output.

The student understands the pathophysiology of increased intracranial pressure.

The student understands the cross-sectional anatomy of the spinal cord.

The student knows the longitudinal anatomy of the spinal cord and nerve roots and can translate that knowledge into an understanding of dermatomes, myotomes, and sphincter innervation.

The student understands the relationship between the anatomy of the spinal column and the spinal cord and nerve roots.

The student understands the structure of a peripheral nerve and has knowledge of the sensory and motor functions of major limb nerves and plexuses.

The student has knowledge of the normal pediatric anatomy and understands the ascent of the spinal cord during childhood.

OBJECTIVES

INTRACRANIAL DISEASE

1. Develop a common vocabulary so that the clinical findings and sites of localization can be described accurately to consultants and colleagues.
2. Apply the Glasgow coma scale to levels of consciousness.
3. List and explain the indications and contraindications for a lumbar puncture.
4. List the steps, explaining their significance, in the determination of brain death.
5. Recognize and list the early symptoms and signs of raised intracranial pressure.
6. Recognize and manage transtentorial herniation.
7. List the features that distinguish focal mass, cerebral swelling, and hydrocephalus as causes of increased intracranial pressure. Understand the methods for monitoring and treating each of them.
8. Describe the initial evaluation of the comatose, head-injured patient.
9. Describe the management of scalp lacerations and penetrating injuries.
10. List the types of skull fracture; describe the steps in their management and their complications.
11. Describe common subacute and chronic head injury problems.
12. List the clinical and radiological features that differentiate ischemic from hemorrhagic stroke; list the disorders that can produce each.
13. Define TIA, RIND, and completed stroke.
14. List the indications for carotid surgery.
15. Describe the diagnosis and management of intraparenchymal bleeding and subarachnoid hemorrhage.
16. List the common brain tumors that afflict adults and children, the prognosis of each, and the symptoms that herald a brain tumor.
17. On the basis of the history and physical examination, choose and interpret the diagnostic tests needed to establish the site and nature of the tumor.
18. List the indications for stereotaxic biopsy, open surgical excision, radiation, and chemotherapy of brain tumors.
19. Describe the symptoms, evaluation, and treatment of a patient with a brain abscess.

INTRASPINAL DISEASE

1. List the early and late symptoms and signs of acute spinal cord compression and differentiate them from radiculopathy.

2. Describe the following spinal cord syndromes: acute transverse myelopathy, Brown-Sequard syndrome, anterior cord syndrome, central cord syndrome.
3. Describe the clinical significance of the disparity in growth between spinal cord and column.
4. List the important evaluation and management steps in the care of acute spinal cord injury. Consider (*a*) bodily injuries, (*b*) spinal instability, and (c) spinal cord damage.
5. Describe the indications for external immobilization and for internal decompression and fusion. Include consideration of anterior and posterior approaches.
6. Describe the clinical manifestations, diagnostic workup, conservative management, and surgical indications for a patient with (*a*) cervical disc herniation and (*b*) lumbar disc herniation.
7. List the pathologic features and clinical symptoms and signs of (*a*) spinal stenosis and (*b*) spondylolisthesis.
8. List the common spinal infections, their symptoms and treatment.
9. List the common intramedullary, intradural extramedullary, and extradural tumors and compare their modes of presentation.
10. List the three most common origins of spinal metastases.
11. List the indications for surgery of primary and metastatic spinal tumors.

PERIPHERAL NERVE PROBLEMS

1. Define neuropraxia, incomplete transection, and complete transection and describe the means to differentiate them.
2. Compare the healing of a crushed nerve, a transected nerve, and a surgically joined nerve.
3. List the factors that enter into the timing of peripheral nerve repair.
4. Describe the features that distinguish carpal tunnel syndrome, tardy ulnar palsy, and cervical disc disease.

FUNCTIONAL NEUROSURGERY

1. List the indications for surgical relief of pain and the surgical options available.
2. List the indications for epilepsy surgery.
3. Describe the symptoms of normal pressure hydrocephalus.

CONGENITAL DEFECTS

1. Describe the symptoms and evaluation of a patient with suspected hydrocephalus.
2. List the clinical and radiological indications for shunt placement in hydrocephalus.
3. Describe the complications of ventricular shunting.
4. Differentiate between meningocele and myelomeningocele according to deficits and appearance. Describe and compare them with respect to associated neural and other problems.
5. List the complications associated with a dermal sinus tract.
6. Describe the shape of the head with premature closure of (a) the sagittal suture, (*b*) one coronal suture, (c) both coronal sutures, and (*d*) the lambdoid suture.

Intracranial Disease

Anatomy

In the central nervous system, cells are organized uniquely at different levels permitting regional and lateralized specialization of function. The brain is thus unlike other organs (such as the liver, lungs, kidneys, and muscles) that have cells organized into repetitive identical units (such as lobules, alveoli, or glomeruli). The pattern of specialization in the central nervous system is both segmental and hierarchical. Activity at each segmental level can be modified by successively higher levels. Knowledge of this segmental and hierarchical organization, as well as of the regional specializations that occur at each level, enables accurate interpretation of neurologic and radiologic findings.

The left and right cerebral hemispheres sit atop the brain stem in the anterior and middle fossae of the cranium. The two hemispheres, connected by the corpus callosum, are composed of an outer layer of gray cortex (containing neurons), a middle layer of white matter (consisting of axons), and an inner mass of gray matter (containing neurons) (Figs. 8.1, 8.2, and 8.3). The cortical gray matter is folded into gyri separated by sulci; especially prominent sulci are called *fissures*. The Sylvian fissure separates the frontal from the temporal lobe while the Rolandic fissure separates the frontal from the parietal lobe (Figs. 8.2, 8.5**A**). The frontal lobes lie in the anterior fossa on the orbital roof. The temporal and occipital lobes lie in the middle fossa on the temporal bone and the tentorium.

Lesions in the cerebral hemispheres produce focal neurologic signs reflecting regional segregation of function. Thus, lesions of the anterior frontal lobes cause loss of restraint and flattening of affect. The motor and sensory cortex lie more posteriorly, just anterior and posterior to the Rolandic fissure (Fig. 8.2); consequently, posterior frontal lobe lesions cause contralateral hemiparesis and hyperreflexia, whereas lesions of the anterior parietal lobe cause contralateral hypesthesia with loss of fine sensibility. Lesions in the left and right hemispheres often differ in the symptoms they produce. Left hemisphere lesions can cause language problems in right- and most left-handed subjects. Such lesions are usually situated adjacent to the Sylvian fissure (Fig. 8.2). Thus, a posterior inferior frontal lobe lesion just over the left Sylvian fissure causes expressive

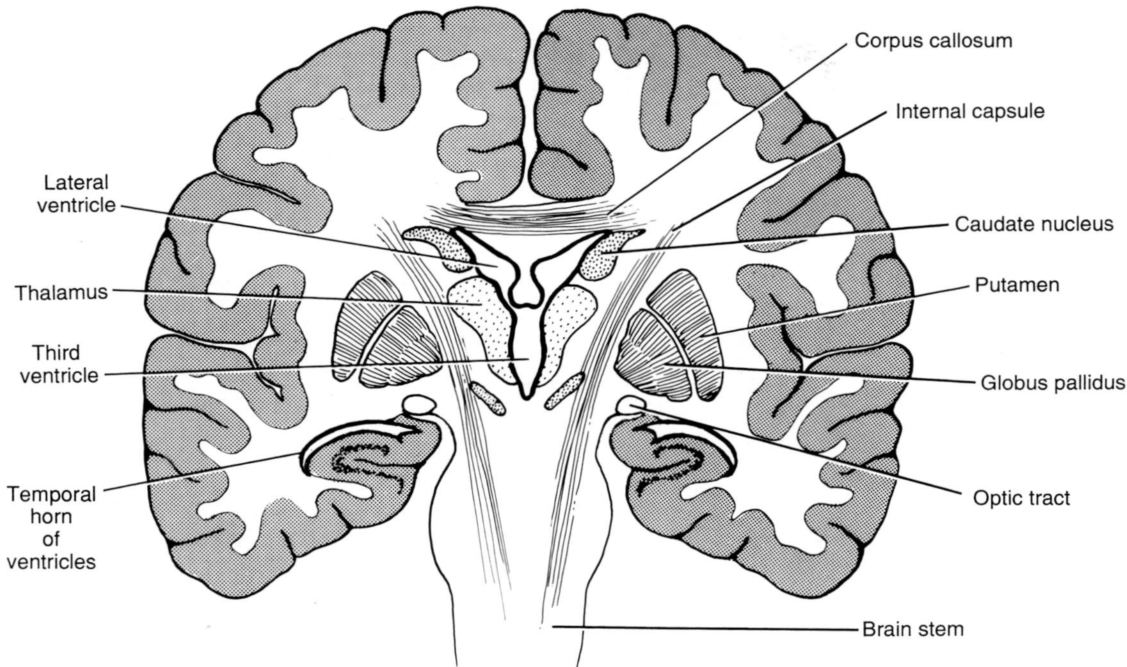

Figure 8.1. Coronal section of the brain (gray matter stippled).

(nonfluent) aphasia with sparse speech. A lesion behind this site in the left inferior parietal lobule or below the fissure in the superior temporal lobe produces both loss of speech comprehension and unintelligible utterances (receptive or fluent aphasia). Correspondingly, the right hemisphere is more specialized for both cognitive and executive spatial functions.

The olfactory nerves (first cranial) extend from the nasal mucosa up through the cribriform plate to synapse in the olfactory bulbs. Each tract (erroneously called the olfactory nerve) extends posteriorly from the olfactory bulb back under the frontal lobe to the hippocampal gyrus and amygdala in the medial temporal lobe. Lesions in and about the amygdala may cause olfactory seizures characterized by an unusual smell at the onset. The hippocampal formation lies buried in the medial temporal lobe. Along with the hippocampal gyrus, it forms the limbic system. Lesions of the hippocampus can lead to difficulty with memory, changes in affect, and temporal lobe (partial complex) seizures.

The internal capsule is the major channel for motor and sensory pathways connecting the cerebral hemispheres with the lower centers in the brain stem and spinal cord (Figs. 8.1, 8.9**E**). The internal capsule passes between the basal ganglia: the putamen and globus pallidus lie lateral, whereas the caudate head lies medial to the internal capsual.

The thalami lie atop the brain stem behind and medial to the basal ganglia and internal capsule (Figs. 8.1, 8.9**E**, 8.10). The nonspecific nuclear groups, extensions of the reticular formation, are involved with arousal and alertness. When they are damaged, as with a thalamic hemorrhage, coma occurs. The thalamus acts as a relay point for sensation. Somatosensory input from the spinal cord and brain stem is processed in the ventral posterior thalamus and relayed to the parietal lobe. Special sensory afferent information is relayed to the cortex from the posterior thalamus—hearing from the medial geniculate nucleus to the temporal lobe and vision from the lateral geniculate nucleus to the occipital lobe. Input from the limbic system related to memory and emotion is also processed in the thalamus: the anterior nuclei receive limbic input from the mamillary bodies (a site to which the hippocampus projects) and project in turn to the medial cortex of the frontal lobe (the cingulate gyrus).

The hypothalamus lies beneath the thalamus on either side of the third ventricle. The hypothalamus integrates cortical input to coordinate emotional, autonomic, and neuroendocrine responses. Inferiorly, the floor of the third ventricle contains the median eminence covered by the pars tuberalis of the pituitary. Together these give rise to the pituitary stalk that descends into the sella to end in the neural (posterior) lobe of the pituitary stalk, which in turn ends as the neural lobe of the pituitary gland. This lobe together with the pars distalis (anterior lobe) forms the pituitary gland within the sella turcica (Fig. 8.11).

The optic nerves (second cranial) originate in the retina, the only portion of the central nervous system that can be visualized with an ophthalmoscope. In the optic chiasm the medial fibers of each nerve cross the midline to join the lateral fibers from the opposite nerve to form the optic tracts. Each tract projects to the lateral geniculate nucleus of the thalamus. The visual output from the geniculate continues as the optic radiations that pass through the parietal and temporal lobes to the occipital lobe. It should be evident to all students, then,

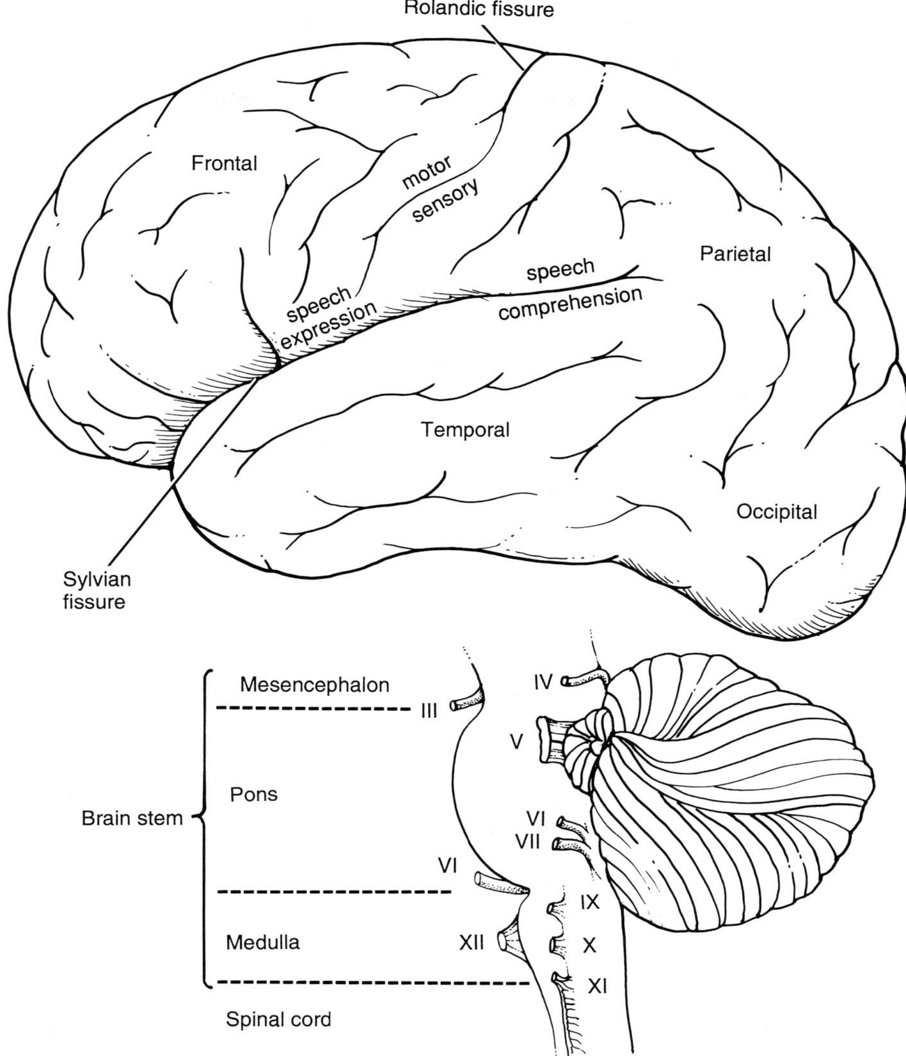

Figure 8.2. Medial aspect of left brain with brain stem displaced caudally for purposes of illustration.

that unilateral blindness is caused by a lesion in the globe, retina, or optic nerve; bitemporal hemianopia is caused by a lesion of the optic chiasm; and homonymous hemianopia is caused by a lesion in the optic tract, radiations, or the occipital lobe opposite the side of visual loss.

The posterior fossa of the skull lies beneath the tentorium and contains the cerebellum and the brain stem. The brain stem is subdivided into mesencephalon (midbrain), pons, and medulla (Figs. 8.2, 8.3, 8.11). It is continuous rostrally with the thalamus and internal capsule and caudally with the spinal cord. Like the spinal cord it is a modified tube that is bilaterally symmetrical. Unlike the spinal cord, its cavity is displaced dorsally and varies in size from the narrow aqueduct of the mesencephalon and upper pons to the large fluid-filled fourth ventricle of the lower pons and medulla.

The dorsal brain stem, the tegmentum, contains the reticular formation, brain stem nuclei, and lemniscal sensory tracts. The tegmentum rests upon a great ventral system of motor fascicles descending from the cerebral hemispheres to the cerebellum, brain stem, and spinal cord. Penetrating the sides of the tegmentum are the cranial nerve roots. The motor nerves (fifth, seventh, ninth, 10th, 11th) innervating the derivatives of the branchial arches (glands, pharynx, larynx) leave the lateral surface of the tegmentum with the sensory nerve roots to form mixed cranial nerves (Fig. 8.3). Of the somatic motor (eye and tongue) cranial nerves (Fig. 8.3), the third, sixth, and 12th exit ventrally near the midline, while the fourth exits dorsally. The brain stem reticular formation controls respiration, heart rate, blood pressure, and consciousness.

Most of the long tracts passing between the spinal cord and brain stem cross from side to side at the spinomedullary junction. At this level, the right medial lemniscus receives its fibers from the left pair of dorsal columns. It projects to the right ventral posterior thalamus and from there to the right parietal lobe. Motor tracts also cross at this level. The ventrally located mo-

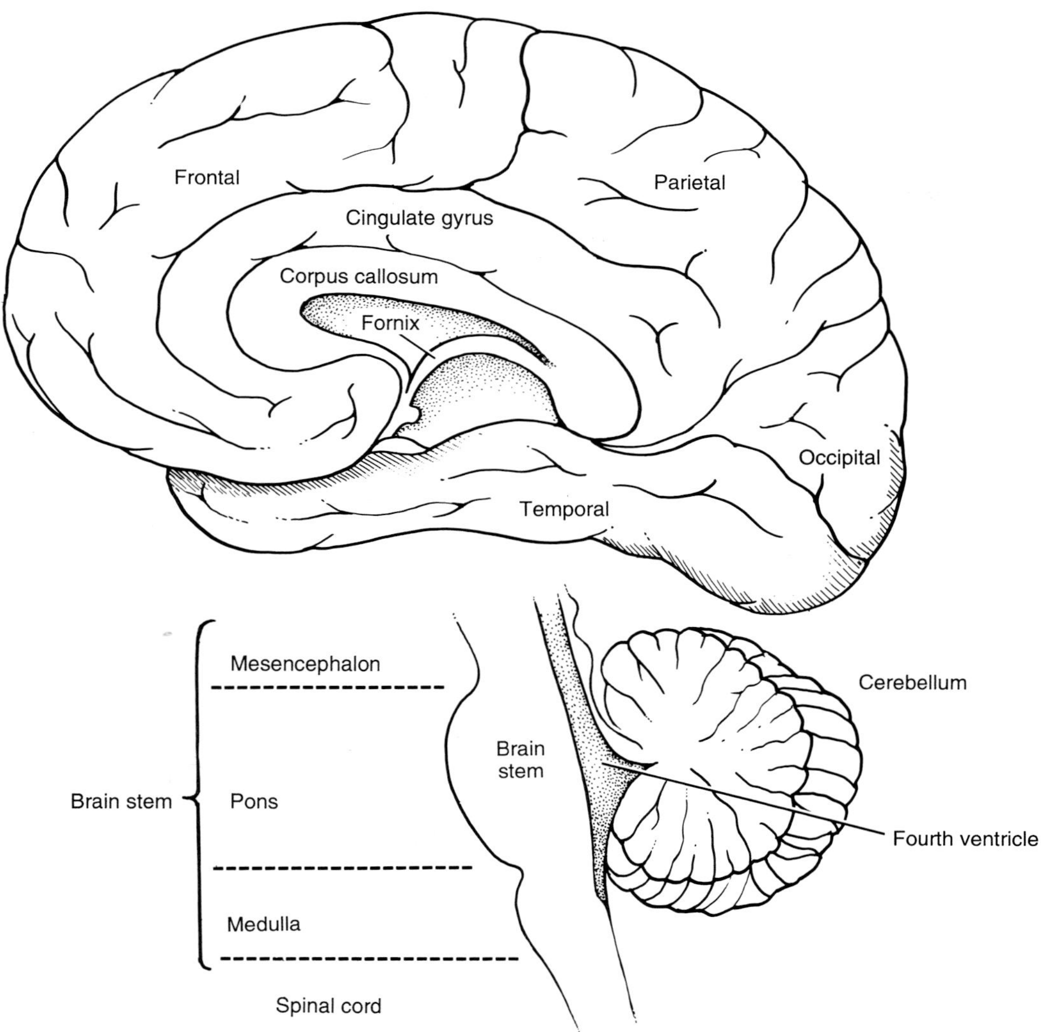

Figure 8.3. Lateral view of left brain with brain stem displaced caudally for purposes of illustration.

tor (corticospinal) tracts form the medullary pyramids that decussate (form an X) at the junction of the spinal cord and medulla. The left pyramid of the medulla becomes the right corticospinal tract in the spinal cord. Thus, a lesion of the motor or sensory system on one side of the brain causes weakness or sensory symptoms on the opposite side of the body.

The cerebellum connects to the brain stem by three pairs of peduncles that provide input and outflow (Figs. 8.2, 8.11). It consists of two lateral hemispheres united by a narrow middle portion, the vermis. Hemisphere lesions produce limb ataxia on the same side as the lesion, while vermis lesions cause truncal ataxia. A small region of the cerebellum (the vermian nodulus and the hemispheral flocculus) is connected to the vestibular nuclei of the brain stem. If a lesion involves the vestibular apparatus, the vestibular nerve or nuclei, the nodulus, or the flocculus, nystagmus can develop.

Blood Supply. The major blood vessels supplying the brain can be visualized by arteriography and often show clearly on MRI scans. The circle of Willis, lying at the base of the brain, receives blood flow from each internal carotid artery and from the basilar artery. The branches of the internal carotid artery that can easily be seen on the arteriogram are the posterior communicating, middle, and anterior cerebral arteries of the anterior portion of the circle of Willis. The posterior communicating arteries join the proximal portion of the posterior cerebral arteries to form the posterior portion of the circle. Anatomical variations determine whether the connections between different portions of the circle of Willis are of sufficient caliber to provide collateral circulation. The arteries of the circle of Willis supply the cerebral hemispheres. In the posterior fossa, the vertebral arteries give rise to the basilar artery, which proceeds upward, anterior to the brain stem, until its ultimate division into paired posterior cerebral arteries at the level of the mesencephalon. Major venous channels include the sagittal, transverse, and sigmoid dural sinuses and their confluence at the torcula.

Cerebrospinal Fluid Circulation. The cerebral hemispheres are hollow and contain the lateral ventri-

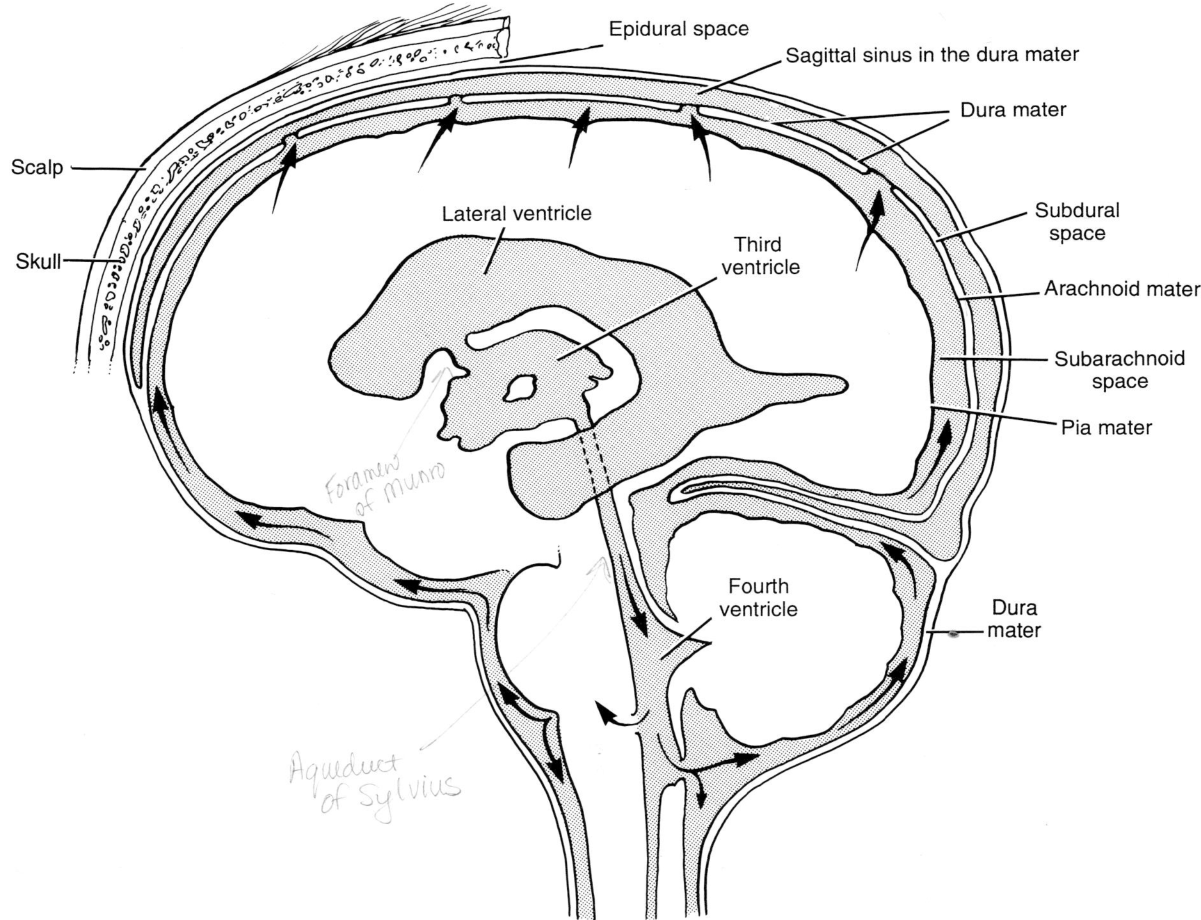

Figure 8.4. The cerebrospinal fluid circulation.

cles. These begin as a pair of vesicles evaginating to each side from the anterior third ventricle. The foramen of Monro marks the site of that evagination and permits cerebrospinal fluid secreted by the choroid plexus of the lateral ventricles to enter the third ventricle (Fig. 8.4). Fluid leaves the third ventricle through the aqueduct of Sylvius and enters the fourth ventricle before entering the subarachnoid space. Some subarachnoid fluid flows down the spinal canal but most travels up through the tentorial incisura over the cerebral hemispheres to the arachnoid villi where it is absorbed into the dural venous sinuses.

The dura mater encases the brain, lines the inner surface of the skull, and projects between (falx) and beneath (tentorium) the cerebral hemispheres. At surgery, after the skull has been removed, the epidural space is entered. After the dura has been opened, the subdural space is entered and the brain exposed. The arachnoid is opened to enter the subarachnoid space, which contains the cerebrospinal fluid and overlies the pia mater on the brain surface (Fig. 8.4).

Evaluation

The Neurological Examination. The neurological examination should be performed in the same order for each patient so that relevant portions are not omitted.

The *mental status examination* includes level of consciousness; orientation to person, place, and time; speech expression and comprehension; drawing; mental arithmetic; remote, current, and immediate memory. Of these, level of consciousness is the most significant in the severely ill patient. Written descriptions should include the nature of the stimulus applied and the response obtained (e.g., reaction to voice or pain). Descriptions such as stuporous or comatose are inadequate. The Glasgow coma scale is useful as a summary statement if the patient's consciousness is altered (Table 8.1). Scores of 8 or less on this scale coincide well with the clinical description "unconscious."

The *cranial nerve examination* must test olfaction in the conscious patient. The complete neurologic examination tests visual acuity, visual fields, and the pupillary size and reactivity in each eye when only one eye is stimulated. The optic discs are evaluated for papilledema, hemorrhages, exudates, and pallor. Extraocu-

Table 8.1.
Glasgow Coma Scale

Activity	Score
Eye opening	
Spontaneous	E4
To speech	3
To pain	2
Nil	1
Best motor response	
Obeys	M6
Localizes	5
Withdraws	4
Abnormal flexion	3
Extensor response	2
Nil	1
Verbal response	
Orientated	V5
Confused conversation	4
Inappropriate words	3
Incomprehensible sounds	2
Nil	1
Glasgow coma score (E + M + V) = 3 to 15	

lar motion is evaluated to see if the eyes move fully and conjugately. Examination of facial sensation includes testing the corneal reflex. Care should be taken to distinguish facial weakness that involves only the lower two-thirds of the face from that which also includes the forehead. The former almost invariably is caused by a contralateral cerebral (supratentorial) lesion, whereas the latter usually is caused by a facial nucleus (brain stem) or facial nerve (peripheral) lesion. Application of a vibrating tuning fork to the forehead and mastoid bones can be used to supplement the evaluation of hearing in each ear. The lower cranial nerves are examined by testing voice, palatal elevation, gag reflex (9th and 10th nerves), sternocleidomastoid strength (11th nerve), and tongue protrusion (12th nerve).

The *motor examination* of the conscious patient includes tests of strength, observation of gait, and search for drift in the outstretched supinated upper extremities (a test that picks up the subtlest degrees of motor weakness). In poorly responsive and unconscious patients, responses to painful stimuli require assessment. Purposeful movement to pain should be distinguished from flexor (decorticate) or extensor (decerebrate) posturing in each of the upper extremities.

The *sensory examination* includes all four modalities: pin, touch, position, and vibration perception. The last is usually spared by intracranial processes. Vibration and position sense (and ankle jerks) are often diminished in the feet in many medical conditions with peripheral neuropathy (including old age and diabetes) and in patients receiving chemotherapy.

Reflexes are usually heightened by intracranial disease, though sudden severe brain damage such as stroke may lead to hyporeflexia of the paralyzed extremities for a day or two. Patients with central nervous system lesions commonly have pathological reflexes associated with muscle weakness, including the Babinski and Hoffmann responses as well as ankle clonus.

The *cerebellar examination* must include gait (width, length, steadiness), balance, and finger-to-nose testing with eyes open and shut. Gait is altered with a hemispheral cerebellar lesion, with the patient tending to veer or fall to the side of the lesion. Balance also is affected by a cerebellar lesion. Normally, balance is maintained by the convergence of three sensory systems (visual, positional, and vestibular) upon the cerebellum. Only two are necessary to preserve the upright position. Because shutting the eyes eliminates one sensory system, a patient with impaired vestibular or position sense will lose balance with eyes shut, but will not do so when they are open. If two of the three sensory paths or their common destination, the cerebellar vermis, are impaired, the patient will lose balance with the eyes open as well as closed. Analogously, finger-to-nose testing will be impaired only with the eyes shut if there is a problem with position sense in the upper extremities; impairment with the eyes open is likely to be caused by a lesion in the ipsilateral cerebellar hemisphere. Nystagmus can be caused by cerebellar or vestibular (brain stem) disease. The slow eye movement tends to be toward the side of the lesion.

In the comatose patient, examination of reflex eye motion helps assess the integrity of the brain stem. Cold irrigation of one ear canal (caloric testing of the oculovestibular reflex) depresses its vestibular function, thereby revealing the function of the opposite ear as conjugate deviation of the eyes toward the irrigated ear. This occurs if the irrigated ear canal is open and if nerve pathways from the labyrinth into and through the brain stem (medial longitudinal fasciculus) and out to the extraocular muscles are intact. Because the brain stem pathway lies in the reticular formation, an intact response implies that the integrity of the reticular formation is also maintained. The same pathways are evaluated by testing for doll's eyes (oculocephalic reflex): when one turns the head of a supine, unconscious patient, normally the eyes will continue to look at the ceiling rather than follow the head from side to side.

The neurological examination permits distinction between unilateral supratentorial (cerebral) and infratentorial (brain stem and/or cerebellar) lesions. Since most neurosurgical lesions are unilateral, this distinction is important. With unilateral *cerebral* disease all observed lateralized deficits are contralateral to the lesion (unless there is herniation as discussed later). In contrast, with unilateral *cerebellar* disease all observed lateralized deficits are ipsilateral to the lesion. With *brain stem* lesions deficits related to lemniscal and motor tracts are manifested contralateral to the lesion, whereas cranial nerve function is disturbed ipsilateral to the lesion of their motor nuclei or sensory root entry zone. Thus, posterior fossa brain stem lesions can produce crossed deficits: ipsilateral (cranial nerve or nuclei) deficits above the shoulders and contralateral (long tract) deficits below.

Lumbar Puncture. Lumbar puncture is an excellent and readily available tool for the investigation of central nervous system disease. It provides information about cerebral spinal fluid (CSF) pressure, protein, sugar content, cell count, and sterility. It is therefore helpful in the diagnosis of such conditions as pseudotumor cerebri (increased intracranial pressure), multiple sclerosis (electrophoretic changes), Guillain-Barre syndrome, meningitis, and subarachnoid hemorrhage. Furthermore, lumbar puncture is a useful means of introducing radiological contrast material for a variety of studies, such as myelography (to define the contents of the spinal canal) and radionuclide CSF flow (e.g., for suspected normal pressure hydrocephalus or CSF leak). Spinal taps are usually performed at L3-4 or below in order to avoid the spinal cord, which normally ends at L1-2.

Lumbar puncture is sometimes used inappropriately, to the detriment of the patient. When lumbar puncture is performed caudal to a mass lesion inside the cranium or spinal canal, dangerous shifts may be induced. Fluid withdrawn or leaking at the puncture site decreases the spinal fluid pressure below such a mass, whereas the pressure in the region of the mass or of the CSF and tissues above it may remain unchanged. The resultant pressure gradient can shift the mass caudally. Such rapid shifts occurring over seconds or hours are poorly tolerated and lead to acute neurological deterioration. When a spinal lesion is involved, there may be irreversible or poorly reversible paralysis below the level of the lesion; when an intracranial mass is involved, brain herniation may occur. Consequently, the presence of a mass lesion or mass effect must be ruled out on clinical and radiological grounds before performing a lumbar puncture. Computerized tomographic (CT) or magnetic resonance imaging (MRI) scans should be performed before any lumber puncture if there is reason to suspect a mass.

Brain Death. Brain death is accepted widely as equivalent to death of the individual. The determination is best made by a neurologist or neurosurgeon, one not part of the transplant procurement or surgical team. The cause of brain death should be known, and there should be no evidence of significant hypothermia or drug overdose. Brain stem reflexes (pupillary, corneal, oculovestibular, caloric, and gag) should be absent. There should be no responses to painful facial stimuli and no more than local motor responses (spinal) to body or limb stimulation. Disconnection of the respirator to test for the absence of spontaneous respiration is essential. The determination of brain death should be carried out after a period of ventilation that allows the P_{CO_2} to become normal. When the respirator is disconnected, adequate steady flow of oxygen is delivered through a catheter introduced well down the endotracheal tube. The patient should be observed for absence of spontaneous respirations and the determination should be carried out until the arterial P_{CO_2} measures greater than 59 mm Hg.

Laboratory tests (electroencephalographic silence; radionuclide, angiographic, or possible transcranial Doppler confirmation of absent cerebral blood flow) are considered optional unless hypotension forces apnea testing to be discontinued. Usually, two complete examinations separated in time that reveal no evidence of brain activity by the above criteria are performed before the patient is pronounced dead.

Increased Intracranial Pressure

Pathophysiology and Clinical Manifestations. Unlike the infant cranium with its open sutures, the adult cranium forms an unyielding container for the brain. As a result, increases in intracranial volume raise intracranial pressure (ICP). Usually, small increases in intracranial contents are compensated for easily by venous compression and CSF displacement, producing only small increments in ICP (high compliance). Each further increase in intracranial contents renders the compensatory mechanisms less able to accommodation, resulting in ever larger increases in ICP (low compliance). Thus, the further ICP rises the more dangerous is each small addition to the intracranial volume. Increases in intracranial contents are tolerated to a point but then result in significant compression and displacement of cerebral structures within the skull.

The adequacy of cerebral perfusion depends upon perfusion pressure, the difference between cerebral arterial and venous pressure. Cerebral venous outflow ultimately passes through veins bridging the subarachnoid space from the brain to the cerebral venous sinuses. With increases in intraparenchymal and CSF pressure, these bridging veins are compressed, ultimately obstructing venous outflow from the brain. Venous obstruction elevates venous pressure to the level of subarachnoid pressure, at which point blood again exits from the brain. Hence, under conditions of abnormally elevated intracranial pressure, perfusion pressure equals the difference between arterial and intracranial (parenchymal, CSF) pressure. For cerebral perfusion adequate to prevent brain ischemia, mean systemic blood pressure should be at least 45 mm Hg greater than ICP. Monitoring arterial blood pressure and ICP permit determination of whether perfusion pressure is acceptable.

Cerebral autoregulation is a mechanism that normally keeps cerebral blood flow constant over a wide range of blood pressure (40–140 mm Hg) by varying cerebrovascular resistance in parallel with arterial blood pressure. Repeated or prolonged rises of ICP interfere with cerebral autoregulation. When this mechanism is disrupted, cerebral blood flow varies as a function of blood pressure. If hypotension occurs, cerebral ischemia may result; if hypertension occurs, small conductance vessels and capillaries receive its full impact and the blood-brain barrier can be disrupted. The combination of increased hydrostatic pressure in the small cerebral vessels and the loss of the blood-brain barrier promotes cerebral edema.

Aside from its effects upon the cerebral circulation, elevated ICP exerts a mass effect that results in displacement of and pressure upon adjacent, less affected portions of the brain. As a result, many brain lesions produce symptoms and signs from brain regions that are affected only secondarily. The most devastating

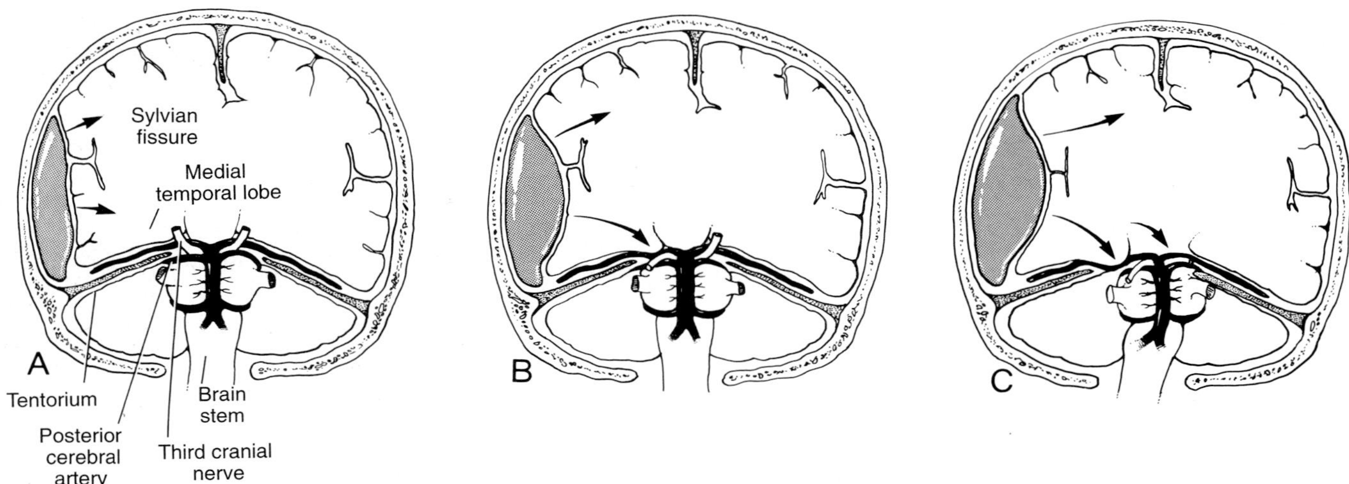

Figure 8.5. **A**, Extracerebral clot with local brain compression. **B**, Early transtentorial herniation. **C**, Late stage of herniation.

forms of brain displacement are those that produce downward herniation of brain through the tentorium or foramen magnum.

Transtentorial herniation, a common form of extreme brain damage from increased ICP, occurs when the etiology of the increase is supratentorial. One or both medial temporal lobes are displaced through the tentorial incisura and press upon the brain stem. With progression, hemorrhagic infarction occurs, resulting in irreversible brain stem dysfunction and death.

The initial effects of a space-occupying cerebral lesion are largely those of local pressure (Fig. 8.5**A**). Because the responsible lesion usually is located on one side, its initial effects are to produce unilateral cerebral dysfunction and contralateral paresis. Some decrease in level of consciousness occurs because of the generalized increase in pressure. As the lesion increases in size or produces more edema, the affected cerebral hemisphere shifts in two directions: across the midline and down through the tentorial notch. Early changes associated with transtentorial herniation include further alteration in the level of consciousness and pressure upon the ipsilateral third nerve, resulting in dilatation of the ipsilateral pupil (Fig. 8.5**B**). As herniation progresses, the brain stem is pushed over and crushed against the opposite tentorial edge (Fig. 8.5**C**). Because this edge is sharp, the resulting deformation produces hemiparesis or decerebration contralateral to the tentorial edge but ipsilateral to the patient's primary lesion. This secondary motor loss due to herniation is falsely lateralizing and occurs after the pupil dilates. Consequently, one should lateralize the primary lesion on the side of a dilated pupil rather than on the side opposite the hemiparesis. Ultimately, damage to the brain stem causes both pupils to dilate, and the patient becomes bilaterally decerebrate or flaccid. Apnea ensues and brain death occurs.

In contrast to a unilateral lesion, a lesion located more centrally or bilaterally produces symmetrical transtentorial herniation. In such cases pupillary size may be equal and dilation may not occur until it is too late to help the patient. Initially, the patient is drowsy with mid-range or small pupils. Breathing progresses from periodic (Cheyne-Stokes respiration) to rapid and deep (central neurogenic hyperventilation). Flexor (decorticate) and then extensor (decerebrate) posturing develop. The patient becomes flaccid and respiration appears normal but shallow. Eventually, both pupils become fixed and dilated, respiration ceases, and the patient is brain dead.

Herniation through the foramen magnum occurs with lesions of the cerebellar hemispheres or vermis. It rapidly causes coma, extensor posturing, pupillary dilatation, ophthalmoplegia, respiratory arrest, and death. Compression of the brain stem or spinomedullary junction interrupts neural control of respiration, causing breathing to cease. Respiratory system failure is in contrast to circulatory system preservation: denervation of the heart causes it to assume a slower idioventricular beat but not to stop functioning. Consequently, large increases in ICP lead to respiratory arrest, with cardiac arrest occurring as a secondary phenomenon. Even before respiration ceases, the effects of increased ICP upon the patient's vital functions are evident: respirations become less effective (often slow but sometimes rapid and shallow), and blood pressure rises while the heart rate falls (Cushing phenomenon).

Diagnosis and Monitoring. To prevent irreversible damage, increased ICP must be recognized early and treatment instituted. Symptoms include headache, nausea, vomiting, and diplopia. An altered level of consciousness (irritability, lethargy, stupor, and coma) is caused by brain displacement and early transtentorial herniation. Physical findings are those associated with local brain disturbances and brain herniation. If the process has been acute, examination of the optic fundi may reveal venous engorgement; if pressure has developed over a longer period of time, papilledema may also be evident. As with other neurologic illnesses, the tempo of the disease is important. Mass lesions that develop

Table 8.2.
Medical Treatment of Increased ICP

Method	Treatment
Osmotic diuretics	Mannitol 20%, 1 g/kg i.v. single dose or 1/4 g/kg q.8h. p.r.n. for repeated usage
and/or	
Renal diuretics	Furosemide 1 mg/kg i.v. single dose or 1/4–1/2 mg/kg q.8h. or more p.r.n.
Fluid restriction	Half maintenance with hypotonic or normal electrolyte solutions
Hyperventilation	P_{CO_2} 25–30 mm Hg

acutely over minutes or hours are less well tolerated than those that develop over weeks, months, or years: the latter develop to a much larger size before causing the same severity of symptoms or signs. The cause of intracranial hypertension—mass, edema, or hydrocephalus—should be identified, as treatment depends on the cause. Computerized tomography or magnetic resonance imaging greatly aid the diagnosis.

When present, intracranial hypertension should be monitored to ensure adequate treatment. If the ventricles are normal or enlarged, a ventricular catheter is inserted (external ventriculostomy). If the ventricles are normal or small, an intraparenchymal or subdural bolt, sensor, or catheter is preferable. These devices are placed using sterile techniques at the bedside or at the time of an intracranial procedure. Lumbar puncture is contraindicated because it can precipitate or accelerate downward herniation of the involved brain.

Treatment. Acute or persistent elevations of ICP can be treated as described in Table 8.2. Sometimes pharmacological paralysis with muscle relaxants combined with controlled respiration may be necessary to prevent additional rises in ICP because of coughing and straining. Steroids are helpful if pressure rises are due to tumors or blood clot but not for stroke or trauma. Surgical removal or decompression is usually advisable for mass lesions. Hydrocephalus is decompressed by means of a shunt, an external ventriculostomy, or removal of the obstructing lesion. Careful attention is given to maintenance of normal blood pressure, oxygenation, and electrolyte balance. If the above measures fail, the patient may be placed in barbiturate coma to protect the brain. While most clinicians try to keep ICP under 15 mm Hg, higher pressures sometimes must be accepted. Every attempt should be made to maintain cerebral perfusion pressure above 45 mm Hg.

Head Injury

Acute Problems

Types of Injury. Of concern in acute head trauma are brain injury, intracranial hematomas, and skull fractures (closed and open). Direct brain injury can cause concussion, a condition in which there is brief loss of consciousness at the moment of impact followed by a rapid return to normal. A pathologic lesion has not been identified in human beings, but in primates experimental studies have identified diffuse axonal injury in the brain stem after concussion. More severe trauma to the brain results in more extensive axonal injury, damage to the microcirculation, and disruption of the blood-brain barrier. The resultant cerebral edema raises ICP, which in turn produces further barrier disruptions and edema, thereby further increasing ICP. This tendency for self-perpetuating increases in ICP should be interrupted as early as possible, thus preventing secondary brain injury.

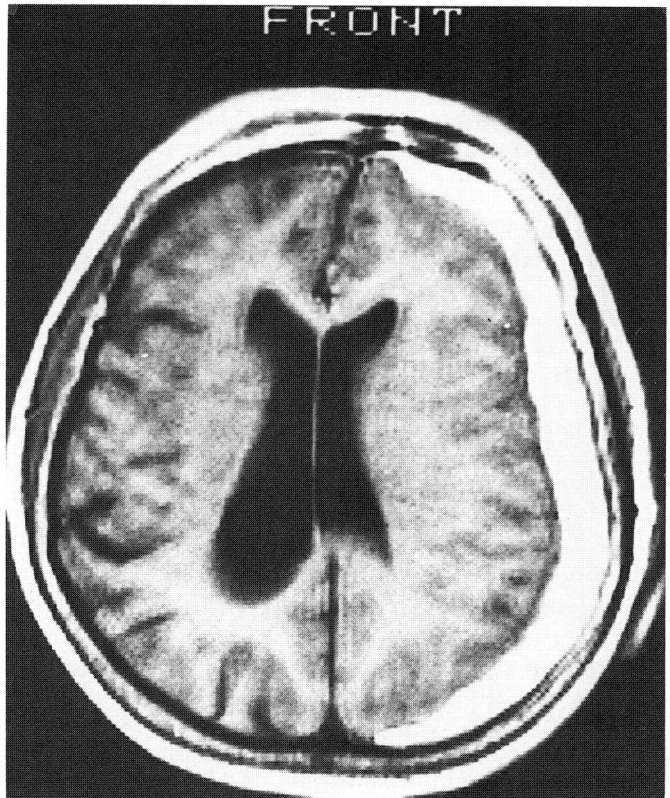

Figure 8.6. MRI of subacute subdural hematoma.

Traumatic intracranial hematomas may be epidural (Fig. 8.5), subdural (Fig. 8.6), or within the brain substance (intraparenchymal). While severe head injury often produces cerebral contusions, large focal intraparenchymal clots are unusual and suggest the head injury may have occurred after the bleed. Epidural and subdural hematomas, which are much more common, require evacuation unless they are very thin. Patient outcome depends upon the rapidity with which ICP elevation is relieved, the preoperative neurological deficit, and the amount of underlying direct brain damage. The most common hematomas and brain contusions involve the temporal and frontal regions where the brain strikes the skull base. Contusions are frequently bilateral, hematomas only occasionally so.

Skull fractures are one indication of the force of impact. Significant hematomas or other complications of head injury are more common when fractures are present. Compound fractures of the cranial vault occur when the overlying skin is lacerated or the fracture extends into the skull base and involves the paranasal sinuses or mastoid air cells. Since the inner table of a depressed fracture often is displaced to a greater extent than the outer table, simple inspection or palpation of the depression through a skin laceration will not reveal its true extent. A benign appearance is no assurance that the dura has not been lacerated, thereby exposing brain to infection.

Basilar fractures can connect the mucosa-lined cavities of the skull (paranasal sinuses, mastoid air cells) with the intracranial cavity, providing an opportunity for intracranial infection if the dura is torn. If CSF leakage occurs, or if intracranial air is evident on x-ray or CT scan, the dura has been breached. In rare instances air accumulates intracranially under pressure (tension pneumocephalus), producing intracranial hypertension and brain displacement. CSF leakage also can occur when head trauma causes an avulsion of the olfactory bulbs and filaments through the cribriform plate. The resultant opening of channels between the cranial and nasal cavities can also serve as a conduit for intracranial infection.

Evaluation. The evaluation attempts to determine the presence and degree of brain and other injuries, the presence of clots, degree of intracranial hypertension, occurrence of simple or compound skull fractures, and whether there is potential or demonstrable CSF leak. A careful history should be obtained to determine how the injury occurred, whether there may have been some predisposing medical event (e.g., myocardial infarction, drug ingestion), and whether the patient has improved or deteriorated since the time of the accident.

As with all trauma, the patient first should be evaluated for *airway, respiratory, and circulatory* problems. These problems, requiring management in their own right, also exacerbate the effects of brain damage and intracranial hypertension by producing secondary brain injury. Conversely, head injury results in circulatory and respiratory abnormalities. An increased ICP can produce a slow pulse and/or elevated blood pressure. These changes are opposite to those occurring after blood loss. Since the head-injured patient is often the victim of multiple system trauma, the presence of hypotension *cannot* be attributed to the head injury unless there are severe scalp or facial lacerations, there is an open fracture with sagittal or transverse sinus injury, or the patient is an infant with open sutures. In almost all cases, hypotension in a head-injured patient is caused by significant blood loss elsewhere in the body. Extracranial sites of blood loss should be sought diligently even if the blood pressure has returned to normal or is above normal, because initial hypotension caused by blood loss subsequently can be masked if ICP rises sufficiently to produce reflex hypertension.

Respiration is often abnormal after head injury. Hypoxia secondary to hypoventilation can accompany brain injury with a depressed level of consciousness or result from local airway obstruction. Occasionally, hypoxia or hypotension can cause a depressed level of consciousness in a trauma victim who has escaped head injury. Airway obstruction can be caused by local trauma to the larynx or trachea or as a result of loss of consciousness with loss of motor tone of the tongue and larynx. Careful inspection is necessary to reveal the nature of the problem and determine whether intubation is necessary. Intubation of the comatose head-injured patient is preferably done after cervical spine radiographs and/or cervical CT scans reveal no fractures. If intubation is indicated emergently, orotracheal intubation with in-line neck stabilization is used if a cervical fracture cannot be ruled out. Placement of a nasogastric tube to empty the stomach contents should be avoided if a cribriform plate or paranasal skull base fracture is suspected. Attempts at nasotracheal or nasogastric intubation in such cases risks introducing the tube inside the cranial cavity.

Blood pressure is evaluated next. If hypotension is present, its cause should be determined and corrected rapidly. From the neurosurgical point of view, it probably is preferable to expand a depleted circulatory volume with colloid rather than crystalloid solutions. Rapid infusion of salt solutions, and especially of pure dextrose solutions, may exacerbate cerebral edema and increase ICP.

The *neurological* evaluation should assess the level of consciousness, pupillary response, and motor function. A rapid examination may be necessary if pharmacological paralysis is urgently required for respiratory control. If increased ICP is suspected or demonstrated, it should be treated as outlined in the section on elevated ICP. CT scan will identify the cause of raised intracranial pressure and demonstrate intracranial clots requiring evacuation. Seizures increase intracranial pressure and hemorrhage. They should be treated emergently with intravenous diazepam (0.2 mg/kg) followed by an infusion of phenytoin (15 mg/kg at 0.6 mg/kg/min or less).

If the patient is poorly responsive, brain stem function can be evaluated by testing oculocephalic (doll's eyes), corneal, and gag reflexes. The doll's eyes maneuver should not be attempted unless cervical spine films and/or CT scan of the neck show no injury. Caloric testing can be substituted if necessary (provided the tympanic membranes are intact). The Glasgow coma scale score should be tallied (Table 8.1). The duration of coma (lack of voluntary responses to others) and of posttraumatic amnesia are measures of injury severity and good indicators of the eventual outcome.

Other pertinent portions of the neurosurgical examination include careful examination of the nose, eyes, and ears. Clear fluid behind the eardrum and clear or bloody drainage from the nose or ear that forms a central red and peripheral pink "target sign" on a paper towel strongly suggests a CSF leak. If the fluid is colorless, it can be tested for sugar by inserting coated test strips into the nares or ears. The presence of sugar indicates CSF. The following signs indicate basal skull fracture and hence potential CSF leak: blood in the external ear canal with a ruptured ear drum or blood behind an intact one, an ecchymosis over the mastoid process, a perfectly round black eyelid, loss of sense of smell, or loss of hearing and facial motion on one side.

The scalp should be examined for lacerations. Careful inspection and palpation of the skull through the laceration may reveal a fracture; however, absence of a palpable fracture does not rule out a skull fracture. A circumscribed, raised area of scalp without any laceration may be caused by an underlying cephalhematoma—hemorrhage between the pericranium and the outer table. The step-off at the edges of the hematoma gives the illusion of palpating a depression. A depressed skull fracture cannot be diagnosed by palpating a cephalhematoma.

Further evaluation is *radiological*. Before the neck is moved for examination or intubation, a lateral and preferably also an anteroposterior cervical radiograph is taken to ensure there is no fracture or dislocation. In cases of severe trauma, intubation is usually necessary before the cervical spine can be evaluated radiologically, and intubation must be carried out without moving the neck. Skull films may be taken at the same time to check for fracture (increased association of intracranial hematoma), air in the head (CSF leak), or clouding of the paranasal sinuses (potential CSF leak). A fracture that extends across the groove of the middle meningeal artery or a dural venous sinus suggests the potential for an intracranial hematoma. A *computerized scan* of the head is performed in patients with progressive neurologic deficit; progressive decrease in consciousness; poor responsiveness to commands; lateralized neurologic deficit; significant headache; temporal, occipital, or vertex fractures; or the prospect of a long anesthetic for repair of some other injury. In many practices, any patient with loss of consciousness undergoes a CT scan. If a scan is to be done, skull films may be unnecessary. The cranial scan should be checked for midline shifts, hematomas and contusions, clouding of the paranasal sinuses or mastoid air cells, and calvarial fractures. If the lateral neck film does not demonstrate the cervical spine down through the top of the first thoracic vertebra, a scan of this region should be performed as well. Finally, an intracranial pressure monitor may be inserted. Monitoring is done in most patients with scores of 8 or less on the Glasgow coma scale.

Other Treatment Considerations. The alert patient with a history of recent concussion but with no abnormal findings requires only a decision as to whether observation should be carried out at home or in the hospital. Factors that might justify hospitalization include a severe headache, prolonged period of unconsciousness, lack of responsible observers, or associated injuries. If the patient is sent home, a responsible adult should be advised to check the patient at regular intervals and instructed on how to evaluate the patient. The patient should return to the hospital if there is hemiparesis, pupillary inequality, increase in headache, or decrease in consciousness.

Patients with more *severe head injuries* have a poorer outcome. Patients with Glasgow coma scale scores of 3 or 4 on admission have a 50–100% mortality rate; patients with scores of 5 or 6 have a 25–65% mortality rate; patients with scores of 7 or 8 have a 10–25% mortality rate. If present and producing mass effect, acute epidural or subdural hematomas are removed as soon as possible. Most intraparenchymal bleeding is in the form of a contusion and usually does not warrant surgery. Whether surgery is required or not, medical management of increased intracranial pressure is carried out (Table 8.2) as dictated by the patient's clinical picture and ICP measurements.

Simple *scalp lacerations* require early irrigation, sometimes debridement, and single layer skin closure. Since the blood vessels of the scalp lie superficial to its deepest layer, the galea aponeurotica, scalp lacerations are closed by placing sutures deeply enough to include the galea.

Closed linear skull fractures of the cranial vault are covered by an intact scalp and require no direct treatment. However, fracture location over a vascular channel (meningeal artery or dural venous sinus) may indicate a potential for intracranial bleeding. While closed depressed fractures may require elevation in the operating room, there is debate as to whether this procedure accomplishes much for the patient other than cosmetic improvement. Continued pressure of a depressed fragment upon the underlying brain does not appear to predispose the patient to future seizures or persistent neurologic deficits. Instead, these problems are the result of the immediate impact at the time of injury. Elevation of closed depressed fractures is usually limited to depressions greater than the thickness of the skull that are not located over major dural venous sinuses.

Compound linear skull fractures are inspected for trapped hair or foreign bodies and are debrided, along with devitalized soft tissues. Cultures should be performed when the patient is first seen and antibiotics begun. If there is a depressed fracture beneath a laceration it is elevated and debrided in the operating room as soon as feasible. If the dura is torn, the brain must be inspected and damaged regions debrided lest they act as a culture medium for infection. The dura must have waterproof closure, if necessary with a graft of periosteum or galea. It may be possible to cleanse and replace bone fragments, including the galea and the cuticular layer, before skin closure.

Penetrating injuries require debridement and are treated similarly to open depressed fractures. Bone fragments and foreign bodies also should be removed if feasible. Bone fragments are a clue to the extent of foreign body penetration. Compound depressed skull fractures and penetrating wounds require urgent surgery to prevent brain abscess and meningitis.

Basilar skull fractures have the potential for CSF leak and intracranial infection. In contrast to patients with compound depressed skull fractures or penetrating injuries, patients with basilar fractures are not operated upon emergently, even if CSF leakage is evident. Such patients are kept at bed rest with the head at a constant modest elevation. Activities that vary the intracranial to atmospheric pressure difference, such as changes in position or coughing, are avoided. Prophylactic antibiotics are often used, although there is some debate as to whether this treatment is helpful. If there is no evidence of CSF leakage after 5 or more days, the patient is permitted to ambulate. If CSF leakage persists, lumbar spinal subarachnoid drainage may be used to enhance healing of the leak. Should this prove unsuccessful, surgical closure is necessary. The leak is localized by physical examination, radionuclide subarachnoid scanning, subarachnoid contrast CT scan, or skull tomography.

Subacute and Chronic Head Injury Problems. Subacute and chronic problems after head injury include chronic subdural hematoma, spinal fluid leak, growing fracture, cervical carotid injury, carotid-cavernous fistula, and symptomatic residua (such as epilepsy and posttraumatic syndrome).

Chronic subdural hematomas usually occur in very young children or the elderly. They arise from rupture of a vein bridging the surface of the cerebral hemisphere and the skull. The clot liquefies and becomes bounded by a thick, friable, vascularized outer membrane and a thin, lucent inner membrane. Recurrent bleeding from the outer membrane leads to expansion of the hematoma, increased ICP, shift of the cerebral hemispheres, transtentorial herniation, and death.

In childhood, chronic subdural hematomas are most common in infancy. Affected children present with an enlarged head, symptoms of intracranial hypertension (vomiting, irritability, lethargy), and sometimes seizures. Often there is no history of trauma and the child is thought to have hydrocephalus. Ultrasound or computerized tomographic scanning establish the diagnosis. The child should be carefully screened for abuse. Regular removal of hematoma fluid by means of subdural taps usually eliminates the need for surgical drainage or a shunt procedure.

In older children or adults, chronic subdural hematomas also present with symptoms of increased ICP or seizures. However, they are much more common in the elderly, the demented, or the alcoholic because their brains are atrophic. In adults they may produce a progressive dementia, gait problem, or focal deficit. As the hematoma enlarges, the patient becomes obtunded. Signs of transtentorial herniation develop and the patient quietly dies. It is characteristic of this disease that obtundation is out of proportion to focal neurological deficit. Again, a history of trauma is often absent or very minor. CT scanning establishes the diagnosis, revealing these lesions to be quite lucent relative to brain tissue. Occasionally, these hematomas have not lost all density; they are isodense and indistinguishable from brain tissue, although a midline shift is evident. Enhancement of their inner membranes with intravenous contrast may help to visualize isodense subdural collections. Burr hole drainage usually is sufficient to effect a cure since chronic hematomas are liquid, unlike acute and subacute hematomas.

Occasionally, a head-injured patient suffers from an undetected chronic *CSF leak* and meningitis occurs. If such a patient has a history of head injury, especially if there have been repeated episodes of meningitis or pneumococcus is cultured from the CSF, a persistent or recurrent traumatic CSF leak should be suspected. Diagnostic measures and surgical treatment previously outlined for this problem must be pursued after the meningitis has been successfully treated with antibiotics.

Skull fractures are usually not long-term problems. However, wide linear fractures, especially in children under the age of 3 years, merit follow-up skull films in 6 months. Rarely, such a fracture is associated with a dural tear that permits an arachnoid hernia to pulsate through the defect, preventing healing and gradually widening the fracture line. Such *growing fractures* require surgical repair. Occasionally, a delayed cranioplasty is necessary to repair a skull defect after removal of a compound depressed skull fracture or a decompressive craniectomy.

A subacute problem that may be associated with head injury and mimic its effects is *cervical carotid injury*. It may take the form of thrombosis, dissection, or aneurysm formation and is often complicated by embolization. Thrombosis, embolization, and dissection produce their symptoms early but not immediately after the injury: onset is almost always more than 12 hours after the injury and usually more than 24. While neurological deficit opposite the damaged carotid may be mild, massive cerebral infarction with severe deficits—including coma with hemiparalysis or decerebration—can occur. With carotid injury, damage to the surrounding sympathetic nerves often produces a small pupil on the side of injury and contralateral to the side of major motor weakness. This response contrasts with the large pupil of brain herniation. Some evidence of direct trauma to the neck is often visible. Treatment of the injured cervical carotid artery is debated. In cases with mild neurological deficit, anticoagulation therapy or carotid surgery have been advocated. If symptoms are severe, ICP elevations should be treated medically.

Injury to the carotid artery as it passes through the cavernous sinus before becoming intradural can produce a *carotid-cavernous fistula*. Within the cavernous sinus the carotid is entirely surrounded by venous channels; a tear in the arterial wall or in a small venous branch produces an arteriovenous fistula. Arterial blood shunted into the venous plexus of the cavernous sinus drains through multiple channels, including the ophthalmic veins. Pulsatile blood of arterial pressure in this channel produces a pulsating exophthalmos with a bruit, a vasodilatory chemosis of the conjunctiva, visual loss, extraocular muscle paresis, and glaucoma in the affected eye.

Potential residua of head injury include motor deficits (these serve as an early clue to ultimate functional ability), cognitive deficits, behavioral changes, and a constellation of disturbing complaints lumped under the term *posttraumatic syndrome*. This syndrome is largely accepted as being organic in origin. It includes a variety of symptoms that may occur in the absence of any neurologic deficit: headache, dizziness, vertigo, fatigability, and inability to concentrate. It is often, but unfortunately not always, self-limited. Subtle cognitive and personality changes may be the only residua, but may be sufficient to interfere with employment and social activities.

Cerebrovascular Disease

Stroke is defined as the sudden or rapid (seconds to hours) occurrence of neurological dysfunction or loss of consciousness due to cerebrovascular disease. Stroke may arise from hypertension, carotid atherosclerosis with emboli, intracerebral atherosclerosis, heart disease, coagulopathies, polycythemia, drug abuse, or diabetes mellitus. Entities that may mimic stroke are seizure, syncope, multiple sclerosis, migraine, and brain tumors. In this chapter we will discuss structural lesions and masses amenable to a surgical approach, including obstructive vascular lesions, vascular anomalies, and hematomas.

Fundamental to stroke diagnosis and management is the distinction between ischemic and hemorrhagic stroke. Ischemic strokes result from vascular obstruction while hemorrhagic strokes follow vascular rupture. On occasion, both occur together as a hemorrhagic infarction. Ischemic strokes (cerebral infarctions) are usually characterized by the rapid onset (seconds) of focal neurological deficit with little or no headache and without loss of consciousness. In contrast, hemorrhagic strokes are slower in onset, evolving over minutes to hours. They usually are accompanied by headache, nausea, or vomiting and produce marked disturbance of consciousness as an early symptom. Unlike many ischemic events, the effects of hemorrhage almost never resolve quickly, if at all. The immediate mortality rate from ischemic stroke (infarction) is 25%, whereas that from hemorrhage is 70%.

Confirmation of the ischemic or hemorrhagic nature of the lesion should be obtained by CT scan, since MRI scan very often fails to disclose subarachnoid hemorrhage. Intracerebral hemorrhage is readily apparent. If the CT scan is normal, ischemic stroke or subarachnoid hemorrhage still remain as possibilities and can be distinguished clinically. The CT scan will often show evidence of infarction in several days. The sudden, painless onset of neurological deficit is common with cerebral infarction. Sudden severe headache, usually accompanied by meningismus, is characteristic of subarachnoid hemorrhage. In patients with this presentation, the diagnosis of subarachnoid hemorrhage should be pursued even if the CT scan is normal. A lumbar puncture should be performed. Other diagnoses such as migraine, temporal arteritis, acute sinusitis, or thunderclap headache should also be considered.

Risk factors for stroke, especially hypertension, cardiac sources of emboli, diet, and smoking, should be sought and corrected.

Ischemic Stroke (Cerebral Infarction). Patients may have focal symptoms that are transient (<24 hours) with complete recovery (transient ischemic attack—TIA) or reversible after a day (reversible ischemic neurological deficit—RIND); they may recover partially, fail to recover, or progress (completed stroke). The risk of cerebral infarction occurring after a TIA is about 5% per year, increasing if there are multiple, frequent TIAs or a lingering partial deficit.

The vascular distribution of the stroke determines prognosis and influences therapy. Stroke in the intracranial internal carotid artery distribution is often caused by arteriosclerosis in the cervical internal carotid artery at the carotid bifurcation. Infarction occurs when debris or clot dislodges from the arteriosclerotic plaque and embolizes into the carotid artery territory in the brain, or when regional cerebral blood flow is decreased by progressive stenosis or thrombosis of the cervical internal carotid artery lumen. Either abrupt monocular visual loss or loss of function limited to the ipsilateral hemisphere suggests the cervical carotid artery as the source of the problem. Stroke in the vertebrobasilar distribution, however, rarely is caused by disease of the cervical portion of the vertebral arteries and is much less often amenable to surgical intervention. Bilateral symptoms and signs and crossed deficits indicative of posterior fossa disease and/or ataxia suggest vertebrobasilar disease.

Evaluation. A history of sudden onset of neurological deficit establishes a preliminary diagnosis of stroke, particularly if physical examination demonstrates a focal neurologic deficit. In addition, the optic fundi should be examined for signs of hypertension, arteriosclerotic change (narrowing, arteriovenous (A-V) nicking), and emboli. The carotid and subclavian arteries should be palpated and checked for bruits, which occur in a significantly narrowed vessel and suggest the site of the pathology. However, bruits can also occur in the vessel opposite an occlusion or in a relatively normal but tortuous vessel, or they can radiate from a diseased aortic valve. Duplex sonography (Doppler waveform analysis plus B-mode imaging) of the cervical vessels is often helpful in establishing the source of the bruit. Echocardiography and Holter monitoring help to establish the heart as the source of emboli. If cervical carotid disease is suspected and surgery is being considered, contrast angiography should be performed. In the future, it is expected that sufficient definition of the suspected pathology will be able to be obtained from noninvasive techniques such as MRI or sonography. Studies for hypercoagulability and arteritis should also be considered.

Treatment. Carotid surgery is prophylactic: while it decreases the future incidence of stroke it does not improve an existing stroke. There is currently vigorous debate over whether it produces a better outcome than judicious medical care alone. Patients with atherosclerotic disease of the cervical carotid artery that are suitable candidates for endarterectomy include those with carotid distribution TIAs, RINDs, or completed but not severe strokes having a deeply ulcerated plaque, or >70% stenosis. In such patients surgery can be considered if there are no other major health problems and if the surgeon's combined morbidity and mortality of angiography and surgery is less than 5%. A recent prospective randomized study showed that patients with TIA's and a >70% ipsilateral carotid stenosis had a

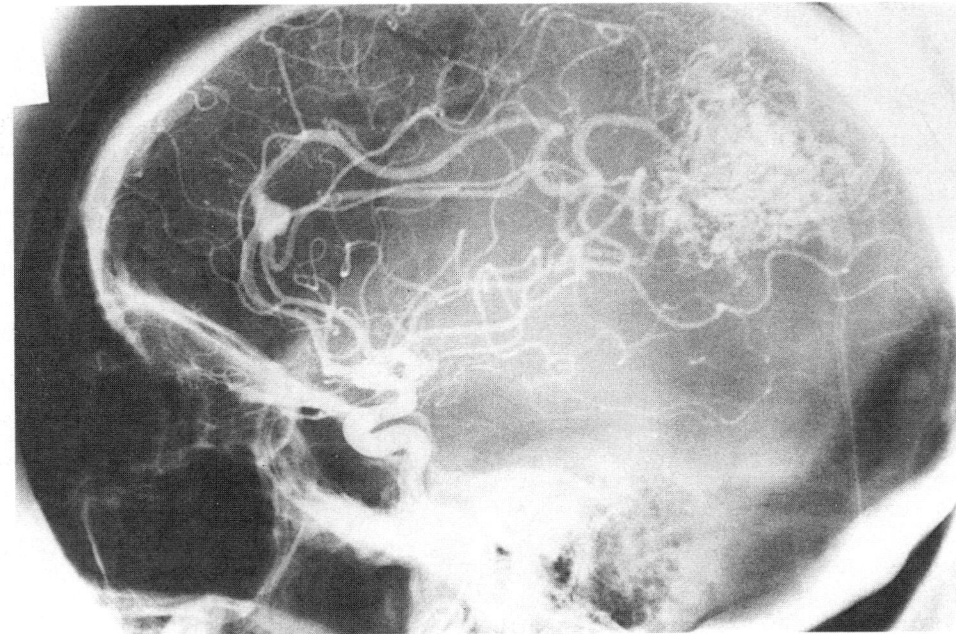

Figure 8.7. Lateral angiogram of parietal AVM with aneurysm located proximally on an enlarged feeding vessel.

much lower stroke rate and mortality with carotid endarterectomy than those treated medically. Except for patients with tight stenosis of the carotid lumen (1–2 mm), patients with an asymptomatic cervical carotid lesion have not been demonstrated to benefit from carotid endarterectomy, although prospective clinical trials are currently underway. Occlusions are not usually correctable. The major alternative to surgery is antiplatelet therapy with aspirin, a regimen often used in postoperative patients as well. Long-term follow-up of unoperated or operated lesions should include repeated clinical evaluation and duplex sonography.

Hemorrhagic Stroke

Types. Two types of nontraumatic intracranial hemorrhage should be distinguished because their etiology and therapy differ: *intraparenchymal bleeding* and *subarachnoid hemorrhage*(SAH). Sudden death is common with either. Hypertension is the most common cause of spontaneous intraparenchymal bleeding, but anomalies of the cerebral vessels (aneurysms and arteriovenous malformations—AVMs) are the most common causes of spontaneous SAH. Intraparenchymal bleeding destroys local tissue, elevates ICP, and shifts the brain. The cause of the ill effects of SAH is less clear. Sudden death or neurologic devastation occurs in almost 50% of spontaneous SAH cases. New onset of severe headache, acute neurological deficit, or diminished alertness are common signs of intracranial hemorrhage and are signals to perform a CT or MRI scan.

An intraparenchymal hemorrhage can burst into the subarachnoid space or a SAH can have an intraparenchymal component. When subarachnoid and intraparenchymal hemorrhage occur together, it is usually the intraparenchymal hemorrhage that dominates the clinical presentation because of the mass effect of the hematoma. Hypertensive hemorrhage typically occurs in the basal ganglia, thalamus, pons, or cerebellum rather than the white matter of the cerebral hemispheres. It results from weakening of the wall of medium-sized penetrating arterioles. Except for the cerebellar hemorrhage, hypertensive hemorrhage usually occurs in the deep gray matter masses of the brain. Lobar hemorrhage occurs in the white matter of the cerebral hemisphere. Its cause is often unknown, but small, occult AVMs or cerebrovascular amyloidosis are suspected.

Arteriovenous malformations are usually congenital and consist of multiple arteriovenous communications forming a knot of feeding arteries and draining veins within brain tissue (Fig. 8.7). Because of the abnormal structure of the vessel walls and the direct communication between the feeding and draining vessels, clinical signs of rupture are a common presentation. Bleeding is typically intraparenchymal rather than subarachnoid. Rapid shunting of blood through the AVM and away from the adjacent brain is equally common; small bleeds cause local brain damage with fluctuating neurological deficits or seizures.

Intracranial aneurysms most often occur as saccular dilatations at branch points of major vessels at the base of the brain (berry aneurysm). At these points there appears to be a defect of the media and elastica. The etiology is debated and may involve both congenital and atherosclerotic elements. Most aneurysms occur at branch points of the anterior circle of Willis, especially at the posterior internal carotid-communicating artery junction (Fig. 8.8), at the anterior communicating artery, or the middle cerebral artery bifurcation. Another 15% occur in the posterior circulation, especially at the basilar artery bifurcation into the posterior cerebral ar-

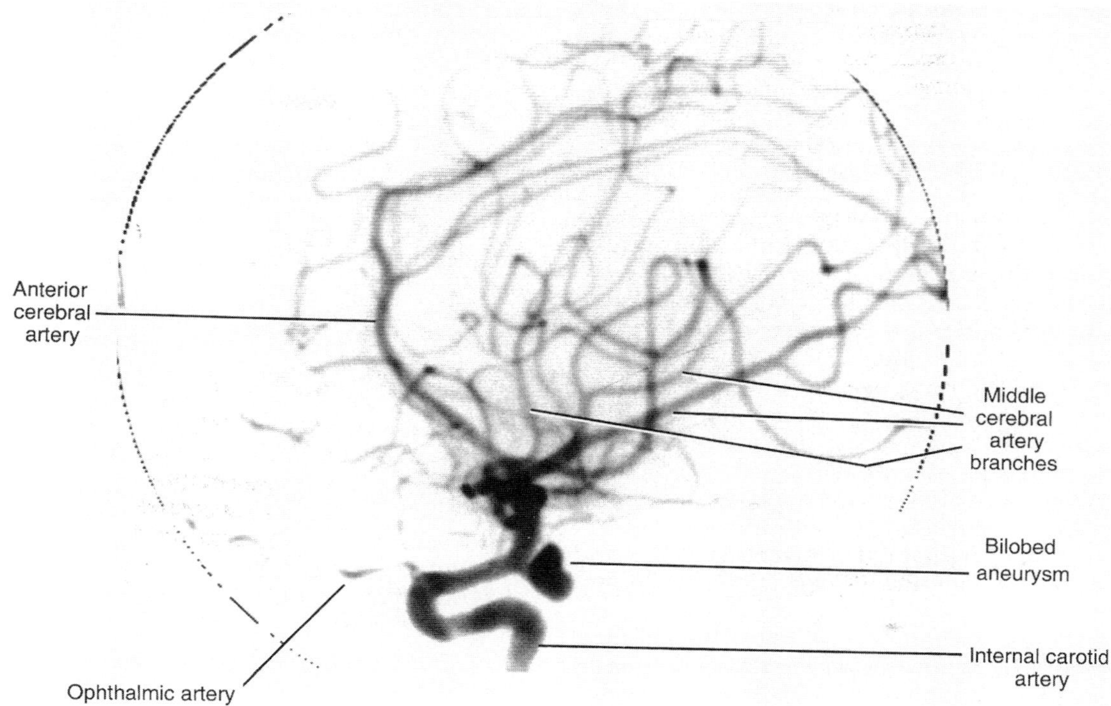

Figure 8.8. Internal carotid-posterior communicating artery aneurysm.

teries. Aneurysms are multiple in 20% of cases, often making it difficult to decide which lesion bled. Hemorrhage is typically subarachnoid. Symptoms are similar to those of any intracranial hemorrhage, though meningismus is often present.

Evaluation. Intracranial hemorrhage can be suspected in cases of (*a*) sudden severe headache occurring in a patient without a long previous history of such headaches and (*b*) sudden unconsciousness. Nausea and vomiting frequently accompany these symptoms. If the hemorrhage has a subarachnoid component, neck stiffness usually is evident, though it may not be present during the first hours. Initial evaluation by CT or MRI scan confirms and localizes the lesion. If an intraparenchymal hematoma is found, enhanced CT or MRI scans may reveal an AVM. Aneurysms usually will not be identified but should be suspected if the clot borders upon the anterior circle of Willis or Sylvian fissure. These cases and those that demonstrate an AVM on scan should undergo angiography.

Most patients with *aneurysms* present with bleeding. The hemorrhage is usually subarachnoid, but at times it produces an intracerebral clot. Secondary neurological deterioration may occur as a result of rebleeding, vasospasm, or hydrocephalus. Because an aneurysm is likely to rebleed early, rapid diagnosis is critical. Vasospasm is a severe complication of aneurysmal subarachnoid hemorrhage and often leads to brain infarction with morbidity and death. Diagnosis is made by arteriography and/or transcranial Doppler studies. Hydrocephalus secondary to adhesions blocking the subarachnoid spaces is another complication that can occur over the ensuing days and weeks.

Occasionally, aneurysms produce other symptoms with no bleeding or with only mild bleeding. An example is the unilateral third nerve paresis (pupillary dilatation with lid droop and loss of medial gaze in the same eye) produced by some internal carotid-posterior communicating artery aneurysms (Fig. 8.8). These patients remain alert with mild or no headache. The paresis is caused by the aneurysmal expansion pressing upon the adjacent third nerve. Since expanding aneurysms are likely to rupture, emergency angiographic confirmation is necessary.

Other aneurysms may be mycotic or traumatic. Mycotic aneurysms secondary to septicemia arise more peripherally, well beyond the circle of Willis. Such cases are usually discovered after they bleed. Since these aneurysms are friable, they can rarely be obliterated without sacrificing their vessels of origin. Consequently, initial management consists of systemic antibiotics and serial angiography to detect enlargement. Traumatic aneurysms are rare and are usually caused by penetrating injury, though a rare fracture can also produce one. Delayed posttraumatic epistaxis, especially after fractures involving the orbit, is one manifestation of these lesions.

Unlike aneurysms, only half of symptomatic arteriovenous malformations present with bleeding; most other symptomatic AVMs present with seizures. Because AVMs presenting with seizures have a significantly lower rate of future bleeding, they are resected less frequently. A small percentage of adult AVMs without seizures or bleeding present as mental deterioration or migraine. In infancy, intracranial AVMs may have high output cardiac failure (because of the low resistance shunt) or obstructive hydrocephalus (secondary to dilated venous drainage channels) as their initial symptoms.

Treatment. Treatment of an *intraparenchymal hematoma* depends upon its location. Patients with moderate or large lobar hematomas frequently benefit from early hematoma evacuation, because the clot separates white matter fibers without a great deal of destruction. Evacuation is usually by open craniotomy, but stereotaxic needle aspiration has been used. Open evacuation of deep hematomas in the basal ganglia and internal capsule is more controversial. Neurologic deficits usually are severe and irreversible; surgery risks further injury. Stereotaxic aspiration may have a role in the management of these lesions. Supplementary treatment consists of reducing marked rises in ICP and reversing brain herniation with diuretics and hyperventilation.

Among patients with posterior fossa hematomas, those with cerebellar hemorrhage uniquely benefit from surgical evacuation. The history of headache, diplopia, ipsilateral conjugate gaze palsy, Babinski's sign, and cerebellar deficits with evolving lethargy and coma is almost diagnostic of a lesion both potentially fatal and fully correctable. Evacuation of the hematoma frequently leads to complete recovery.

Regardless of etiology, the outcome of surgery for hematoma strongly depends on the preoperative status of the patient. The better the patient's general status and neurological function before surgery, the better the outcome.

Because an *aneurysm* is likely to rebleed early, surgical obliteration of the aneurysm within the first few days is recommended by clipping of the aneurysmal neck. In neurologically intact patients, operative mortality or morbidity is very low, but among those who are moribund few survive with or without surgery. The short-term rebleeding risk of an aneurysm is 35–45% within 4 weeks, with a mortality rate of 50%, After 6 months, the long-term rebleeding risk of an unoperated aneurysm is only 3% per year, but approximately half of these patients die.

Treatment of vasospasm, a complication of aneurysmal subarachnoid hemorrhage, consists of hemodilution, hypervolemia, and elevation of blood pressure by pharmacologic manipulation. Since this regimen risks aneurysmal rupture, it is used most often after the aneurysm has been obliterated. In addition, a calcium channel blocker, such as nimodipine, may be helpful as a cerebral vasodilator and is often given to patients as soon as the diagnosis is suspected. Vasospasm usually occurs about 3–9 days after subarachnoid hemorrhage.

Some aneurysms present without hemorrhage. In patients with the isolated onset of a unilateral third nerve paresis but no evidence of hemorrhage, angiography is urgent. An expanding posterior communicating artery aneurysm may be present. If this proves true, surgery should follow urgently. Similarly, atherosclerotic aneurysms enlarge without bleeding and gain attention by producing other focal neurological deficits peculiar to their location. Their treatment is usually not emergent. Treatment of asymptomatic aneurysms is a matter of debate. There is a 1.5% annual bleeding rate of unruptured aneurysms, with death in half of patients whose aneurysms bleed.

Unlike the risk following aneurysmal subarachnoid hemorrhage, the risk of an AVM rebleeding is spread evenly over time with a much lower morbidity and mortality per bleed. Consequently, if the clot is judged not to pose immediate danger, surgery is delayed until the patient stabilizes and edema subsides. Surgery is done to prevent rebleeding, especially if the lesion is readily accessible, does not involve eloquent areas of the brain, and is not excessively large. Alternative and supplemental treatment options include interventional endovascular radiological approaches with glues and embolic materials and, in the case of smaller lesions, stereotaxic radiosurgical treatment.

In some patients, an aneurysm produces an intracerebral clot. Unless the clot is accompanied by intracranial hypertension or significant brain shift, surgery will not improve the patient's condition. Surgery is prophylactic and intended to prevent rebleeding. Early management is medical and includes sedation, reduction of increased ICP, treatment of hypertension, and adequate pain medication to relieve headache. Adjuvant management includes measures to prevent the patient from straining, such as giving stool softeners. Rectal examination should be avoided.

Brain Tumors and Brain Abscess

Brain tumors often are categorized by their relationship to brain tissue (extrinsic versus intrinsic), site (supratentorial versus posterior fossa), and age of presentation (pediatric versus adult). Each of these factors is of practical significance in diagnosis and management: extrinsic tumors are more often benign and totally excisable than intrinsic ones; infratentorial tumors more often present with hydrocephalus and rapid onset of increased ICP than supratentorial tumors; and pediatric tumors are more often infratentorial (60%), whereas adult tumors are usually supratentorial (85%). Furthermore, while all histological types of tumors occur in both age groups, certain types are much more common in one than another, as will be discussed subsequently.

Symptoms of brain tumors can be divided into three broad categories: (*a*) those due to stretching or irritation of surrounding nonneural structures, (*b*) those due to generalized increase in intracranial pressure, and (*c*) those due to focal displacement or destruction of neural tissue. Headache is the most common presenting complaint (54%) of patients with a brain tumor. However, although many people have a headache, only a few (about 1%) have a brain tumor. Therefore, the physician must look for additional symptoms and signs. Headache heralds the presence of an intracranial mass

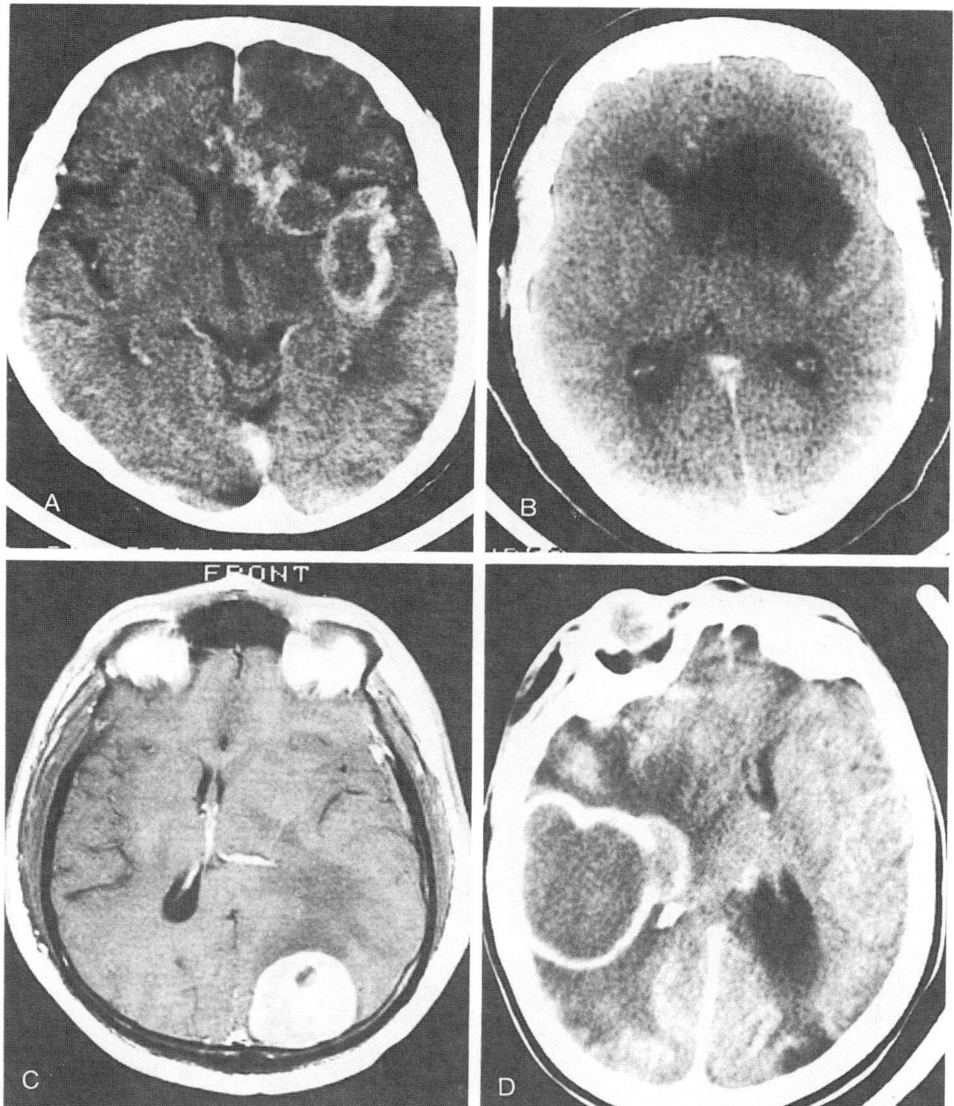

Figure 8.9. **A**, Glioblastoma multiforme (enhanced CT scan). **B**, Low-grade astrocytoma (enhanced CT scan). **C**, Metastatic melanoma (enhanced CT scan). **D**, Brain abscess (enhanced CT scan).

if it is accompanied by neurological deficit, change in affect, intellectual loss, seizure onset, papilledema, or endocrine dysfunction. Focal neurological deficit or mental change is manifest in 68% of patients with brain tumor by the time of diagnosis, while seizures will have occurred in 26%.

Signs of focal neurological dysfunction and of ICP are determined by location of the tumor. Increased ICP occurs more rapidly from obstruction of CSF flow than from pressure exerted by growth of the tumor. Because CSF pathways are narrowest at the aqueduct of Sylvius, they are often occluded at this site by pressure from tumors in the posterior fossa. Since tumors of the cerebellum often grow without causing much focal deficit, hydrocephalus occurs early in the course of their presentation. Consequently, many posterior fossa tumors present with hydrocephalus and the accompanying symptoms and signs of increased intracranial pressure.

For all brain tumors, diagnosis is established by CT or MRI scan, with and without intravenous contrast enhancement. Such scans indicate whether the tumor is intrinsic or extrinsic to the brain, reveal its location, and suggest its histology (Fig. 8.9). Stereotaxic biopsy is often a helpful option to establish the cell type and confirm the diagnosis (Fig. 8.10).

Treatment of all brain tumors involves surgery and radiation. The relative success rates for each specific tumor are discussed below. If there is significant disturbance of consciousness or of neurological function, steroids are given as a temporizing supplementary measure to reduce cerebral edema and maintain neurologic function until treatment has been instituted.

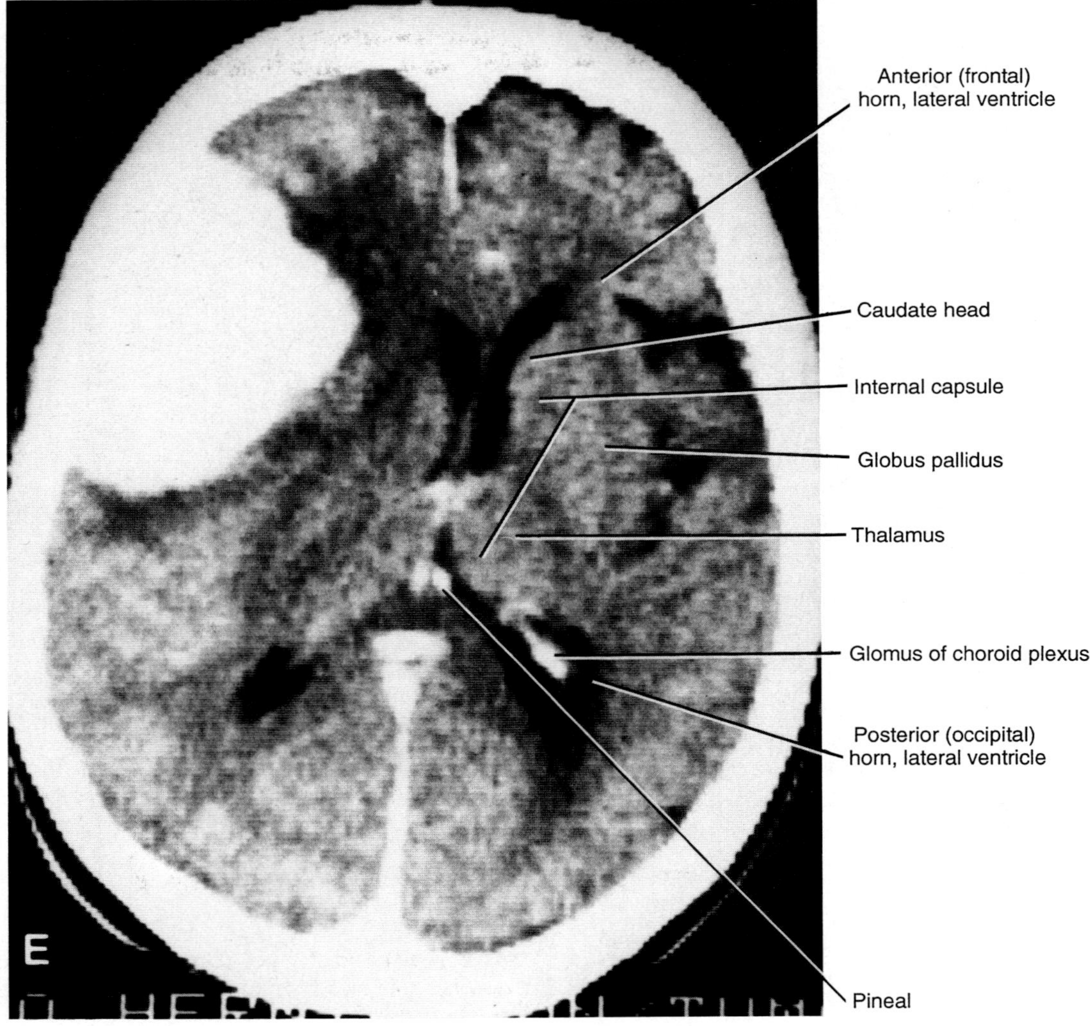

Figure 8.9. *(continued)* **E**, Meningioma (enhanced CT scan).

Adult Brain Tumors

Intrinsic Tumors. Intraparenchymal brain tumors account for about 60% of primary intracranial tumors. Most occur above the tentorium. Glial tumors arise from the supporting cells of the brain and are divided into (*a*) glioblastoma, (*b*) anaplastic astrocytoma, (*c*) astrocytoma, (*d*) oligodendroglioma, and (*e*) ependymoma. Metastatic tumors are also intrinsic and account for about 50% of all brain tumors. Cerebellar hemangioblastomas, although benign, also require removal. Neuronal tumors are rare.

Glioblastoma multiforme is highly malignant and the most common glial tumor of adults (Fig. 8.9**A**). These poorly differentiated tumors are characterized by the presence of hyperplasia with nuclear pleomorphism, necrosis, pseudopalisading, and endothelial proliferation. Though they metastasize infrequently, they grow rapidly, recur locally after apparent total excision, and can extend widely throughout the brain. They are uniformly fatal. Only 10% of affected patients are alive at 18–24 months. The 5-year survival rate is zero and the mean duration of life after diagnosis is about 12 months.

Anaplastic astrocytoma is only slightly less aggressive. It is characterized by the presence of hyperplasia and anaplasia with nuclear pleomorphism, but lacks the necrosis and other features characteristic of glioblastoma. The 5-year survival rate is 18%; the mean duration of life after diagnosis is about 28 months.

Astrocytoma (low grade) is a benign tumor of astrocytes that can occur anywhere in the brain. It accounts for about one-fifth of gliomas and also occurs in children. It is characterized by mild to moderate hyperplasia with little if any abnormality in nuclear morphology. The 5-year survival rate is 50–75%. Young patients do better than older ones; those with cystic or microcystic changes do better than ones with solid lesions. Gross total removal results in a better survival rate than biopsy or subtotal removal. Prognosis is much worse if the tumor harbors small foci of anaplastic cells. Occasionally, some tumors with a benign histology dediffer-

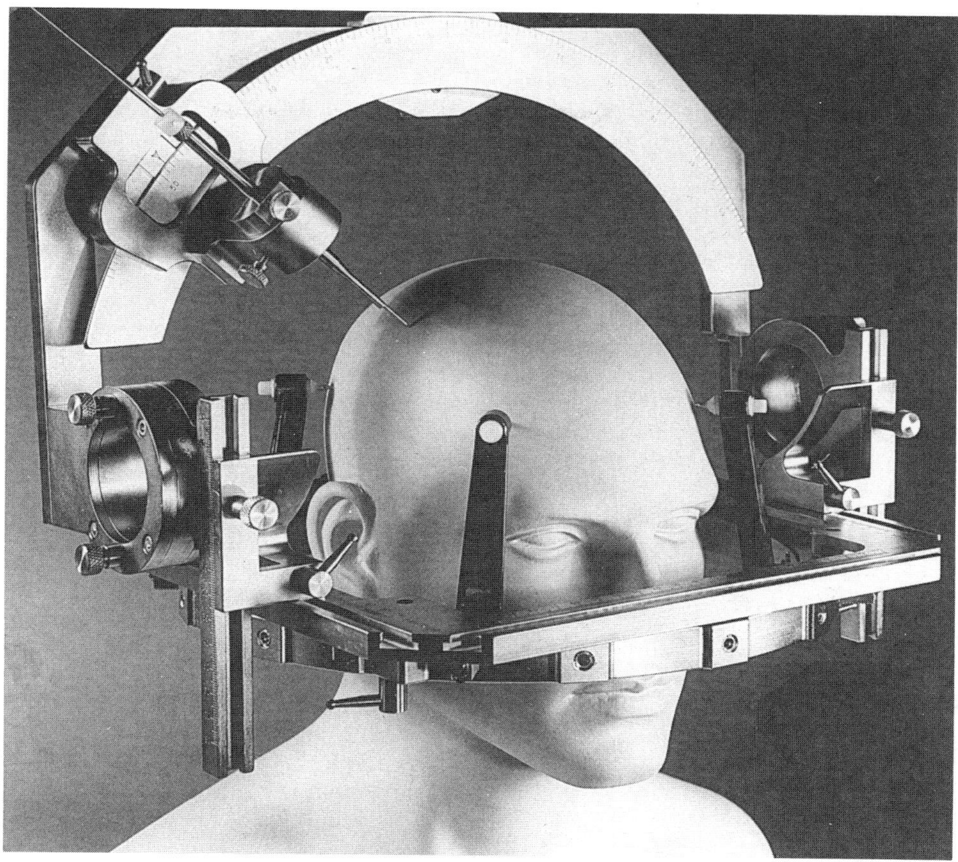

Figure 8.10. Stereotaxic biopsy.

entiate into anaplastic astrocytoma or glioblastoma. About 20% of glioblastomas are believed to begin as low-grade astrocytomas.

Oligodendroglioma comprises about 5% of gliomas. They frequently contain calcium, which forms a distinctive pattern on CT scan. Patients harboring these tumors commonly present with seizures (60%). The length of survival after surgery is said to be inversely proportional to the duration of the symptoms before surgery. The 5-year survival rate after surgery and radiation is 60–85%.

Ependymoma comprises about 5% of gliomas. In adults ependymomas occur with equal frequency above and below the tentorium. The 5-year survival rate after surgery and radiation of patients with ependymoma is only 35%, even though histologically the tumor is benign.

Cerebral metastases occur in about 25–30% of patients afflicted with cancer and are among the most common types of brain tumor (Fig. 8.9**C**). The most frequent origins are from lung, breast, kidney, gastrointestinal tract, skin (melanoma), and thyroid. A cancer patient presenting with headache and seizures or a focal neurologic deficit should be suspected of having a cerebral metastasis, even though all cancer patients with focal neurologic signs do not have metastases. Spinal metastasis, carcinomatous meningitis, and remote effects of carcinoma need to be considered if an intracerebral mass is not found. Even if the patient is not known to have cancer, the presence of a solitary lesion within the brain must lead to a consideration of metastases. If there are multiple mass lesions, the diagnosis of metastasis is more assured. The median survival of patients with brain metastases is only 6 months, but is influenced by the tumor's histology, location, and treatment.

Hemangioblastoma is a benign tumor that most commonly arises in the cerebellum and is composed of pericytes, endothelial cells, and stromal cells arising from blood vessels. About one-third of cases occur in patients with von Hippel-Lindau disease (retinal angiomatosis with hemangioblastomas of the neuraxis as well as visceral tumors, including clear-cell carcinoma of kidney and pheochromocytoma). Surveillance should be maintained after complete removal since tumors recur. In patients with von Hippel-Lindau disease, multiple or new tumors are common.

Diagnosis of Intrinsic Tumors. Evaluation of patients suspected of having a brain tumor includes a careful history and physical examination as well as a chest film to look for a primary source of cancer. Inherited diseases such as von Hippel-Lindau disease, neurofibromatosis, or tuberous sclerosis, should be sought. CT or MRI scan with and without enhancement shows whether the lesion is intrinsic and what its characteristics are. For example, glioblastoma frequently enhances irregularly and shows marked enhancement at the periphery with low attenuation values in the center. On CT scan astrocytomas (low grade) frequently have a low signal and show little enhancement with contrast injection. Focal areas of abundant high CT signal without enhancement suggest the presence of calcium and hence an oligodendroglioma. A spherical, solid, intraparenchymal lesion that enhances is suggestive of a metastasis, as are multiple lesions. Arteriography may be desirable to evaluate the vascularity of the lesion and delineate associated vascular structures.

Surgery is necessary to establish a diagnosis and constitutes an important, sometimes essential, treatment for many intrinsic brain tumors. CT or MR-guided stereotaxic needle biopsy is useful in eliminating the need for a more extensive procedure and in reaching an otherwise inaccessible site such as the thalamus. However, the targeted lesion should not be excessively vascular since hemorrhage may complicate the procedure. Such a biopsy can be done under local anesthesia.

Treatment of Intrinsic Tumors. If needle biopsy or clinical impression indicates glioblastoma, the surgeon should consider performing an internal decompression by debulking the tumor prior to instituting radiotherapy. Opinion differs as to whether open surgery is necessary or helpful. The same considerations apply for a more benign glioma lying in a particularly eloquent or vital area. If the biopsy demonstrates an accessible benign glioma, radical surgical excision is the treatment of choice.

Surgical excision aims to achieve "a gross total removal" of the tumor. On most occasions it is necessary to enter the tumor and aspirate it (compare with the techniques of tumor removal in general surgery). Even benign gliomas do not usually have a distinct plane between tumor and surrounding brain. A tumor-free margin is thus difficult to obtain without causing unacceptable damage. The gross margins about metastatic tumors are more clearly defined. Single metastases, especially if symptomatic, are considered candidates for excision. Recent studies have demonstrated considerable benefit from a combination of surgical removal and postoperative radiation of solitary metastasis, resulting in prolongation of functional life beyond 1 year. Vascular tumors such as hemangioblastoma or metastatic renal cell carcinoma should be excised without biopsy because bleeding can be severe.

Radiation therapy has a clearly demonstrated but often limited benefit in the treatment of most gliomas and metastatic disease. Its use in low-grade adult astrocytomas is debated. Chemotherapy is of limited efficacy in treating these brain tumors.

Extrinsic Tumors. In adults, extrinsic brain tumors occur almost as frequently as intrinsic ones. Because these tumors invaginate into the brain rather than arise from within it, they frequently can be totally excised, especially when they are small. The most frequently occurring types are meningioma, pituitary adenoma, and acoustic neuroma.

Meningiomas are benign tumors that arise from arachnoid cap cells. They are found at sites of arachnoid granulations, such as over the convexity, along the sagittal or other dural sinus, along the falx, or at the base of the skull (Fig. 8.9**E**). Such tumors frequently cause seizures because of pressure upon the underlying cortex. Occasionally invasion of the overlying skull produces a visible protuberance beneath the scalp. They account for about 20% of primary brain tumors. Most occur as discrete masses (globoid) but a few can form sheets of tumor (en plaque). Meningiomas recur with a frequency of only 12% after apparently complete removal, but not all tumors are amenable to gross total removal. In general, the outlook is good, with one series reporting 50% of patients alive and free of disease at 20 years. The subtypes of meningiomas are similarly benign, except for angioblastic meningioma, which is much more likely to recur.

Because meningiomas usually attach to the dura, they receive their principal blood supply from meningeal branches of the external carotid. Angiography will demonstrate this characteristic blood supply. As meningiomas grow they invaginate into the brain and gain an additional blood supply. Preoperative embolization of the external carotid artery reduces the dural blood supply, thereby limiting blood loss during surgery.

Meningiomas of the cranial base can arise from many sites, most commonly from the olfactory groove beneath the frontal lobe, about the sella turcica, and along the sphenoid ridge. Less commonly tumors arise from the tentorium or posterior fossa. Tumors at each site have unique manifestations that can be deduced with an adequate knowledge of neuroanatomy. For example, bitemporal hemianopia with loss of the sense of smell suggests a tumor of the olfactory groove that has grown back to involve the optic chiasm; bitemporal hemianopia with sparing of endocrine function and no anosmia suggests a tuberculum sella meningioma; unilateral optic atrophy with proptosis suggests a sphenoid wing meningioma.

Pituitary adenomas, arising from the gland's anterior lobe (in the sella turcica), comprise about 15% of primary brain tumors. Most pituitary tumors are functional: they secrete a hormone capable of causing endocrine symptoms. Because most patients with functioning tumors present clinically with a positive symptom or sign, rather than with the loss of a normal function, they are diagnosed early, when the tumor is a microadenoma. Nonfunctioning tumors either do not secrete hormones or secrete biologically inactive ones. These tumors are diagnosed later, when the tumor is large enough (macroadenoma) to destroy normal pituitary function or press upon neighboring neural structures (Fig. 8.11). Hormone-containing tumor cells can be identified by immunohistochemistry.

The most common functional tumor is prolactinoma, which causes amenorrhea-galactorrhea syndrome in females and impotence in males. Somatotroph tumors secrete excess growth hormone, causing acromegaly. In

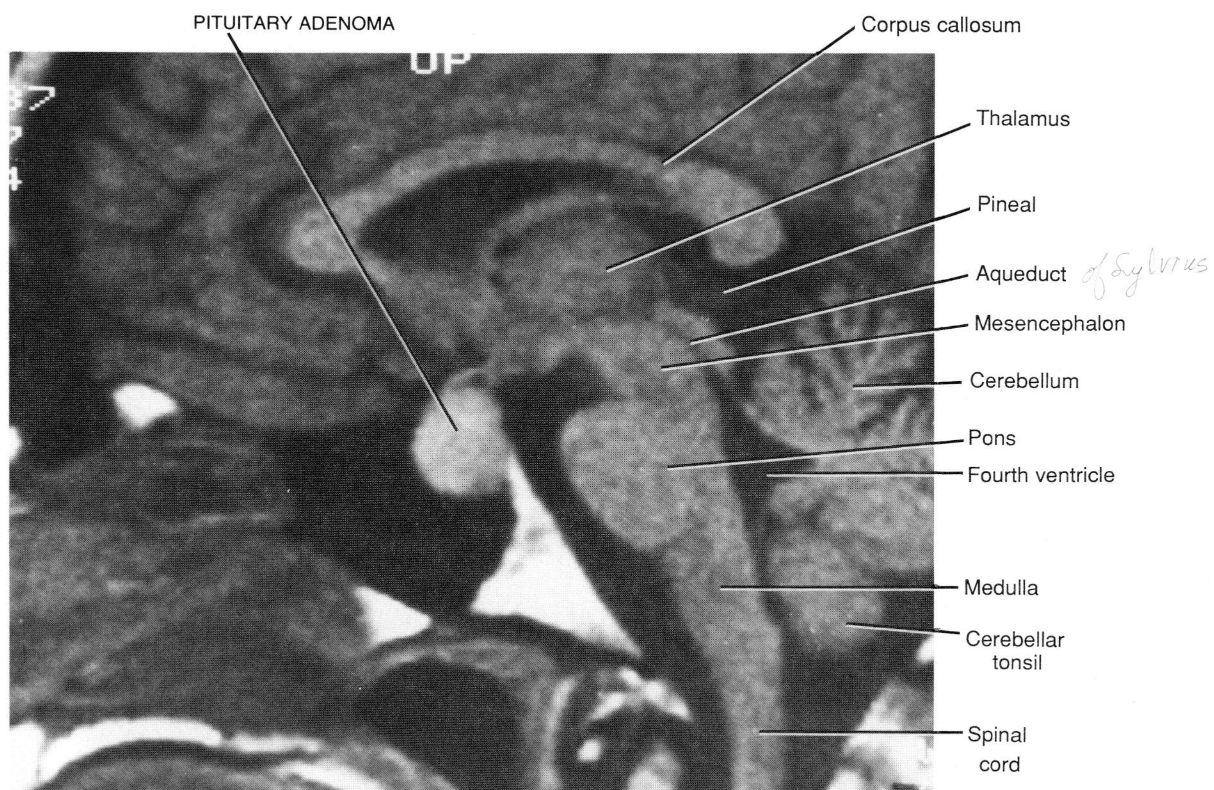

Figure 8.11. Pituitary adenoma (midsagittal, enhanced MRI scan).

addition to outward changes of coarsened features, prognathism, and hand and foot growth, the patients develop hypertension, diabetes mellitus, and myopathy including cardiomyopathy. Corticotroph tumors secrete adrenocorticotropic hormone (ACTH), causing Cushing's disease. In addition to visible changes of truncal obesity, a buffalo hump, striae, and easy bruising, these patients develop hypertension, diabetes mellitus, and myopathy. These changes are due to an excess of circulating cortisol that in turn is caused by the excess of circulating ACTH. Tumors of gonadotrophs secrete follicle-stimulating hormone (FSH) or luteinizing hormone (LH). They are rare and cause sterility, loss of libido, and impotence.

As pituitary tumors enlarge, pressure on the normal portions of the gland produces hypopituitarism. Further growth results in neurological deficits due to compression and even invasion of adjacent structures. Upward (suprasellar) expansion compresses the overlying chiasm producing bitemporal hemianopia. Extreme upward growth can obstruct the foramen of Monro and cause hydrocephalus with papilledema. On occasion expansion is lateral into the cavernous sinus, causing diplopia due to pressure upon the third, fourth, or sixth cranial nerves. While small pituitary tumors (microadenomas) fail to enlarge or distort the sella turcica, large ones not only produce pituitary and neurologic deficits but expand and erode the sella to produce changes that are evident on ordinary skull x-rays.

Acoustic neuromas arise from Schwann cells of the vestibular nerve at or inside the internal auditory canal and comprise about 5% of primary brain tumors (Fig. 8.12). The history is usually one of unilateral tinnitus with vertigo that disappears as the vestibular nerve is destroyed. With tumor growth into the cranial cavity at the cerebellopontine angle, pressure upon the auditory nerve renders the ear deaf. The function of the adjacent, equally stretched facial nerve (motor) is preserved. The finding of unilateral sensorineural hearing loss with impairment of taste on the same side is highly suggestive of acoustic neuroma. As the neuroma grows, it involves the fifth cranial nerve, causing loss of the corneal reflex and eventually facial numbness. Ultimately, there are cerebellar signs (staggering gait and veering toward the side of the lesion) and ninth and 10th cranial nerve deficits (hoarseness of voice, dysphagia, and aspiration).

Diagnosis of Extrinsic Tumors. Evaluation of the patient with a brain tumor begins with the history and physical examination. While symptoms and signs such as headache, seizures, hemiparesis, hemianopia, and aphasia occur with extrinsic tumors arising from the dura of the cranial vault, they also occur with intrinsic tumors and thus are relatively nonspecific. In contrast, presentation with pure cranial nerve or pituitary dysfunction suggests an extrinsic tumor at the cranial base. Tumors are characterized according to their site. Subfrontal tumors present with mental change and

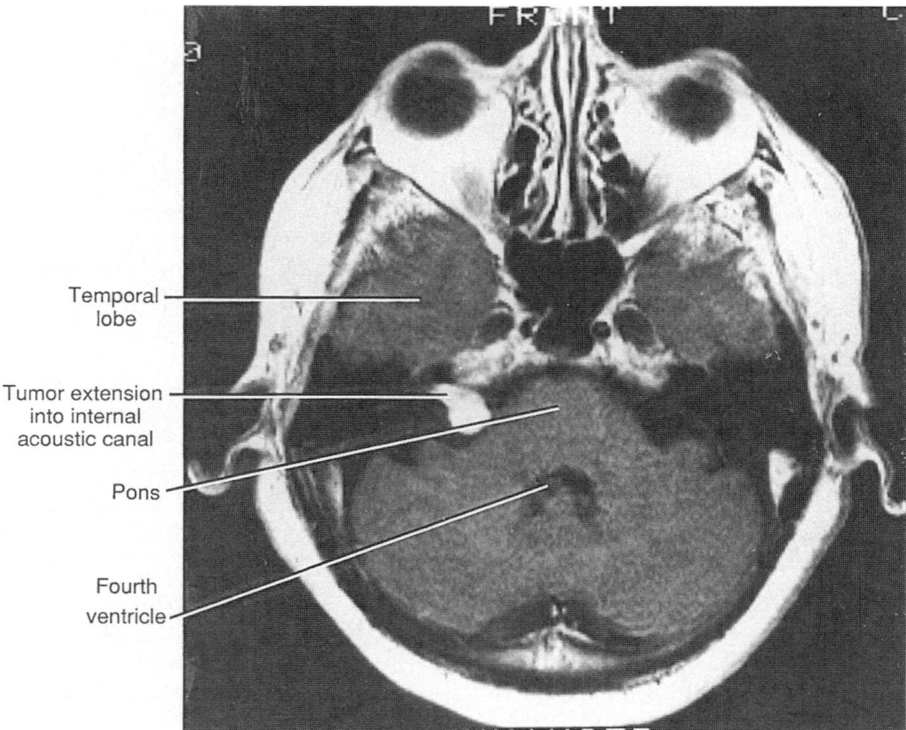

Figure 8.12. Acoustic neuroma (enhanced MRI scan).

seizures; testing will reveal anosmia. Sellar tumors are heralded by pituitary and/or visual dysfunction as described in the sections on meningiomas and pituitary tumors. Parasellar tumors are manifest by oculomotor dysfunction, optic atrophy, and facial numbness. Cerebellopontine angle tumors usually present with unilateral deafness and are acoustic neuromas.

Patients presenting with hyperpituitarism can be presumed to have a pituitary tumor even if the neurological examination, CT scan, and MRI are normal. Removal of the tumor will cure the disease in a high percentage of such patients. An elevated pituitary hormone level helps substantiate the diagnosis. Acromegaly with elevated growth hormone is presumptive evidence of a pituitary adenoma because ectopic tumors secreting growth hormone/releasing hormone are rare. In other presumed states of hyperpituitarism, the decision is not as easy. Amenorrhea and galactorrhea with hyperprolactinemia frequently are caused by a pituitary adenoma. If radiographic studies of the sella are normal, other conditions such as excessive breast stimulation, pregnancy, phenothiazines, or simply too much exercise must be ruled out. Cushing's syndrome with a relative excess of circulating ACTH despite elevated cortisol levels can be caused by excessive ACTH (or even corticotropin-releasing hormone) secretion from ectopic sites. Exploration of the sella in the absence of radiographic signs of a pituitary tumor should proceed only after these other conditions have been excluded.

As in the case of intrinsic tumors, CT or MRI scan will establish the presence of a tumor (except for some small secreting pituitary adenomas). Contrast-enhanced CT or MRI scans are essential for diagnosis and planning. For example, gadolinium-enhanced MRI scans will reveal tiny acoustic tumors missed on unenhanced studies. Enhancement will reveal meningiomas otherwise indistinguishable from brain tissue on noncontrast MRIs and help define arterial displacements or venous sinus invasion characteristic of many of these tumors. The pattern of MRI enhancement also provides a clue as to the type of tumor (for example, a suprasellar tumor versus an aneurysm). Arteriography provides even greater definition of vascular involvement.

Surgery can be expected to cure a patient with an extrinsic brain tumor if the tumor can be removed completely. However, complete removal may incur significant risk. Radiological studies help in evaluating this risk preoperatively and in planning the operation. Surgery has been facilitated by various techniques: use of the operating microscope to improve visualization, new surgical dissecting instruments employing ultrasound to cavitate tumors, or laser light to vaporize the tumor without disturbing neighboring structures. New monitoring techniques (evoked potentials) enable the surgeon to monitor visual, somatosensory, auditory, cerebral, and brain stem function.

Although meningiomas are benign and many can be totally removed, the physician advising patients and their families needs to be aware that many factors often limit total removal (such as vascular or cranial nerve involvement). Such tumors, however, can be resected when they recur.

Most pituitary adenomas can be removed transsphenoidally, a direct approach that avoids the brain retraction necessary with craniotomy. The incidence of recurrence varies with the extent of the tumor. Apparent complete removal of microadenomas can be accomplished about 85% of the time with a recurrence rate of about 20% 5 years after surgery. Larger lesions are less often completely removed; if suprasellar extension occurs, the 5-year surgical cure rate falls to about 50%. Craniotomy is used for tumors that herniate laterally beyond the reach afforded by the transsphenoidal approach, or where the intrasellar component is small but the suprasellar component is large.

Total removal of most acoustic neuromas can be accomplished successfully. A translabyrinthine approach can be used but will destroy whatever hearing is left. A posterior fossa retromastoid craniotomy can also be performed, and in selected patients with small tumors it is possible to preserve hearing. The approach chosen depends upon the disposition of the tumor and the expertise of the surgical team. Facial nerve function can be preserved in about 80% of patients with small intracanalicular tumors, and in about 50% of patients with large tumors mushrooming into the posterior fossa as far as the brain stem.

Medical therapy for benign extrinsic tumors is limited to prolactinomas. Treatment with bromocriptine frequently shrinks these tumors and usually suppresses their growth and secretory activity.

Radiotherapy is employed to eradicate or control residual tumor. The symptomatic recurrence rate of pituitary tumors large enough to enlarge or destroy the sella can be reduced by half. Sometimes radiation therapy is employed to treat residual basal meningioma. While x-ray beams focused by linear acceleration or the gamma knife have been used to treat some tumors, results of this treatment are uncertain.

Pediatric Brain Tumors

Intrinsic Tumors. Intrinsic primary brain tumors in children most frequently are found below the tentorium. The four most common are medulloblastoma, cerebellar astrocytoma, ependymoma, and brain stem glioma. All of these originate from glia except for medulloblastomas, which derive from neurons. The most malignant tumors arising above the tentorium are the primitive neuroectodermal tumors. These may be the supratentorial equivalent of cerebellar medulloblastomas. Other intrinsic supratentorial tumors include cystic or solid astrocytomas and ependymomas. Less common are pineal and choroidal tumors.

Diagnosis of Intrinsic Tumors. Evaluation of a child with intrinsic brain tumor is often limited. Since very young children are not likely to complain of headache, failing vision, clumsiness, or weakness, the physician must rely upon reports of family members and upon the physical examination. In contrast to brain tumors in adults, most brain tumors in children are infratentorial and evidence posterior fossa involvement (signs of hydrocephalus and cerebellar dysfunction). Focal neurological deficit is often absent (Figs. 8.13, 8.14**B**, 8.14**C**). The ability to recognize increased intracranial pressure is vital to diagnosis. An exception is the patient with a brain stem glioma, presenting with an eye turning inward (unilateral esotropia) and an ipsilateral facial weakness (Fig. 8.14**A**).

If a tumor is suspected, a CT or MRI scan is done. As in adults, the scan can provide helpful clues as to tumor type and degree of malignancy. However, with the exception of a brain stem glioma (revealed by marked enlargement of the pons on MRI scan) or an optic glioma (revealed by unilateral enlargement of the optic nerve or enlargement of the chiasm), a tissue sample is necessary to confirm the diagnosis.

Medulloblastomas account for about 30% of posterior fossa tumors. They arise from granule cells in the cerebellar vermis and are, like retinoblastoma and pinealoblastoma, truly neuronal tumors. They are composed of small cells with scant cytoplasm and hyperchromatic nuclei. Primitive glial elements may also be present. There is a 3:1 male preponderance, and peak incidence is at age 3–4 years. Growth down into the fourth ventricle or obstruction of the aqueduct produces the hydrocephalus that makes the patient ill. These malignant tumors tend to recur locally after removal and often disseminate throughout CSF pathways. Treatment consists of tumor removal and chemotherapy. Ten-year survival rates of 43% have been reported.

Cerebellar astrocytomas account for about 30% of posterior fossa tumors (Figs. 8.13, 8.14**C**). They arise from astrocytes and may be cystic with a mural nodule, solid with many microcysts or, rarely, solid with malignant features such as mitosis, pleomorphism, or necrosis. The peak age of incidence is 4–9 years. As with medulloblastoma and ependymoma, cerebellar symptoms tend to be mild and it is usually obstruction of the fourth ventricle with hydrocephalus that prompts the parent to seek medical attention. If the tumor is cystic with a mural nodule, only the mural nodule need be removed. Solid tumors should be completely removed if possible. Surgery results in permanent cure of almost all cystic and most solid benign cerebellar astrocytomas and should be expected unless the tumor also involves the brain stem. Radiation therapy is not indicated except in those rare instances of malignant histology or subtotal excision.

Ependymomas account for about 10% of posterior fossa tumors in children (Fig. 8.14**B**). They arise from the ependyma in the floor of the fourth ventricle, which they come to occupy and obstruct, producing noncommunicating hydrocephalus. The peak age of incidence is 3–5 years. The histology is deceptively benign and does not differ from that of the supratentorial ependymomas found in adults. During surgery a small amount of tumor usually has to be left at the point of tumor origin, because attempted removal causes dangerous changes in vital signs. As in adults, the 5-year survival rate is about 35%. Ependymomas can also arise in the cerebral hemispheres but are associated with the ventricular system only in about 50% of cases. The

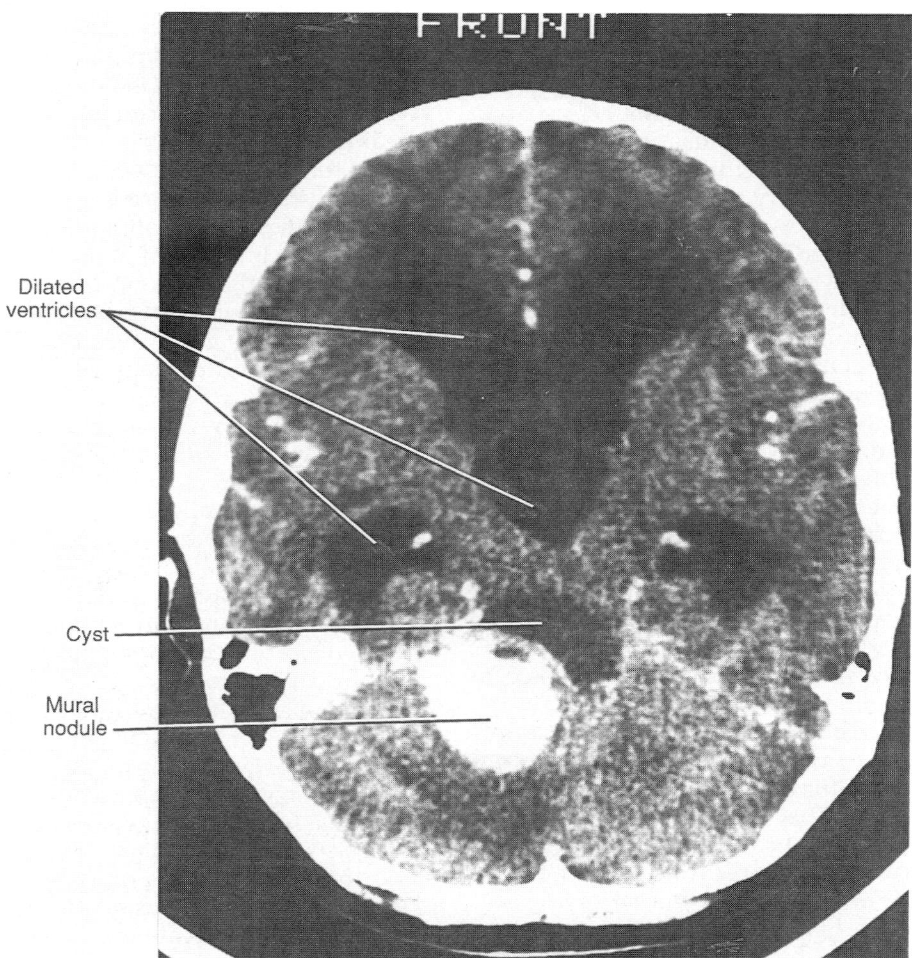

Figure 8.13. Cerebellar astrocytoma (enhanced CT scan).

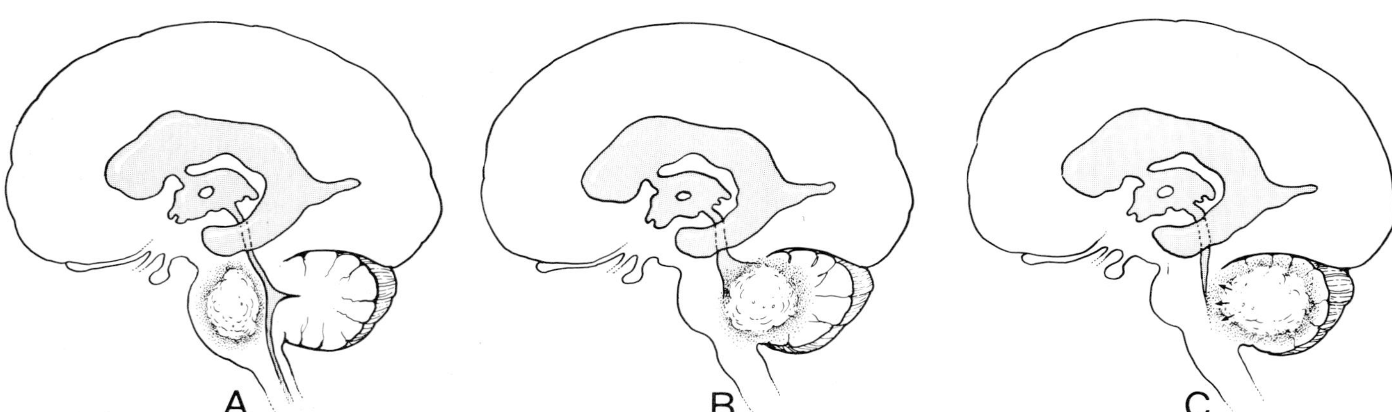

Figure 8.14. **A**, Brain stem tumor infiltrating up and down, displacing but not occluding fourth ventricle (cranial nerve and long tract signs). **B**, Fourth ventricular tumor displacing cerebellum and obliterating fourth ventricle (hydrocephalus and cerebellar signs). **C**, Cerebellar tumor compressing and displacing the cerebellum so as to obliterate the fourth ventricle (hydrocephalus and cerebellar signs).

long-term outlook for this subset of ependymomas is poor.

Brain stem gliomas, accounting for about 20% of posterior fossa brain tumors, arise from astrocytes in the pons (Fig. 8.14**A**). The peak age of incidence is 7–8 years. Because these tumors usually infiltrate the brain stem, their location generally makes surgery unwise. Early symptoms often include diplopia due to unilateral sixth nerve paresis and frequently an accompanying ipsilateral facial weakness. Examination may disclose contralateral hemiparesis or Babinski's sign. Life expectancy is about 18 months.

Primitive neuroectodermal tumors, most frequently found above the tentorium in the cerebrum, arise from glial and neuronal precursors. These tumors grow rapidly, treatment is palliative, and only short-term survival is expected.

Cerebral astrocytomas in children may be cystic or solid. The pathologic findings are the same as in adults. Like the cerebellar astrocytomas of childhood, these tumors are usually indolent. The patient can expect a long life after gross total resection. When these tumors occur in certain locations they are not resectable: hypothalamic astrocytomas, while histologically benign, cannot be removed safely. Astrocytomas may produce failure to thrive and cachexia (Russell's syndrome) or precocious puberty. Optic gliomas can originate either in the optic nerve or chiasm. They grow slowly and, if limited to the optic nerve, can be resected (albeit with unilateral visual loss). Gliomas of the optic chiasm have a more dismal outlook because their resection would cause blindness and damage the hypothalamus. Optic and often other low-grade astrocytomas occur with increased frequency in patients with neurofibromatosis.

Treatment of Intrinsic Tumors. Surgery provides tissue for histologic examination and a means to remove the tumor. CT-guided stereotaxic biopsy provides a convenient method for diagnosis. If the tumor is benign and resection feasible, it should be removed. If the tumor is malignant, it usually also should be removed as completely as possible within the limits imposed by the structures involved. Among posterior fossa tumors, complete surgical removal of benign cerebellar astrocytomas is curative but removal of medulloblastomas and ependymomas is not. In the case of cerebellar and fourth ventricular tumors, shunting for hydrocephalus is often necessary as well. Resection without CT-guided stereotaxic biopsy is used for most cerebellar tumors. Stereotaxic biopsy is sometimes chosen when evaluating patients believed to harbor a brain stem glioma. However, surgical resection of brain stem lesions is attempted only rarely, and then usually only for cystic or exophytic lesions.

Radiation and chemotherapy may help to extend useful survival when surgery is not curative. Unfortunately, the prognosis for children with primitive neuroectodermal tumors treated with radiation is the same as that of adults with glioblastoma. Patients with ependymoma are treated with radiation to the tumor bed and to the entire neuraxis if the tumor borders the ventricles. The prognosis is poor, with only a few patients breaking Collins' law (surviving their age in years once again plus 9 months). Medulloblastoma has also been treated postoperatively with radiotherapy, including supplementary radiation of the entire neuraxis. Such therapy, however, usually is not curative and has severe side effects (especially in very young children), including mental retardation, loss of pituitary function including growth hormone secretion, and direct suppression of growth from spinal (vertebral) irradiation. These adverse sequelae have led to a new interest in chemotherapy. Radiation alone is the primary treatment of brain stem, chiasmatic, and hypothalamic gliomas, but the outlook is poor.

Extrinsic Tumors. Extrinsic brain tumors in children most frequently arise in the suprasellar region from congenital rests and lie in the midline. They include craniopharyngiomas, epidermoids, dermoids, and teratomas, of which craniopharyngiomas are by far the most common.

Craniopharyngiomas arise in the sellar and suprasellar regions of the pituitary (pars distalis and pars tuberalis) from ectodermal rests. Their histology frequently resembles that of the primitive tooth bud or skin. Like other epithelial structures, these tumors desquamate and secrete a sebaceous substance that can collect in cysts. While rare, release of this material into the subarachnoid space can cause a sterile meningitis. They grow either as a firm, solid mass containing calcium that adheres to the hypothalamus, or as a cystic lesion with gossamer membranes that insinuate themselves into recesses between major vessels and cranial nerves. Although benign, they are difficult to remove completely. The natural history of the condition is unpredictable, making treatment decisions difficult.

Evaluation of a child with a craniopharyngioma often suggests an endocrinologic problem rather than a brain tumor. Stunted growth frequently brings the child to medical attention, and in an older child delayed pubescence is apparent. Diabetes insipidus may occur and, less commonly, visual complaints. Diagnosis is remarkably easy if this tumor is considered. Physical examination confirms short stature and delayed pubescence. A visual examination may reveal decreased visual activity, optic atrophy, or a bitemporal hemianopia, confirming the central nervous system (CNS) origin of what appears to be an endocrinologic problem. Radiographic bone age is delayed. Growth hormone levels are depressed as are gonadotropins if the patient is of pubertal age. Plain skull x-rays demonstrate suprasellar calcification in 90% of pediatric cases. CT or MRI scan better defines the cystic and solid components of the lesion and demonstrates calcium in the tumor.

Surgery is the primary treatment, if feasible. About 40% of tumors lie at least partially within the sella and can be removed through the transsphenoidal route. Other cases are approached by a craniotomy. Resection is frequently limited by involvement with the carotid arteries, hypothalamus, and optic apparatus. Radiation therapy is employed to treat patients with residual or recurrent disease. For cystic recurrence, stereotaxic implantation of a radiation source can be helpful.

Brain Abscess

Etiology. Pyogenic brain abscesses evolve over about a 2-week period. At first a localized cerebritis occurs with the inoculation of bacteria into the brain. As polymorphs and lymphocytes invade, necrosis progresses centrifugally. Initially, the process is not walled off and cerebral edema is maximal. About 10 days later, a reticulin matrix develops and walls off the central zone of necrosis (pus) and inflammation. Two weeks or more after inoculation a mature collagen wall forms about the pus. Such intracranial abscesses are found most frequently in the cerebrum but can also be cerebellar. Less common are extrinsic abscesses (subdural or epidural empyema). Fungal and tuberculous abscesses evolve more slowly than pyogenic ones and may contain either pus or granulation tissue.

The source of infection is identifiable in about 80% of cases. Previous surgery and penetrating head trauma account for about 10%, while 20% represent extensions from adjacent localized cranial infections such as sinusitis, mastoiditis, or dental infection. Another 20% have a cardiac source such as valvular or congenital heart disease. A right-to-left shunt in congenital heart disease (or a pulmonary AVM) is a frequent predisposing cause since the filter of the lungs is bypassed. Hematogenous spread from infected loci elsewhere in the body account for 30%. Another group, 5% but rapidly increasing in size, is immunocompromised because of organ transplants or acquired immunodeficiency syndrome (AIDS).

The agent of infection depends upon the source, and multiple organisms are common. Abscesses that arise after surgery or penetrating trauma most frequently are due to *Staphylococcus aureus*, *Staphylococcus epidermidis*, or *Streptococcus*, although an increasing number of Gram-negative infections are being seen. Brain abscesses arising from distant hematogenous sources or from paranasal sinus, mastoid, or inner ear infections are caused most commonly by anaerobic *Streptococci*, although *Bacteroides* or other species often are present as well. *Toxoplasma* and to a lesser extent *Aspergillus* and *Candida* are the most frequent causative agents in immunocompromised patients, including AIDS cases (although lymphoma must be considered).

Symptoms and Signs. The classic symptoms of brain abscess are headache, fever, and focal neurological deficits, but this triad is found in less than 50% of those affected. Headache is the most common symptom (70–90%) and may be accompanied by nausea and vomiting. Fever occurs in less than 50% of patients and is usually low grade. There is usually little or no elevation of the sedimentation rate or peripheral white blood cell count. Increased intracranial pressure produces obtundation or confusion, and focal neurological deficits depend upon the location of the abscess. Seizures occur in about 30% of patients. Symptoms are those of a brain tumor, but evolve more rapidly, with 75% of patients having symptoms for less than 2 weeks. Intraparenchymal abscesses tend to extend toward the ventricles. Intraventricular rupture as well as increased ICP and local brain destruction are the major causes of disability and death.

Evaluation. Evaluation of the patient presenting with a headache and neurological change must begin with the realization that the suspected mass lesion could be a brain abscess or a tumor. A history or findings of sinus, middle ear, lung, or other infections, recent head trauma, or cranial surgery should be sought. Inquiry and examination should include the possibility of rheumatic and especially congenital heart disease, prior cardiac surgery, hemoptysis, immune compromise, or drug abuse. The presence of one or more of these factors favors the suspicion of a brain abscess rather than brain tumor. The presence of a fever should alert the examiner to the possibility of a brain abscess, but its absence should never lead one to dismiss the diagnosis.

CT scanning has helped decrease the mortality rate from 30–40% to about 5–10%. CT scanning permits rapid diagnosis, localization, and identification of multiple abscesses. A uniform, thin, enhancing wall surrounding a low density core (Fig. 8.9**D**) suggests but does not prove the diagnosis. MRI scanning promises to be equally as effective. Lumbar puncture plays no role in diagnosis or management because the puncture lowers the pressure beneath a mass lesion and encourages transtentorial herniation. Furthermore, the spinal fluid usually is sterile with few or no white blood cells.

Treatment. Surgery is performed to remove pus, determine the organism involved, reduce mass effect, and speed sterilization of the abscess. If there is only cerebritis, surgery is not indicated. Once an abscess forms, it may be aspirated or surgically excised if it is readily accessible and not in a vital or eloquent region. Real time ultrasound helps localize the lesion at surgery. Care is taken not to enter the abscess and thus soil the surrounding brain. CT-guided stereotaxic aspiration is the treatment of choice if the abscess is not readily accessible, is small, lies in an eloquent or vital region, is associated with congenital heart disease, or if there are multiple lesions. This procedure, done under local anesthesia, evacuates the pus and provides material for culture to establish a bacteriologic diagnosis. Aspiration can be repeated to remove reaccumulated pus or to ascertain whether antibiotic treatment has sterilized the abscess.

Antibiotic therapy is begun after material has been obtained for culture. Preliminary choice of antibiotics is based upon judgment of which organisms are involved, and coverage is modified as culture results become available. The abscess is much more likely to be sterilized if the offending organism is identified and pus evacuated. Antibiotic therapy is continued for about 6–8 weeks following aspiration, or until the abscess has almost disappeared on CT (or MRI) scan. Corticosteroid therapy reduces the mass effect of cerebral edema surrounding an abscess. However, it also decreases the phagocytic effectiveness of leukocytes and the capacity of fibroblasts to wall off the infection. Consequently steroids usually are reserved for cases with significant mass effect and edema.

Intraspinal Disease

Anatomy

The spinal cord lies within a canal formed by the bones of the spinal column (Fig. 8.15**A**, **B**). The spinal cord and spinal column are organized into repetitive segments that are longitudinally stacked. Each cord segment receives sensory input from paired left and right dorsal roots and sends its output through a pair of ventral roots. On each side of the spinal cord the dorsal and ventral roots of each level join to form a segmental nerve within the neural foramina of the spinal column.

Each cord segment is bilaterally symmetrical and innervates a specific body segment (dermatome, sclerotome, and myotome) through its paired segmental nerves. Each segment relays the sensory information it receives from its dorsal nerve roots up to the brain through ascending reticular and lemniscal systems. Correspondingly, the segmental motor output through the ventral roots is brought under voluntary control by descending suprasegmental systems to the motor neurons of each cord segment. Section of the spinal cord (transverse myelopathy) thus leaves the patient insentient and paralyzed below the level of the lesion. Movement can occur in the paralyzed limbs, but it is reflex, not voluntary movement.

Spinal cord lesions at any level tend to produce sensory and motor loss over large areas of the body below the lesioned level. In contrast, the effects of nerve root lesions at one level are restricted to a single dermatome and myotome. However, should many nerve roots be affected (e.g., lumbar canal lesions affecting the cauda equina or polyneuropathies), the extent of neurological dysfunction will mimic that of spinal cord damage. The two can still be distinguished because spinal cord dysfunction (unless acute) usually will produce hyperreflexia, spasticity, and confluent sensory loss below the level of the lesion, while nerve and nerve root lesions result in hyporeflexia, hypotonia, atrophy, and often nonconfluent areas of sensory loss. Furthermore, while nerve root lesions often cause pain, spinal cord lesions rarely do. However, any spinal column lesion can cause local pain or tenderness in and about the spine.

The cross-sectional anatomy of the spinal cord explains the effects of unilateral cord lesions (Fig. 8.15**A**). Position and vibration sense pass upward to the brain by way of the ipsilateral dorsal columns, whereas pain and temperature sensation are relayed contralaterally in the anterolateral spinothalamic tracts. Touch sensation is transmitted bilaterally. Voluntary movement requires that messages from the brain travel down the lateral corticospinal tract of the cord ipsilateral to the motor neurons and muscles involved. Thus, hemisection of the cord (Brown-Sequard syndrome) causes loss of pain perception on the body side opposite the lesion but loss of position and vibration sense as well as paralysis and hyperreflexia on the same side as the lesion.

Lesions in the center of the spinal cord (intramedullary tumors, syringomyelia) cause a loss of pain and temperature sensation at the level of the lesion. An island of hypalgesia lies suspended between regions of normal sensation. This loss, due to destruction of second order fibers that cross from the root entry zone to the contralateral anterior spinothalamic tract, is typical of the central cord syndrome. Sphincter dysfunction, spastic weakness, and dorsal column deficits below the level of the lesion occur as the lesion expands.

An acute anterior cord syndrome arises from central disc herniation or posterior dislocation of a vertebral body directing pressure against the anterior two-thirds of the spinal cord. Sparing of column function is the hallmark of this syndrome. All function below the level of the lesion is lost, except light touch, proprioception, and vibratory sense.

The spinal cord extends from the foramen magnum to the lowest lumbar level in the newborn. As the child ages, the greater growth rate of the spinal canal results in the relative ascent of the spinal cord within the canal. By adulthood the tip of the cord reaches only as far as the top of the L1-2 vertebra. If the cord is tethered at its distal end during development, it will be stretched as the child grows and neurological deficit can result.

Below the level of the conus, in the mid and lower lumbar as well as the sacral spinal canal, there are only nerve roots. These supply lower extremity, sphincter, and sexual function. Because lesions at these levels affect only nerve roots, their prognosis is better than that of lesions in the cervical or thoracic canal which affect the spinal cord, a structure easily damaged irreversibly. It is thus important to diagnose and treat higher level lesions before they have produced marked symptoms.

The longitudinal organization of the spinal cord also has clinical implications. Lesions at any given level are capable of producing functional loss at all levels below the lesion (see Table 8.3). Consequently, one can best think of the possible effects of a spinal lesion in terms of the functions controlled by successively higher levels of the cord beginning at the conus and progressing up to the level of the lesion.

Loss of sphincter function predisposes to urinary tract infection and necessitates bladder catheterization. Lesions also affecting the lower extremities can produce both anesthesia and immobility. Consequently, such lesions or those higher up predispose the patient to decubitus ulcers, necessitating frequent positional changes or special bedding. Lesions at or above the midthoracic level interrupt half or more of the sympathetic outflow and frequently produce hypotension. Such hypotension, usually resolving over several days, is treated with a peripheral vasoconstrictor rather than fluid loads. Higher lesions disrupt respiratory motion of the chest wall to a degree that may predispose to pneumonia. Lesions at C5 to T1 can disrupt upper extremity function. Those at or above C3 to C5 result in varying degrees of diaphragmatic paralysis as well. Since complete lesions at these levels also eliminate control of

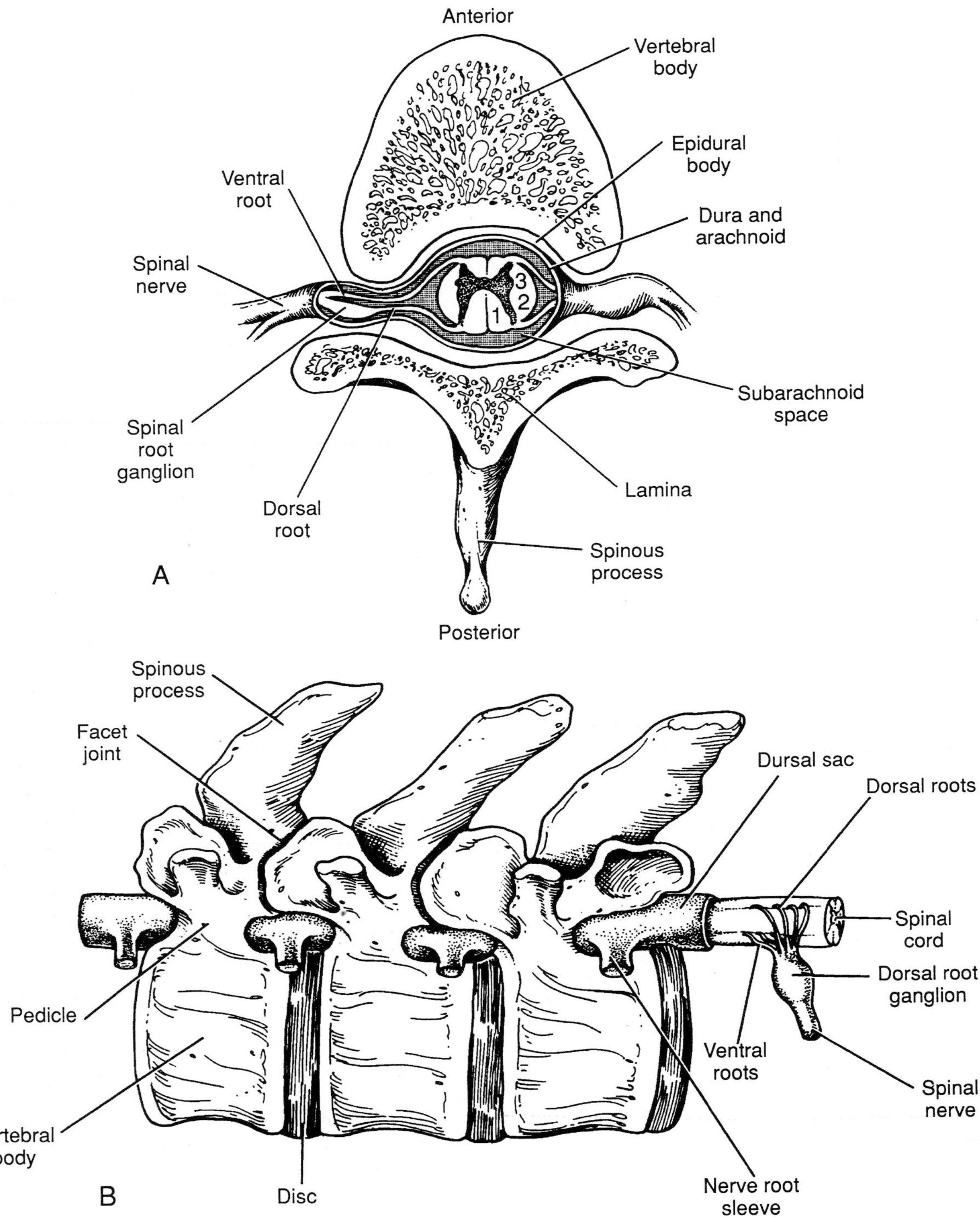

Figure 8.15. **A,** Spinal cross-section. 1 = Posterior column (position and vibration sense); 2 = Posterolateral column (motor); 3 = Anterolateral column (pain and temperature). **B,** Lateral view of vertebral column and its contents.

chest wall musculature, respiration is compromised severely if not completely, requiring intubation with ventilatory assistance.

The spinal canal (Fig. 8.15**A**, **B**) is defined by the vertebral bodies and their intervening intervertebral discs anteriorly, by the paired pedicles and facets laterally, and by the paired lamina and their junction at the base of the spinous process posteriorly. The posterior longitudinal ligament lines the anterior portion of the canal, while the laminae and their intervening ligamenta flava form the posterior aspect. Lesions in the canal can affect the spinal cord or its nerve roots. The neural foramina lie lateral to the canal and provide the conduit through which pass the segmental roots and nerves (Fig. 8.15**B**).

Table 8.3.
Signs of Disc Herniation

Level	Root	Weakness	Reflex Loss	Numbness
C4-5	C5	Deltoid	—	Over deltoid
C5-6	C6	Biceps	Biceps jerk	Thumb/index
C6-7	C7	Triceps	Triceps jerk	Index/middle
L3-4	L4	Quadriceps	Knee jerk	Pretibial
L4-5	L5	Ant. tibialis extensor hallicus	Hamstrings	Medial foot/toes
L5-S1	S1	Gastrocnemius	Ankle jerk	Lateral foot/toes

The foramina are formed by the pedicles of the vertebra above and below; posteriorly by the joint formed by the superior and inferior facets at the lateral portion of the disc and adjacent vertebral bodies. Lesions extending into the foramina damage nerve roots.

Evaluation

All spinal disease of potential surgical significance should be viewed as a combination of two problems: neurological affliction (spinal cord and nerve root) and mechanical stability (vertebrae, discs, joints, and ligaments). The importance of the latter largely is due to its potential for producing the former, although instability may be a cause of pain or other disability as well.

Examination of the spinal column includes palpation for deformity, tenderness, and spasm, as well as tests of mobility. The latter should not be performed unless one is certain there is no spinal instability. Tests of mobility include flexion, extension, rotation, and tilting of the neck and back. The neurological examination permits evaluation of nerve root and spinal cord function.

Radiographs of the spine provide information regarding vertebral anomalies, displacement, destruction or remodeling, and disc space narrowing. If no change is obvious but the patient has significant symptoms or findings, or if there are changes that seem to merit further investigation, CT or MRI scans are performed. An alternative study is myelography with or without subsequent CT scan. Myelography requires lumbar puncture and risks increasing a neurological deficit if there is significant spinal canal compromise because of tumor or abscess. In such instances no CSF should be removed, and the amount of contrast injected should be small. MRI, including an enhanced study, is preferable in such cases.

Spinal Trauma

Unfortunately, spinal trauma often produces spinal cord injury with resulting paralysis. People in their teens, 20s, and 30s are most commonly devastated. There have been strong calls for heightened awareness of preventive measures, including the use of seat restraints and air bags in cars, the observation of precautions before diving into the water (feet first the first time), and an increase in the protection of and instructions for athletes. When injury damages the spinal cord, recovery is usually very limited. Most medical efforts are directed toward prevention of further injury and care for its complications. Occasionally, treatment can promote the return of function.

Mechanically, the spinal column is composed of three columns. Disruption of two of the three columns causes spinal instability. The anterior column is made up of the anterior longitudinal ligament, the anterior one-half of the vertebral body, and the anterior half of the intervertebral disc. The middle column consists of the posterior half of the vertebral body, the posterior half of the intervertebral disc, the posterior longitudinal ligament, and the paired pedicles. The posterior column is composed of the paired facets and lamina, the spinous processes, and the interspinous and interlaminar ligaments.

Severe spinal cord injury follows a pattern of progression after the impact. Slowing of the cord circulation centrally at the level of impact with stasis and edema is followed by blood leaking through disrupted capillaries. Swelling and extravasation of vasoactive peptides and amines into the extracellular space produce vasoconstriction and ischemia. Central necrosis with hemorrhage ensues, spreading both outward from the center and rostrocaudally away from the injury site. Spinal column elements as well as the spinal cord are injured. Instability of the spinal column with displacement narrows the canal and compresses the spinal cord. Bone or intervertebral disc fragments may also compromise the cord.

Symptoms and Signs. Symptoms and signs after acute trauma differ from those described for chronic or slowly evolving lesions. In acute, complete spinal cord injury, there is flaccid hypotonic paralysis with loss of deep tendon reflexes, rectal tone, and all sensation below the level of the lesion, a condition called spinal shock. The reappearance of reflex activity and of simple reflex movements usually does not signal improvement. It means only that the segments of spinal cord below the level of the injury, now disconnected from the central nervous system above, are acting autonomously. The reappearance of reflexes during emergence from spinal shock does not imply that the patient will regain voluntary control of paralyzed limbs.

Evaluation. Spinal injury often results in permanent paralysis. Initial evaluation at the site of injury should include assessment of limb motion without moving the patient's head or body. A sturdy cervical collar should be applied and maintained in every patient in whom the possibility of significant neck injury

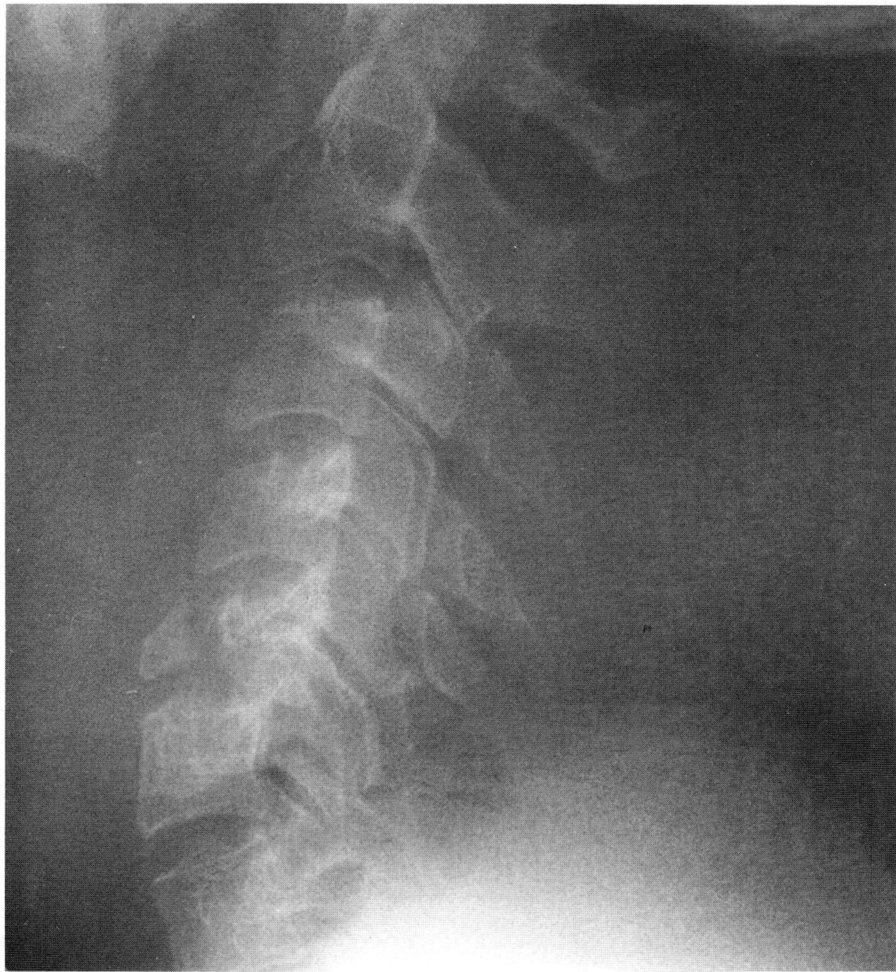

Figure 8.16. Fracture dislocation, C5 on C6.

cannot be excluded. Subsequent transfer should maintain the patient's spinal alignment from head to buttock. Upon arrival in the emergency room the patient should be evaluated for multiple trauma with the realization that at least one useful sign of focal injury, local pain and tenderness, will not be present in areas of sensory loss. Furthermore, cervical spinal cord lesions at or above the midthoracic level can produce loss of sympathetic tone. It may be difficult to distinguish the hypotension that accompanies spinal cord injury from that which occurs with blood loss. When hypotension is present, bradycardia, warm extremities, and normal capillary refill following pressure on the skin suggest that spinal cord injury rather than blood loss is responsible for the low blood pressure. Higher lesions at the mid and upper cervical levels also impair respiration and often require ventilatory assistance. Subsequent spinal evaluation includes neurological examination to localize the level and degree of the lesion. Palpation of the spine for deformity or tenderness is done without moving the patient. X-rays are then taken (Fig. 8.16). Depending upon features of the patient's other injuries and the facilities available, areas of the spine that are thought to be possible sites of trauma on the basis of clinical and x-ray examination should be studied further with CT or even MRI or x-ray tomography. While a myelogram may detect an acutely herniated disc, MRI—if available—will usually suffice to demonstrate any significant spinal cord compression.

Management. Initial therapy is directed at minimizing further effects of the injury by (*a*) assuring respiratory and cardiovascular support to avoid hypoxia and ischemia and (*b*) immobilizing the patient to protect the spinal cord from further injury. Intubation, if needed, must be accomplished without neck motion lest a cervical spine injury dislocate and produce additional cord damage. The cause of hypotension, if present, should be determined and sympathomimetic amines, fluids, or blood administered, depending on the cause of hypotension. In the case of cervical spinal cord injury, rapid reduction of spinal column displacement (and hence spinal cord compression) with external traction should be attempted. New evidence suggests that massive doses of steroids begun within 8 hours of injury may help alleviate at least a small but significant portion of spinal cord paralysis. An indwelling urinary catheter should be inserted during the patient's initial management.

When spinal dislocation produces significant narrowing of the spinal canal, the spinal cord is often compressed (Fig. 8.16). Usually, such compression produces complete paralysis at and below the level of dislocation from which the patient seldom recovers, regardless of treatment. Consequently, treatment of such cases focuses on early operative fixation and fusion rather than decompression. The aim is to promote rapid mobilization and rehabilitation.

On the other hand, patients with stationary partial neurological deficits and those with progressive deficits deserve urgent radiographic identification of the lesion and appropriate decompression. The situation is emergent if the deficit has progressed. When the offending pathology is anterior, an anterior decompression (vertebrectomy and/or discectomy) is indicated; when it is posterior, the spinal canal should be decompressed from the back (laminectomy). The operation usually includes some form of internal stabilization even if an external fixation device has already been applied. On occasion, spinal canal compromise can be corrected without operative decompression. In the cervical region, traction or external fixation with a halo vest may be sufficient to decompress the cord. However, if the efficacy of obtaining and maintaining decompression is uncertain, internal fixation and fusion are performed.

Management also should consider existing neurological sequelae and mechanical instability. If there is spinal paralysis, the bladder should be catheterized very soon after the patient's arrival to avoid overdistension and ensuing loss of bladder tone, which heightens the chance for infection. Spinal paralysis requires early and regular monitoring of the skin for signs of redness and incipient decubitus ulcers, as well as an immediate program for regular turning or placement upon a special bed. Within the first days, physical therapy, a bowel program, and intermittent catheterization are begun. In the long term excessive spasticity can develop, necessitating medication, spinal nerve root or peripheral motor nerve section or injection, spinal myelotomy, or other maneuvers. Autonomic hyperreflexia with hypertension in response to stimulation (e.g., bladder catheterization) below the level of a complete lesion with potential brain hemorrhage is another late complication.

Radiographic studies show areas of actual or potential instability. The type and location of bony and ligamentous damage determine the management of the instability. The neck is often stabilized with skull traction. Longer term stabilization is achieved with external braces, a skeletal fixation device (halo vest), and/or surgery with internal fixation and fusion. Potentially unstable fractures and dislocations of the thoracic and lumbar spine usually are treated surgically. The patient may then be placed in a brace or body cast. Bed rest and postural reduction are less-favored alternatives.

Spinal Disease

Included in degenerative diseases of the spine are disc herniation, spinal osteoarthritis and stenosis, and spondylolisthesis. Low back and neck strain present in a similar fashion. While some of these conditions—such as intervertebral disc disease and spinal osteoarthritis—are related to either acute or chronic trauma, they are discussed here because they often have a degenerative component and share many features of the other entities discussed. For similar reasons, rheumatoid disease of the spine is included.

Disc Disease. The intervertebral disc is composed of the nucleus pulposus and the surrounding annulus fibrosis. Degeneration of the disc occurs when the nucleus pulposus becomes desiccated with age or recurrent trauma. In contrast, herniation of a disc occurs when the nucleus pulposus is extruded through a tear in the annulus. Extrusion usually occurs posterolaterally and often results in compression of a nerve root. When it occurs centrally in the cervical or thoracic spinal canal, it can compress the spinal cord. Unlike disc herniation, disc degeneration is often asymptomatic. In disc herniation, symptoms may be local in the back or neck, radicular (from nerve root compression), or myelopathic (from spinal cord compression).

Most symptomatic disc herniations occur in the lumbar region, 95% of them at the L4-5 and L5-S1 levels. Cervical disc herniation is also common, especially at C5-6 and C6-7. Symptomatic thoracic discs are quite uncommon but may produce paraplegia. Disc herniation with extrusion beneath or through the posterior longitudinal ligament is likely to produce radicular pain and even neurological deficit (Fig. 8.17). Disc protrusion caused by bulging of the disc posteriorly beneath the posterior longitudinal ligament often does not cause symptoms. Excision of a bulging disc is not likely to provide pain relief. Furthermore, even with frank extrusion, radicular pain is more likely to be relieved than back or neck pain.

Symptoms of disc herniation are almost always pain, both in the spine and down one extremity. This pain is often exacerbated by straining, coughing, or sneezing and by motions of the affected portion of the spine. Herniated discs and other cervical spine problems produce neck pain and often refer pain to the scapular region as well as to the arm and hand. Lumbar disc herniations produce low back and leg pain, usually worse on weight bearing. Such leg pain is characteristically sciatic, radiating down the posterior or lateral leg into the calf or even to the foot. Signs of disc herniation include numbness and weakness in a radicular pattern and reflex loss (see Table 8.3).

Herniation of an L4-5 disc usually compresses the L5 nerve root, although it is the L4 nerve root that exits the spinal canal between the L4 and L5 vertebra. The roots of the cauda equina exit just above the corresponding disc, but it is the root exiting the foramen below that is at risk from the usual lateral lumbar disc herniation, explaining the apparent discrepancy.

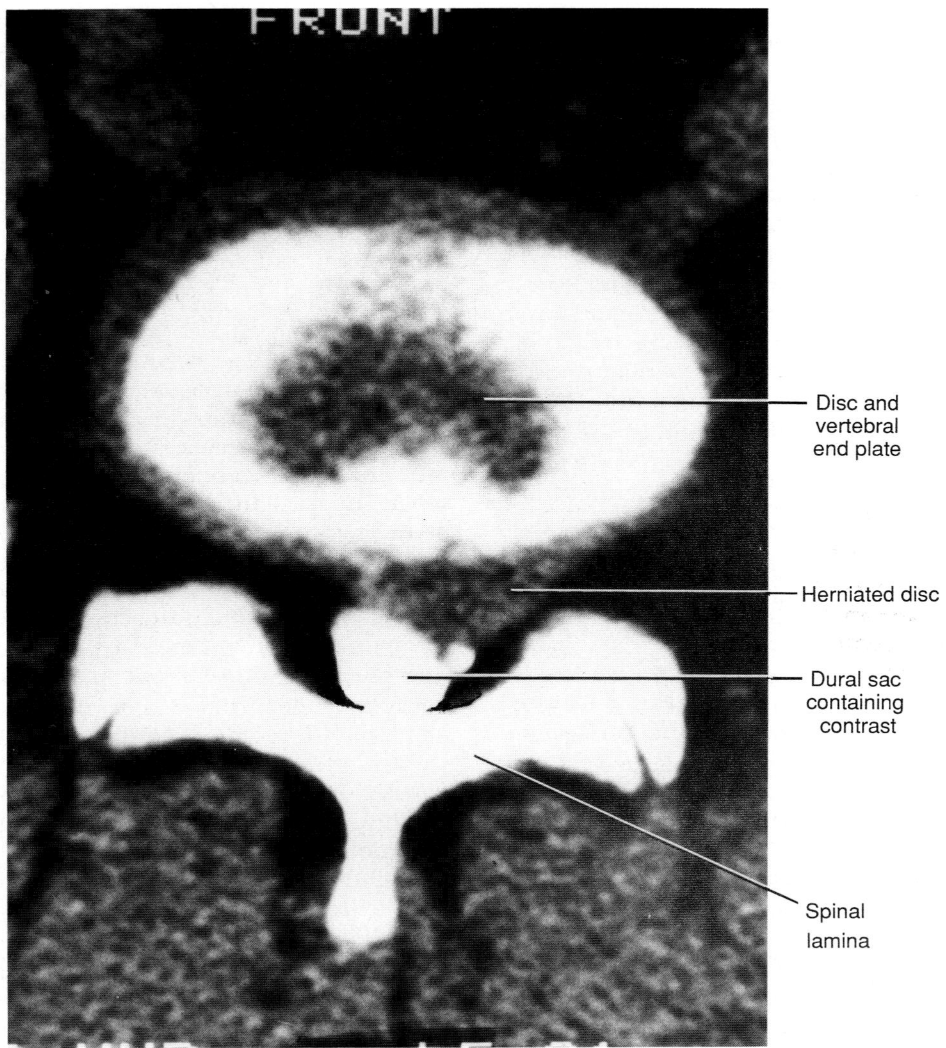

Figure 8.17. Herniated nucleus pulposus L5-S1 (positive contrast CT scan).

Differential diagnosis of cervical disc disease (neck or arm pain) includes angina if there is left arm pain, cervical osteoarthritis and stenosis, upper limb nerve entrapments, tumors or infections within or adjacent to the spine, as well as shoulder and elbow disease. Corresponding considerations in the lumbar region include vascular claudication, hernia, gynecological disease, abdominal aortic aneurysm, spinal and retropelvic tumors or infections, lumbar osteoarthritis and stenosis, lower limb nerve entrapments, and hip and knee disease.

Evaluation. Signs sought in evaluating complaints of neck, back, or radicular pain include point tenderness of the lumbar spine, paraspinal muscle spasm, and limited range of spinal motion. The straight-leg-raising sign should be tested; if the patient experiences pain, especially sciatic pain, as the examiner attempts to raise the affected leg straight up from the lying position, the patient is exhibiting a sign characteristic of lumbar disc herniation. A crossed straight-leg-raising sign, which is pain in the affected leg when the asymptomatic leg is raised, is pathognomonic. Gait should be observed. Neurological examination localizes the radicular compression.

Radiological diagnosis and surgical treatment are emergent if acute or subacute spinal cord compression causes paraparesis or sphincter dysfunction. Similar urgency attends those cases with sudden bilateral leg pain or numbness with associated weakness in both feet and disruption of bladder function caused by massive lumbar disc extrusion. In either instance, other diagnoses should be pursued vigorously if radiological studies fail to reveal a disc herniation. For apparently uncomplicated cases, a spine film usually is not revealing. With chronic spine disease, CT scans do not demonstrate many cervical disc herniations well. They often reveal lumbar disc herniations but occasionally fail to distinguish these from the dural sac and its contents. MRI scans and CT myelograms are more informative in both the lumbar and cervical regions. If there is reason to suspect a diagnosis other than a simple disc herniation,

MRI scans are probably the best initial means of obtaining a comprehensive evaluation of spinal pathology.

Treatment. Initial treatment of most patients is conservative and usually requires no diagnostic radiological studies unless there is reason to suggest another diagnosis. Treatment consists of rest for the symptomatic spinal segment, analgesics, anti-inflammatory agents, and possibly muscle relaxants. In the cervical region treatment includes a collar (to limit motion) and possibly traction. In the lumbar region treatment consists of at least 3–4 days of strict bed rest with very gradual increase of activity as tolerated. As improvement occurs, the patient may resume normal activities but should avoid excessive lifting or bending. If progress is slow, physical therapy may be added to the regimen. Only if there is no further progress over a period of weeks, if the condition worsens, or there is marked weakness should surgery be considered.

Surgical treatment of disc herniation consists of excision, using the microscope. While percutaneous techniques have been developed, their efficacy is debated. Standard techniques for lumbar or cervical discectomy include a posterior approach with limited removal of the adjacent lamina on the side of herniation, excision of the ligamentous flavum, gentle retraction of the nerve root, and removal of the underlying disc herniation. In the lumbar region disc material also is removed from the intervertebral space. For cervical disc herniation an anterior approach with or without spinal fusion is a common alternative. It is approached between the trachea and esophagus medially and at the carotid sheath laterally. The disc is excised through the anterior longitudinal ligament, back to and through the posterior longitudinal ligament with removal of the herniated fragment. Good results follow surgery in 95% of patients with radicular pain and clear-cut radiographic findings. Surgery is successful less often if these conditions are not met or if the patient has had a previous operation.

Spinal Osteoarthritis and Stenosis. Both congenital factors and degenerative changes can produce narrowing of the neural foramina laterally or the spinal canal centrally. Achondroplasia is the most common congenital cause of canal stenosis. In spinal stenosis the canal is narrowed by osteoarthritic vertebral end plates, disc protrusion, and hypertrophy of the facets and ligamentum flavum. The neural foramina can be narrowed by similar processes. In the cervical region both myelopathy and radiculopathy can occur, but in the lumbar region only radiculopathy is possible. Multiple vertebral levels are often involved and changes are frequently bilateral. Thoracic stenosis is rare.

Symptoms and Signs. Cervical spinal stenosis involving the foramina causes arm pain, numbness, and weakness. These symptoms are usually chronic, bilateral, and diffuse, reflecting nerve root compression at several spinal levels rather than at the single level usually seen in cervical disc herniation. However, the process may be sufficiently limited to affect only one nerve root severely and mimic a soft disc herniation. If osteoarthritis compromises the cervical spinal canal, myelopathy with lower extremity weakness, gait ataxia, and sphincter disturbance will result. As the same process encroaches upon the nerve roots in the neural foramina, associated changes in the upper extremities help direct attention to the cervical spine. Signs typical of severe cervical spondylosis include lower motor neuron weakness and radicular pain or numbness in the arms, and upper motor neuron weakness in the legs. Other conditions such as a cervical cord tumor must also be considered.

Lumbar stenosis may produce leg pain mimicking disc disease. However, leg pain, numbness, and weakness are usually more chronic, more often bilateral, and more widespread in stenosis than in disc herniation. Furthermore, in lumbar stenosis the straight leg raising test is usually normal (70% of cases). Patients frequently assume a somewhat anteflexed position when standing or walking; their pain worsens on bending backwards. These mechanical signs are caused by infolding of the ligamentum flavum, which further compromises the spinal canal in the neutral and especially the extended position. A few patients describe increase in pain or numbness of the legs after walking a fixed distance, with relief at rest. These symptoms resemble those of intermittent claudication of vascular origin. If these patients are found to have no evidence of lower extremity arterial compromise, neurogenic claudication should be suspected and they should be evaluated for lumbar spinal stenosis.

Evaluation and Treatment. Evaluation and treatment for spinal stenosis are similar to those for a herniated disc. Surgery for cervical spinal stenosis may be carried out from either the anterior or posterior approach, often requiring operation at multiple levels. Procedures for relieving foraminal stenosis are similar to those for disc disease. If spinal canal stenosis is present, however, a limited approach is often insufficient and laminectomy over multiple levels may be required. While this approach is satisfactory in the lumbar region, in the cervical region there a potential for late instability after extensive laminectomies. Consequently, many patients with cervical stenosis receive anterior operations. If the stenosis is not limited to the region of the discs and adjacent end plates, considerable portions of the vertebral bodies and discs must be removed. After a fusion is performed, the patient is maintained in an external fixation device or support.

Spondylolisthesis. Forward slippage of one vertebral body upon another, or spondylolisthesis, is found most commonly at the L4-5 or L5-S1 level. Bilateral defects (spondylolysis) across the spinal lamina diagonally just below the pedicle allow the most rostrolateral part of each lamina with the attached pedicle and vertebral body to separate and shift anteriorly, sometimes compromising the spinal canal. These shifts, most common in children and adolescents, tend to stabilize. Back pain and nerve root compression symptoms can present in this younger age group. Adults, especially older ones, can develop spondylolisthesis sometimes without spondylolysis. In such cases, ligamentous laxity accompanying osteoarthritic change permits slippage of adjacent vertebral bodies upon one another to produce stenosis of the spinal canal. CT and MRI scans are extremely helpful in evaluating the patient and planning surgery. Operative stabilization and fusion may be necessary and decompression should be performed if there is neurological deficit or radicular pain.

Rheumatoid, Traumatic, and Congenital Atlantoaxial Dislocations. Rheumatoid arthritis compromises the spine, usually in the cervical region, especially at the atlantoaxial (C1-2) level. Lesions at any cervical level may cause neural compression secondary to infiltration of vertebral bodies with collapse, to ligamentous and disc degeneration with angulation and dislocation, or to pannus (granulation tissue membrane) formation with mass effect. Such changes, especially ligamentous laxity at the C1-2 level, result in chronic anterior dislocation of C1 on C2, compressing the spinal cord between the odontoid and the posterior arch of C1. Myelopathy can result but tends to progress slowly or not at all. The resultant neurological deficits are difficult to distinguish from the more common neuropathies, motor degeneration, contractures, and arthritic deformities. Repeated evaluation, cervical collars, and surgical decompression, fixation, and fusion are all important treatment considerations.

Similar considerations govern congenital C1-2 dislocations, though symptoms tend to be more episodic. Surgical stabilization is commonly performed even if there is no neurological deficit. Traumatic C1-2 dislocations are associated with fractures of the odontoid. They are treated with external halo fixation devices when the dislocation is not marked and the fracture is down into the vertebral body rather than beyond it. Otherwise, surgical fusion is performed because external fixation alone often fails to produce bony fusion, leaving the spine unstable.

Spinal Infection

Infection of the spine may involve the vertebral body, disc, or epidural or subdural space.

Vertebral body involvement usually is due to tuberculosis, and the infection is chronic. It begins beneath the two vertebral end plates bordering a disc space and ultimately extends to involve both vertebral bodies. Collapse of the vertebral bodies leads to angulation of the spine and kyphotic deformity. Infection may spread to form an epidural abscess. Angulation, epidural abscess, and even disc prolapse can compromise the spinal cord and lead to paralysis. Associated paraspinal abscess is common and gives a telltale radiographic appearance. Pyogenic osteomyelitis presents and progresses similarly but usually evolves more rapidly and is associated with more spinal pain and tenderness.

Discitis is far more common than osteomyelitis of the spine. It usually occurs in a setting of diabetes, immunocompromise, intravenous drug abuse, or previous disc surgery. Infection is pyogenic (usually staphylococcal) in origin. There are complaints of back or neck pain and sometimes radicular pain as well. Local tenderness is often present. Spinal cord or cauda equina compromise is rare. Within several months, spinal x-rays show dissolution of the vertebral endplates bordering the disc space. Disc collapse and destruction follow. Ultimately, adjacent vertebral body collapse and angulation occur. MRI and even CT scans reveal changes earlier than do x-rays. As in all forms of spinal infection, the sedimentation rate is elevated and provides a measure of response to therapy. Fever and leukocytosis are uncommon since most cases are subacute or chronic and pursue an indolent course.

Treatment of discitis and osteomyelitis is with appropriate antibiotics and external immobilization. Advanced osteomyelitis requires operative debridement and bone grafting as well.

Epidural or subdural abscess may result from hematogenous spread or direct extension from an abscess of the vertebral body, disc, or paraspinal tissues. Such abscesses usually are pyogenic (most staphylococcal) and occur in the thorax. Acute abscesses present with neck or back pain, fever, and spinal tenderness. Progression is similar to that of epidural tumors, with subsequent onset of radicular pain followed by spinal cord paralysis. Chronic abscesses progress more slowly and usually fail to develop fever or leukocytosis. MRI scan is especially helpful in revealing the lesion. Treatment requires both appropriate antibiotics and surgical drainage.

Spinal Tumors

Spinal tumors are divided into three groups that differ somewhat in age of presentation and prognosis: (*a*) intramedullary tumors arise from the glial element of the spinal cord or trapped ectodermal elements; (*b*) intradural extramedullary tumors arise from the dural sheath about the spinal cord or the Schwann cell sheath about the spinal roots; (*c*) extradural tumors arise from the osseous element of the spinal column (Figs. 8.18, 8.19).

Types

Intramedullary Tumors. Lying within the substance of the spinal cord, intramedullary tumors are more frequent in children than adults. Some may be associated with a large cyst, causing them to be confused with a simple syrinx. Astrocytomas of the spinal cord are the most common intramedullary tumor of childhood (Fig. 8.19**A**). Their biological behavior resembles that of low-grade cerebral astrocytoma; malignant forms are rare. In some regions the tumors blend with the spinal cord, limiting the extent of surgical excision.

Ependymomas of the spinal cord are the most common intramedullary tumor of adults. They arise from the ependyma of the central canal. They usually are well demarcated, making gross total excision feasible.

Hemangioblastomas of the spinal cord comprise less than 10% of intramedullary tumors. Sometimes cystic, these tumors are fairly circumscribed and do not extend over many segments.

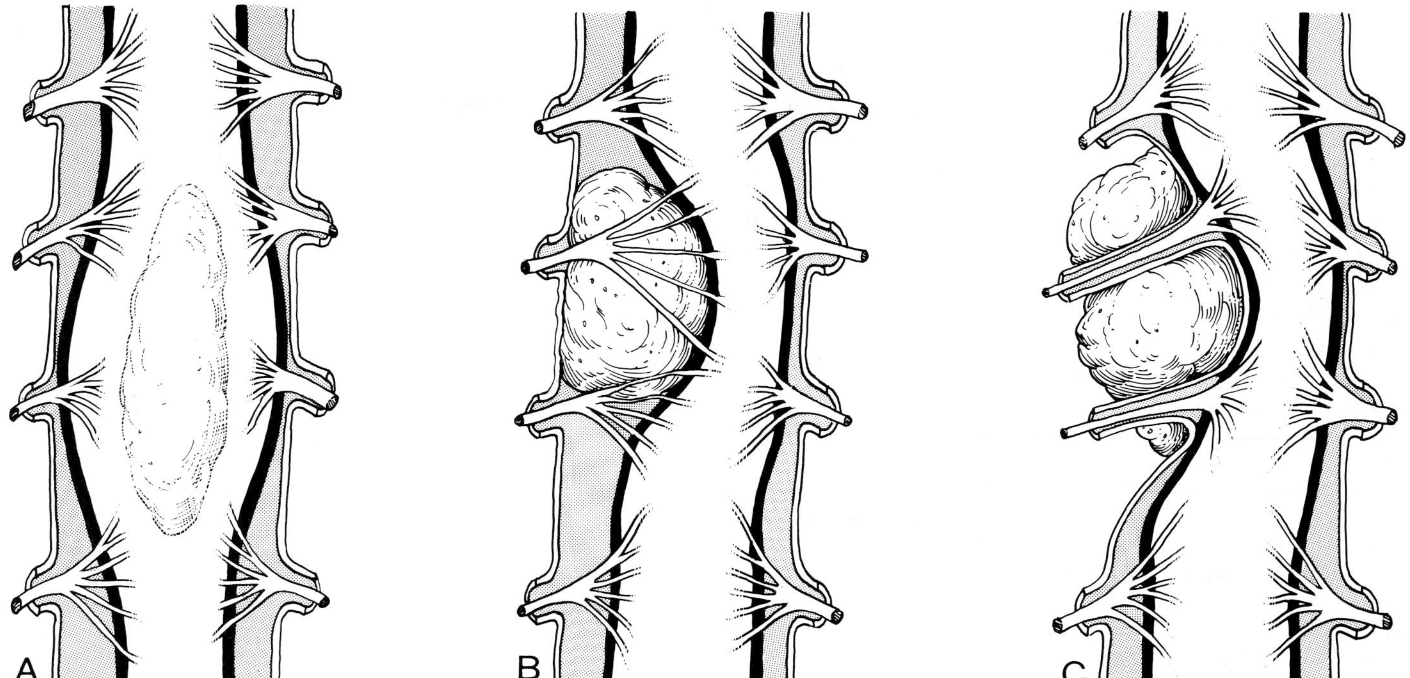

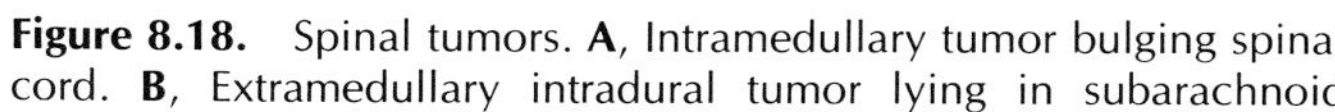
Figure 8.18. Spinal tumors. **A**, Intramedullary tumor bulging spinal cord. **B**, Extramedullary intradural tumor lying in subarachnoid space, displacing and compressing spinal cord. **C**, Extradural tumor lying in epidural space, displacing dural sac and spinal cord.

Dermoids, epidermoids, and lipomas can also be found within the spinal cord, most commonly at or below the conus. A dermoid frequently is associated with a dermal sinus tract in the skin overlying the spine, which leads to the intraspinal tumor. Likewise, a lipoma involving the conus or filum usually is in continuity with an overlying subcutaneous extension.

Intradural Extramedullary Tumors. Intradural extramedullary tumors lie within the dural tube but outside the confines of the spinal cord. In the cervical and thoracic spine they lie adjacent to the spinal cord and local nerve roots, which they often distort and compress to produce symptoms and signs of root or cord dysfunction. In the lumbar canal they lie among the roots of the cauda equina and produce polyradicular symptoms and signs. These tumors are well circumscribed and do not extend over many segments. Since they are usually benign, the history is often long.

Neurofibromas are the most frequent intradural extramedullary tumors. Each typically arises from a single dorsal root. Multiple tumors are found in neurofibromatosis patients. Neurofibromas can extend through an intervertebral foramen and grow out extradurally into the retropleural or retroperitoneal space. This dumbbell extension can become very large and may be the first portion of the tumor identified. For this reason, masses close to the spine should have additional radiological evaluation to determine whether they extend into the spinal canal.

Meningiomas are almost as common and are based on the dura. They occur four times as frequently in women as men.

Extradural Tumors. The most frequently encountered spinal tumors in adults are extradural and usually metastatic (Fig. 8.20). Metastases grow rapidly, usually presenting with symptoms of spinal cord compression of hours' to a week's duration. Most are carcinomas. Common primary lesions are located in the lung, breast, prostate, and kidneys. With the exception of lymphoma, these tumors usually destroy bone. They compress the spinal cord in one of two ways: (*a*) by growing in the epidural space or (*b*) by causing collapse of the involved vertebra, resulting in distortion, narrowing, and instability of the spinal column.

Symptoms and Signs. Symptoms of spinal tumors can be divided into four broad categories: local pain, radicular pain, weakness and numbness in the legs or arms, and sphincter disturbances. Local pain in the back or neck, frequently the first complaint, usually does not signal alarm unless the patient is known to have cancer. Spinal tenderness to percussion may be present. The onset of radiating pain, however, especially if in the chest or abdomen, should alert the physician to the seriousness of the underlying cause. Spinal (or radicular) pain at night suggests tumor rather than spinal arthritis or disc disease. Weakness or numbness of the extremities below the level of spinal or radicular pain suggests the presence of a neoplasm. Autonomic dysfunction with impotence and urinary or fecal incontinence indicates severe loss of function. Total paralysis and loss of sensory function below the lesion is rarely reversible.

Signs of neurologic dysfunction depend upon the site of the tumor along the spinal axis. If it is in the cer-

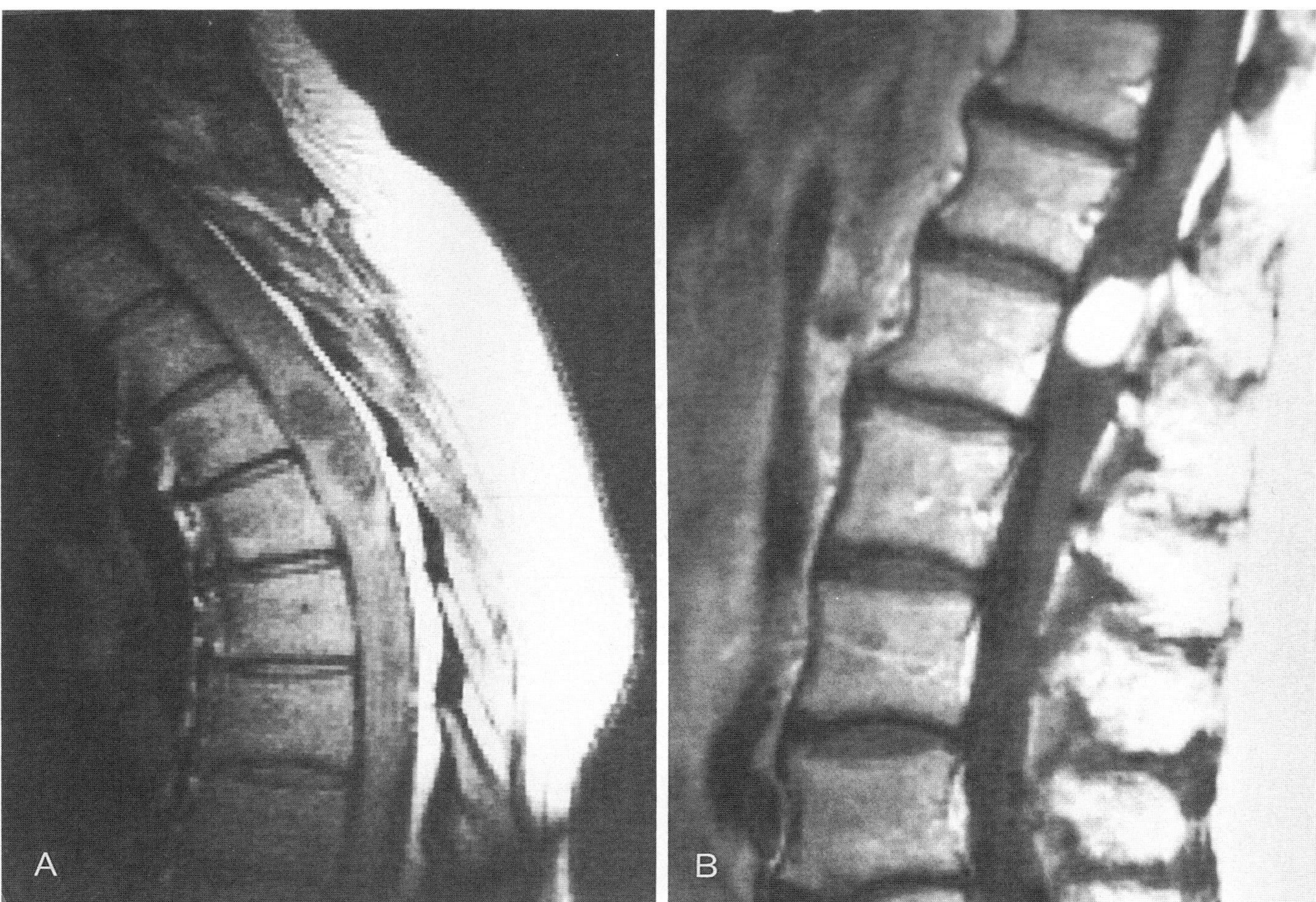

Figure 8.19. **A**, Spinal cord astrocytoma (intramedullary tumor—enhanced MRI scan). **B**, Spinal neurofibroma (extramedullary intradural tumor—enhanced MRI scan).

vical spine, the arms and legs will be affected. Tumors below T1 spare the arms. If the tumor is lumbar, only nerve root signs (segmental motor, sensory, and reflex loss) may be found. With cervical or thoracic lesions, the spinal cord is involved and hyper- rather than hyporeflexia is found. The pattern of neurological involvement also depends upon whether the tumor is extradural, intradural extramedullary, or intramedullary.

Tumors in Adults

Evaluation. In the adult, evaluation begins by suspecting the presence of a neoplasm and assessing the relative possibilities. Extradural tumors occur most often and hence most are metastatic. Progression is rapid with extradural tumors but intradural tumors are slow to affect the spinal cord.

Radiologic evaluation starts with plain spine films. Extradural (metastatic) tumors destroy bony elements. X-rays may show vertebral collapse that spares the disc spaces but not the cortical end plates. Often there is loss of one or more pedicles (Fig. 8.20**A**). Intradural extramedullary lesions may cause widening of a neural foramen (if a neurofibroma). Intramedullary lesions can enlarge the spinal canal with a resultant increase in the interpedicular distance. CT-myelography and especially MRI scanning increasingly are used to evaluate these patients. While avoiding the danger of lumbar puncture, MRI visualizes the lesions, their effects upon the spinal cord, and changes in the vertebra. Gadolinium enhancement of the MRI scan increases the definition of many spinal tumors. An MRI scan is the most useful early step when a patient presents with spinal cord symptoms and is especially urgent if there is a history of cancer.

Treatment. The goal in treating an adult with a spinal tumor is to relieve pain, maintain or restore ambulation, and, if possible, cure the patient. Steroids are helpful as a supplemental measure to other therapy, especially in cases with significant deficits. Extradural tumors are treated surgically for palliative decompression of the spinal cord. Metastatic cancer, myeloma, lymphoma, and chordoma are not cured by surgery. The location of the compression dictates the type of operation performed. If the compression is from the back of the spinal canal or in the lateral gutters, laminectomy with tumor removal from the extradural space should

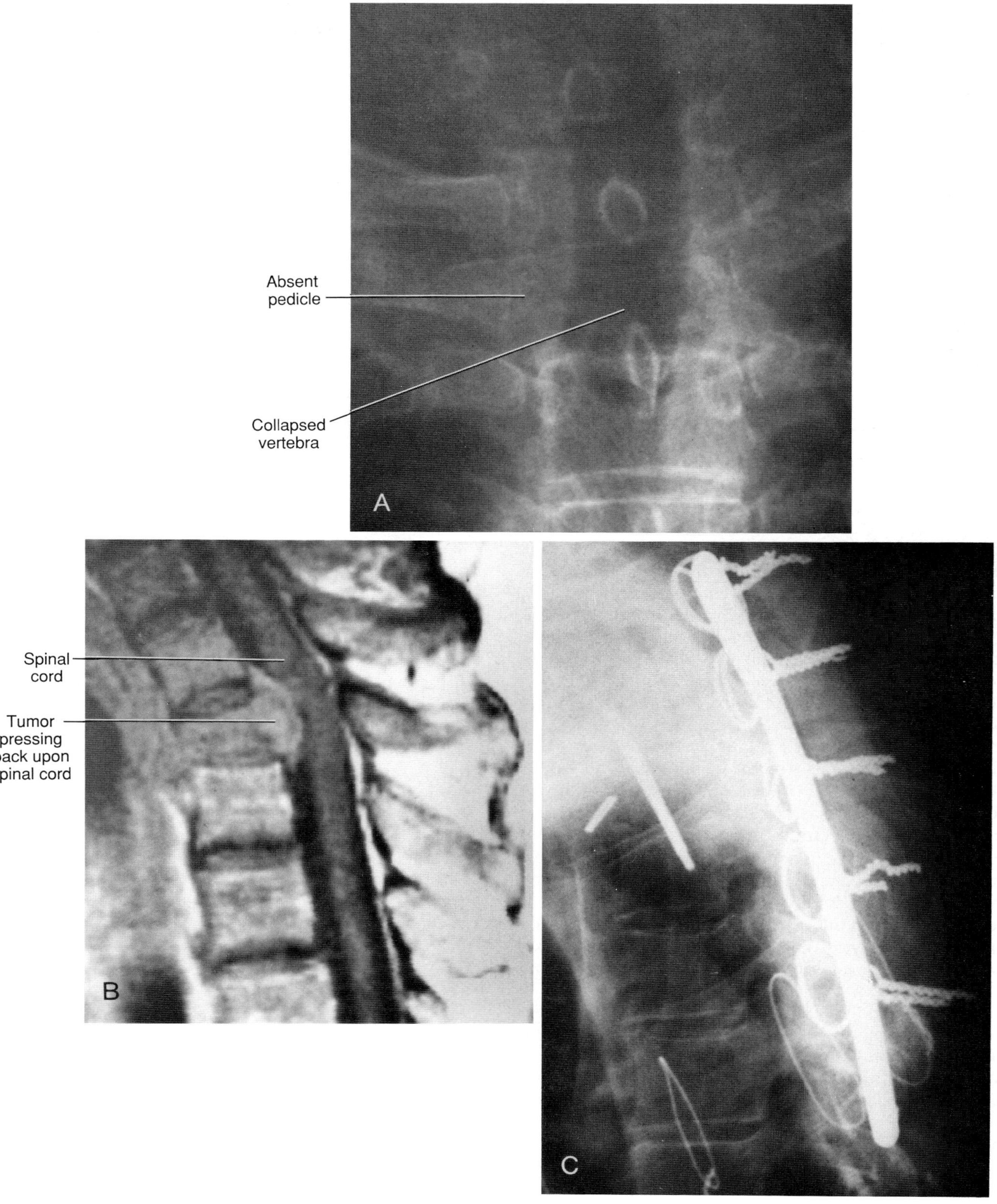

Figure 8.20. **A**, Metastatic tumor to spine. **B**, Metastatic spinal tumor (enhanced MRI scan). **C**, Metastatic spinal tumor (lateral spine film following anterior decompression and fusion with posterior stabilization and fusion).

suffice. Fusion is seldom necessary. If the compression is from the front due to vertebral collapse with angulation or as a result of tumor anterior to the cord, operation is more difficult. Although a lateral posterior (costotransversectomy) approach has been advocated, the approach used most frequently is anterior decompression and fusion (Fig. 8.20**C**). Tumor surgery is most effective for patients without complete loss of spinal cord function. The ability of the patient to walk out of the hospital is related most directly to whether the patient walked in. Average survival following surgery for metastatic disease is 6 months. Surgery is most useful if the tumor type is unknown or if the primary tumor has already been identified and is not especially radiosensitive.

Intradural extramedullary tumors can be cured because they usually can be removed completely. Various techniques facilitate removal: before the dura is opened the tumor is localized by means of real time ultrasound; the operating microscope and microsurgical techniques, including the laser and ultrasonic aspirator, are used to remove the tumor; neurological function can be monitored by repetitive testing of somatosensory evoked responses. Recurrence rates of only 6% after 15 years have been reported for meningioma, and similar or better results are expected for neurofibroma. Of patients, 80% improve and 50% become completely normal.

Intramedullary tumors are treated surgically in an attempt to remove the tumor and prevent further neurologic deterioration. Unlike intracranial ependymomas, ependymomas of the spinal cord often are removed completely. The lack of a clear cleavage plane between an astrocytoma and the spinal cord hinders attempts at complete removal; only about 50% of spinal astrocytomas can be removed relatively completely. Microsurgical technique has greatly facilitated resection. Although the majority of patients improve following surgery, recent reports suggest that spinal cord astrocytomas tend to recur with increasing disability and even death.

For spinal metastases that produce spinal cord compression, surgery plus radiation is the treatment of choice. Radiation alone is preferred if the tumor is known to be quite radiosensitive (such as a lymphoma). Radiation is also an important adjunct in the management of patients with chordoma. Radiation plays no role in the management of patients with the usual intradural extramedullary tumors. Its role in managing patients with incompletely removed intramedullary astrocytomas is uncertain, but it is probably helpful for residual ependymomas.

Tumors in Children

Evaluation. The distribution of spinal tumors in children differs from that in adults. Intramedullary tumors (sarcomas and neuroblastomas) are most often seen. Two complaints bring the child to medical attention: walking usually has deteriorated and enuresis is common. Neck or back pain may be present. The differential diagnosis is the same as for adults—astrocytoma, ependymoma, lipoma, and dermoid. Other lesions are uncommon.

Intramedullary tumors of the conus medullaris are especially frequent in children. These lipomas, dermoids, or ependymomas extend caudally out of the conus or from the filum terminale into an intradural extramedullary location among the nerve roots of the cauda equina. Examination of the back may reveal a superficial extension of the tumor in the form of a dermal sinus, hypertrichosis (tuft of hair), or a subcutaneous lipoma in or close to the midline of the low lumbar spinal region.

Radiologic evaluation and findings resemble those described for adult tumors. In addition, spina bifida occulta may be present. MRI scanning is the most valuable study.

Treatment. The rationale and treatment is similar to that for the corresponding adult tumors. Intraspinal lipomas are difficult to remove completely without damaging spinal cord function. However, cavitation of intramedullary and exophytic tumor with marked reduction of its bulk seems to provide adequate therapy. Intraspinal dermoids are also difficult to remove completely because often they have very thin capsules and tend to adhere to surrounding structures. Capsule remnants show little propensity to regrow.

Spinal Vascular Malformations

Spinal vascular malformations are uncommon but almost always are arteriovenous malformations or cavernous angiomas. The latter occur within the cord but AVMs can be on the cord or within it. This relationship to the cord defines the type and hazards of their surgical treatment. Similar to tumors, lesions within the cord are more difficult to excise, and operation risks spinal paralysis to a far greater degree than with extramedullary AVMs. In many of the latter, division of the feeding arteries entering along the nerve root is sufficient to stop circulation within the AVM and effect a cure. Vasular malformations of the cord often present with repeated attacks of spinal cord dysfunction or progressive spinal cord deficit. Less frequently, vascular malformations cause significant subarachnoid hemorrhage in the spine.

Peripheral Nerve Problems

Anatomy

Peripheral nerves are covered with an external connective tissue layer, the epineurium; within this sheath are multiple nerve fascicles, each covered by its own connective tissue layer, the perineurium. The fascicles branch, repeatedly interchanging axons with one another over the length of the nerve. Within the fascicles are motor axons from the spinal cord that end upon effectors (muscles, blood vessels, glands, and other organs) and sensory axons that conduct messages to the spinal cord from skin, joints, and other soft tissue receptors.

Each peripheral nerve is the simple extension of spinal nerve roots from a single segmental level (chest and abdomen) or the conjoined extension of roots from a number of adjacent levels (limbs). Limb nerves form as the ultimate extension of multiple recombinations of these nerve root contributions in the brachial and lumbosacral plexus. As a result of the simple segmental innervation of the trunk, myotomes and dermatomes are successively oriented in almost parallel fashion, with each receiving the overlapping contribution of several spinal roots centered on that region. Radicular and peripheral nerve distributions are similar. In the limbs this simple radicular arrangement is oriented about a median axis: the progress of the dermatomes (and of the myotomes to a much less recognizable extent) in sequential fashion down one aspect of each extremity to the large digit and up the other aspect from the smallest digit is reflected in their innervation by successive overlapping spinal roots. In contrast to nerve roots, the peripheral nerves innervating limbs are composed of less orderly contributions from a variety of spinal roots. Consequently, lesions of peripheral nerves innervating the limbs usually produce neurological deficits recognizably different from those due to spinal root disease. Thus, the median nerve carries sensation from the palmar aspect of the radial 3 1/2 fingers of the hand and adjacent palm; the corresponding dorsal aspects are largely the responsibility of the radial nerve; sensation from the ulnar 1 1/2 fingers is transmitted by the ulnar nerve. By contrast, the sensory innervations of the sixth, seventh, and eighth cervical roots center respectively upon all aspects of the thumb, long, and small fingers.

Nerve Injury

Trauma. Complete nerve transection leads to degeneration and loss of all axons beyond the point of transection. Reinnervation can occur by regeneration. Axonal sprouts from the proximal cut surface cross the gap and progress down the preserved Schwann cell sheaths of the transected axon. This outgrowth is provided by axoplasmic flow from the nerve cell bodies down the length of the regenerating axon. Axonal regrowth averages 1 mm per day. Since injury causes architectural disruption of the proximal and distal nerve stumps at the point of transection, many new axons find their growth blocked or travel down paths that lead them to inappropriate terminals (e.g., motor instead of sensory). The problem is minimized when the transected nerve stumps are cleanly severed and accurately approximated.

In crush or blunt nerve injury without transection, internal damage to the nerve can be sufficient to disrupt the axons and fascicular architecture even though the nerve remains in continuity. Some axons may cross the injury site and grow down the distal segment; others do not and pile up blindly because fibroblasts have invaded the injured area. This fibrous tissue scar can prevent functional recovery. When this occurs the neuroma must be resected and the resulting nerve ends sutured together to permit adequate regeneration.

With minor injuries, only axons may be disrupted. Axons distal to the injury site degenerate but Schwann cell sheaths and fascicular architecture are preserved. Consequently, regenerating axons will migrate down their original or adjacent channels and reinnervate the effectors and receptors they originally supplied. Regeneration is possible without surgical intervention, and the prognosis for satisfactory spontaneous recovery is excellent. In even milder cases, axons may remain intact but fail to function (neuropraxia). Such a conduction block may be a component of nerve entrapment syndromes or posttraumatic epineural scarring. Minor nerve injuries may have a component of axonal disruption as well.

Evaluation. The etiology of the trauma indicates whether the injured nerve is likely to be in continuity. Penetrating trauma with a clean sharp object is apt to cause transection and is amenable to repair. The outcome of injury caused by bullets and missiles is harder to predict. Missiles traveling close by nerves may produce damage without transection; such lesions in continuity may or may not recover satisfactorily. Closed injuries tend to produce neuromas in continuity. Stretch injuries of peripheral nerves can produce irreparably long segments of intraneural scar, while traction on nerve roots of the brachial plexus often results in irreparable root avulsion.

With nerve injury, Schwann cell damage and demyelination are common. If an axon is preserved but loses its myelin sheath, it becomes quite sensitive to mechanical stimuli. Tapping over the portion of the nerve containing unmyelinated axons produces an electrical sensation (Tinel's sign) experienced within the skin regions normally supplied by the nerve. With progressive regeneration, Tinel's sign can be elicited further down the course of the nerve.

The neurological evaluation localizes the site of the lesion. Electromyography and nerve conduction studies are of supplementary value. If either the neurological examination or the electrical studies shows evidence of preserved innervation, the injured nerve cannot have been totally transected. A conservative approach is to delay exploration of lesions that appear to be in continuity in order to determine whether there will be evidence of axonal regrowth distal to the site of injury (progressive Tinel's sign, electrical or clinical evidence of recovery of function). If clinical and electrical testing reveal no function distal to the lesion, the continuity of the nerve cannot be determined with certainty. Only direct visualization of the nerve can confirm continuity.

Lack of function beyond the point of injury presents a clinical dilemma. Sufficient time should be permitted to allow detection of axonal growth beyond the site of injury (14 days for regeneration plus several months to permit it to extend 5–6 cm beyond the site of damage). Exploration can be delayed if signs of regeneration can be expected within 3 months. However, if the injury is located far from the nearest site of potential reinnervation, early nerve exploration should be considered, since atrophy or contractures of denervated muscle and changes in denervated skin receptors occur over time.

Evaluation of brachial plexus stretch injuries should include MRI scan or myelography to determine if pseudomeningoceles indicative of root avulsion have formed in the cervical spinal column. Electromyography (EMG) and nerve conduction studies are helpful in following the course of the injury.

Neuromas forming at the site of a nerve transection or other injury can be the source of a great deal of pain. The free nerve endings embedded in a fibrous scar are easily traumatized. Sometimes, repeated nociceptive (pain-transmitting) input into the spinal cord gives rise to a central pain syndrome.

Treatment. Sharply transected nerves should be repaired immediately; macerated nerves are not repaired until the extent of irreparable damage becomes evident. At surgery the severed ends are cut back sharply to normal fascicular architecture and then connected. While fascicular repair with perineurial sutures has been advocated, joining the cut stumps with epineural sutures appears to be just as effective. Other techniques such as tissue glues and laser repairs are occasionally used. If exploration reveals the nerve to be in continuity, the surgeon must decide whether to divide and reconnect the nerve or simply free it from scar (external neurolysis). Electrical stimulation is carried out proximal and distal to the lesion. The action potential is recorded far distally. Proximal stimulation across the injury site should reveal a conduction block with either no conduction (neuroma in continuity) or an increase in latency and decrease in amplitude (partial neuroma and/or external scar). Distal stimulation should determine whether viable axons are present distal to the lesion. If a neuroma in continuity is resected after detection of a complete conduction block, the remaining gap may be too long to be bridged without undue tension. Bridging the stumps with an interposition nerve graft is then necessary.

Stretch injuries pose particular problems. A common example is injury to the peroneal nerve at the fibula head caused by a fall in which the leg twists. Traction injuries also commonly involve the brachial plexus. These injuries are sometimes seen in the newborn after difficult deliveries, as well as in adults with trauma to the shoulder girdle. When traction or stretch injuries are irreparable, techniques that may provide some substitute for lost function are used. These include muscle transfers when the lesion is incomplete or suture to the proximal portions of the spinal accessory or intercostal nerves.

Painful neuromas occurring after trauma or surgical amputation may be resected once. If failure occurs, as is likely, repeated, more proximal resection of the nerve is not to be considered, since further failure is probable and the cost in terms of lost proximal nerve function is unjustified.

Compression Syndromes. Nontraumatic causes of nerve compression in the extremities are most commonly caused by further narrowing or compression of normal passages through which nerves travel. This compromise may occur spontaneously but frequently is promoted by conditions that affect the nerve or the tissues surrounding it. Thus, entrapment syndromes are more common in diabetes, connective tissue disease, myxedema, acromegaly, edema associated with menses or pregnancy, and as a late complication of focal trauma (e.g., Colles' fracture). If the problem is severe, surgical release of the nerve is required.

The most common nerve entrapment is *carpal tunnel syndrome,* caused by compression of the median nerve as it enters the hand beneath the carpal ligament. Symptoms include pain or paresthesia in the palmar aspect of the hand and fingers, especially at night or upon awakening. Symptoms may extend above the wrist into the arm but are not as pronounced as in the hand. Eventually, numbness and difficulty with fine motor tasks occur. Diagnosis depends upon the presence of these pain characteristics and finding a Tinel's or Phalen's sign (reproduction of symptoms after a minute of maintained wrist flexion) at the wrist. It is supported by electrical studies showing slowed conduction in the median nerve at the wrist—although these studies occasionally are normal. Treatment should be directed at any underlying pathology. Diuretics help in cases of edema. Splints and local steroid injections may provide relief, but such relief is often only temporary, and simple division of the carpal ligament often is necessary.

Patients with *tardy ulnar palsy* present not with pain but with numbness and weakness. For this reason, the condition often is far advanced by the time the patient is seen; both physical signs and electrophysiological abnormalities of muscle activity and nerve conduction are readily evident. There is a Tinel's sign on tapping medially to the elbow, sensory loss in the ulnar distribution, as well as weakness and wasting of the interossei muscles. Treatment is transposition of the ulnar nerve anterior to the medial epicondyle, or other technique that prevents compression.

Thoracic outlet syndrome, when it produces nerve rather than vascular compression, shares some of the features of tardy ulnar palsy in that it includes compression of the lower portion of the brachial plexus, which in turn supplies the ulnar nerve. The compression occurs where the brachial plexus emerges into the axilla through a narrow passage beneath the clavicle and between the anterior and middle scalene muscles while resting upon the first rib. Abnormality of the anterior scalene is sometimes blamed for the production of symptoms, but it is not the only cause. While the presence of a cervical rib may compromise the underside of the plexus and cause symptoms, asymptomatic cervical ribs are frequent and one should not insist upon ascribing symptoms to them in patients with arm pain. Pain or neurological deficit occurring in the ulnar distribution, and especially numbness extending up the ulnar forearm, may be caused by any demonstrable cervical rib or especially prominent transverse process of C7. Surgical resection helps many of these patients. If no cervical rib is present but the pain and neurological deficit are in the ulnar distribution with no other source of the problem identified, first rib resection sometimes is helpful.

The differential diagnosis of ulnar nerve entrapment and thoracic outlet syndrome should include lesions of the lower cervical spine, such as cervical disc herniation. In addition, a tumor at the apex of the lung, usually metastatic from the pulmonary hilum, must be considered. Such tumors, producing Pancoast syndrome, affect the lower brachial plexus and may mimic thoracic outlet syndrome. Such a tumor should be suspected when arm pain is accompanied by a smaller pupil and ptosis of the ipsilateral eye (Horner's syndrome)—an unusual finding in thoracic outlet syndrome. Diagnosis usually can be made from an apical lordotic chest x-ray.

Lower extremity nerve entrapments, less common, include entrapments of the lateral femoral cutaneous nerve to the anterolateral thigh by the inguinal ligament, the ilioinguinal nerve supplying the medial thigh, or the genitofemoral nerve supplying the uppermost medial thigh and scrotum.

Nerve Tumors. Tumors of peripheral nerves are usually benign and present with swelling and/or pain. Neurilemomas (schwannomas) arise within the nerve, displace the nerve fibers around the tumor, and are amenable to removal; neurofibromas arise within a nerve but grow between and around the nerve fibers so that any excision necessitates sacrifice of the nerve. If a nerve tumor expands rapidly, seems fixed to surrounding tissues, or becomes newly painful, malignancy should be suspected. With time, malignant tumors extend along the nerve and into surrounding tissues. They can metastasize. Radical excision with or without radiotherapy is the treatment of choice. Multiple benign nerve tumors of both types are found in patients with neurofibromatosis with a correspondingly high proportion of patients in whom a malignant transformation occurs.

Functional Neurosurgery

Pain

Pain is treated by determining and removing its cause. When this course is not possible and pain medication fails, pain can be treated neurosurgically. Possible approaches include:

- Ablating the pathways carrying the sensation of pain to the brain rather than the underlying cause (e.g., anterolateral cordotomy, dorsal root entry zone lesions, sensory root section)
- Stimulating large fibers in the spinal cord or peripheral nerve to block painful input over small fibers (e.g., dorsal column or peripheral nerve stimulator implantation)
- Delivering opiates directly to the spinal cord by means of implanted epidural catheters

Several specific pain syndromes commonly are treated with neurosurgical procedures even though their etiology is only partly understood. Examples are trigeminal neuralgia and causalgia. *Trigeminal neuralgia* (tic douloureux) occurs as repetitive, transient attacks of pain in the maxillary or mandibular region of one side of the face. Attacks may be brought on by touching specific trigger areas of the face or mouth peculiar to each person afflicted. There is no neurological deficit. Medication (especially carbamazepine) usually is effective in ablating these symptoms. If medication is not tolerated or is not ineffective, symptoms may disappear following percutaneous, fluoroscopically guided procedures that permit compression (balloon), thermal injury (electrode), or chemical damage (glycerol) of the trigeminal ganglion. Open operations include posterior fossa craniectomy with decompression or partial section of the proximal trigeminal nerve root. *Causalgia* is a peculiar burning pain that may occur after the partial injury of a major limb nerve. The pain is heightened by stress and usually begins some months after trauma. It may resolve spontaneously after a year or two. Repeated local anesthetic injections into sympathetic ganglion or sympathectomy may be necessary to relieve this problem.

Movement Disorders

Spasticity was discussed under spinal trauma. Infrequently, *Parkinson's disease, dystonias, and athetosis* are treated with stereotaxically placed brain lesions. Unlike seizures, *hemifacial spasms* consist of repetitive but unevenly spaced unilateral facial twitching. Treatment consists of partial facial nerve section or botulinum injection. In recent years a less destructive approach, microvascular decompression of the facial nerve in the posterior fossa, has provided satisfactory results without producing facial nerve (motor) paralysis.

Epilepsy

Seizures are a manifestation of disease affecting the cerebral cortex. They usually are treated by a variety of anticonvulsant medications. However, if the seizures are focal or of new onset, a brain tumor, abscess, or AVM should be considered. Even when such lesions have been removed, residual changes in the brain may cause seizures to persist and necessitate anticonvulsant therapy in patients after neurosurgery.

Surgery is considered for any patient whose seizures become disabling despite prolonged drug therapy. When a focus of seizure origin can be determined and hemiplegia is not present, focal brain resection has a 50–85% chance of controlling seizures. Such surgery is especially helpful for unilateral temporal lobe epilepsy. The focal origin of seizures is determined by (*a*) scalp electroencephalogram (EEG) with or without subdural or depth electrode recordings and (*b*) videotaped observations of seizure activity. Additional evaluation, including neuropsychological testing and speech evaluation during intracarotid Amytal injection, helps to determine cerebral dominance and define the risks of surgery.

When no single focus of seizure origin is identifiable, there is little that can be done surgically unless the seizures are generalized. If they are, section of the corpus callosum usually reduces their frequency and intensity. If the patient already has profound hemiparesis, as occurs in some cases of epilepsy originating in childhood, a modified hemispherectomy may be preferable to callosal section. This operation helps to alleviate behavioral disturbances and cognitive impairment as well as to control the epilepsy.

Dementia

Most causes of dementia are not of neurosurgical concern. As has been discussed, brain tumors, brain trauma, epilepsy, or chronic subdural hematomas diminish mentation, including memory. One other surgically remediable cause of dementia deserves mention—*normal pressure hydrocephalus* (NPH). While it is readily evident that hydrocephalus with elevated ICP can produce mental slowing, it is possible for hydrocephalus exerting average or high-normal pressure to do so as well. NPH occurs within the setting of other brain compromise—the brain atrophy of the elderly or previous brain insults, such as subarachnoid hemorrhage and trauma. Presumably, such a brain is susceptible to the effects of ventricular pressure within the normal range.

When hydrocephalus develops following head injury or SAH, the patient's condition often plateaus or regresses after a period of improvement. In the elderly, the onset of spontaneous NPH is even more insidious. With NPH, a sequence of symptoms develops: gait disturbance, memory loss, and urinary incontinence. Diagnosis depends upon CT or MRI scans revealing ventricles that are disproportionately enlarged relative to the cortical sulci. While cerebral atrophy produces a proportionate enlargement of both the ventricles and the sulci, hydrocephalus enlarges only the ventricles. The hydrocephalus is communicating in that there is communication between the ventricular system and the subarachnoid space. Radionuclide scans (with tracer injected by lumbar puncture) demonstrate entry of tracer from the subarachnoid space into the ventricles with delayed emptying because of a subarachnoid block. For the same reason, tracer does not accumulate early or to a large degree in the subarachnoid spaces over the cerebral convexities that normally provide access to the main absorption sites, the arachnoid granulations. There is debate over the best method of establishing the diagnosis so as to increase the chances for a satisfactory surgical outcome. Treatment consists of placing a lumboperitoneal or ventriculoperitoneal shunt with a low-pressure valve. Complications include a low incidence of subdural hematoma caused by tearing of a bridging vein as the ventricles diminish in size and the cortex separates further from the inner surface of the skull.

Congenital Defects

Infants, children, and even adults present with congenital defects. Common ones are hydrocephalus, spina bifida (including spina bifida occulta, meningocele, myelomeningocele, lipomeningocele, intradural lipomas and dermoids), Chiari malformations and syrinx, Dandy-Walker syndrome, encephalocele, and craniosynostosis.

Hydrocephalus

Hydrocephalus is a dilatation of the ventricular system that is almost always caused by obstruction of the flow of cerebrospinal fluid. Because obstruction of CSF flow does not greatly alter its production, intracranial pressure increases with obstruction. The situation is similar to blowing up a balloon: a high initial intraluminal pressure is necessary to begin expansion, but with further ventricular dilatation enlargement continues at lower pressure. Expansion occurs at the expense of normal brain structure and therefore of function.

Noncommunicating hydrocephalus occurs when obstruction prevents CSF from flowing out of the ventricular system into the subarachnoid space. The obstruction may be caused by an intraventricular hemorrhage (common in premature infants) or tumor. The cause may also be a congenital defect, most commonly aqueductal stenosis, that blocks the flow of CSF from the third to the fourth ventricle.

Communicating hydrocephalus occurs when obstruction in the subarachnoid space prevents CSF from flowing into the venous system by way of the arachnoid villi. Some infants are born with the condition, which is thought to be caused by intrauterine subarachnoid hemorrhage or sterile meningitis. Others develop it as a result of spontaneous traumatic subarachnoid hemorrhage or inflammatory changes following meningitis, which obstruct CSF flow into the subarachnoid space or out through the arachnoid villi.

Symptoms and Signs. Symptoms and signs of hydrocephalus vary with the age of the patient. Because infants have open cranial sutures, their heads enlarge with expansion of the ventricles. The fontanelle becomes enlarged and tense, even when the child is in a sitting position. Though irritability and vomiting often develop in children with hydrocephalus, it is not uncommon for an infant to appear to be normal except for excessive head enlargement. Hydrocephalus in infants is usually caused by one of the congenital malformation discussed earlier, but may be caused by intraventricular hemorrhage in premature infants, neonatal meningitis, and—rarely—congenital brain tumors. Evaluation begins with a neurologic history and examination that includes measuring the circumference of the head. The measurement is compared to normative data. In this age group, transillumination of the head is helpful, since it rapidly discloses those cases with extreme cortical thinning. It is important to realize that in the newborn, and especially in the premature, the brain gives way to the hydrocephalus far more easily than the skull. The enlargement of the head may thus be surprisingly small compared to that of the ventricles.

Older children, in whom the cranial sutures have closed, present with signs of irritableness. Headache, nausea, and vomiting are common. Vision may be affected if papilledema occurs and becomes severe. Sixth nerve paresis or even deficient upward gaze may occur. With progressive ventricular enlargement, developmental milestones are delayed. Because childhood hydrocephalus presenting after the first year of life is caused at least as often by the presence of a posterior fossa tumor (Fig. 8.12) as by a congenital defect, an especially careful examination of cerebellar function should be carried out.

Adults also present with symptoms and signs caused by hydrocephalus. Tumor, previous trauma, subarachnoid hemorrhage, or meningitis are frequent causes. Occasionally, the hydrocephalus is secondary to a congenital defect. Headache, nausea, vomiting, and mental slowing are the most common symptoms. While they raise the suspicion of increased ICP—and possibly of hydrocephalus—they do not disclose its underlying etiology.

Evaluation. CT scanning (or ultrasound in infants) indicates the size of the ventricles and confirms the diagnosis of hydrocephalus. The scan is useful in determining whether hydrocephalus communicates with the subarachnoid space or if the block is in the ventricular pathways and there is noncommunication. If it is noncommunicating, the ventricular system rostral to the site of obstruction is dilated while more caudal sites are not. For example, in aqueductal stenosis the lateral and third ventricles are large while the fourth is small. On occasion, evaluating the fourth ventricle with CT may be difficult. If there is doubt, an MRI scan can be performed. If the clinical presentation or scans suggest that a tumor is the cause of noncommunication, an enhanced CT scan or MRI should be done. Evaluation of the patient with hydrocephalus ends only when the cause of hydrocephalus has been determined.

Treatment. Treatment for hydrocephalus consists of placing a ventriculoperitoneal shunt that allows the flow of CSF from the ventricular system to the peritoneal cavity, where the fluid will be resorbed. An alternative ventriculoatrial shunt places the distal tubing in the right cardiac atrium through the jugular vein. A shunt consists of a ventricular catheter exiting the skull to a reservoir, pump, and one-way valve in line with a catheter extending down into the abdomen or right atrium. The ventricular catheter is connected to a reservoir that can be tapped to sample the fluid.

Hydrocephalus secondary to intraventricular hemorrhage in the premature infant may respond to conservative measures or to a period of decompression through an external ventriculostomy. Shunting is a problem when these infants are very small because the skin may break down over the shunt. Long-term outlook is affected by the amount of intraparenchymal bleeding and damage.

Complications. The two most common complications are shunt malfunction and shunt infection. Complications from ventriculoatrial shunting, more frequent and more severe than those from ventriculoperitoneal shunting, include infection and obstruction. In growing children operations to lengthen the atrial catheter are frequent. Other complications include recurrent pulmonary emboli, hemolytic anemia, and shunt nephritis. For these reasons, ventriculoperitoneal shunts usually are preferred.

Evaluation of shunt function is often necessary. Symptoms of shunt malfunction are those of hydrocephalus with increased ICP—headache, irritability, nausea, vomiting, or even coma. Upward gaze may be impaired due to ballooning of the suprapineal recess. Papilledema may occur in patients whose cranial sutures have closed. Pumping the shunt can be helpful. If the pump chamber does not compress easily, the distal end is blocked. However, it is well to remember that the results of pumping the shunt can be misinterpreted. The finger pressing on the pump exerts a far greater pressure than does the normal flow of CSF. A shunt that pumps does not necessarily function. A shunt that refills slowly may be functioning so well that the ventricular wall has collapsed about it and slowed its filling. (At times function is sufficiently excessive CSF drainage to produce headache.) If poor shunt function is suspected, x-rays over the extent of the shunt (shunt series) may demonstrate it to be too short or reveal breaks or disconnections. A CT scan demonstrates ventricular size. Comparison with a previous scan taken when the shunt was functioning often is helpful. If there is doubt, a shunt tap is done to measure ventricular pressure.

The speed with which symptoms of shunt malfunction develop can vary tremendously. Some patients tolerate obstruction for days; others tolerate it for only short periods before pressure elevates markedly and consciousness, vision, or life is lost. It is thus advisable to revise the shunt rapidly once the diagnosis of malfunction has been established.

Shunt infection is suspected when a treated hydrocephalic patient develops malaise and fever. The shunt may or may not be malfunctioning. Repeated shunt malfunction should lead to suspicion of infection. Shunt infection is diagnosed by tapping the shunt and sampling the CSF. To avoid the small risk of infecting the shunt, it should be tapped only after other sources of infection have been excluded. Infection occurs in about 7% of shunted patients, and 90% of shunt infections occur within one year of placement. The organism is usually indolent, most commonly *S. epidermidis*, and there is usually only low-grade fever.

Revisions. Surgery to revise the shunt consists of either finding the site of obstruction and clearing it or replacing the entire shunt. Surgery to cure infection consists of replacing the shunt after the CSF has been sterilized with intravenous antibiotics. Replacement is necessary because antibiotics often fail to sterilize the shunt even though they may sterilize the CSF.

Spina bifida encompasses a spectrum of dysraphic states ranging from spina bifida occulta through meningocele and myelomeningocele. It is usually lumbar or lumbosacral in location and is characterized by deficient closure of the neural tube, vertebral column, and over-

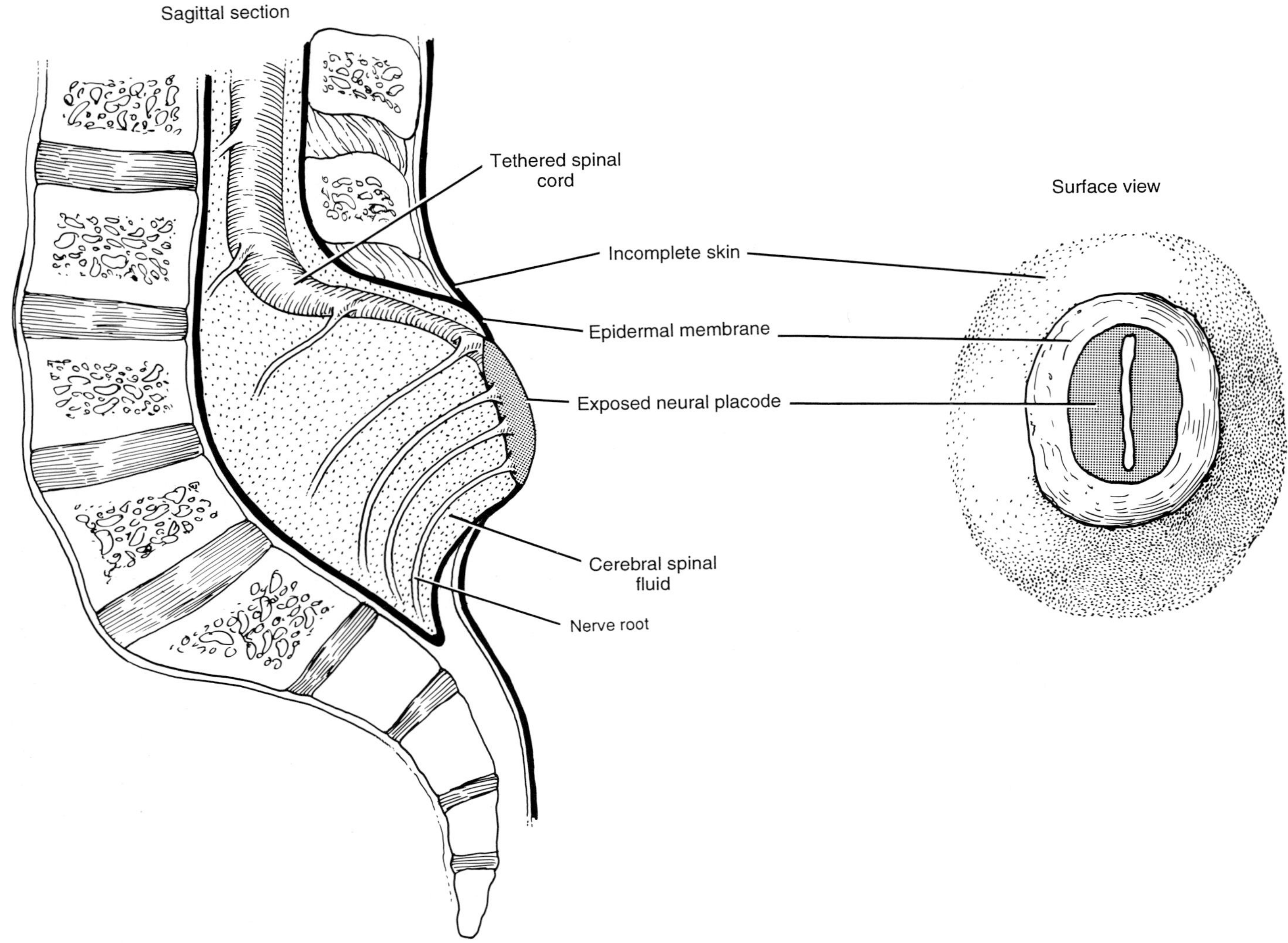

Figure 8.21. Myelomeningocele.

lying soft tissues. The most common but least severe form, *spina bifida occulta*, usually occurs without an underlying neural defect and presents as an incidental x-ray finding of an incomplete lamina (commonly at S2 or even L5). In some cases it is associated with an occult lipomeningocele (spinal lipoma) or intraspinal dermoid. A more severe defect without neural malformation, a *meningocele*, results when most of the elements dorsal to the spinal canal fail to close: the dural sac protrudes through the vertebral defect to form a bulging sac beneath the skin. While most common in the lumbosacral region, meningoceles can occur anywhere along the midline neuraxis, including the forehead and occiput. Neural elements are not present within the sac except insofar as they float up into it. Since the neural elements are not deformed, affected children have no neurological deficits.

When the malformation is more marked (about 1:500 births), neural tube closure is incomplete and a *myelomeningocele* forms, consisting of a protrusion of a central plaque of malformed neural elements posteriorly through a defect in the dura and vertebral lamina (Fig. 8.21). Usually the neural elements are not covered by epidermis and the myelomeningocele is said to be open. The sac lies below the midthoracic region and usually is lumbar. Most children have hydrocephalus as well as significant sphincter and lower extremity function deficits. The sibling of a child with myelomeningocele is at a twentyfold increased risk for having the condition.

As mentioned earlier, the normal spine grows more rapidly than the spinal cord, resulting in the ascent of the tip of the spinal cord from L5 at birth to L1 by adulthood. In myelomeningocele, the cord is tethered to the skin ectoderm. With growth, the spinal cord is stretched and distorted, leading to progressive scoliosis and delayed neurologic deficit above the static deficit. Tethering may also occur after a repair because of scarring.

Other dysraphic states, such as *lipomeningocele* (spinal lipoma) and *intradural dermoids* have been discussed in the section on spinal tumors. While delayed onset of neurologic deficit usually occurs because the cord is tethered, it may also be caused by the slow growing tumor compressing neural elements. Lumbar intradural lipomas often communicate with the subcutaneous tissue of the same dermatome as the spinal site of origin. Similarly, intradural dermoids are often connected to the skin by a dermal sinus tract. Lipomas and dermoids can consequently have an extensive intradural course. In other cases, subcutaneous lipoma and dermal sinus tracts extend from the skin surface down only through the dermis or subcutaneous layers. The location of the skin dimple of a *dermal sinus* distinguishes it from a *pilonidal sinus*. The latter lies within the top of the buttock crease while the former lies above it.

Meningitis is a dangerous complication of dermal sinus because the sinus tract can be colonized by skin bacteria. Staphylococci are the usual invaders. However, if the sinus orifice lies in the lumbosacral region, there is a danger that Gram-negative bacteria from the anus can gain access to the subarachnoid space. In addition, accumulation of dermoid desquamation debris in the intraspinal portion of a tract can produce pressure upon neural structures or rupture of the dermoid with resultant sterile meningitis. An infant, child, or even adult who has had either staphylococcal or recurrent meningitis should be thoroughly examined for the presence of a midline dermoid sinus over the back, neck, or head.

Evaluation. Evaluation of spina bifida occulta is necessary if patients manifest sensory problems, weakness in the lower extremities, or bladder or bowel dysfunction. X-rays reveal the laminal defect; such patients should be carefully examined for skin changes and undergo MRI scan or CT myelogram to screen for such tumors as lipomeningocele, spinal lipoma, or dermal sinus tract.

Evaluation for myelomeningocele may begin in utero. Sampling of maternal blood for α-fetoprotein during the first trimester provides an adequate screen for the presence of an open myelomeningocele. If the test is positive, amniotic sampling for α-fetoprotein and ultrasound examination of the fetus in utero are employed to confirm the diagnosis. Evaluation for neonatal hydrocephalus can also be accomplished with ultrasound.

Meningoceles and myelomeningoceles are evident in the newborn. The examiner should record the site and dimensions of the lesion, whether it is open or closed, the level of any motor deficit, and the extent of reflex activity. The sensory level often is difficult to determine and depends upon the infant's response to pain. The anal wink reflex and rectal tone should be tested and plain x-rays of the spine taken. If the lesion is a myelomeningocele, a cranial CT scan or ultrasound determines whether hydrocephalus is present and visualizes associated brain malformations. Early urologic consultation is requested to evaluate bladder function. Orthopedic evaluation is necessary because dislocated hips and lower extremity deformity are frequently associated with myelomeningocele. High lesions are associated with scoliosis.

Treatment. Surgery is required to repair meningoceles and myelomeningoceles. The meningocele is repaired according to the same principles as a hernia: the sac is dissected free, opened, divided, and closed level with the dura. The overlying soft tissue is closed in layers. Myelomeningoceles generally are repaired as soon after birth as feasible, on the premise that early surgery avoids meningitis or ventriculitis if there is an open meningocele. While appearing rational, this approach is debated as it places a significant strain upon the parents, one of whom is recovering from childbirth and may not be in the same hospital as the newborn undergoing surgery. However, if CSF leakage is present, closure should not be delayed unnecessarily. Myelomeningocele repair requires dissection of the neural tissues from the surrounding cutaneous elements with reconstruction of a dural tube about the neural tissue. A fascial layer may be mobilized to reinforce the closure. Skin closure often requires the development of cutaneous or myocutaneous flaps.

Follow-up. Repeated follow-up is required to evaluate the many problems encountered in these patients. Expertise in a variety of fields is necessary: neurosurgery, urology, orthopedics, ophthalmology, developmental neurology, rehabilitation, and social services. Such expertise can best be provided in a clinic setting that focuses on the care of children with myelomeningocele. Continued surveillance for the development of hydrocephalus (if not initially present) or shunt malfunction is necessary. Should leg function deteriorate or scoliosis progress, MRI of the spinal cord to search for tethering or syrinx formation is warranted.

Other Malformations

Chiari Malformations and Syrinx. The *Chiari II (Arnold-Chiari) malformation* is uniquely associated with myelomeningocele. The posterior fossa is small with the caudal portions of the medulla, cerebellum, and fourth ventricle extending below the foramen magnum into the cervical spinal canal. There is buckling of the brain stem at the pontomesencephalic junction. The brain is maldeveloped with hypoplasia of lower cranial nerve nuclei as well as both cerebellar and cerebral microgyria and heterotopias. There is hydrocephalus because the fourth ventricular outlet foramina are obstructed and because aqueductal stenosis is common. *Syringomyelia* may occur. The onset of symptoms from Chiari II malformation may occur in infancy, childhood, or even adult life.

The *Chiari I malformation*, less complex, is marked by tonsillar descent into the cervical spinal canal without displacement of medulla and fourth ventricle. Syringomyelia is frequent (Fig. 8.22). Symptoms and signs occur when enough tissue is crowded into the foramen magnum and adjacent cervical spinal canal to compress the caudally displaced medulla and the uppermost cervical spinal cord. In infants, symptoms include opisthotonos, difficulty swallowing, stridor, and apnea. In childhood and adulthood the manifestations can be classified as brain stem (dysphagia and bulbar speech),

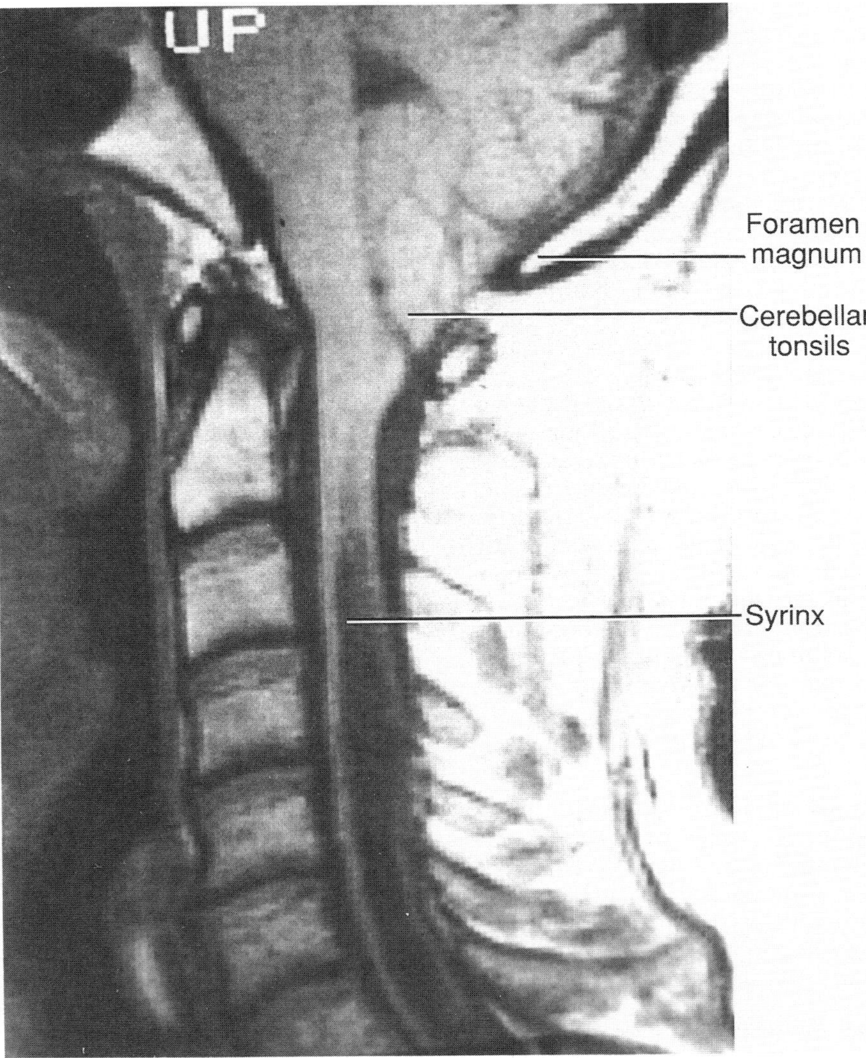

Figure 8.22. Chiari I malformation (MRI scan).

cerebellar (nystagmus, oscillopsia), and upper motor neuron (hemiparesis or quadriparesis). In addition, if present, the syrinx can become symptomatic and cause lower motor neuron weakness in the upper extremities, with a hanging sensory deficit in the shoulders that can extend to the arms and chest.

Surgery is performed to reverse progression of neurologic deficits. There is some controversy as to what constitutes adequate surgery. Most neurosurgeons agree the basic procedure involves decompression of the foramen magnum, with opening of the dura, lysis of arachnoidal adhesions, and widening of the dural sac. Opening the foramen of Magendie, and/or amputating herniated cerebellar tissue are additional options. Opening the syrinx several cord segments lower and shunting the syrinx to the subarachnoid space or pleura is advocated by some surgeons.

Encephalocele. Encephaloceles are herniations of malformed brain through defects in the skull and usually are covered with skin. Like myelomeningoceles, they probably arise from failure of somites to close. Occipital and cerebellar encephaloceles, the most common, are readily apparent. Nasofrontal encephaloceles may not be recognized, but they should be suspected if a soft tissue swelling is found at the medial canthus, in the nasal region, or even in the palate. Encephaloceles can even present as a nasal polyp. Evaluation has been simplified by CT and especially MRI scanning, which demonstrates connection of the contents of the sac with the brain. Surgery is performed to amputate or reduce the sac contents and repair the defect. For patients with cerebellum or brain stem contents in the sac, the outlook for satisfactory existence is limited. For patients with nasofrontal encephaloceles, the prognosis is good if the hypothalamus has not herniated into the sac.

Craniosynostosis

Craniosynostosis is the premature closure of one or more cranial sutures. Early closure, usually a primary intrauterine event, can occur secondary to early shunting of hydrocephalus or the presence of microcephaly. Primary craniosynostosis can be sporadic or inherited. Normally, fibrous union of the sutures begins around age 2 and is completed by age 8. With premature suture closure, continued brain growth causes compensatory growth of the skull at the remaining open sutures, while growth is halted in the direction perpendicular to the line of premature closure. Cosmetic deformities result.

When craniosynostosis involves the sagittal suture, the head is long and thin; when it involves the bilateral coronal sutures, it is short and wide. Premature closure of the metopic suture results in a keel-shaped skull. When it involves one coronal suture, the skull is asymmetrical with flattening of the forehead and supraorbital ridge on the involved side and compensating contralateral frontal bossing. Corresponding changes occur posteriorly if one lambdoid suture is stenosed.

The appearance of the child prompts the parents to seek medical attention. Rarely, signs of increased ICP are present. In such cases, several or all the cranial sutures are prematurely closed and the skull is small. If mental development is slow and all sutures are closed prematurely, and if there are no signs of increased ICP, microcephaly and not primary craniosynostosis is probably the correct diagnosis.

Evaluation includes skull x-rays and even radionuclide bone scans to identify the closed sutures. Additionally, CT scans with bone windows are helpful in evaluating facial bones and sutures at the skull base. If good correction is to be obtained, surgery is best performed between 3–6 months of age. The closed suture is excised or opened throughout its length until a normal suture on each end of the abnormal one is crossed. A closed sagittal suture is thus opened over its entire length across both the coronal and the lambdoid sutures. Coronal craniosynostosis involves freeing not only the coronal suture but also the frontosphenoidal suture and advancing the ipsilateral supraorbital ridge and frontal bone. Often there are accompanying facial deformities, requiring a team of neurosurgeons and plastic surgeons to effect reconstruction.

SUGGESTED READINGS

DeMyer W. Technique of the neurologic examination. New York: McGraw Hill, 1980.

Gatz AJ. Clinical neuroanatomy and neurophysiology. Philadelphia: FA Davis, 1966.

Wilkins RH, Rengachary SS. Neurosurgery. New York: McGraw Hill, 1985.

Youmans JR. Neurological Surgery. Philadelphia: WB Saunders, 1990.

Skills

ANATOMY AND NEUROLOGICAL EXAMINATION (INTRACRANIAL)

1. Given an adult patient with hemiparesis, complete a history and an examination (including neurological) and localize the lesion(s) responsible.
2. Given a nontrauma patient who is obtunded to the degree that there are no responses to verbal questions or commands, record the obtainable history and do a physical examination (including neurological) and localize the lesion(s) responsible.
3. For the patient in Statement 2, write a set of admission orders.
4. For either or both patients in Statements 1 and 2, provide a list of diagnostic tests to be obtained.
5. Interpret the CT scan or MRI scans obtained on the above or comparable patients.
6. Describe and diagram a spinal puncture.
7. Examine any patient or fellow student and carry out the examination of the brain stem reflexes omitting tests of respiration.

HEAD INJURY

1. Given a patient with head injury and poor or no verbal responsiveness, obtain a history and perform a physical examination (including neurological).
2. Determine the Glasgow coma score for several head-injured patients of differing levels of consciousness.
3. Interpret a skull x-ray from a patient with severe head trauma.
4. Interpret a CT scan from a patient with severe head trauma.
5. Write a set of admission orders for a patient with severe head trauma (Glasgow coma score = 5) who is not going to require surgery.
6. Write appropriate daily follow-up notes in the chart for the patients in Statement 2. Include your current examination and assessment.

NONTRAUMATIC INTRACRANIAL DISEASE

1. Perform a history and physical examination of patients being seen as outpatients or being admitted for neurological deficit.
2. List a differential diagnosis in order of likelihood.
3. Write daily follow-up notes in the charts of at least two inpatients. Include your current examination and assessment.
4. Interpret CT scans and MRI scans of patients with nontraumatic intracranial disease.

SPINAL DISEASE

1. Perform a history and physical examination of patients being seen as outpatient or being admitted for neck or back pain with neurological deficit.
2. Perform a history and physical examination of at least one patient with significant paresis or paralysis from spinal disease and localize the lesion on this basis.

3. Write a set of orders for the patient in Statement 1.
4. Write a set of orders for the patient in Statement 2.
5. Interpret spine x-rays and any myelograms or scans performed on the patient in Statement 1 or comparable patients.
6. Interpret spine x-rays and any myelograms or scans performed on the patient in Statement 2 or comparable patients.
7. Write daily progress notes in the charts of patients in Statement 5.
8. Write daily progress notes in the charts of patients in Statement 6. Include examination and assessment.

CONGENITAL DEFECTS

1. Examine and describe the observable malformation in a child with myelomeningocele.
2. Do a proper head circumference measurement and interpret the result on a normal growth curve for a full-term and a premature infant.
3. Examine and determine the motor deficits and the anal sphincter function in a child with myelomeningocele.
4. Interpret an ultrasound and a CT scan from a normal child and one with hydrocephalus.

Study Questions

ANATOMY AND NEUROLOGICAL EXAMINATION (INTRACRANIAL)

1. During a duel, one of the antagonists is struck in the left orbit with a 1-inch wide sword. On x-ray the blade is seen to pass through the orbital apex horizontally and medially with its tip centered in the midline just above and 1 inch behind the top of the posterior wall (dorsum sella) of the sella turcica. The flat of the blade lies parallel to the floor of the skull. The swordsman dies instantly.
   a. Describe which nerve, brain and vascular structures are found to be injured at autopsy.
   b. Describe the deficit associated with each structural injury.
2. Discuss the difference in the visual fields of patients with unilateral blindness, bitemporal hemianopia, and homonymous hemianopia and their localizing significance. Describe any deficits that might occur if the lesions producing each of these were large enough to press on structures adjacent to the part of the visual pathway affected.

LUMBAR PUNCTURE

1. List three conditions in which lumbar puncture might provide helpful information. List a condition in the differential diagnosis of each of these for which lumbar puncture might prove dangerous.

BRAIN DEATH

1. List the conditions that must be satisfied or excluded before any examination and determination of possible brain death can be carried out with validity.

INCREASED INTRACRANIAL PRESSURE

1. List the stages of transtentorial herniation, contrasting the effects of central and lateral hemispheric masses.
2. Describe the circumstances and significance of (*a*) respiratory arrest and (*b*) hypotension in the patient with increased intracranial pressure.

HEAD INJURY

1. A head-injured patient arrives comatose (Glasgow coma score = 5) in the emergency room with a dilated right pupil and left hemiparesis. General surgical consultation reveals that there are no other injuries except to the head.
   a. Describe pathological anatomical changes responsible for this picture.
   b. List the diagnostic steps in managing such a case, including the historical details you would like to elicit and the tests you would order.
   c. Describe therapeutic management for such a patient and how it might be affected by the test results.
2. Discuss which skull fractures require urgent surgical treatment, nonurgent surgical treatment, medical care, or no treatment, and explain the rationale for the treatment you choose.

NONTRAUMATIC INTRACRANIAL DISEASE

1. A 60-year-old right-handed woman presents with sudden but transient difficulty speaking.
   a. Contrast other symptoms and those physical findings that might be present in this patient that would favor each of the following diagnoses:
      i. Carotid stenosis
      ii. Meningioma
      iii. Vertebral artery disease
      iv. Hypertension with focal hematoma
      v. Chronic subdural hematoma
      vi. Cerebral embolus of cardiac origin
   b. Describe differences in management of each of these circumstances.
2. A 2-year-old child was febrile and irritable 2 months ago because of a purulent otitis media. Fever abated after antibiotic treatment and the ear cleared. She now presents with lethargy and papilledema. A CT scan reveals lateral and third ventricular dilation, but the posterior fossa is not well seen because of the child's small size, artifact, and difficulty with sedation.
   a. Discuss the differential diagnosis.
   b. Discuss the management of this case: how would you arrive at a diagnosis; how would you manage each diagnostic possibility; what about the hydrocephalus?

SPINAL DISEASE

1. A 55-year-old man presents with a complaint of difficulty walking and right arm pain.
   a. Contrast the aspects of the history and the physical findings that might be present in this patient if the problem were due to:
      i. Cervical disc
      ii. Cervical osteoarthritis
      iii. Neurofibroma
      iv. Metastatic carcinoma
   b. Describe the diagnostic radiological tests and the findings peculiar to each.
   c. Describe differences in management for each.
   d. Discuss why it is unlikely that the lesion is intracranial, is a syrinx, is a spinal cord astrocytoma, or is a congenital dislocation of C1 on C2.
2. A 24-year-old woman is brought to the emergency room by ambulance following an automobile accident in which she was rendered numb from the mid-anterior thighs down (including the buttocks) and is without any ability to contract any muscles in her lower extremities. Examination confirms total loss of sensation and flaccid paralysis.
   a. Describe the level of the lesion.
   b. Give an initial management plan, including diagnostic procedures and therapy of the lesion and its complications.
   c. Discuss factors affecting the prognosis.

PERIPHERAL NERVE DISEASE

1. A 30-year-old skier executing a rapid turn falls on his back, twisting but not striking his right leg. He has immediate low back pain, right lateral calf pain, right foot numbness and weakness. Examination reveals weakness of dorsiflexion at the ankle and toes.
   a. Discuss the possibility that this is due to a nerve injury or a lumbar disc herniation. Which nerve and which disc might be involved and how can you differentiate the two problems of physical examination?
   b. Describe the type of nerve injury that might be involved and its prognosis.
   c. If incomplete recovery occurs, how would you manage the patient?

FUNCTIONAL NEUROSURGERY

1. List ablative procedures that might be used for:
   a. Pain
   b. Spasticity
2. List nerve conditions that might respond to each of the procedures listed in answer to Question 1 and mention other treatment alternatives.
3. Describe the complications and drawbacks of each of the procedures listed in answer to Question 1.
4. List reversible causes of dementia and their treatment.

CONGENITAL DEFECTS

1. The mother of a 2-month-old child complains that tops that are the correct fit for her child's chest no longer slip over the infant's head. The child's weight has increased steadily and is appropriate for age.
   a. Discuss the examination of the child.
   b. List the differential diagnosis.
   c. Describe the treatment of each of the possibilities.
   d. List the follow-up measures for each possible treatment.
2. Head shapes vary when congenital defects are present. Such heads may present as:
   a. symmetrical but smaller than usual in one or more dimensions;
   b. asymmetrical without focal protrusion;
   c. symmetrical with a midline focal protrusion;
   d. symmetrical except for lateralized focal protrusion.

   Discuss causes, treatment, and prognosis for each.
3. Birth defects of the spine may present with various visible abnormalities.
   a. Describe the skin and soft tissue changes with meningocele, myelomeningocele, dermal sinus tract, lumbosacral lipoma, and pilonidal sinus.
   b. Describe the underlying changes in the spinal canal and its contents that may accompany each of these conditions.
   c. Discuss treatment prognosis and follow-up of each.

9 Urology: Diseases of the Genitourinary System

William J. Somers, M.D., Robert A. Badalament, M.D., Jeffrey P. York, M.D., Joseph A. Smith, Jr., M.D., Bruce E. Woodworth, M.D., and John A. Nesbitt, M.D.

ASSUMPTIONS

The student knows the anatomy and physiology of the genitourinary system: prostate, kidneys, bladder, testes and peritesticular organs, urethra, and penis.

The student has performed a physical examination of the normal prostate. The student is familiar with pathology that occurs in the kidneys, including infections and neoplasms.

The student understands the concept of the hypothalamic pituitary gonadal axis and understands basic testosterone synthesis and spermatogenesis.

OBJECTIVES

PROSTATE

1. Define the anatomy and physiology of the prostate gland.
2. Describe the clinical presentation, work-up, and management of a patient with acute and chronic prostatitis compared with a patient with non-bacterial prostatitis.
3. Define the clinical presentation, workup, and management of a patient with benign prostatic hypertrophy.
4. Describe how one can distinguish between benign prostatic hypertrophy and prostate cancer by clinical evaluation and diagnostic studies.
5. Discuss the use of prostate specific antigen determinations in evaluating patients with carcinoma of the prostate and benign prostatic hypertrophy.
6. Outline the staging and management of prostate cancer, both localized and advanced.

KIDNEYS

1. Discuss the types of renal trauma, mechanisms involved, and the appropriate management for each.
2. Discuss two congenital urinary tract anomalies requiring intervention.
3. Discuss the etiology and management of inflammatory renal disease; outline the treatment of pyelonephritis.
4. Describe the workup for a renal mass lesion; discuss the characteristic findings in a common benign and a malignant renal mass.
5. Describe the workup and treatment options in the management of patients with calculous disease of the urinary system.

URETER

1. Describe the etiology, clinical presentation, sequelae (if untreated), and management of ureteral obstruction.
2. Outline the management of iatrogenic ureteral injuries.

BLADDER

1. Describe the different tests used in a urodynamic evaluation.
2. Describe the pathophysiology of vesicoureteral reflux, its evaluation, and modes of treatment.
3. Discuss the evaluation and treatment of bladder trauma.
4. Describe the pathophysiology, diagnosis, and treatment of bacterial cystitis and interstitial cystitis.
5. Describe the symptoms, evaluation, and treatment of bladder fistulae.

6. Discuss the physiology of normal bladder function and disorders of micturition (incontinence, neurogenic bladder).
7. Discuss the etiology, presentation, and treatment of bladder cancer.

PENIS

1. Describe the etiology, clinical presentation, evaluation, and management of penile trauma.
2. Describe the etiology, clinical presentation, evaluation, and treatment of penile cancer.
3. Describe the clinical presentation and management of four acquired penile disorders.
4. Describe the clinical presentation and management of three congenital penile anomalies.
5. Discuss six sexually transmitted diseases. Demonstrate a knowledge of their causative pathogens, clinical presentation, evaluation, and treatment.
6. Discuss the indications for and complications of circumcision.

URETHRA

1. Describe the etiology, clinical presentation, evaluation, and management of urethral trauma.
2. Describe the natural history, evaluation, and treatment of male and female urethral cancer.
3. Discuss the etiology, presentation, evaluation, and management of urethral stricture disease.
4. Describe the clinical presentation, evaluation, and management of the two congenital disorders, posterior urethral valves and hypospadias.
5. Name the common pathogens responsible for urethritis.

TESTES, MALE INFERTILITY, IMPOTENCY

1. Discuss three congenital anomalies involving the testes.
2. Discuss the evaluation and differential diagnosis of the patient with acute testicular pain.
3. Describe three scrotal infections.
4. Describe the evaluation of a patient with a scrotal mass.
5. Discuss germ cell tumors of the testicle, their staging, and their treatment.
6. Provide a concise evaluation plan for the infertile male.
7. List the four major categories of erectile impotency.

Prostate

Anatomy and Physiology

The normal prostate gland is located just distal to the neck of the urinary bladder and surrounds the urethra for a distance of 2–3 m. The ejaculatory ducts empty into the prostatic urethra at the verumontanum (Fig. 9.1). The prostate gland anatomically is divided into zones that can be distinguished both histologically and grossly. The central zone accounts for only 5–10% of prostate volume and surrounds the ejaculatory ducts. The transition zone surrounds the urethra and enlarges substantially in men with benign prostatic hyperplasia. The peripheral zone is the origin of nearly 90% of prostatic cancers. A thin fibromuscular capsule surrounds the peripheral zone (Fig. 9.2).

The blood supply to the prostate originates primarily from branches of the hypogastric artery which enter the prostate posterolaterally (Fig. 9.3). A large dorsal vein complex is located on the anterior surface of the prostate. The puboprostatic ligaments anchor the prostate gland anteriorly to the pubic bone. Microscopically, the prostate gland is composed of glandular epithelium contained within a fibromuscular stroma.

Secretions from the prostate gland account for a major portion of the volume of a normal ejaculate. The prostatic fluid provides nutrients that are necessary for normal sperm motility and function. The prostate remains relatively dormant from birth until puberty and then begins to function as an exocrine gland. Enlargement begins in the fourth decade of life but usually is not functionally significant until the sixth or seventh decade.

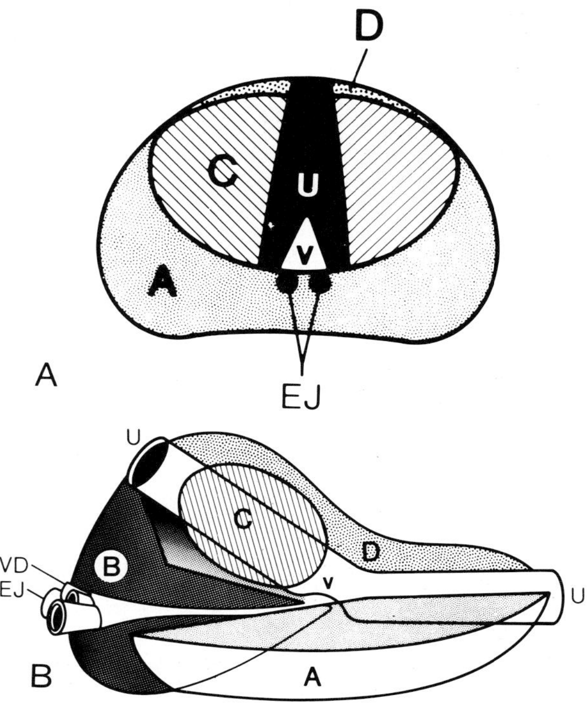

Figure 9.1. **A,** Schematic transverse image of the mid-portion of the prostate. A = peripheral zone; C = central zone; V = verumontanum; EJ = ejaculatory ducts; D = anterior fibromuscular stroma. **B**, Schematic longitudinal representation of the prostate. A = peripheral zone; B = central zone; C = transition zone; D = anterior fibromuscular stroma; U = urethra; V = verumontanum; EJ = ejaculatory ducts; VD = vas deferens.

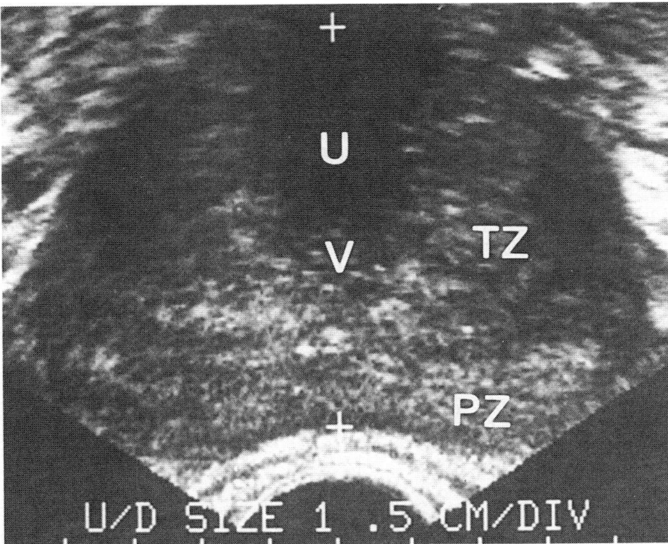

Figure 9.2. Transverse ultrasound image of the prostate gland showing the homogenous peripheral zone (PZ), the transition zones (TZ) around the urethra (U) and the entrance of the ejaculatory ducts at the verumontanum (V).

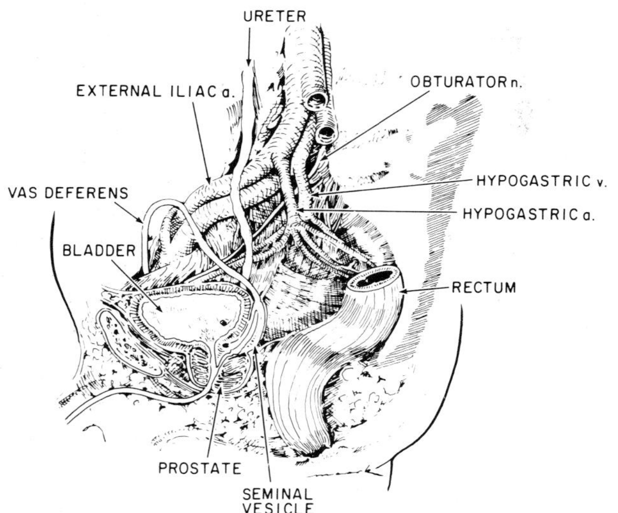

Figure 9.3. Sagittal view of male pelvic anatomy showing the relationship of the prostate gland to adjacent pelvic structures.

Prostatitis

The term *prostatitis* refers to an inflammatory condition of the prostate that may be bacterial in origin but often has no defined etiologic agent. *Prostatodynia* or *prostatosis* define a symptom complex that consists of an aching perineal discomfort, urinary frequency, urgency, and dysuria. More classic obstructive symptoms such as urinary hesitancy, dribbling, or difficulty emptying the bladder may occur. A distinction between bacterial and nonbacterial prostatitis can not be reliably made based upon symptoms alone.

Acute Prostatitis. Acute prostatitis is a relatively unusual bacterial infection of the prostate that may have protean manifestations. The disease occurs typically anytime after the second decade of life and is characterized by fever, back pain, chills, and dysuria. The symptoms are usually of relatively rapid onset. On physical examination, the prostate gland is swollen and often described as "boggy," sometimes warm to the touch because of inflammation, and frequently exquisitely tender. The urine sediment shows white blood cells and the serum white blood cell count may be elevated. Patients may present in acute urinary retention because of prostatic edema.

The infectious agent is usually a Gram-negative bacterium, most often *Escherichia coli*. Treatment consists of broad spectrum intravenous antibiotics. Bed rest is also frequently recommended.

Chronic Prostatitis. Chronic prostatitis has a more indolent clinical course than acute prostatitis. It is uncertain whether chronic bacterial prostatitis is a consequence of recurring independent infections or of failure to eliminate adequately an initial infection. Most often, there is no antecedent history of acute prostatitis. Patients typically present with discomfort in the perineum, back, or pelvis associated with urinary frequency, hesitancy, and dysuria. A voided urinalysis usually shows white blood cells. Prostatic fluid obtained after digital prostatic massage characteristically has greater than 10 white blood cells per high powered field. Cultures of the prostatic fluid should be positive for bacteria before assigning a diagnosis of chronic bacterial prostatitis. Treatment consists of oral broad spectrum antibiotics such as trimethoprim-sulfamethoxazole, quinolones or carbenicillin. The voiding symptoms usually resolve promptly on antibiotics but may recur rapidly after antibiotics are discontinued.

Non-bacterial Prostatitis. A common and frequently frustrating problem for patients and physicians is the symptom complex of nonbacterial prostatitis. The subjective manifestations may be indistinguishable from those associated with chronic prostatitis. However, no bacterial or other etiologic agent is consistently identified, although *Chlamydia trachomatis* has been isolated in some patients. Frequently, there are no objective findings and the prostatic fluid is normal to microscopic examination. Antibiotic therapy often is not beneficial unless an etiologic agent has been identified. Appropriate therapy consists of reassurance of the patient as well as symptomatic treatment consisting of sitz baths and, occasionally, nonsteroidal anti-inflammatory drugs.

Benign Prostatic Hyperplasia

Epidemiology. Benign prostatic hyperplasia (BPH) defines a process of progressive prostatic enlargement that consists of both hyperplasia (proliferation in the number of cells) and hypertrophy (enlargement in size of the prostate). The pathologic process occurs primarily in the transition zone and can be demonstrated histologically as early as the third decade of life. Symptomatic manifestations of BPH are uncommon before the age of 50. There is no apparent causal association between BPH and other pathologic conditions of the prostate such as prostatitis or cancer. The natural history of BPH is poorly understood and variable. Significant spontaneous symptomatic improvement is relatively uncommon, but not all patients have progressive symptoms if left untreated. Histologic evidence of BPH is almost universal in aging men but there is no direct correlation between prostate size and symptomatology.

Signs and Symptoms of BPH. Because of its anatomic position surrounding the urethra, enlargement of the prostate typically results in a relative bladder outflow obstruction. Classic obstructive symptoms are hesitancy in initiating voiding, a decrease in the force of the urinary stream, terminal dribbling, and a feeling of incomplete bladder emptying. Because of bladder irritability that may result from obstruction, typical irritative voiding symptoms such as frequency, urgency, and nocturia are also common. The symptoms are usually of gradual onset but may progress to the point of acute urinary retention.

Digital rectal examination of the prostate shows palpable enlargement. There may be some asymmetry of the prostate but BPH characteristically has a smooth contour and a soft consistency. In the absence of infection, a voided urinalysis is normal. A urine flow rate shows diminished force of the urinary stream (usually less than 15 mL/sec in symptomatic patients). An abnormal amount of urine in the bladder after voiding (post-void residual) may be demonstrable either by direct catheterization or ultrasonography. Intravenous pyelography may show thickening of the bladder detrusor muscle (trabeculation) and "J-hooking" of the distal ureters as they are displaced cephalad by the enlarged prostate. A decompensated bladder with poor emptying is a relatively unusual manifestation of longstanding BPH but may result in hydronephrosis and renal failure because of the chronically increased intravesical pressure.

Treatment. Although occasional patients may present with objective indications for treatment such as renal failure or poor bladder emptying resulting in recurrent infection, the most common reason to pursue treatment of BPH is for symptomatic relief. Patients should be counselled that symptomatic improvement can be achieved with treatment in the majority of patients but that progressive symptoms or detrimental consequences from untreated BPH are not inevitable.

Medical Therapy. Medical treatment for BPH can provide symptomatic benefit in some patients. α-1-Adrenergic blocking agents which are marketed for treatment of hypertension are sometimes used and are undergoing clinical trials. They exert a beneficial effect in some patients through relaxation of the smooth muscle component of the prostatic capsule and bladder neck.

Finasteride (Proscar) is a 5-α-reductase inhibitor recently approved by the FDA for the treatment of symptomatic BPH. The usual dose is 5 mg daily. 5-α-Reductase converts testosterone to the active intracellular metabolite dihydrotestosterone. Consequently, Proscar exerts its effect through blocking androgenic activity on the prostate cells. A modest decrease in prostatic size (20–30%) occurs and some patients have mild symptomatic improvement or a small increase in urinary flow rates. The drug is well-tolerated with very few side effects.

Surgical Therapy. The surgical removal of obstructing prostatic tissue can be performed via either an open or transurethral route. An open surgical approach is usually chosen for patients with a very large (> 60 g) prostate size. The prostate is approached through a lower midline abdominal incision or, in special cases, a perineal incision. The enlarged prostatic adenomatous tissue is enucleated by sharp dissection with scissors and blunt finger dissection through either the bladder (suprapublic prostatectomy) or the prostatic capsule (retropubic prostatectomy).

More often, the transurethral route is chosen for the performance of transurethral prostatectomy (TURP). An electrocautery loop is used to successively remove prostatic tissue under direct visualization. The resection is usually carried to the level of the prostatic capsule and all obstructing tissue is removed. Alternatively, a transurethral incision of the prostate (TUIP) can be performed in patients with smaller glands. With either technique, hemostasis is obtained with electrocautery.

Usually, one or two nights of hospitalization are required after TURP and patients should be voiding well at the time of hospital discharge. The risk of incontinence is low (1–2%) and treatment related impotence occurs in fewer than 10% of patients. In properly selected patients, treatment results are excellent and there is usually a substantial increase in urinary flow rate.

Carcinoma

Epidemiology. Carcinoma of the prostate is the most common cancer in men in the United States and the second leading cause of cancer death. Over 95% of prostatic cancers are adenocarcinoma arising from the prostatic acinar structures. The incidence of prostate cancer increases with age. A familial pattern has been identified and the disease is more common in African-Americans than in Caucasians.

Histologically, adenocarcinoma can be identified at autopsy in over 30% of men over the age of 50. Thus, there is a large discrepancy between the microscopic presence of the disease and the clinical incidence and death rate from prostate cancer.

Most men with early-stage prostate cancer have no disease related symptoms. Prostate cancer and BPH may occur simultaneously, but there is no apparent causal relation. Obstructive voiding symptoms may be from BPH or, as the cancer enlarges, from malignant tissue. Patients with advanced disease may present with pelvic pain, ureteral obstruction, or bone pain from distant metastasis.

Early Detection

Digital Rectal Examination. Digital rectal examination has been the primary method for early detection of prostate cancer. A normal prostate is smooth, symmetric, and has a consistency similar to the muscles of the thenar eminence. Most prostate cancers arise in the peripheral zone and, once they attain sufficient size, are palpable as an area of induration or nodularity within the substance of the prostate (Fig. 9.4).

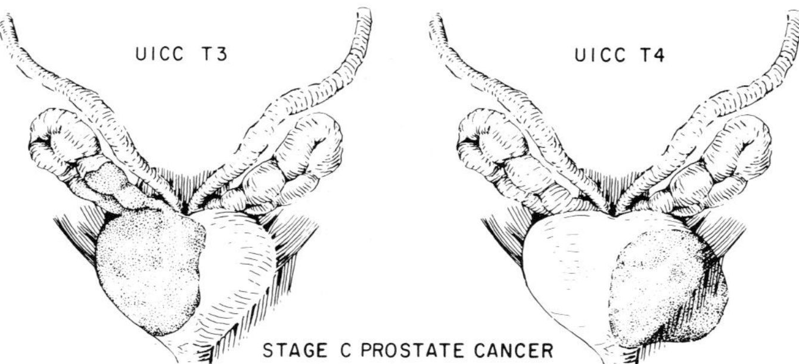

Figure 9.4. Schematic representation of a palpable prostate cancer with extension into the seminal vesicle (left) and the levator ani muscle (right). Most prostate cancers arise in the peripheral zone and, once they attain sufficient size, are palpable by digital rectal examination as an area of induration or nodularity.

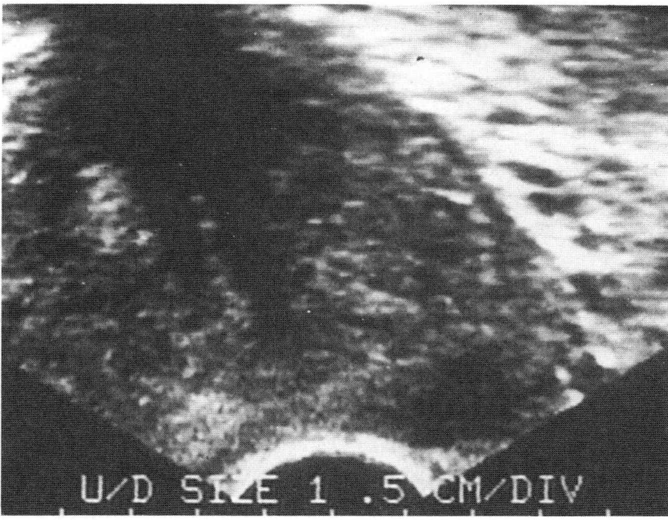

Figure 9.5. Transverse ultrasound image of the prostate showing a hypoechoic area in the peripheral zone and the left base which is characteristic of prostate cancer. Ultrasound can help direct biopsies to specific areas of the prostate that may be suspicious for cancer.

For digital rectal examinations, patients are either placed in the knee-chest position or are standing while bending forward at the waist. A gloved and lubricated index finger is inserted into the rectum. The prostate gland is palpable beneath the anterior rectal wall. Normal seminal vesicles are not palpable on digital rectal examination. The margins of the prostate should be distinct and any areas of induration, nodularity, or asymmetry should be noted.

Prostate Specific Antigen. Prostate specific antigen (PSA) is a serine protease enzyme whose function is to cleave the proteins in the postejaculatory semen. Serum PSA is specific for the prostate but is secreted by both benign and malignant prostatic epithelial cells. PSA may be elevated in men with prostatitis, BPH, or prostate cancer.

PSA levels of less than 4.0 ng/mL (Hybritech assay) are considered normal. Modest elevations in PSA are usually from BPH rather than cancer, but nearly one in five men with an abnormal PSA are found to have cancer on biopsy. PSA is elevated in over 95% of men with metastatic prostate cancer and should fall to undetectable levels after radical removal of the entire prostate.

Acid Phosphatase. Acid phosphatase levels are elevated in most men with metastatic prostate cancer but are less sensitive than PSA and less specific. Acid phosphatase is usually normal in men with localized disease, so it is not useful for early detection. Elevated acid phosphatase in a man with a diagnosis of prostate cancer but no demonstrated metastatic disease is a poor prognostic sign and usually indicates the presence of subclinical metastasis, often to lymph nodes.

Transrectal Ultrasonography. The best imaging test for prostate cancer is transrectal ultrasonography (TRUS). TRUS can distinguish the zonal anatomy of the prostate and is an accurate measure of prostate size. Prostatic cancers typically are located in the peripheral zone and have a hypoechoic pattern (Fig. 9.5). Because of its lack of sensitivity and specificity, TRUS is usually performed only in patients with an abnormal PSA or a palpable abnormality of the prostate.

Prostate Biopsy. Biopsy for detection of prostate cancer can be accomplished through the perineum but more often is performed via a transrectal route. Ultrasonography facilitates accurate needle placement. A spring-loaded automatic gun is used to obtain cores of tissue from suspicious areas of the prostate or for random sampling. Patients are premedicated with a broad spectrum antibiotic which is continued for 48 hours after the biopsy.

Staging of Prostate Cancer. Staging of prostate cancer defines the local, regional, and distant extent of disease. The Whitmore modification of the Jewett system has been used frequently in the United States to define local tumor extent. The tumor-node-metastasis (TNM) system is being used increasingly, however, and allows categorization of nonpalpable tumors detected because of PSA or ultrasound abnormalities (Table 9.1).

The primary staging modality for local disease is digital rectal palpation. Transrectal ultrasonography may provide useful information in some patients. Serum prostate specific antigen levels correlate only roughly with disease extent. However, bone metastasis is quite uncommon in patients with a PSA of less than 20 ng/mL. Radionuclide bone scanning is the most sensitive method for detection of bone metastases (Fig. 9.6). Prostatic cancer typically affects the axial skeleton and forms osteoblastic metastases on plain radiograph (Fig. 9.7). Soft tissue metastasis may also occur but are unusual without concomitant bone metastasis.

Lymph node staging is of critical importance in selecting patients for therapy. Computerized tomography scanning may show enlarged lymph nodes in patients with high volume or high grade primary tumors. Laparoscopic pelvic lymphadenectomy is technically feasible and can provide adequate sampling of the pelvic lymph nodes. Most often, though, lymph node dissection is performed through an open incision immediately prior to radical prostatectomy. The anatomic limits of a staging lymph node dissection for prostate cancer are the

Table 9.1.
Staging for Prostate Carcinoma

T—Primary Tumor		
TX	Primary tumor cannot be assessed	
T0	No evidence of primary tumor	
T1	Clinically inapparent tumor not palpable nor visible by imaging	
	T1a	Tumor incidental histologic finding in 5% or less of tissue resected
	T1b	Tumor incidental histologic findings in more than 5% of tissue resected
	T1c	Tumor identified by needle biopsy (e.g., because of elevated PSA)
T2	Tumor confined within prostate[a]	
	T2a	Tumor involves half of a lobe or less
	T2b	Tumor involves more than half of a lobe, but not both lobes
	T2c	Tumor involves both lobes[b]
T3	Tumor extends through the prostatic capsule	
	T3a	Unilateral extracapsular extension
	T3b	Bilateral extracapsular extension
	T3c	Tumor invades seminal vesicle(s)
T4	Tumor is fixed or invades adjacent structures other than seminal vesicles	
	T4a	Tumor invades any of: bladder neck, external sphincter, rectum
	T4b	Tumor invades levator muscles and/or is fixed to pelvic wall

[a]Invasion into the prostatic apex or into (but not beyond) the prostatic capsule is not classified as T3, but as T2
[b]Tumor found in one or both lobes by needle biopsy, but not palpable or visible by imaging is classified "T1c"

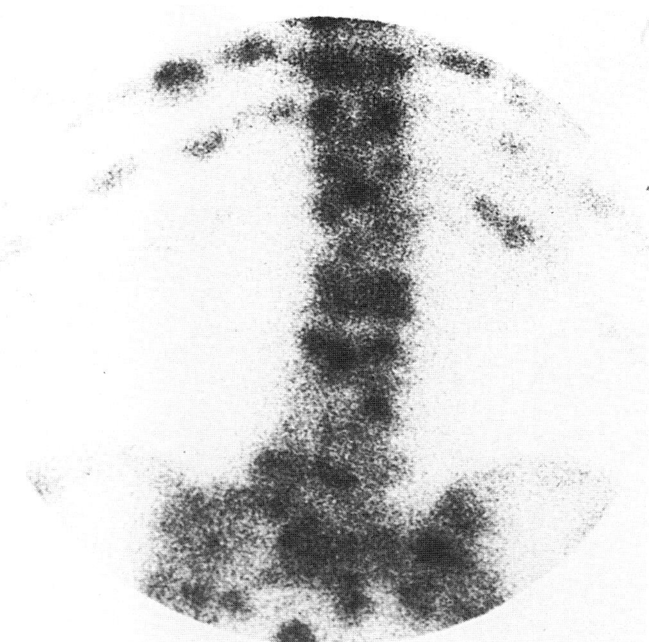

Figure 9.6. Radionuclide bone scan showing multiple areas of abnormal uptake in the pelvis and spine, typical of metastatic prostate cancer.

bifurcation of the common iliac artery proximally, the circumflex iliac vein distally, the midportion of the external iliac artery laterally, and the bladder wall medially. The dissection is carried posteriorly to the obturator nerve (Fig. 9.8).

Treatment

Localized Disease. For patients who otherwise have an anticipated life expectancy of greater than ten years, treatment of localized prostate cancer is indicated. External beam irradiation can provide adequate disease control in some patients but there are concerns about positive biopsies after radiation that may be identified in over half of patients. Most often, when the disease is felt to be intracapsular, radical prostatectomy is recommended.

Radical prostatectomy can be performed via a perineal approach (Fig. 9.9). An inverted U-incision is made anterior to the rectum and the dissection continues in the plane between the prostate and rectum. The posterior layer of Denonvilliers's fascia is opened and the prostate gland including the capsule and the seminal vesicles are dissected free entirely. The perineal route is associated with minimal postoperative pain but does not allow simultaneous lymph node dissection.

More often, radical prostatectomy is accomplished by a retropubic route. An incision is made from the umbilicus to the pubis. Usually, pelvic lymphadenectomy is performed. During radical retropubic prostatectomy, the entire prostate including the prostatic capsule is removed along with the seminal vesicles and ampullary portion of the vas deferens. After removal of the prostate, a direct anastomosis is performed between the reconstructed bladder neck and the urethra (Fig. 9.10). In patients who are sexually active before therapy, potency can be retained in nearly two-thirds by preservation of the neurovascular bundle that lies immediately posterolateral to the prostate and urethra. In patients with negative surgical margins, a 15-year, disease-free survival of nearly 50% can be anticipated. In patients with positive surgical margins or histologically positive lymph nodes, adjuvant radiation treatment or hormonal therapy may be used.

Metastatic Disease. Prostate cancer is a partially androgen dependent disease. Therefore, the primary treatment for metastatic carcinoma of the prostate is deprivation of androgens from the cancer cell. Suppression of serum testosterone can be achieved by bilateral surgical orchiectomy. Alternatively, medical therapy may be considered. Oral administration of estrogens effectively lowers serum testosterone but is associated with cardiovascular side effects in up to one-fifth of patients. When given in high doses, luteinizing hormone-releasing hormone (LHRH) analogs effectively suppress testosterone to the castrate range within 1 month of administration. LHRH analogs are associated with few serious side effects but do cause vasomotor hot flashes in around two-thirds of patients. Loss of libido and impotence are a consequence of either orchiectomy or LHRH administration.

Less than 10% of circulating androgens in men are of adrenal origin. The contribution of these androgens to the growth of prostate cancer is uncertain. Flutamide

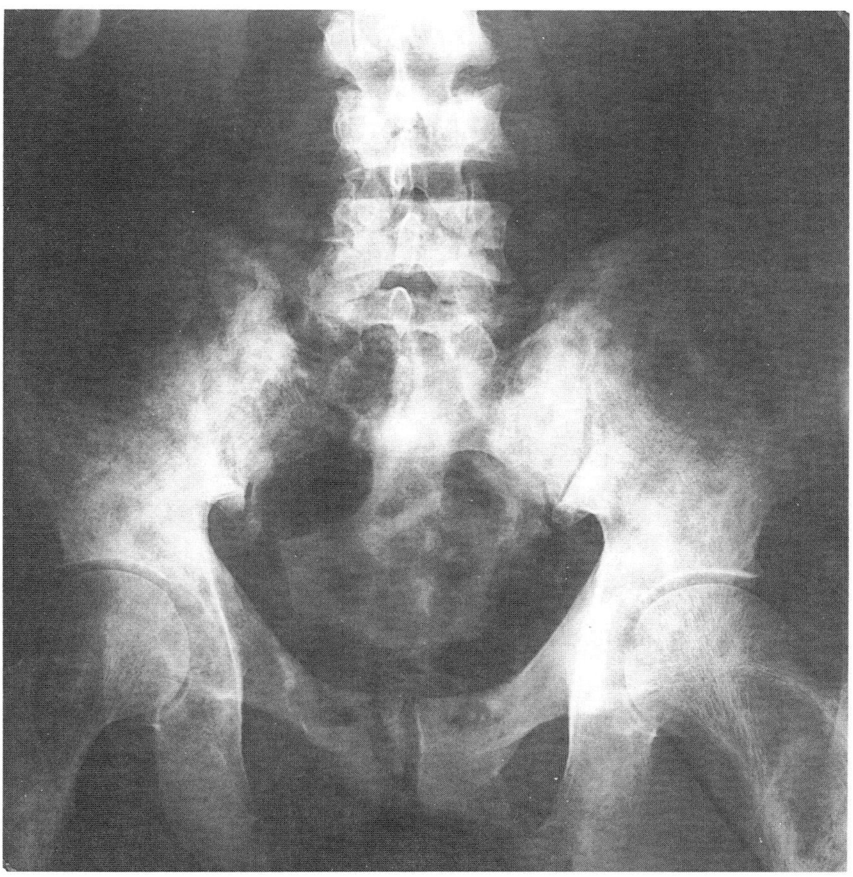

Figure 9.7. Radiograph of the pelvis showing characteristic osteoblastic metastases from prostate cancer.

(Eulexin) is a nonsteroidal pure antiandrogen. Some studies have shown that Eulexin can prolong the duration of response when used in conjunction with LHRH analogs or orchiectomy. However, other studies have shown conflicting results. Flutamide is administered orally and causes some degree of gynecomastia in most patients and gastrointestinal side effects (usually diarrhea) in 15–20% of patients.

The duration of response to hormonal therapy in patients with metastatic prostate cancer is usually around 18–24 months. After that time, disease progression occurs. There are no treatments known to favorably alter the course of the disease after hormonal therapy. Radiation can be effective for isolated sites of bone metastasis. Most patients with metastatic carcinoma of the prostate die within 2 to 3 years of the time of diagnosis.

The Kidneys

Anatomy

The kidneys are paired retroperitoneal organs that lie on either side of the vertebral column, opposite the 12th thoracic and the 1st through 3rd lumbar vertebrae. They are bordered by the diaphragm posteriorly and superiorly, and by the psoas and quadratus lumborum

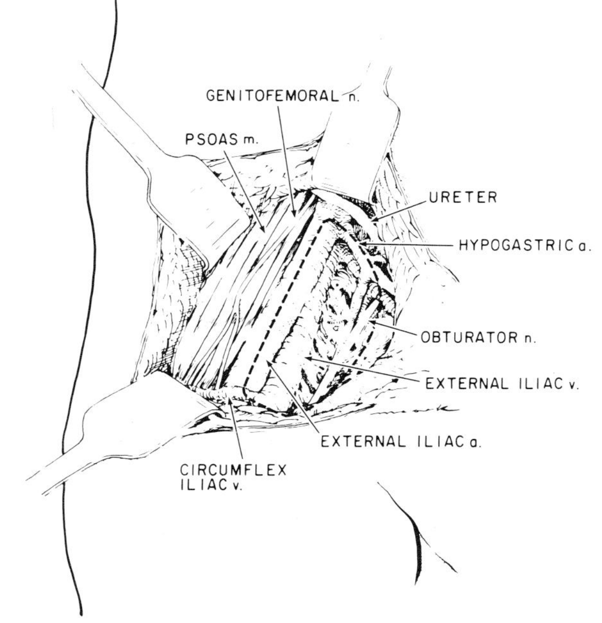

Figure 9.8. Anatomic boundaries of a staging pelvic lymph node dissection for prostate cancer.

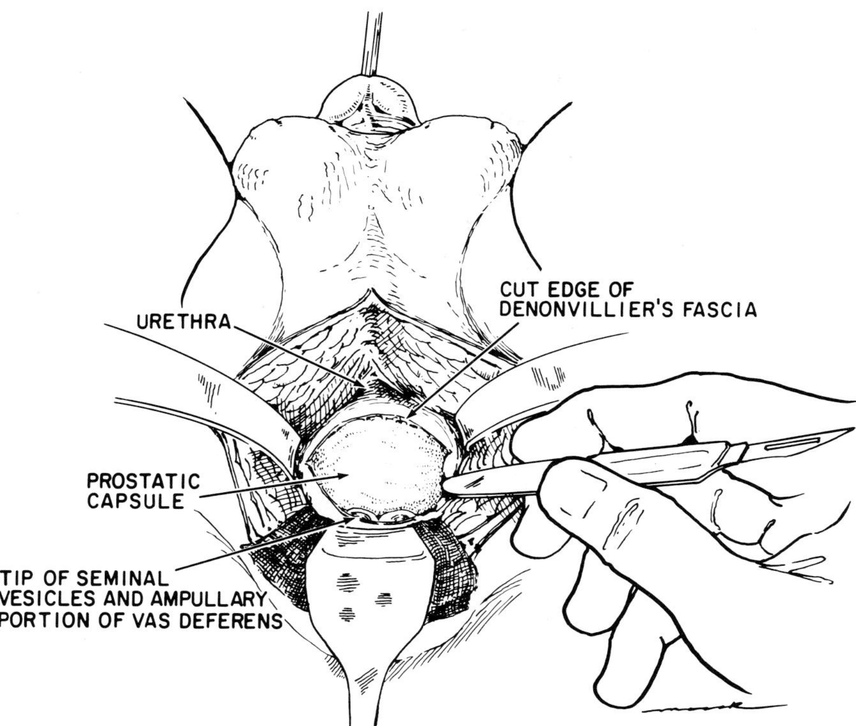

Figure 9.9. Radical perineal prostatectomy. The rectum is retracted posteriorly and the posterior layer of Denonvilliers' fascia has been incised to expose the prostatic capsule.

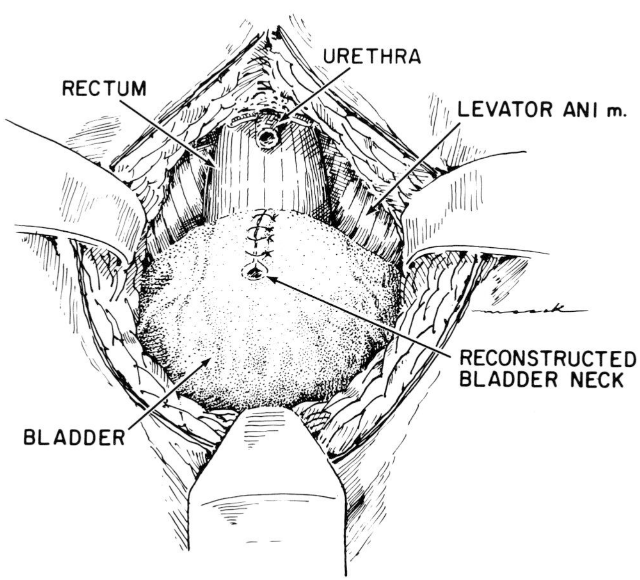

Figure 9.10. Radical retropubic prostatectomy. The surgical specimen has been removed and the bladder neck reconstructed. A direct anastomosis is performed with the stump of the urethra.

muscles posteriorly. The right kidney is bordered by the right lobe of the liver anteriorly and superiorly and by the right colon inferiorly (Fig. 9.11). The duodenum lies over the anteromedial portion of the right kidney. The left kidney lies adjacent to the spleen with left colon over its anterior lateral surface. The stomach borders the anterior surface of the upper pole, the jejunum overlies the anterior lower pole, and the tail of the pancreas overlies the hilum. Normally, the left kidney lies more cranially than the right one. The dimensions of the average kidney are approximately 11 cm in length, 6 cm in breadth, and 3 cm in anteroposterior thickness. The kidney typically weighs 150 g in the male and about 135 g in the female.

The kidney is covered by a renal capsule composed of fibrous tissue that is closely applied to the renal cortical surface. At the hilum this layer becomes continuous with the fibrous sheaths of the renal and great vessels. The capsule is easily stripped from the parenchyma. The layer of adipose connective tissue surrounding the kidney and its vessels, the perirenal fat, is thickest at the borders of the kidney. Surrounding the perirenal fat is a layer of fibroareolar connective tissue, the renal fascia or Gerota's fascia. The anterior layer of Gerota's fascia is termed the fascia of Toldt, and the posterior layer is known as the fascia of Zukerkandl. Superiorly, the fascial layers envelop the adrenal glands. Inferiorly, the layers remain separate and surround the ureters. Medially, the layers fuse and adhere to the renal vessels and kidney pelves, limiting any extravasation of urine, blood, or purulence.

Renal Physiology. The kidneys maintain water and electrolyte balance. They are also responsible for elimination of waste products and reabsorption of important solutes. They have an influence on maintaining blood pressure, and they help maintain acid-base balance in the body. Additionally, the kidneys function as an en-

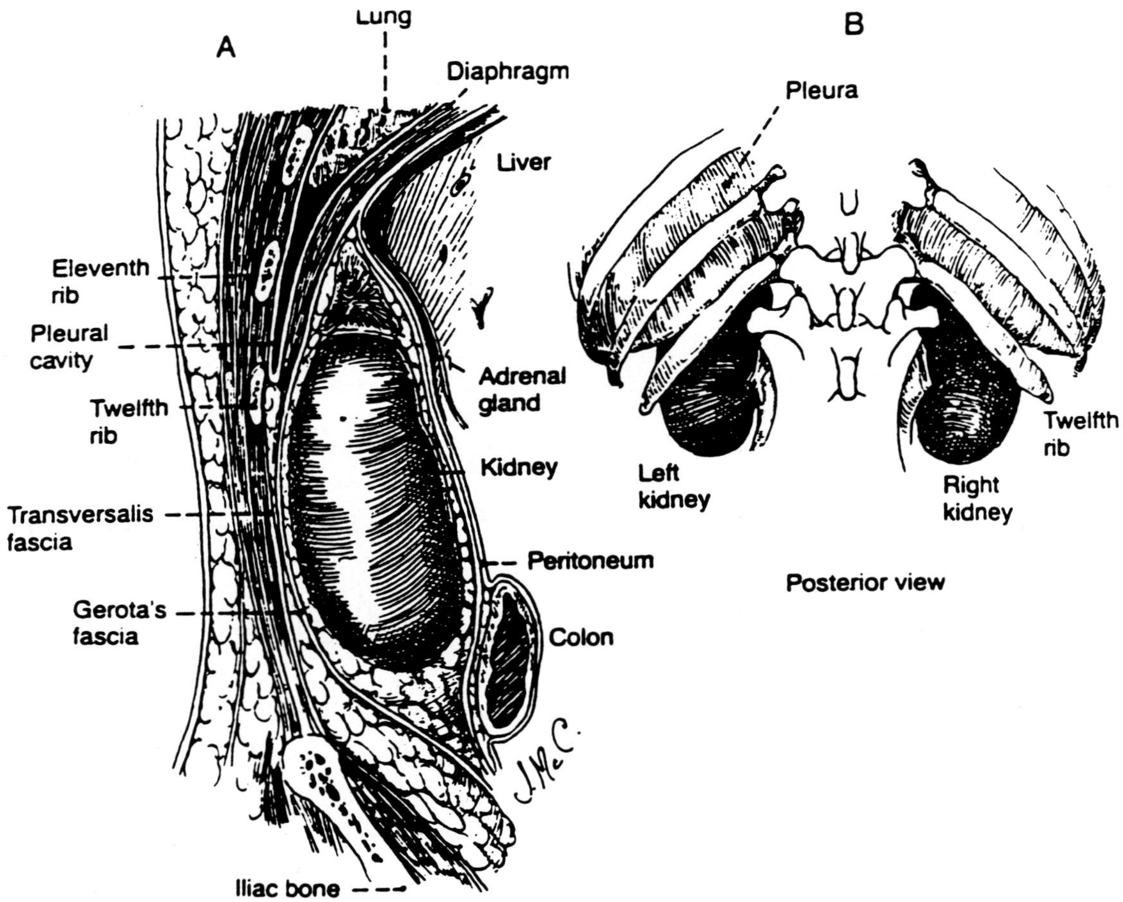

Figure 9.11. Anatomic relationship of the pleural cavity and some intra-abdominal structures to the kidneys.

docrine organ and as the site of renin production and of vitamin D_3 synthesis.

The basic functional unit of the kidney is the nephron, of which there are approximately 2 million per renal unit located in the outer region of the cortex and in the inner medullary region. Each nephron is composed of Bowman's capsule, a proximal tubule, loop of Henle, a distal tubule, and collecting ducts. A fine capillary system surrounds each nephron. The outer cortical nephrons have a short loop of Henle that only minimally penetrates the medulla. The juxtamedullary nephrons have a larger glomerulus and a longer loop of Henle. The surrounding capillary system, called the *vasa recta*, descends into the medulla adjacent to the loop of Henle.

The formation of urine begins in the glomerulus where blood is filtered under pressure to form an ultrafiltrate that is similar to plasma. Glomerular filtration is regulated by Starling forces. Two of these forces promote ultrafiltration (intracapillary hydrostatic pressure and interstitial oncotic pressure) and two forces oppose it (plasma oncotic pressure and tissue turgor). In addition, glomerular capillary wall pressure, total surface area of the capillary, and the rate at which plasma flows into the kidney also regulate filtration. Glomerular filtration rate (GFR) is measured by the concept of clearance, where

$$\text{Clearance} = \frac{\text{(urine concentration of substance) (volume of urine flow)}}{\text{plasma concentration of that substance}}$$

Normal GFR is between 75 and 125 mL per minute, a rate that is actually a measure of creatinine clearance. Creatinine clearance is the most commonly used method for determining renal function in clinical patients. A simple formula for creatinine clearance is:

$$\frac{(140 - \text{age})\ (\text{body weight in kilograms})}{72 \times \text{creatinine}}$$

After the ultrafiltrate passes into the proximal tubule, 70–80% of the sodium and water is reabsorbed, resulting in an isoosmotic filtrate. Osmotic diuretics can interfere with sodium and water reabsorption in this segment. As the filtrate passes into the ascending loop of Henle, sodium and chloride are absorbed, resulting in dilute filtrate. The next segment of nephron collecting tubule is the site of the final regulation of sodium and water reabsorption. Antidiuretic hormone stimulates water elimination or absorption in this segment, depending upon the plasma concentration. ADH increases tubule permeability, allowing increased water absorption, and it also causes vasa recta contraction, preventing the removal of solutes from the medulla. In this way either a concentrated or dilute urine is produced. Urine concentration can be used as a measure of renal function. A low urinary concentration of <20 mEq/L can indicate sodium conservation in the kidney. This measurement is seen in some patients before the onset of renal failure.

The fractional excretion of sodium (FENa) is a more accurate measure of renal function. It is calculated as follows:

$$\text{FENa} = \frac{\text{amount of sodium entered}}{\text{amount of sodium filtered}}$$

A FENa less than 1% is seen in hypervolemia, CHF, and hypertension. A FENa greater than 1% is seen in renal damage, as from acute tubular necrosis.

The kidney also has a vital role in maintaining the body's acid-base balance. Approximately 70 mEq of metabolic acid is produced daily by the body and must be eliminated. The lungs and kidney participate in buffering and eliminating this acid load. Although the renal response to an increased acid load may take from hours to days to occur, it plays a vital role. The kidneys perform this function by reabsorption and excretion of bicarbonate. Reabsorption of bicarbonate occurs in the proximal tubule. Here, filtered bicarbonate combines with hydrogen ions, forming carbonic acid that disassociates into carbon dioxide and water. Carbonic acid rapidly disassociates into a bicarbonate and hydrogen ion, and the bicarbonate ion moves into the peritubular fluid. Bicarbonate is generated through a similar process in the distal tubule. The kidney is also able to secrete such substances as uric acid, metabolic waste products, weak acids and bases, and drug metabolites. In addition, tubular secretion is responsible for potassium elimination.

The kidney is the site of a number of endocrine functions. Renin is produced by the juxtaglomerular cells located adjacent to the afferent arteriole of the glomerulus. Renin acts on angiotensinogen to cleave a peptide bond, forming angiotensin I, which is then converted to its physiologically active form, angiotensin II. Angiotensin II is a potent vasopressor and is responsible for stimulating release of aldosterone and catecholamines. It causes increases in systolic and diastolic pressures and increases in sodium reabsorption from the ascending loop of Henle. Platelet-activating factor is also produced by the renomedullary interstitial cells of the kidney. This factor causes aggregation of platelets and is a hypotensive agent. Erythropoietin is produced in the renal cortex in response to hypoxia and is responsible for erythrocytosis. Finally, the proximal tubule is the site of conversion of calcidiol to calcitriol, one of the most potent stimulators of intestinal calcium absorption and a metabolite of vitamin D_3 (calcidiol).

The Renal Blood Supply. The blood supply to the kidneys, about 20% of cardiac output, is about 20 times greater than that to any other organ. The renal vascular pedicle is anterior to the renal pelvis, entering at the hilum (Fig. 9.12). Usually, a single renal artery supplies each kidney, entering at either the upper or lower pole. Later it divides into branches that supply the various kidney segments. Variation in number and configuration of the renal arteries is extremely common. In one study, 65% of kidneys examined had at least one aberrant vessel. Interruption of these vessels may result in ischemia and infarction of that portion of the kidney, since aberrant vessels typically do not form anastomotic channels with other renal arteries. The potential long-term sequela of this type of injury is hypertension. Additionally, aberrant lower pole arteries may be associated with congenital ureteropelvic junction (UPJ) obstruction. Because the blood supply to anomalous kidneys is unpredictable, angiography is recommended before surgery is performed.

Evaluation and Treatment of Renal Trauma

Renal injury may result from either blunt or penetrating abdominal trauma. Many cases of blunt renal trauma may be managed expectantly, if diagnostic studies provide adequate information on the extent of the injury. Virtually all cases of penetrating renal trauma require surgical exploration. However, the diagnostic studies used in blunt trauma are of value in these cases as well.

Blunt Renal Trauma. Blunt trauma, accounting for about 70–80% of all renal injuries, usually results from motor vehicle accidents and less commonly from accidental falls or contact sports. The mechanism of injury is from either forces of rapid deceleration or actual impact upon the upper abdomen, flank, or back. Hematuria is found in most patients. Associated injuries include rib fractures, vertebral body and transverse process fractures, as well as flank contusions and abrasions. Retroperitoneal hematoma must be considered in patients who present in shock. These patients often have sustained a rapid deceleration injury and present with a palpable abdominal mass.

Diagnosis. Patients in whom gross or microscopic hematuria is detected must be evaluated for injury to the genitourinary tract, even though 20% of patients with significant renal injury do not have hematuria. The importance of obtaining a good history and performing a careful physical examination cannot be overemphasized. Elucidating the mechanism of injury may lead to the suspicion a renal injury has occurred.

In patients who have sustained lower abdominal trauma in addition to flank trauma, a cystogram followed by intravenous urography should be considered. Urethral injury must be excluded especially in males by retrograde urethrography before a cystogram is performed. The cystogram consists of instilling 300–350 mL of contrast solution into the bladder and then taking a postvoid film. Upper tract evaluation includes an intravenous pyelogram (IVP). Tomographic cuts are obtained as necessary to visualize the kidneys or ureters. Early films and tomograms obtained during the nephrogram phase may demonstrate renal parenchy-

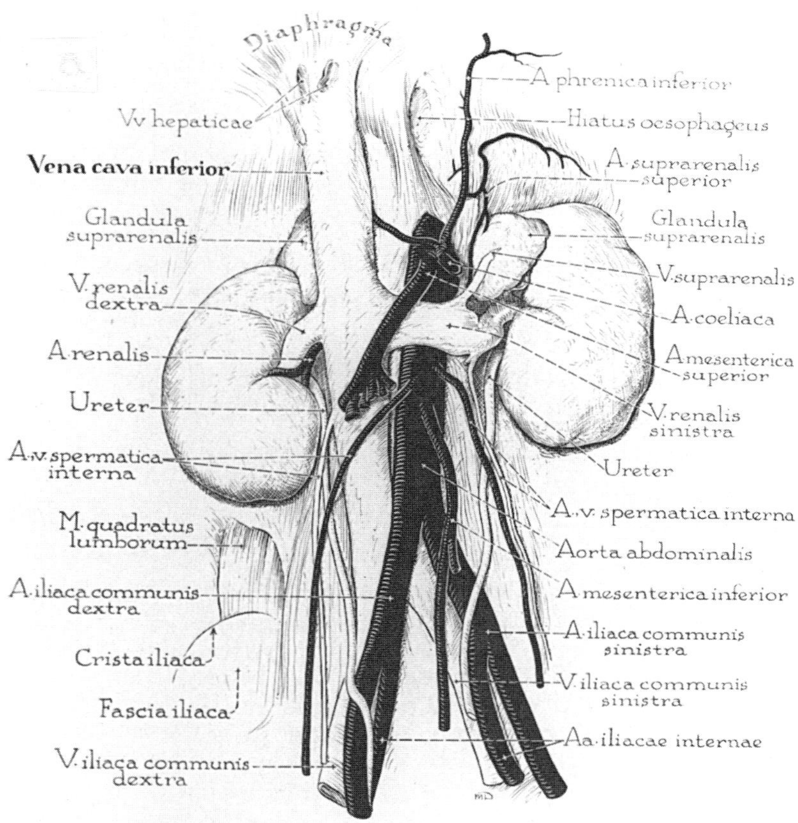

Figure 9.12. Blood supply to the kidneys.

mal injury. Later films (15–30 minutes apart) are good for demonstrating urinary extravasation. An IVP can show the presence or absence of the kidneys, the integrity of the renal outlines, the integrity of the collecting systems, and whether a kidney is delayed in functioning or is nonfunctional. Perfusion may be evaluated grossly (but not quantitatively) with this study as well. In approximately 14% of these patients a kidney may not be visualized. While vasospasm or minor renal injuries may be the cause, a recent series showed 57% of patients with nonfunction had injuries of a magnitude that eventually required nephrectomy.

While intravenous urography coupled with tomography is adequate for staging 85% of renal injuries, computed tomography (CT) may be used as an additional staging modality and is valuable in delineating parenchymal laceration, extravasation, nonviable tissue, size and location of renal hematoma, and adjacent organ injury.

Whenever vascular injury is suspected, an arteriogram should be performed. On the basis of angiographic findings, renal injuries may be subdivided into those that must be managed operatively and those that may be managed expectantly. In one series, only 2% of patients treated conservatively required subsequent operative intervention. As CT improves, it may supplant arteriography in delineating renal vascular injury. Sonography is an alternate imaging modality in renal trauma, but its accuracy is inferior to arteriography or CT.

Classification. Renal injury resulting from blunt trauma falls into several categories (Fig. 9.13). Minor contusions are the most common. Lacerations of the kidney may be minor or major. In minor lacerations the injury extends no further than the renal cortex, there is no urinary extravasation or large hematoma, and the capsule may remain intact. In major lacerations there is a transcapsular rupture through the corticomedullary junction of the kidney and often associated urinary extravasation or large perirenal hematoma. When treated conservatively, multiple lacerations are associated with a higher complication rate. Macerated kidneys are rarely salvageable by any approach.

In severe blunt trauma during rapid deceleration (as in automobile-pedestrian accidents), the ureter may be avulsed from the renal pelvis. While this type of trauma is uncommon, one must suspect this injury in order to make the diagnosis. The right collecting system is injured approximately 2.7 times more often than the left. In about 80% of injuries, the site of avulsion is usually at or within 4 cm of the UPJ. Bilateral ureteral injury from blunt trauma is exceedingly rare.

Treatment. Treatment of these patients depends on clinical findings and not only on x-ray findings.

Penetrating Renal Injuries. Penetrating renal injuries are associated with simultaneous intra-abdominal

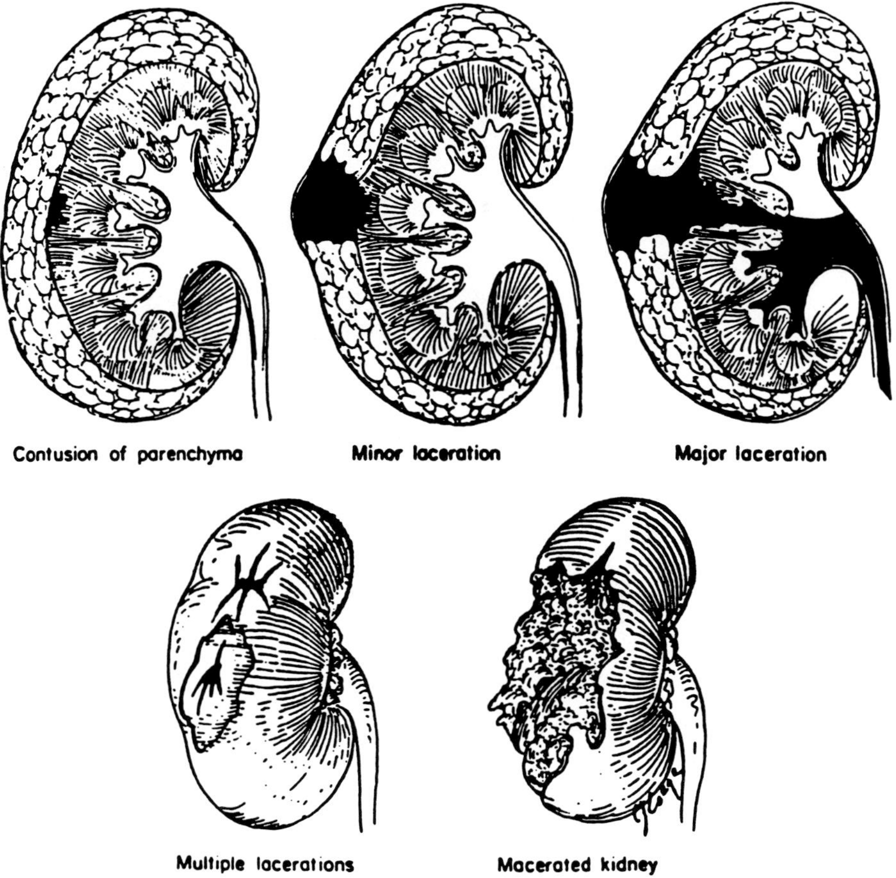

Figure 9.13. Categories of renal trauma.

injuries in excess of 80% in some series. For this reason, these injuries should be explored surgically. Preoperative evaluation should proceed similarly to blunt renal trauma, with IVP routinely performed. In the presence of hematuria, the entire urinary tract should be evaluated, with a retrograde urethrogram and cystogram to be included.

Renal Pedicle Injuries. Because the renal pedicle is anatomically fixed in the retroperitoneum, it is susceptible to injury in blunt trauma. Displacement of the kidney with respect to the upper ureter, by either lateral flexion and hyperextension of the spine or cephalad displacement of the kidney, appears to be responsible for the injury. Avulsion of the ureter may be explained by its anatomical fixation at the UPJ. Primary repair of this injury produces excellent or satisfactory results in approximately 80% of patients.

While renal pedicle injuries occur in association with blunt trauma, they are most frequently associated with penetrating injuries to the abdomen. Multiple vascular injuries are common since the left renal vein crosses the aorta and overlies the left renal artery, the splenic vein, and the superior mesenteric artery. While clinical instability of the injured patient may preclude preoperative studies, an IVP obtained as soon as feasible will confirm the presence of a functioning contralateral kidney. In patients with hypovolemic shock and rapid deterioration, immediate exploration for control of bleeding is essential. Once the patient has been stabilized, contrast studies may be performed.

Patients with renal pedicle injuries associated with multiple system trauma have a mortality rate of approximately 42%. Hematuria is often absent and, because of severe associated injuries, formal evaluation of the renal pedicle may be delayed. Delay in diagnosis reduces the chance of successful repair. The success rate for revascularization approximates 80% at 12 hours, dropping to 57% at 18 hours.

If surgical exploration is required before radiographic evaluation, the renal vessels must be visualized first. Damage may be overlooked if they are explored by palpation alone. If the patient is stable and the renal unit cannot be visualized on excretory urography, immediate arteriography is indicated. This test must be done expediently since renal function recovery is directly related to ischemic time.

Renal Trauma Surgery. A midline incision extending from the xiphoid to the pubis allows for both speed and excellent exposure of the abdominal cavity and renal hilum. The small bowel should be retracted to the right after an incision in the posterior parietal peritoneum (Fig. 9.14). The left hilum is exposed by an inci-

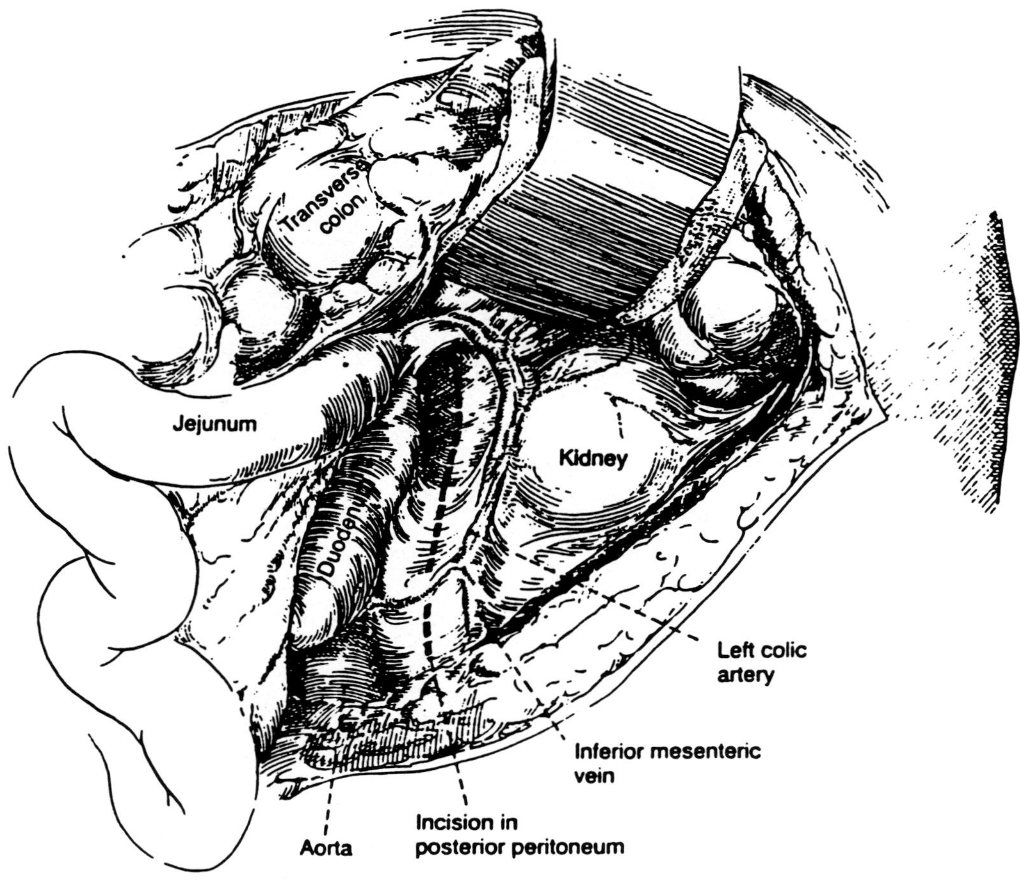

Figure 9.14. Exposure of kidney on left side via transabdominal approach.

sion that begins just inferior to the ligament of Treitz, extends inferiorly along the aorta, and is medial to the inferior mesenteric vein. This approach exposes the splenic vein as well and simultaneous injury to the spleen can be evaluated. The right hilum is exposed with a similar maneuver by medial retraction of the duodenum (Kocher's maneuver see Fig. 9.15).

The etiology as well as the extent of renal injury determines the subsequent surgical procedure. If renal pedicle injury has been previously diagnosed or suspected, the aorta and vena cava may be controlled both above and below the renal vessels using this approach. A retroperitoneal hematoma is usually evident upon opening the abdomen. A good rule of thumb is to observe the hematoma for a few minutes. If it is expanding, then surgical repair with control of the vascular pedicle is necessary. If the hematoma seems stable and if there is no evidence that the kidney is fractured, then observation only may be required. A pulsatile hematoma may indicate continued vascular bleeding.

Once the pedicle has been exposed, the decision to repair it is based upon the type and extent of the injury. Associated injuries and total ischemic time of the kidney may rule against a more complicated repair and for nephrectomy. Nephrectomy not only shortens the procedure time but reduces postoperative morbidity. Local bowel or pancreatic injury may require fresh vascular anastomoses, increasing the risk of postoperative complications: mortality exceeds 50% when pedicle injuries are associated with pancreatic or duodenal injuries. The interposition of omentum or peritoneum between abdominal contents and the vascular repair will minimize postoperative complications. Injuries to the renal pedicle caused by gunshot wounds require extensive debridement of the vessels prior to reanastomosis. If the injury is widespread, an interposition vascular graft may be necessary. Penetrating renal pedicle injuries have a mortality rate approaching 30%, with nephrectomy being required in over one-third of cases.

Congenital Disorders

Scores of congenital anomalies are found in the urinary tract. Some are symptomatic and discovered in children, others are asymptomatic and discovered serendipitously, and yet others do not become symptomatic until adulthood. Two of the more common disorders requiring intervention are discussed below.

Horseshoe kidney occurs in from 1:600 to 1:1800 live births. It is the most common type of renal fusion anomaly and usually occurs at the lower pole. Symptoms, if present, are urinary infection and, less commonly, hematuria. Occasionally, patients describe a vague abdominal discomfort. Diagnosis is usually made

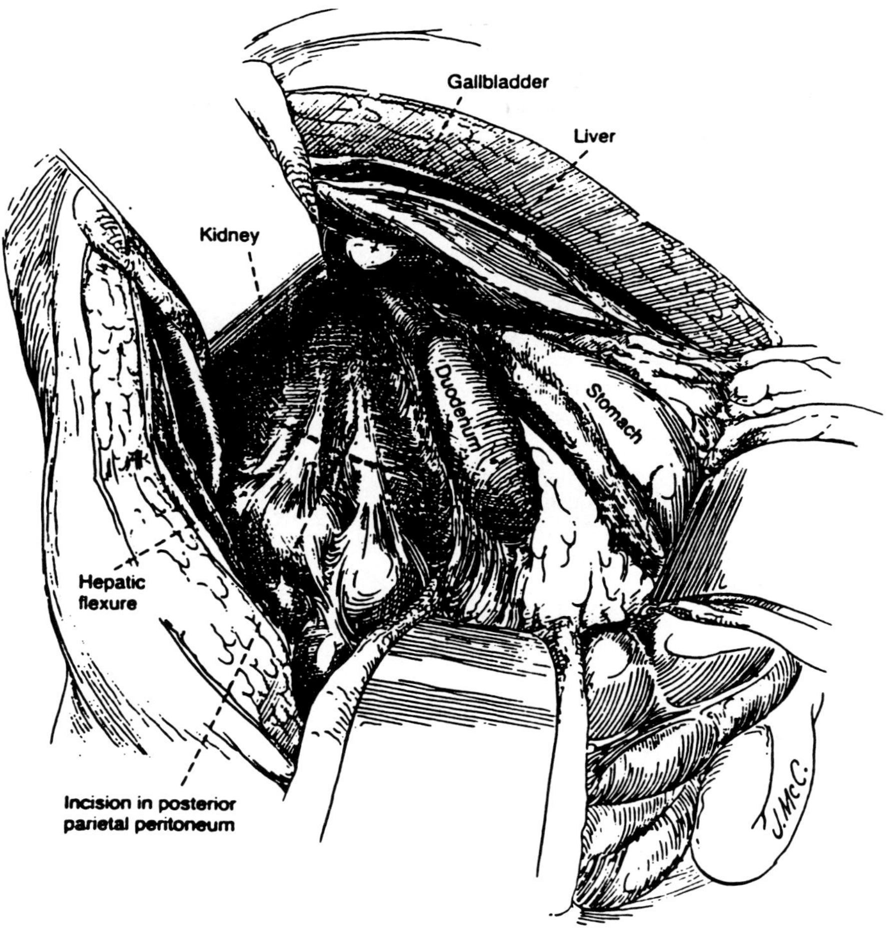

Figure 9.15. Exposure of kidney on right side via transabdominal approach.

by IVP, although ultrasonography and CT are useful as well. When intervention is necessary, the renal isthmus connecting the kidneys is divided surgically. Revision of the ureteropelvic junction may need to accompany the symphysiotomy.

Congenital obstruction of the urinary tract occurs most frequently at the junction between the ureter and the renal pelvis, the ureteropelvic junction. The etiologic factors in this obstruction are myriad, complex, and result in varying degrees of hydronephrosis. Bilateral involvement is frequent early in life, with unilateral involvement presenting later. The leading theory is that an aberrant vessel or band causes constriction of the ureter at the UPJ, interfering with normal development of the intrinsic ureteral muscle fibers. The resulting stenosis or functional obstruction leads to hydronephrosis. Presenting signs and symptoms are palpable abdominal mass, pain, hematuria, urinary infection, fever, hypertension, and renal stones. Diagnosis is by IVP or ultrasonogram. Nuclear scan confirms obstruction. Surgical repair of the obstruction is performed to prevent progressive renal insufficiency and recurrent urinary tract infections.

Inflammatory Diseases

Diseases. Pyelonephritis, currently the most common renal inflammatory disorder, is one of the most challenging diagnostically and clinically. While it can be seen in any age group, it is most often seen in infants (mostly females), in women of childbearing years, and in elderly men (secondary to enlarged prostates). *Escherichia coli* is the predominant organism, with *Pseudomonas* sp., *Proteus*, and *Klebsiella* accounting for recurrent infections. Chronic pyelonephritis often leads to renal failure and, after glomerulonephritis, is the second most common reason for renal transplantation. Findings on IVP, usually nonspecific, include diffuse renal enlargement with calyceal distortion.

Since the introduction of effective chemotherapy, renal tuberculosis is much less common than in the first half of this century. The acid-fast tuberculosis bacteria attack the renal cortex or the glomeruli where they form abscesses that coalesce to form large, caseating granulomas. It is not unusual for the ureter and bladder to become involved because of rupture of these abscesses into the renal collecting system. Since this disease is uncommon, clinical suspicion is the most important step in diagnosis. Typical findings on IVP include scarred, narrowed, and elongated renal infundibula as well as a scarred and strictured ureter. Histologic findings are those of caseating granulomas associated with Langhans' giant cells. With adequate chemotherapy, nephrectomy is rarely necessary.

Two less common inflammatory diseases are malakoplakia and xanthogranulomatous pyelonephritis. Malakoplakia is an inflammatory process found throughout the urinary tract and renal parenchyma. The process, which may be associated with chronic irritation and repeated infection, is identified in females at least 80% of the time. The offending organism is uniformly *E. coli*. Presentation consists of fever, hematuria, pyuria, and flank pain. IVP shows a distorted renal collecting system with renal enlargement. Treatment for this disease is directed toward controlling the chronic infection through long-term administration of antibiotics. Xanthogranulomatous pyelonephritis has been called "the great imitator"; it is frequently misdiagnosed as renal cell carcinoma. The lesions may be quite large and invade adjacent structures. Nephrolithiasis and staghorn calculi are typically present. While the etiology of the disease is unknown, females are affected more frequently (70%). Because of the high mortality rate associated with staghorn calculi, nephrectomy is usually required.

Treatment. Simple nephrectomy is often necessary for nonmalignant renal disease, such as nonfunction, nephrolithiasis, abscess, and chronic hydronephrosis. The preferred approach is through the flank, over the bed of the 11th or 12th rib. If necessary, the rib is partially resected. Before nephrectomy is considered, the contralateral kidney and overall renal function must be evaluated by IVP or nuclear scan to insure adequate residual renal function.

In the pediatric age group, a nonfunctional kidney often is part of a duplicated system. If the lower pole is working, an upper pole nephrectomy is performed. In cases of ureteral pelvic junction obstruction, especially in the neonatal period, every effort should be made to preserve renal function by performing a pyeloplasty. In children, the kidney has a tremendous propensity to recover function.

Renal Masses

Renal masses may be classified as benign or malignant; malignant tumors are either primary or metastatic. The most commonly encountered renal mass lesion is a simple cyst (70% of cases). Tumors metastatic to the kidney are the most common neoplasms but usually are occult. Renal cell carcinoma is the most common primary neoplasm of the kidney and accounts for more than 85% of all primary renal cancers in adults. This chapter will discuss only the most frequently encountered tumors.

Evaluation. With the advent of computed tomography in the 1970s, the evaluation of renal masses has been revolutionized. CT scanning plays a prominent role in the workup of solid renal masses and may be valuable in characterizing some atypical cystic masses. Cystic lesions are frequently identified by IVP and confirmed by ultrasound. A fairly standard algorithm for the evaluation of a renal mass is found in Figure 9.16. Arteriography, once a standard preoperative study, is recommended only in selected cases where the diagnosis is in doubt or aberrant vasculature is expected. In cases of large lesions or right-sided tumors, an inferior vena cavagram is an important preoperative study to determine the extent of involvement and to aid in planning the surgical approach.

Benign Neoplasms. While most cystic lesions are asymptomatic and require no intervention, some are multicystic or complex and require further investigation to rule out malignancy. Cysts may enlarge to the point of compressing abdominal contents and adjacent organs, and they may cause flank discomfort. Cysts may be found in as high as one-third of the population. These cysts have a low incidence (4:1400) of malignancy. Solid tumors may arise from any of the cell types found in the kidney. The most frequently encountered lesions are renal cortical adenomas. Debate exists as to whether these lesions are benign or represent the earliest, confined stage of well-differentiated renal cell carcinoma. While a size less than 3 cm has been suggested to predict whether the tumor is benign, numerous authors have reported metastases in smaller lesions. Because there is currently no agreement on objective parameters to distinguish between a cortical adenoma and a renal cell carcinoma, all renal cortical tumors should be treated as carcinoma and nephrectomy performed. The treatment is discussed later in this section. Recently, interest has been rekindled in partial nephrectomy for small, solid tumors near a renal pole.

Malignant Neoplasms. Renal cell carcinoma is by far the most common primary solid tumor affecting the kidney, but it accounts for only about 3% of adult malignancies. While etiologic factors have not been well documented in human beings, nitrosamines have been implicated in animal studies. Carcinogens found in cigarette smoke have been implicated, but no specific carcinogen has been identified. It has a 2:1 male-to-female preponderance, and a well-documented association with von Hippel-Lindau disease. Typically unilateral, this lesion is spherical with a pseudocapsule of parenchyma and fibrosis.

Hematuria is the single most common sign, occurring in 29–60% of reported cases. Flank pain and palpable flank mass occur next most frequently, but the classic triad of hematuria, flank pain, and a palpable abdominal mass are reported in only 4–17% of cases. Other common signs and symptoms are fever, anemia, and elevated sedimentation rate. While serum lactate dehydrogenase and alkaline phosphatase may be elevated, there are no reliable tumor markers for renal cell carcinoma.

In later stages this tumor invades the renal vein and vena cava and may even extend into the right

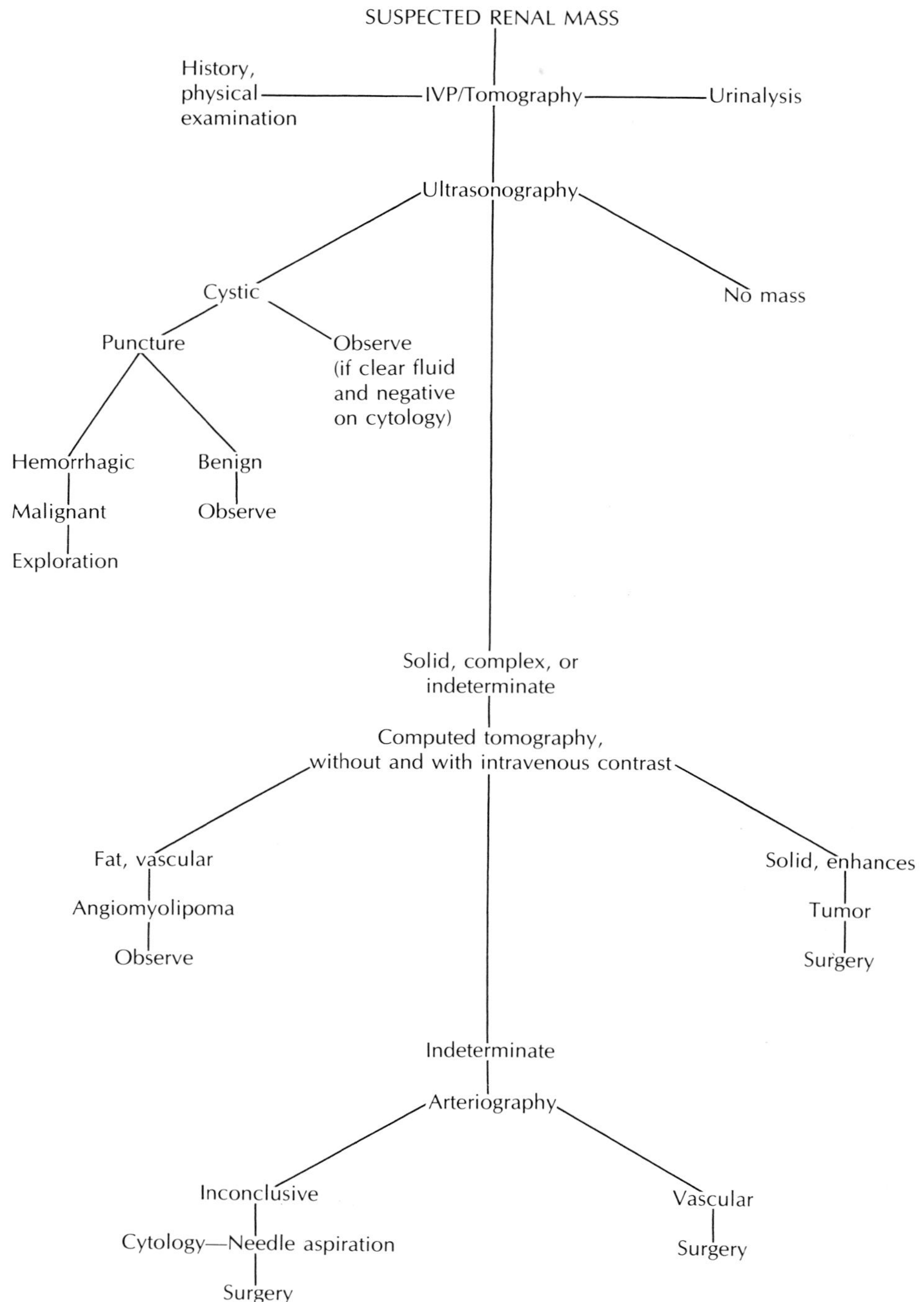

Figure 9.16. Algorithm for evaluation of a renal mass.

atrium. Because the right renal vein is short, vena cava involvement from right renal cell cancers is more frequent. Staging systems, including one proposed by Holland (Fig. 9.17) and a TNM system (Table 9.2), are used to determine the extent of the primary lesion, involvement of contiguous structures, extent of vascular involvement, and whether the tumor has metastasized. Renal cell carcinoma metastasizes most frequently to lungs, bone, and brain, in that order. Metastatic lesions may appear in both the ipsilateral and contralateral kidney, and late metastasis may occur to the liver. Five-year survival rates for stages I and II are 50–60%, and for stages III and IV are 30–40%.

Treatment for renal cell carcinoma, as for other malignant renal tumors, is radical nephrectomy (Fig. 9.18). While small, stage I tumors may be approached through the flank, lesions over 5 cm are better exposed through a thoracoabdominal or transabdominal approach. The kidney, perinephric fat,

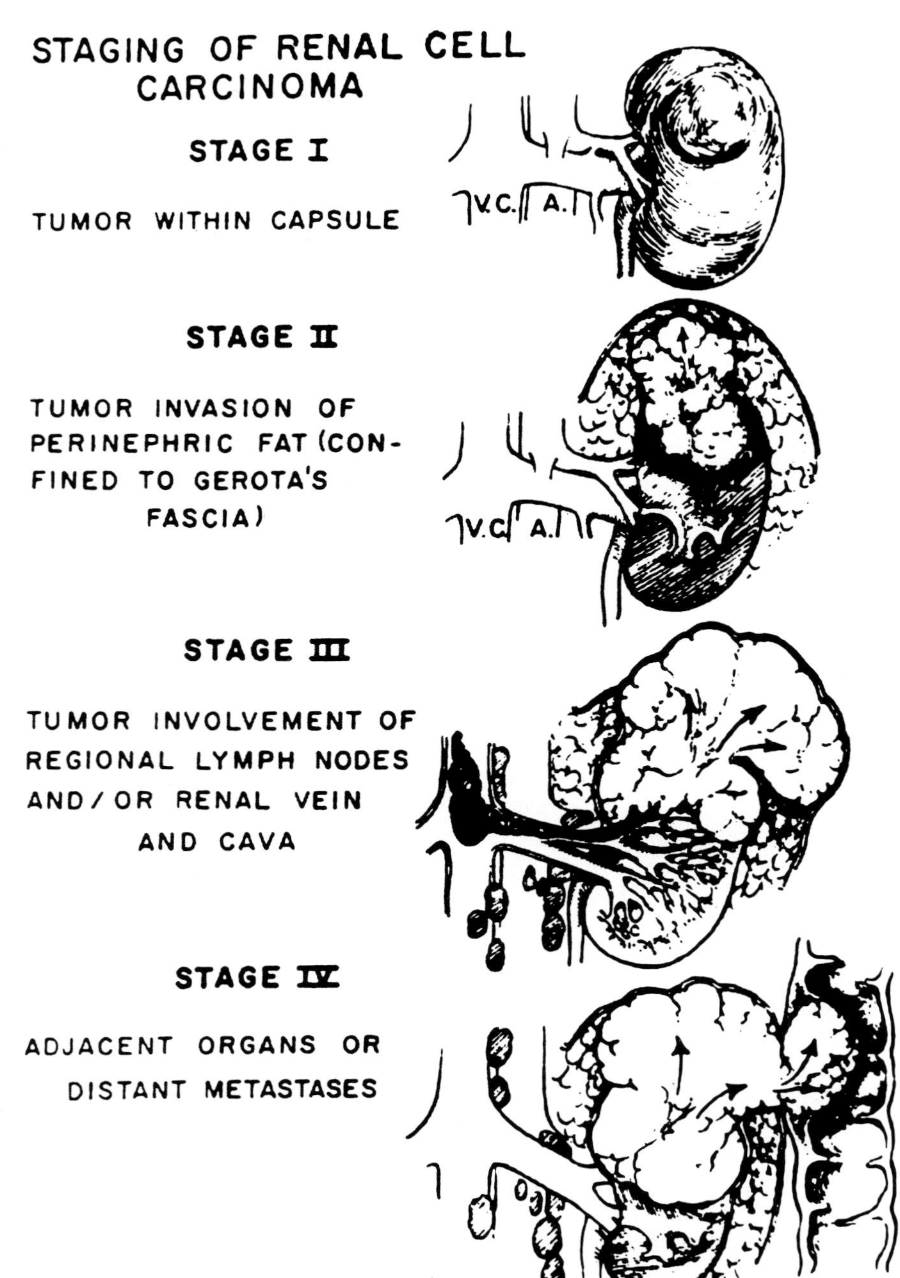

Figure 9.17. Staging of renal cell carcinoma as proposed by Holland, in accord with schemes of Robson, Murphy, and Flocks and Kadesky.

Gerota's fascia, ipsilateral adrenal gland, and ipsilateral regional nodes should all be removed. Large incisions allow for early control of the renal vessels before manipulation and dissection. In cases of vena cava involvement, the incision may need to be extended or a median sternotomy performed in order for adequate exposure. The vena cava, which is controlled superiorly and inferiorly, may be incised in order to remove a tumor thrombus. The lumbar and contralateral renal veins must be controlled as well. Postoperative complications include bleeding, retroperitoneal abscess, ileus, and wound infection, as well as recognized complications of abdominal surgery (e.g., pulmonary embolism).

Transitional cell carcinoma (TCC) of the renal pelvis may present as a renal mass or a filling defect on IVP. Urine cytology may be negative but usually shows abnormal cells. Small lesions are hard to see by computed tomography. Many upper tract lesions seed the lower urinary tract, making upper tract evaluation paramount when TCC is found in the lower tract. Treatment is nephroureterectomy with a partial cystectomy because of the high incidence of ipsilateral ureteral orifice and bladder involvement.

Table 9.2.
TNM Staging Protocol for Renal Carcinoma

T—Primary Tumor	
TX	Minimum requirements of assessment not met
T0	No evidence of primary tumor
T1	Small tumor, minimal renal distortion, surrounded by parenchyma
T2	Large tumor, renal deformity or enlargement
T3a	Large tumor involving perinephric tissue
T3b	Tumor involving renal vein
T3c	Tumor involving renal vein and subdiaphragmatic vena cava
T4	Tumor extending into neighboring organs or abdominal wall
N—Nodal Involvement	
NX	Minimum requirements for assessment not met
N0	No evidence of involvement of regional nodes[a]
N1	Single, homolateral regional nodal involvement
N2	Involvement of multiple regional nodes, contralateral or bilateral
N3	Fixed regional nodes (by exploration)
M—Distant Metastasis	
MX	Minimum requirements for assessment not met
M0	No known distant metastasis
M1	Distant metastasis present (specify site)

[a]Para-aortic and paracaval nodes.

Urinary Stone Disease

Urinary tract calculi represent a significant cause for morbidity in the United States: more than 500,000 people are affected yearly. Males are affected more often than females, and the 30- to 50-year age group has the highest incidence. Risk factors have been associated with specific types of stone formation. Factors leading to formation of calcium oxalate stones include a diet high in calcium intake, hyperparathyroidism, warm tropical climates, sedentary occupation, and a family history of renal tubular acidosis. Risk factors for uric acid stones include high dietary intake of purines, history of gout, and hyperuricosuria. Cystine stones are usually seen in families with a history of cystinuria. Struvite or infection stones develop in patients with urinary obstruction and urinary tract infections.

A number of theories have been proposed to describe the mechanism of stone formation. The most widely accepted theory proposes that urine becomes supersaturated with either calcium oxalate or uric acid. Once supersaturation occurs, spontaneous crystallization follows. These crystals are then either passed harmlessly through the kidney into the ureter or become lodged in the collecting system. Once they lodge, the crystals develop rapidly, forming a stone. If the stone obstructs the UPJ or ureter, hydronephrosis and infection can result. It is believed, but as yet unproven, that individuals who form stones do not possess certain molecular inhibitors, such as citrate, which can prevent stone formation in the urine. The most common stones are composed of calcium oxalate and are thought to be caused by hyperparathyroidism and the absorptive hypercalciurias. The intestines absorb more calcium than the kidneys can handle; the urine becomes hypercalciuric, leading to crystallization. Or, a renal leak can cause a loss of calcium, stimulating the parathyroid to produce parathyroid hormone (PTH), which causes increased absorption of calcium through Vitamin D synthesis in the intestine. Uric acid stones are usually due to a hyperuricosuria, which provokes crystallization through supersaturation. Cystine stones represent a true inherited disorder, in which the renal tubules fail to transport four amino acids. These patients develop stones early in life. Struvite calculi or infection stones are usually composed of magnesium, ammonia, and phosphate. They are described as staghorn calculi and are related to infected urine as well as to a foreign body.

Symptoms and Signs. Urinary tract stones are usually diagnosed in the emergency room. Renal colic is the presenting symptom in most patients with symptomatic stones; it is described as a constant pain in the flank radiating to the groin, accompanied by nausea and vomiting. The pain can be acute and so severe that even large doses of narcotics cannot control it. As the stone moves downward and enters the intramural portion of the ureter, it causes patients to experience urgency and frequency. Actual passage of the stone through the urethra is relatively uneventful. Large nonobstructing renal calculi are usually asymptomatic. These stones are discovered either surreptitiously on urinalysis when hematuria is discovered or on x-rays ordered for an unrelated condition. Large staghorn calculi are usually silent. If left untreated they will cause autonephrectomy of the renal unit.

Evaluation. A workup for renal stones includes serum calcium and parathyroid hormone determinations to rule out primary hyperparathyroidism. In addition, urinary pH must be evaluated to determine whether the patient has renal tubular acidosis, a condition occasionally responsible for stone disease. Urine collections over a 24-hour period can reveal idiopathic hypercalciuria or idiopathic hyperuricosuria. Tests with a calcium load or with a low calcium diet may elucidate whether the renal problem is caused by a GI abnormality, such as short gut syndrome or a primary GI hyperabsorption problem. Additional studies include cyclic adenosine monophospate (cAMP) and PTH as well as determination of the urine creatinine-to-calcium ratios. In a case of acute obstruction, these studies should be made after the patient has passed the stones and is on a normal diet.

Treatment. Treatment of urinary calculi depends on the size, location, and composition of the stones. Calcium oxalate stones less than 5 mm will usually pass spontaneously. These and calcium phosphate stones will not respond to medical management. If the stone is greater than 5 mm and is located in the kidney, extracorporeal shock wave lithotripsy (ESWL—discussed below) is the choice of therapy. A large stone lodged in the ureter for any length of time will require either ureteroscopic removal or ESWL. Uric acid stones, usually nonopaque, are seen on IVP as a filling defect. If the stone is not large, urinary alkalization and increased

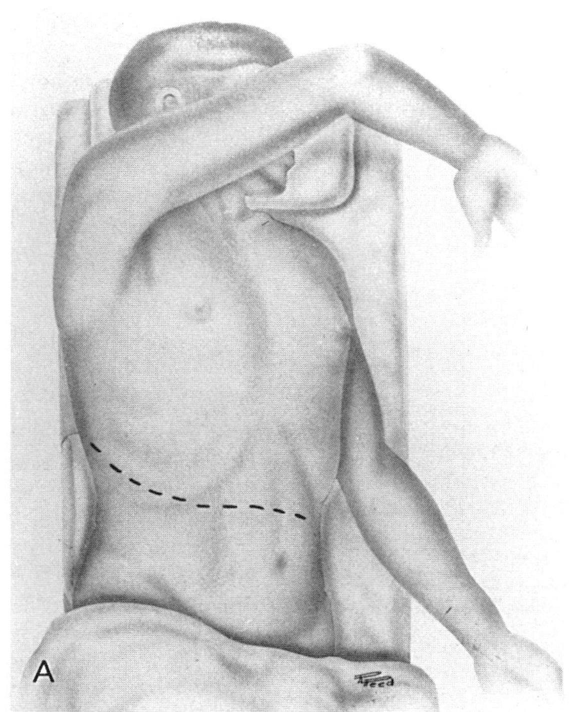

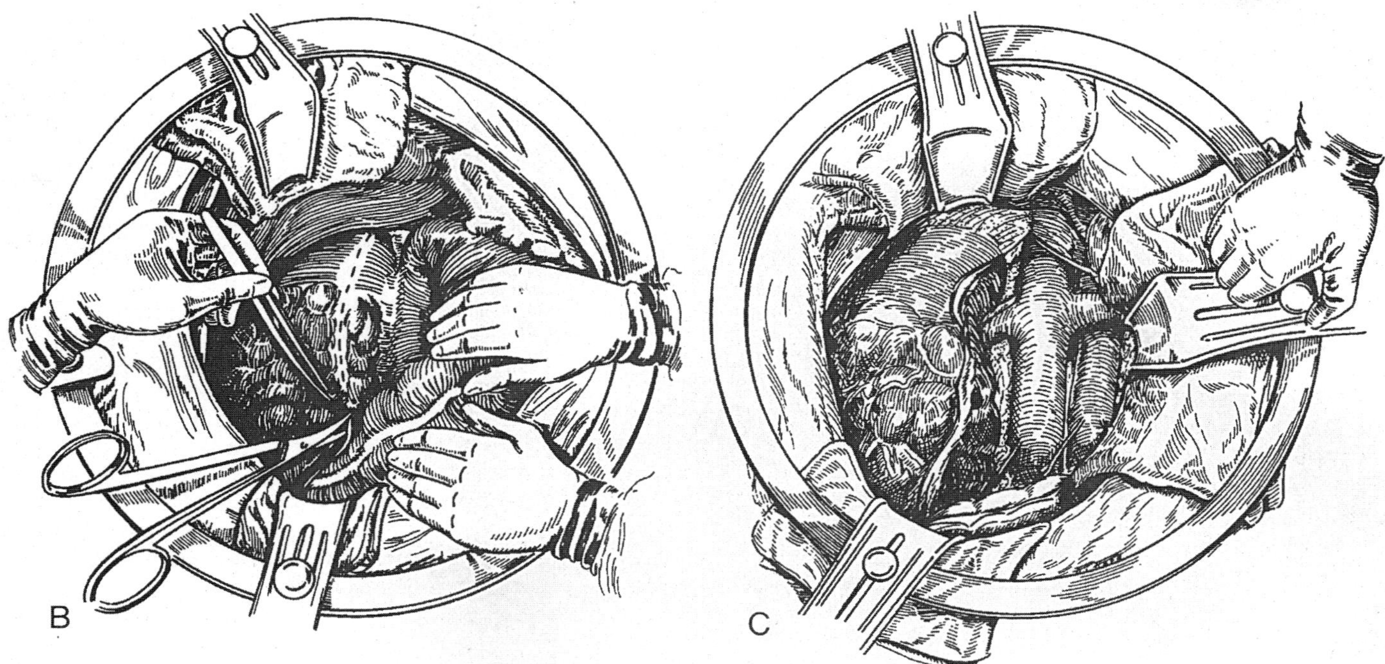

Figure 9.18. **A**, Eleventh rib surgical approach for radical nephrectomy. **B**, Right kidney, renal artery, and tumor identified. **C**, Line of incision in retroperitoneum to expose right kidney.

fluid intake can eventually dissolve it. These stones do not disintegrate well on ESWL. For prophylaxis, the patient can be treated with allopurinol 300 mg once a day and maintenance of an alkaline urine. Cystine stones also resist disintegration so are not amenable to ESWL. These stones can be treated as well with urinary alkalization as well as with d-penicillamine, a chelating agent. Thiola (α-mercaptopropionylglycine) is an alternative for people who cannot tolerate the toxic side effects of d-penicillamine. Struvite stones can be treated by ESWL; however, since most of these stones are large staghorns, percutaneous nephrostomy is required, followed by lithotripsy through the percutaneous tract. Once access is obtained, the stones can be dissolved

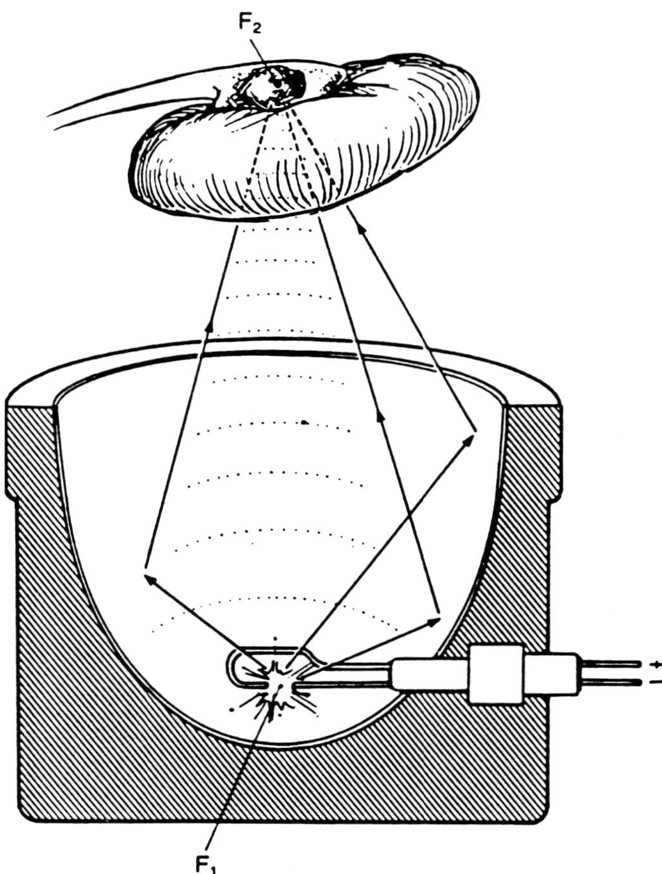

Figure 9.19. Spark gap electrode and semiellipsoid for focusing shock waves. Electrode is placed at first focus inside ellipsoid with stone placed at second focus.

with hemiacidrin and Suby's G solution. Large staghorns usually require multiple treatments with ESWL and percutaneous lithotripsy.

Extracorporeal Shock Wave Lithotripsy. Since its introduction in 1979, ESWL has revolutionized the treatment of renal calculi. There are now over 200 ESWL centers in the United States and Europe, mobile units servicing small hospitals, and second-generation machines available. One-half million patients have been treated successfully and morbidity has been minimal.

The technology involves transmission of a focused shock wave from outside the body to the calculus. A high-voltage underwater spark gap initiates the shock wave. The gap or discharge, occurring in approximately 1 microsecond, results in vaporization of the fluid surrounding the arc, developing a plasma-like state. This explosive vaporization of fluid propagates a high-energy shock wave, which is focused by surrounding the spark gap with a semi-ellipsoid, allowing concentration of the energy at a second focal point, F2 (Fig. 9.19). By placing the calculus at this second focal point, the destructive energy is transmitted to the stone causing it to fragment.

Approximately 85% of patients requiring treatment for kidney stones undergo ESWL. About 75% treated for solitary stones 1 cm or less in size will be stone-free in 3–6 months, while the remainder need more than one treatment. Of treated patients, 96% remain complication-free. Most patients can be treated as outpatients, while others need only an overnight stay. While some tissue damage occurs, there is no evidence that this treatment causes any long-term deleterious effects.

Endourological Treatment. Endourological treatment has become available since the introduction of percutaneous nephrostomy in 1955. Refinements in instrumentation have led to the development of diagnostic and operating ureteonephroscopes. Increased visualization and manipulation capabilities make it possible to perform transureteral resection of ureteral neoplasms, biopsy suspicious ureteral lesions, free impacted ureteral calculi, and fulgurate bleeding points. Direct vision manipulation of ureteral calculi and their fragmentation with either electrohydraulic or ultrasonic lithotriptors is now accomplished safely with little damage to the ureter. The development of intraureteral laser fragmentation techniques, as well as of flexible ureteroendoscopy, will continue to increase the usefulness of endourologic techniques.

For endourological treatment, either an antegrade or a retrograde approach is chosen. In the retrograde approach, stones are removed by either standard cystoscopic techniques (using wire baskets) or by newer ureteroscopic techniques (using baskets, grasping forceps, or either ultrasonic or electrohydraulic lithotripsy). Additionally, stones may be dislodged in a retrograde fashion into the renal pelvis for extracorporeal shock wave lithotripsy. Intraoperative fluoroscopy is necessary with any of these procedures.

The most common complications are infection, hemorrhage, and urine leak. Regardless of treatment modality, complications may occur during manipulation of the stone. The electrohydraulic lithotripter may damage the ureter or pelvis by either heat or concussion. The rigid scope may puncture the renal pelvis or fracture the kidney, especially when torque is applied to the instrument.

Extravasation of fluid during percutaneous renal surgery may occur either extraperitoneally, intraperitoneally, or intrapleurally. Extraperitoneal extravasation should be suspected on noting the following symptoms and signs: marked decrease in the return of irrigating fluid, narrowed pulse pressure, increased central venous pressure, increased systolic and diastolic pressure, dyspnea, and abdominal or flank distention. The clinical picture is one of hyponatremia that may become profound if not treated. Treatment is hypertonic saline and furosemide (Lasix) administration. The symptoms, signs, and effects of extravasation of irrigating fluid intraperitoneally are similar. The patient may experience labored breathing, arrhythmias, vomiting, and a tense, distended abdomen. Treatment consists of a peritoneal lavage catheter or a Stamey suprapubic catheter. A minilaparot-

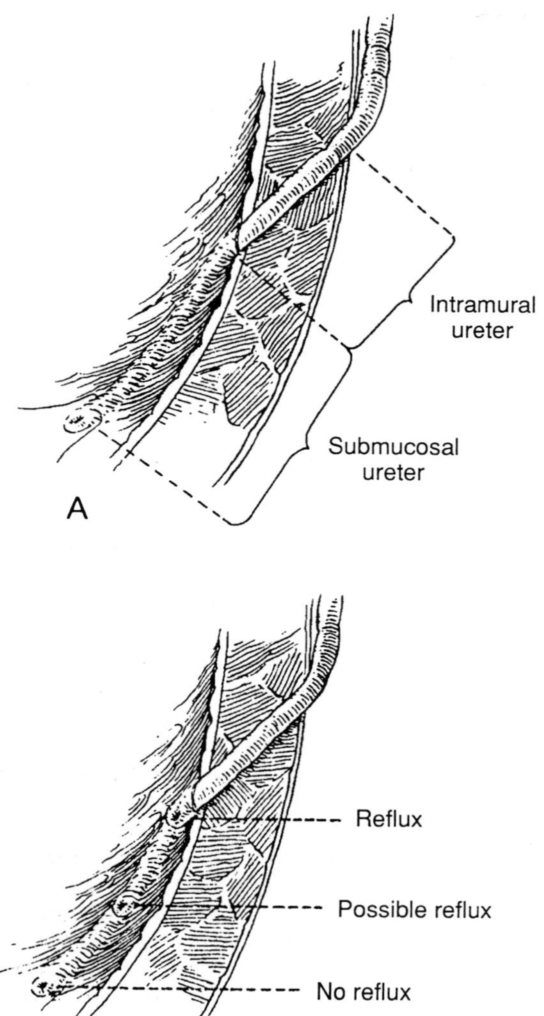

Figure 9.20. **A**, Normal ureterovesical junction, **B**, Refluxing ureterovesical junction and ureterovesical junction showing inadequate submucosal tunnels.

omy may be required if prior abdominal surgery has been performed. The fluid is drained from the peritoneal cavity and the catheter left in place until the majority of the fluid is retrieved and the abdomen is soft. Electrolytes (especially serum potassium and sodium) and hematocrit should be monitored. If intrapleural extravasation occurs, dyspnea, hemoptysis, and elevated systolic pressure ensue. Treatment consists of chest tube placement with ventilatory support until the patient is stabilized.

Surgical Treatment. Surgical treatment is performed in only 4–5% of cases. Pyelolithotomy can be used to remove simple stones from the renal pelvis and occasionally a partial staghorn. An anatrophic nephrolithotomy is reserved for large staghorn calculi. An incision is made along the posterior avascular plane of the kidney. The collecting system is opened, the stone removed, and the kidney closed.

The Ureters

Anatomy

The ureters serve as conduits for urine between the kidneys and the bladder. Each enters the bladder posterolaterally on its inferior portion and courses obliquely for 1.5 cm through the bladder wall. For half that distance the ureter traverses the muscularis; for the other half it is submucosal. The lower portion of the ureter is anchored and supported by special fibromuscular tissue called Waldeyer's sheath. The normal anatomy of the ureter allows free efflux of urine into the bladder but prevents reflux. This one-way flow depends on the complex relationship between the ureteral muscle, the bladder base, and the ureteral route through the bladder wall. In its upper portions the ureteral muscle has an irregular helical pattern, while near the bladder and in its intramural portion the muscle fibers run parallel to the lumen. Peristalsis of the ureteral wall propels urine toward the bladder. As the contraction approaches the bladder, the longitudinal fiber arrangement causes the intramural ureteral lumen to open and shorten, allowing urine to enter. When a ureteral contraction is not present, increasing bladder pressure compresses the submucosal ureteral lumen against the underlying bladder muscle and prevents reflux (Fig. 9.20).

Ureteral Obstruction

Causes for ureteral obstruction include extrinsic masses such as colon tumor, gynecologic malignancy, vascular aneurysm, and inflammatory disease of the colon. Occasionally, the ureters become obstructed with stone fragments following extracorporeal shock wave lithotripsy. If ureteral obstruction is acute, most patients will feel pain and tenderness in the right flank and back. Increased renal pressure and ureteral spasms are believed to cause the pain. If ureteral obstruction is insidious, most patients will not feel much discomfort. It is not uncommon to find an extremely dilated ureter in patients who have long-standing obstruction. Obstruction is cleared by percutaneous nephrostomy, ureteroscopy, stenting, or use of a nephrostomy tube. If left untreated, ureteral obstruction can result in renal parenchymal loss, renal failure, and infection.

Iatrogenic Injuries to the Ureters

Iatrogenic injury to the ureters can occur during general, vascular, and gynecologic surgery. Diverticulitis, aortic or iliac artery aneurysms, and ovarian or uterine tumors exist in close proximity to the ureter, usually the distal third. The ureters are occasionally injured inadvertently during surgery for a large pelvic mass. A preoperative IVP helps the surgeon locate the ureters and avoid them during surgery. Ureteral "stents" may be placed through the bladder prior to surgery to help with intraoperative identification of the ureters. If the ureters are injured in a clean surgical field, they may be repaired with an end-to-end anastomosis and then stented. If they are injured in a contaminated surgical field, however, proximal urinary diversion with percutaneous nephrostomy or open nephrostomy becomes necessary. If the ureter is injured during repair of a ruptured intra-abdominal aortic aneurysm, urine must be kept away from the freshly operated aorta and vascular graft. If the opposite kidney is normal, the surgeon must therefore choose between nephrectomy, incubated ureterostomy, or nephrostomy.

The patient with an unrecognized ureteral injury often experiences flank pain, fever, and chills on the fourth or fifth postoperative day. A workup, including ultrasound or IVP, should be conducted to evaluate the urinary system. If the ureter has been in any way injured, proximal diverting percutaneous nephrostomy becomes necessary followed by a delayed repair. If the ureter has been injured during gynecologic surgery, early surgical exploration is recommended to reimplant the ureter. If there is not enough ureteral length for reimplantation, other techniques outlined elsewhere in this chapter may be necessary.

The Bladder

Anatomy

The bladder is a hollow muscular organ that functions to store urine and evacuate it. When empty, the bladder lies just behind the pubic symphysis. As it fills, its superior portion protrudes into the peritoneal cavity and can be palpated suprapubically. It is lined with transitional epithelium that lies on a loose, elastic connective tissue bed, the lamina propria. The muscle of the body of the bladder, the detrusor, is composed of interlacing smooth muscle bundles with no distinct layers. An exception is the trigone, a triangle-shaped area lying between the ureteral orifices and the urethral opening. In this area the muscle wall has two layers, a superficial one fusing with the ureteral musculature and a deeper one indistinguishable from the detrusor. While only the superior-most portion of the bladder is covered with peritoneum, the entire bladder is covered with the loose fascia of the pelvic cavity. The bladder is firmly attached to the posterior aspect of the pubic bone by condensations of this fascia, called the *puboprostatic ligaments* in males and the *pubovesical ligaments* in females. The median umbilical ligament, the fibrotic remnant of the urachus, attaches the bladder to the anterior abdominal wall. Condensation of the pelvic fascia in the dorsolateral aspect of the bladder also serves as anchor and neurovascular conduit. Blood is supplied by the superior, middle, and inferior vesical arteries, branches of the hypogastric artery. In females, blood is also supplied by the vaginal and uterine arteries. The bladder is surrounded by a rich plexus of veins that drains into the hypogastric veins. Bladder lymphatics drain to the external iliac, hypogastric, common iliac, and sacral lymph nodes.

Evaluation

Endoscopic Evaluation: Cystourethroscopy. The bladder and urethra are evaluated endoscopically by flexible and rigid cystoscopes. These contain an optical fiber-lens system for visualization, fibers to carry illumination, and ports for instruments, catheters, and irrigation fluid. The rigid cystoscope consists of a telescope, a bridge, and a sheath available in various sizes with input and output ports for irrigation. The bridge, forming a watertight connection between the sheath and telescope, may have one or two ports for the introduction of tools, catheters, or electrodes. The telescopes vary in viewing angles from 0° (straight ahead) to 120° (retroview). Flexible cystoscopes have a maneuverable tip for examining the bladder.

An examination regimen is used during cystoscopy to avoid oversights. The entire bladder mucosa is examined systematically for mucosal irregularities, tumors, lesions, or unusual vascularity. Trabeculation (formation of bands of muscle tissue) of the bladder wall, cellule formation (formation of small diverticula that have not yet protruded beyond the bladder wall), and diverticula are noted. Ureteral orifices are checked for position and configuration and their length measured using calibrated catheters. Ureteral urine as it effluxes into the bladder should be observed for color to rule out blood coming from either ureteral orifice. In addition, the bladder neck is evaluated for contracture, the prostatic fossa is checked for mucosal lesions and anatomic obstruction from prostatic tissue, and the urethra is examined for stricture formation, mucosal lesions, and tumors. Retrograde pyelography can be performed through the cystoscope: by inserting a catheter into the ureteral orifice and injecting radiographic contrast to evaluate ureteral and renal pelvic anatomy. Although cystoscopy provides information concerning the anatomy of the lower urinary tract, its ability to assess lower urinary tract function is extremely limited.

Urodynamic Evaluation. Urodynamics, a collection of studies used to evaluate the reservoir and micturition function of the lower urinary tract, is the cornerstone in evaluating neurologic bladder dysfunction. Urodynamic tests include postvoid residual (PVR) urine volume, cystometrogram, flow rate, urethral pressure profile, sphincter electromyography, and fluoroscopic cystography. The PVR is the volume of urine drained from the bladder by catheterization immediately after voiding. Ultrasound can also be used to measure the amount of residual urine. Normal individuals void to completion; residual urine occurs with bladder outlet obstruction, cystocele, and neurogenic bladders. The cystometrogram (CMG) evaluates intravesical pressures during filling and voiding. The CMG measures bladder sensation, capacity, compliance, and voiding pressures; it also can detect premature detrusor contractions. The normal bladder should fill to a capacity of 350–500 mL without a significant rise in pressure or detrusor contraction. The first sensation of needing to void occurs around 150–250 mL of filling, and definite fullness is sensed at 350–450 mL.

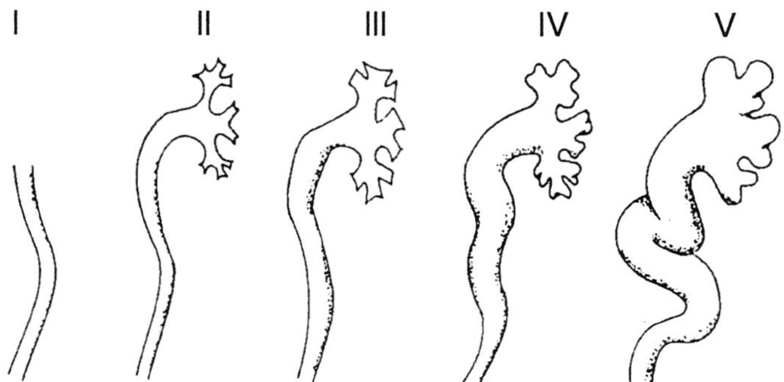

Figure 9.21. Grading of reflux based on findings on voiding cystourethrogram.

Urinary flow rate measures the rate of urine flow from the urethra. Normally, flow rates occur around a tight bell-shaped curve. Males have a peak flow rate of 20–25 mL/sec and females 20–30 mL/sec. Low flow rates indicate either bladder outlet obstruction or poor detrusor function. Intermittent flow rates indicate sphincter spasticity or abdominal straining to aid voiding. Urethral pressure recordings measure intraluminal pressures of the urethra, in order to evaluate sphincter function. Low urethral pressures indicate sphincter compromise. High pressures indicate obstruction from prostatic hypertrophy, stricture, or sphincter spasm.

Electromyography (EMG) is used to evaluate sphincter activity. Normally, sphincter EMG activity rises with filling and drops just before voiding. When pudendal nerve damage has occurred, needle electrodes detect abnormal denervation potentials. Fluoroscopic cystoscopy can visualize the bladder neck and sphincter to determine overactivity or incompetence. It can also detect cystocele, descensus (bladder prolapse), and reflux.

Congenital Anomalies

Vesicoureteral Reflux. Primary vesicoureteral reflux (VUR) is the result of improper development of the longitudinal muscle of the distal ureter with an associated decrease in its intramural length. This anomaly allows potentially infected urine to reflux up the ureter, resulting in damage to the kidneys. The ensuing inflammatory reaction causes permanent tubular damage and loss of renal function. The degree of reflux can be graded to correlate with the possibility of spontaneous resolution or renal damage (Fig. 9.21). Lower grades of reflux (grades I and II) usually resolve as a child grows and the ureterovesical junction matures. Because higher grades of reflux are less likely to resolve spontaneously and present an increased risk of renal damage, surgical correction is recommended. Secondary reflux can occur after resection of the ureteral orifice during removal of an overlying tumor, after ureteral meatotomy to aid in stone removal, after kidney transplantation, or after dilation of the intramural ureter for ureteroscopy. Occasionally, secondary reflux may require operative intervention. During episodes of cystitis, marginally competent ureteral orifices may reflux, but this transient reflux usually subsides after resolution of the bladder inflammation.

Evaluation. Vesicoureteral reflux is most often discovered during the investigation for urinary tract infection (UTI). In children the prevalence of VUR is inversely proportional to age; it is associated with 29–50% of children evaluated for UTIs. The voiding cystourethrogram (VCUG) is the primary diagnostic test for reflux. The bladder is filled with contrast and visualized fluoroscopically to detect reflux as the bladder fills and voids. A VCUG should be performed 2–4 weeks after resolution of a UTI to avoid detecting transient reflux. A voiding cystourethrogram can also be performed using a radioisotope, which allows a smaller total dose of radiation and can detect smaller degrees of reflux. Renal ultrasound and intravenous pyelography detect upper tract dilatation but cannot by themselves diagnose reflux. Cystoscopy is not the usual test performed to demonstrate reflux, but it can be used to measure the intramural ureteral tunnel length with a calibrated ureteral catheter. Patients with longer submucosal tunnels have a better chance of spontaneous resolution.

Treatment. The therapeutic goal in VUR is prevention of urinary tract infections and renal damage. In children with reflux but without dilated ureters (grade I or II reflux), reflux disappears in 20–30% every 2 years with 80% resolving eventually. Continual low-dose antibacterials can be used prophylactically to prevent UTIs and protect the kidneys until reflux stops. It is essential that the antibacterial prophylaxis not be interrupted and that there be careful follow-up. The child should be recultured every 3 months, with each febrile illness, and with urinary symptoms. A VCUG should be performed yearly, along with an upper tract study (intravenous pyelography (IVP) or ultrasound) to detect upper tract scarring or dilation. Serum creatinine, blood-urea-nitrogen (BUN), height, weight, and blood pressure should also be checked yearly.

Surgical repair is undertaken in patients who have severe reflux or in those who fail medical management, either by poor compliance, repeated UTIs despite prophylaxis, or loss of renal function. The goals of ureteral reimplantation include lengthening the intramural portion of the ureter to 4 to 5 times its diameter, immobilizing the ureteral meatus by anchoring it to the underlying detrusor, and supporting the intramural ureter with firm underlying bladder wall. In cases with severe reflux and marked ureteral dilation, the ureter may require plication or tapering before reimplantation.

A new mode of therapy for reflux is the transurethral injection of collagen or Teflon into the bladder wall just below the ureteral orifice. While this method has been effective in milder forms of reflux or after failed reimplants, it is too new to have yielded long-term results or to have received FDA approval for general use.

Currently, there are several techniques used to perform a ureteroneocystotomy, allowing the operation to be tailored to fit the patient's needs and anatomy. Ureteral advancement procedures, such as the Glenn-An-

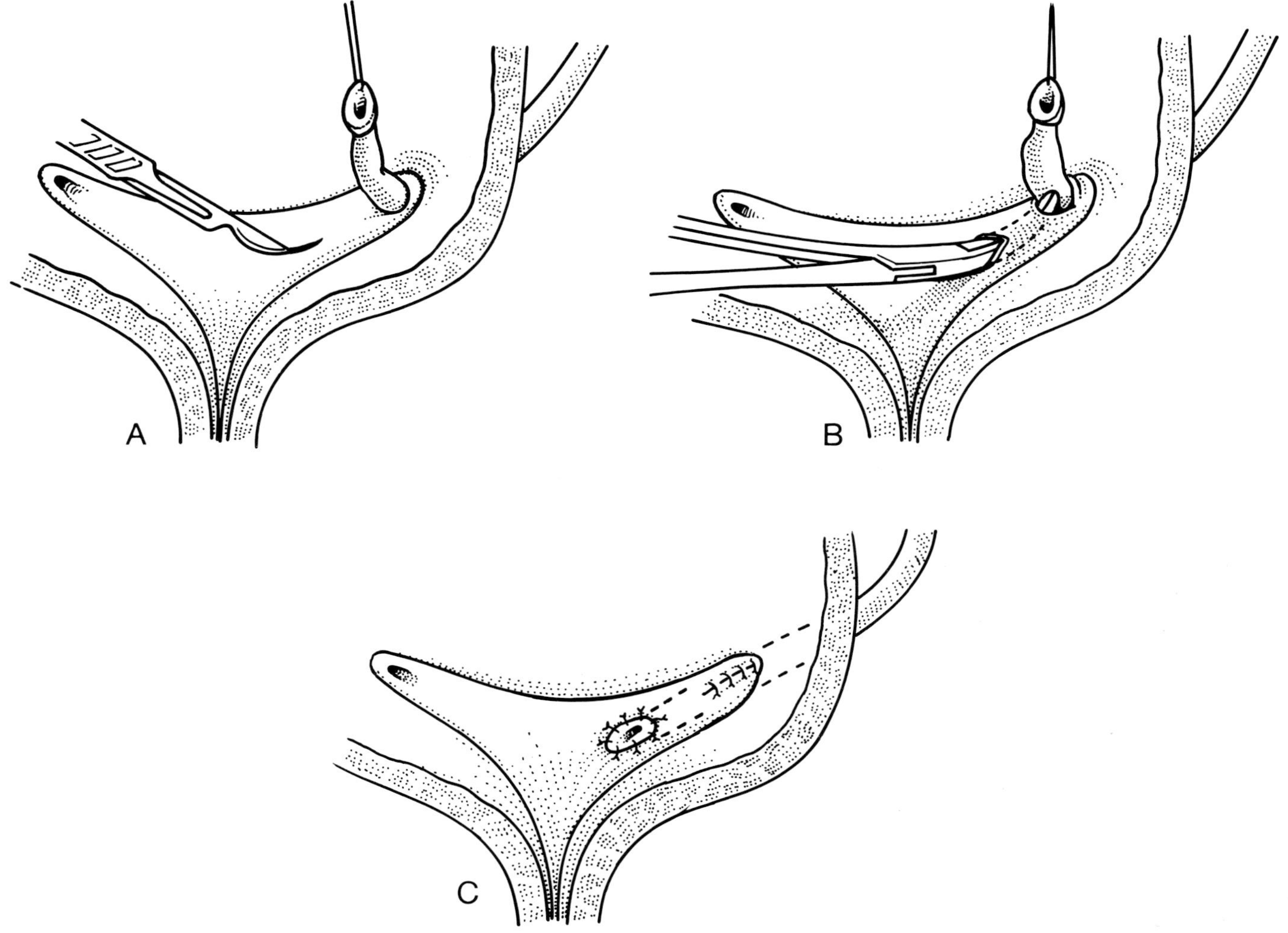

Figure 9.22. Glenn-Anderson Technique. **A**, Ureter has been mobilized and the new site for the meatus is incised. **B**, Ureter is brought through a new, longer submucosal tunnel to the new meatus site. **C**, Completed procedure showing the longer submucosal tunnel.

derson technique, can be applied when the ureteral meatus is high and lateral enough to allow creation of a tunnel of adequate length without placing the new meatus too close to the bladder neck. The ureteral meatus is approached transvesically and the surrounding mucosa circumscribed. A stent is placed up the ureter and sutured to the mucosa next to the meatus (Fig. 9.22). The Cohen procedure is a cross-trigonal advancement of the ureter that can be used when there is insufficient space between the ureteral hiatus and the bladder neck (Fig. 9.23). The Politano-Leadbetter technique is often used when reoperation is required. Although originally a transvesical procedure, it is now most often approached as a combined transvesical and extravesical procedure, in which the ureter is completely mobilized from the bladder. The submucosal tunnel is lengthened by creating a new hiatus superolaterally. The old hiatus is closed and the new orifice is created nearer the bladder neck. The ureter is then brought through the new hiatus and passed submucosally to the new orifice and secured there (Fig. 9.24).

Other Anomalies

Exstrophy of the bladder is the result of improper development of the anterior abdominal wall, pelvic girdle, and anterior wall of the bladder. It results in exposure of the posterior wall of the bladder through the abdominal wall and a separation of the symphysis pubis. It is an uncommon anomaly (1:30,000 births) and has a 3-to-1 male predominance. Besides disfigurement and total incontinence, bacterial colonization and urinary tract infections are common. Surgical attempts to reconstruct the lower urinary system can be successful, especially in milder forms of the disorder. However, total urinary diversion is often necessary to preserve renal function and ease the care of affected individuals. Adenocarcinoma often develops on the site of exstrophic mucosa.

Urachal persistence can occur in the form of an umbilical sinus, abdominal wall cyst, diverticulum at the bladder dome, or fistula from bladder to umbilicus. These are best treated with simple excision. Persistent urachal remnants are also associated with adenocarci-

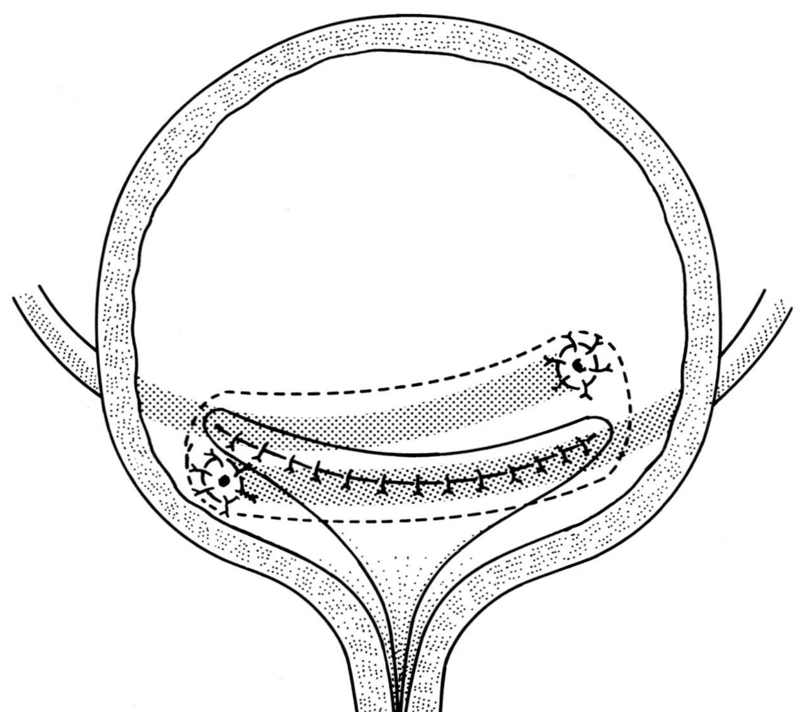

Figure 9.23. Cohen procedure: cross-trigonal ureteral advancement (bilateral reimplants using this technique are shown).

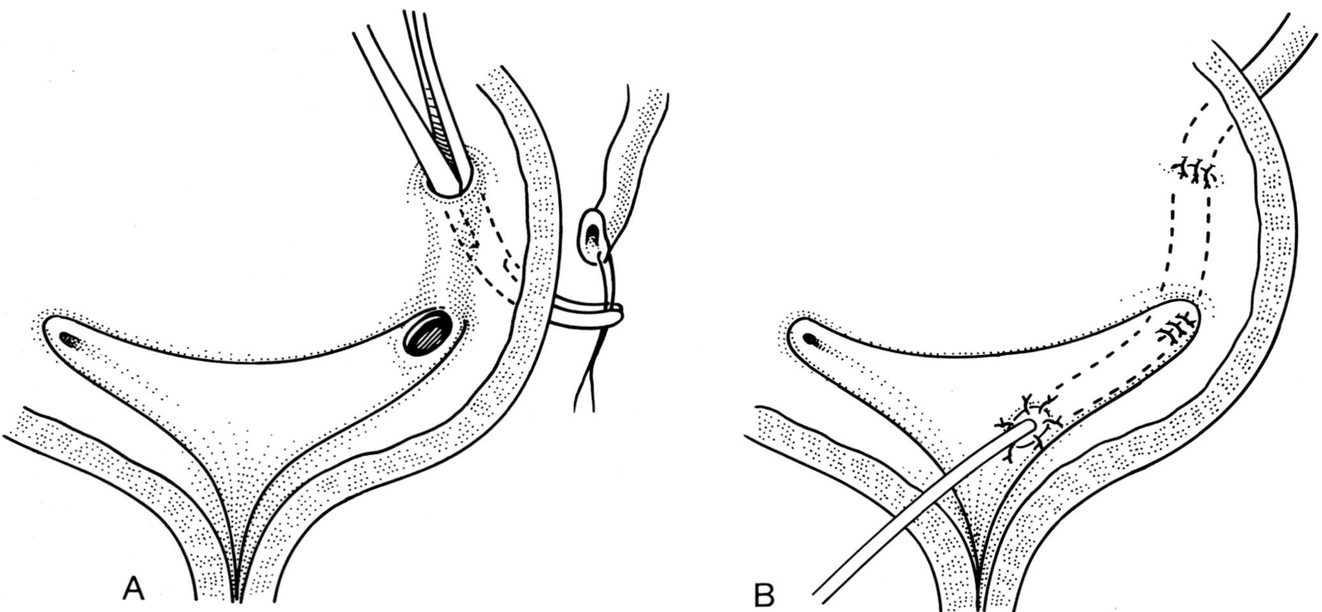

Figure 9.24. Politano-Leadbetter procedure. **A**, The ureter has been dissected completely and a new hiatus made superolaterally. **B**, The finished procedure with stent in place.

nomatous changes. Congenital diverticula are difficult to differentiate from acquired ones. Previously, presence of muscle in the wall of the diverticulum was considered to indicate a congenital origin, but this is no longer held to be true. Excision of the symptomatic diverticulum is the treatment of choice in most situations.

Trauma

Bladder injury can occur as a result of penetrating or blunt trauma. The most common causes of penetrating bladder injuries are gunshot wounds, stab wounds, and instrumentation. Pelvic fractures can cause punc-

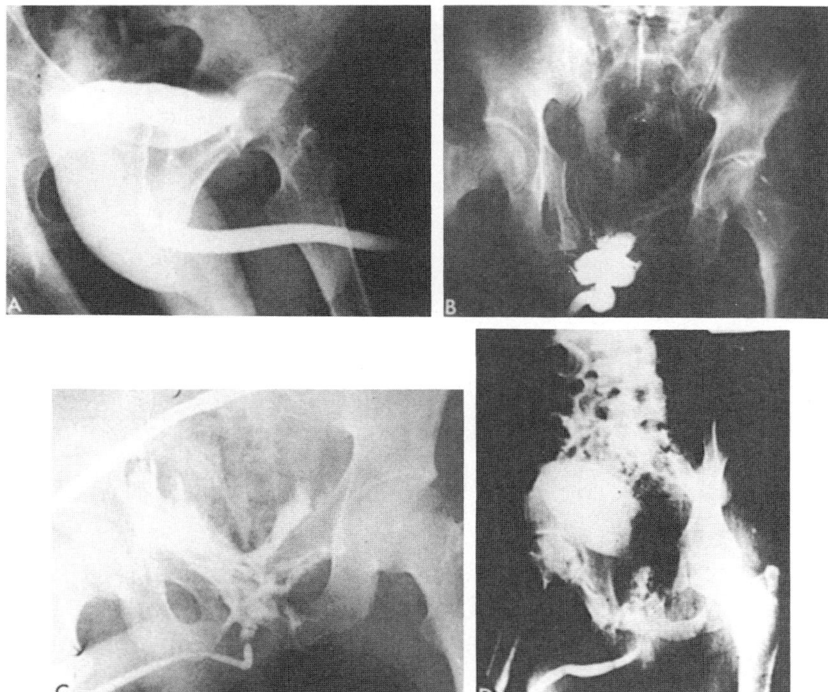

Figure 9.25. **A**, Normal retrograde urethrogram. Note that the contrast material has been injected *during* the exposure to ensure delineation of deep bulbar, membranous, and prostatic urethra. **B–D**, Rupture of urethra superior to urogenital diaphragm in male.

ture of the bladder wall either by sharp fracture edges or fragments. Blunt trauma, as occurs in motor vehicle accidents, causes a sudden rise in intravesical pressure, resulting in a bladder wall contusion or rupture. Bladder contusions often result in hematuria, while bladder tears may result in intraperitoneal or extraperitoneal extravasation. Traumatic bladder ruptures are often associated with damage to other pelvic and intra-abdominal organs.

Evaluation. Conscious patients with a bladder rupture often complain of severe suprapubic or pelvic pain with an inability to void. In unconscious patients, however, a high degree of suspicion is essential to make the diagnosis. Bladder ruptures almost invariably cause hematuria, and if associated with pelvic fractures a urethral disruption must be suspected. The most dependable diagnostic study for a bladder rupture is a cystogram. However, if accompanying urethral damage is suspected (because of blood at the meatus), a retrograde urethrogram must be performed to exclude a urethral tear prior to catheterization (Fig. 9.25). After a scout film has been taken, 200–350 mL of sterile contrast is instilled into the bladder of adults, the catheter clamped, and the necessary AP, lateral, or oblique film taken (Fig. 9.26). A postdrainage film is taken to exclude retrovesical extravasation.

Treatment. Small, extraperitoneal ruptures can be managed with 1–2 weeks of Foley catheter drainage with complete healing anticipated. However, close monitoring is necessary to detect prolonged bleeding or development of a pelvic abscess that requires open drainage and repair. Intraperitoneal bladder ruptures and large or complicated extraperitoneal bladder ruptures require surgical repair.

Repair consists of evacuating fluid and draining the area of extravasation, closing the bladder tear, and providing adequate urinary drainage. Since bladder ruptures are often associated with damage to other intra-abdominal organs, repair is often part of an exploratory laparotomy. Exposure is either through a midline suprapubic or low transverse (Pfannenstiel) incision. The midline is incised, the rectus muscles retracted laterally, the anterior surface of the bladder is freed from surrounding tissue, and the bladder is entered sharply. The bladder tear is inspected, debrided of any necrotic tissue, and closed in two or three layers with absorbable sutures. Absorbable sutures are always used to prevent an exposed piece of nonabsorbable suture from becoming a nidus for stone formation. The extravasated fluid is removed and the area irrigated with copious amounts of saline. If there is extraperitoneal extravasation it is prudent to drain the area externally for several days with Penrose drains. If drains are required in association with a pelvic fracture, a closed drain system should be used for only 24 hours to avoid infection. A suprapubic catheter is placed through a separate incision and the surgical cystotomy is closed. In 7–10 days a cystogram is performed to evaluate healing. The suprapubic tube is left in place until the tear has healed. At one time, peritonitis, abscesses, sepsis, and fistulas from the bladder to the bowel or skin were major causes of morbidity and mortality in patients with bladder perforations. Aggressive drainage, repair, and an-

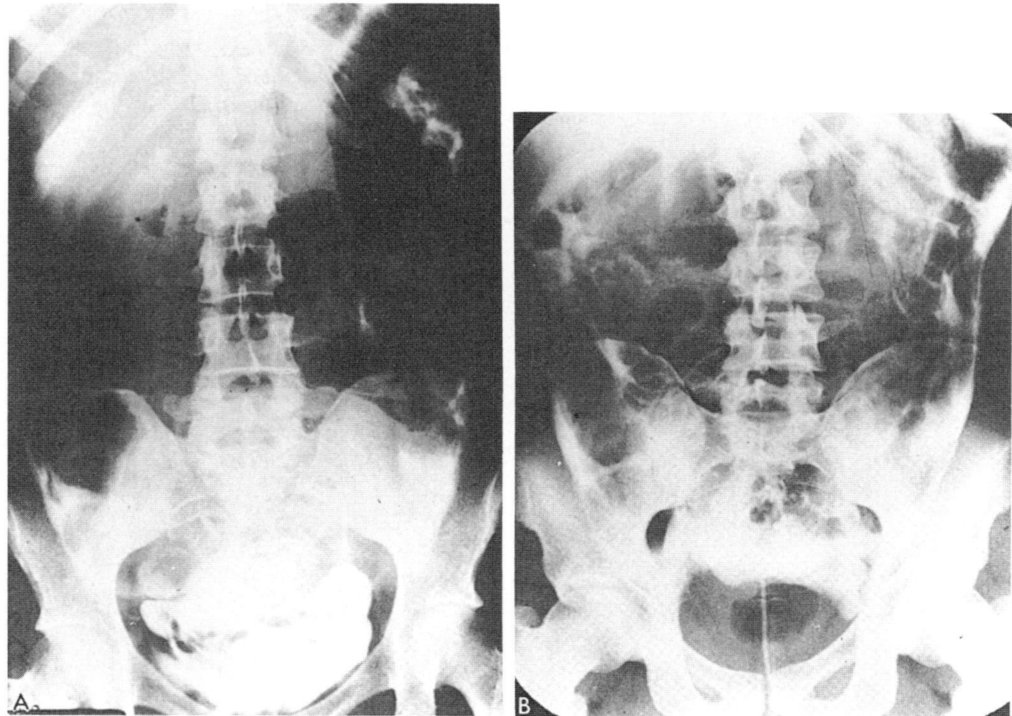

Figure 9.26. Intravesical urinary bladder rupture. **A**, Note pooling of contrast media in right upper quadrant of peritoneum. **B**, The contrast material outlines the peritoneal surface that the bowel interfaces.

tibiotic use have significantly reduced these complications.

Inflammatory Diseases

Bacterial Cystitis. Patients with bacterial cystitis have irritative voiding symptoms, including dysuria, frequency, urgency, nocturia, and, if the inflammation is severe enough, gross hematuria. Fever is not common with uncomplicated cystitis, and if present may indicate the presence of an upper tract infection. Bacterial cystitis is much more common in females, with bacteria ascending to the bladder by way of their shorter urethra. Studies indicate that the vaginal introitus becomes colonized with fecal organisms prior to cystitis. Females prone to recurrent urinary tract infections may be predisposed to infections because of increased vaginal and bladder mucosal bacterial adherence. In males, bacterial cystitis is usually the result of incomplete emptying of the bladder. The most common bacteria involved are the Gram-negative rods of the family *Enterobacteriaceae*. *E. coli* causes over 80% of all urinary tract infections.

Evaluation includes a urinalysis to determine the presence of bacteria, leukocytes, and red blood cells. A properly collected urine specimen (clean catch) for culture and sensitivity is necessary for accurate diagnosis. The initial antibiotic is chosen empirically, usually a drug effective against a broad range of Gram-negative organisms. Antibiotic therapy is then adjusted depending on the culture and sensitivity results. With appropriate therapy, symptoms should resolve in 3–5 days.

Further evaluation of the urinary tract, including cystoscopy and radiologic studies, is indicated in all males and in those females who fail to respond to antibiotic therapy, have multiple recurrent infections, symptoms of obstruction, vesicoureteral reflux, or calculi. The purpose of evaluation is to detect correctable causes of recurrent infections (see Table 9.3). Carcinoma or chronic interstitial cystitis should be considered in patients whose irritative voiding symptoms persist even after sterilization of the urine. To prevent bacteremia, manipulation of the urinary tract should be delayed for at least 7 days after the initiation of therapy and after the acute phase has resolved. Evaluation includes urinary cytologies, voiding cystourethrogram, intravenous pyelogram, or renal ultrasound, and/or cystoscopy. Although cystoscopy aids little in diagnosing bacterial cystitis, it can detect the presence of neoplasm or anatomic bladder outlet obstruction.

Interstitial Cystitis. Interstitial cystitis, a syndrome of no known etiology characterized by lower abdominal pain and irritative voiding symptoms, affects females predominantly. Urinalysis occasionally reveals microhematuria. Typically, urine cultures for bacteria, fungus, and viruses are negative. Cystoscopically, submucosal petechiae (glomerulations) may be seen. Rarely, a mucosal ulceration (Hunner's ulcer) is seen. Interstitial cystitis is a diagnosis of exclusion. Symptoms wax and wane. In some patients the pain and urinary frequency become debilitating. Histologically, the bladder is chronically inflamed, and in severe cases the bladder becomes fibrotic and contracted. Carcinoma in

Table 9.3.
Correctable Urologic Causes for Recurrent Urinary Tract Infections

Prostatic hypertrophy
Urethral stricture
Calculus
Chronic bacterial prostatitis
Ureteral reflux
Foreign body
Infected dysplastic or atrophic kidney
Urethral diverticulum
Papillary necrosis
Vesicovaginal or vesicointestinal fistula
Urachal cyst
Ureteral duplication or ectopy
Perivesical abscess

situ, which can also cause irritative symptoms in patients with sterile urine, is excluded by urinary cytology. Cystoscopy may reveal a Hunner's ulcer or glomerulations after hydrodistention of the bladder. Biopsies often show evidence of chronic inflammation, mast cell infiltration, and fibrosis. Therapy currently consists of bladder dilatations under general anesthesia and instillation of various substances (including dimethyl sulfoxide and oxychlorosene). Such therapy often brings temporary symptomatic relief. A subtotal cystectomy and augmentation with bowel or a cystectomy with diversion may be necessary in patients with a severely contracted bladder whose symptoms are incapacitating.

Degenerative Diseases

Bladder Fistulae. A fistula between the bowel and the bladder most commonly is caused by sigmoid diverticulitis, neoplasm, Crohn's disease, or penetrating abdominal injury. Patients often present with symptoms of urinary tract infection, hematuria, and fecaluria. Diagnosis is made by a combination of radiographs using water-based contrast enemas, cystograms, and/or cystoscopy. Treatment usually involves resection of the involved portion of the bowel, with either reanastomosis or colostomy, depending on the etiology. The edges of the bladder fistula are debrided and closed. Vesicovaginal fistula can occur from pressure necrosis during prolonged labor or from surgical injury. Incontinence, the usual presenting symptom, is typically continuous. The fistula may become apparent immediately after surgery or develop after several days. Diagnosis is made by a cystogram and cystoscopy. Intravenous pyelography is necessary to evaluate the upper tracts for obstruction or a ureterovaginal fistula. Small fistulae may be particularly difficult to delineate and may require additional maneuvers, including instillation of methylene blue into the bladder followed by insertion of a vaginal tampon to detect leakage. Leakage can also be detected by filling the bladder with radiographic contrast and then x-raying the tampon. Examination under anesthesia with distention of the bladder and vaginal inspection for the site of leakage is also helpful.

Repair of a simple vesicovaginal fistula can often be performed by a vaginal approach. With the patient in the lithotomy position, the vaginal portion of the fistula is incised and the edges of the vaginal mucosa mobilized. The fistula is dissected to the bladder and excised. The bladder edges are mobilized and closed with interrupted absorbable suture. The vagina is also closed with interrupted suture. However, if the scar tissue is extensive, the fistula is close to the ureters, or a previous vaginal repair has failed, an anterior abdominal approach is warranted. A midline abdominal incision is preferred. The bladder is opened and the fistula identified. The cystotomy incision is extended to the area of the fistula and the fistula is excised. The posterior surface of the bladder is dissected free from the anterior surface of the vagina. The vaginal defect is debrided and the edges mobilized and closed. The bladder defect is also debrided and closed. The omentum is then mobilized and sutured between the vagina and the bladder. The omentum provides separation of the two suture lines, a readily available vascular supply, and a supple tissue that will not heal with fibrosis. A suprapubic tube and a perivesical drain are placed. The suprapubic tube is removed 7–10 days later, after a cystogram shows healing of the fistula and the cystotomy.

Urinary Incontinence. Urinary incontinence is the involuntary loss of urine. It is caused by a failure of the bladder to store, failure of the sphincter mechanism to function, or a combination of both.

Taking an accurate history is essential in the evaluation of incontinence. The amount of leakage, associated activities, and voiding symptoms should be characterized. A voiding and incontinence diary that records the frequency, timing, and severity of episodes is helpful. The medical history should be reviewed for medications, trauma, pelvic or urinary tract surgery, difficult deliveries, neuromuscular disorders, diabetes, urinary tract infections, and abnormal bowel habits. In males a review of erectile and ejaculatory function may reveal neurologic dysfunction. The physical examination should include special attention to the abdomen, back, pelvis, and rectum. Perianal sensation, anal sphincter tone, as well as lower extremity motor and sensory function and reflexes should be evaluated.

Incontinence is classified by the symptoms associated with the leakage of urine. Stress urinary incontinence is the leakage of urine that occurs as a result of activities that cause a rise in intra-abdominal pressure, such as sneezing, coughing, or straining. Stress incontinence is caused by rotational descent of the bladder neck and internal sphincter from their normal intra-abdominal position. In the normal position, any rise in intra-abdominal pressure is transmitted not only to the bladder but to the bladder neck and sphincter as well. When this increased pressure is added to the intrinsic resistance of the sphincter, the sum is greater than the total intraluminal bladder pressure and continence is maintained. With descensus, intra-abdominal pressure exerts force only on the bladder, not on the sphincter, allowing the intraluminal bladder pressure to overcome the sphincter's resistance, causing leakage.

Detrusor instability has also been called urge incontinence. In patients with this condition, an involuntary contraction of the detrusor overpowers the sphincter and leakage occurs. These uninhibited contractions can be the result of a neurologic lesion or bladder irritation. In a large number of patients with detrusor instability, no cause has been found. Urge incontinence is an inaccurate label for this type of incontinence because patients may have no sensation that a contraction is occurring. These uninhibited contractions can also be precipitated by a change in position or by increased intra-abdominal pressure, making the differentiation between stress incontinence and detrusor instability based on symptoms alone almost impossible. Detrusor instability and stress incontinence are the two most common causes of female urinary incontinence and often occur simultaneously. These conditions have also been observed in men with prostate obstruction.

Incontinence can also be caused by sphincter dysfunction or an inability of the bladder to empty. Sphincter dysfunction can result from damage directly to the sphincter or its innervation from surgery, trauma, radiation, or cancer. Neurologic disorders and congenital anomalies can also affect sphincter function. Overflow incontinence occurs when the bladder overfills and uncontrollably empties. In these patients a large-capacity bladder, often with a weak detrusor, is the result of diabetic autonomic neuropathy, altered mental status, medications, or chronic outlet obstruction.

Evaluation. Females with suspected stress incontinence should be examined in the lithotomy position with a full bladder. About 80% of patients with stress incontinence will leak in this position with coughing; an additional 10% will leak when their pelvis is raised by 45°. A Bonney test is performed by transvaginally elevating the bladder neck to its proper anatomic position and having the patient cough. If there is no leak, incontinence is almost always surgically curable.

Laboratory evaluation should include urinalysis, urine culture, cytology (if indicated), a postvoid residual measurement, and urodynamic evaluation. A CMG is used to detect the presence of uninhibited bladder contractions; it can also differentiate pure stress incontinence from detrusor instability. Urethral pressure studies and sphincter EMG provide evidence of sphincter dysfunction. Fluoroscopic examination of the bladder neck and urethra during voiding documents the descensus of stress incontinence or detects bladder neck and external sphincter incompetence. Radiologic evaluation for incontinence is controversial. Upper tract evaluation should be done when indicated but is not a routine part of an incontinence workup. Cystoscopy cannot evaluate function but is used to rule out intravesical pathology.

Treatment. The cause of incontinence dictates the mode of therapy. Detrusor instability is treated effectively with anticholinergic medications such as propantheline or oxybutynin, which cause detrusor relaxation. Imipramine, a tricyclic antidepressant, is also effective in controlling bladder instability. Mild cases of sphincter dysfunction may be controlled by α-adrenergic medications such as ephedrine, pseudoephedrine, or phenylpropanolamine. Pelvic floor exercises may also be helpful in mild cases. In severe sphincter incompetence, a sling of fascia can be placed under the urethra to coapt its lumen and obstruct the urethra. The bladder is then drained by intermittent catheterization. Another option is an artificial urinary sphincter prosthesis.

Stress urinary incontinence is treated by restoring the bladder neck and urethra to proper anatomic position using any one of a number of procedures. The Marshall-Marchetti-Krantz procedure uses an anterior abdominal approach. The bladder and urethra are dissected off the posterior aspect of the pubic symphysis. Heavy, absorbable sutures are placed into the vaginal fascia on either side of the bladder neck and the urethra. These sutures are then placed in the posterior aspect of the symphysis to reposition and anchor the bladder and urethra superiorly and anteriorly. Usually drains are placed retropubically and a tube placed suprapubically (Fig. 9.27).

Elevation of bladder neck and urethra into proper position can also be accomplished with a suspension procedure using a combined vaginal and suprapubic approach. The Stamey, Raz, and other similar procedures place nonabsorbable sutures through a vaginal incision into the tissue on each side of the bladder neck. In the Stamey procedure, a small piece of Dacron vascular graft placed on the suture near the bladder neck serves as a bolster to prevent the suture from tearing out. In the Raz procedure, the suture is passed several times helically through the connective tissue lateral to the bladder neck. The tissue plane between the anterior surface of the bladder and the posterior aspect of the symphysis pubis that is dissected through vaginal incisions will fibrose and aid the nonabsorbable sutures to hold the bladder in proper anatomic position. In both of these procedures suprapubic incisions are used and a needle ligature carrier is passed from the suprapubic incision immediately behind the pubic symphysis through the vaginal incision. Both ends of the bladder neck sutures are passed by this needle into the suprapubic incision. The suspension sutures are then tied over the anterior rectus fascia with enough tension to correct the anatomy but not kink the ureter. A cystoscope is used during the procedure to confirm proper suture placement and to check for bladder penetration. A suprapubic tube, placed at the time of surgery, serves postoperatively as the primary bladder drainage. Later, as the patient begins to void, it serves to empty any postvoid residuals until normal voiding returns. Success rates of greater than 90% have been achieved with these procedures (Fig. 9.28).

Many times a cystocele (hernia of the bladder) will be present along with stress incontinence. An anterior colporrhaphy can frequently correct the anatomy sufficiently to control associated mild stress incontinence. Occasionally, after a bladder neck suspension there is a persistent cystocele and an anterior colporrhaphy is needed to correct it. An anterior colporrhaphy begins

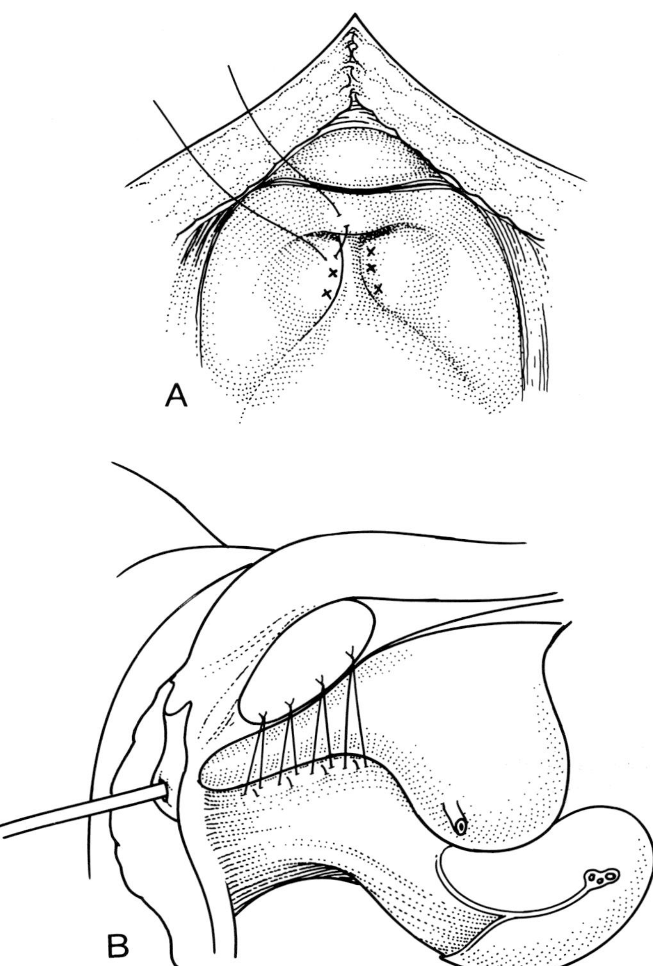

Figure 9.27. Marshall-Marchetti-Krantz procedure. **A**, Placement of absorbable sutures lateral to urethra and bladder neck as seen intraoperatively. **B**, Lateral view of completed repair with bladder neck and urethra in proper position.

with a vertical incision in the anterior vaginal mucosa beginning near the apex of the vagina that is carried down as near as necessary to the urethral meatus. The vaginal mucosa lateral to the incision is dissected off the underlying fascia. This step can be aided by submucosal infiltration with saline. Once the dissection is adequate, the thicker lateral fascia is approximated in the midline using interrupted absorbable sutures. The excess vaginal mucosa is trimmed and closed with care to obliterate any dead space between the fascia and mucosa. A vaginal pack of rolled gauze soaked with povidone and iodine is often used for 18–24 hours to provide mild tamponade.

Overflow incontinence is treated by improving bladder drainage. Relief of obstruction via a transurethral prostatectomy or repair of a stricture can control the incontinence. If bladder atony is present, intermittent catheterization will end the leakage.

Neurogenic Bladder Dysfunction. Micturition is a complex event requiring coordination between different levels of the central nervous system, the somatic and autonomic systems, and the detrusor and sphincter muscles of the bladder. During the storage phase, the bladder accommodates an increasing urine volume by reflex inhibition of detrusor muscle tone. (This ability to store larger amounts of urine without a significant rise in pressure is called *compliance*.) Also, during bladder filling sphincter muscle tone increases. Normal micturition, a voluntary event involving complex coordination of the detrusor and sphincter muscles, begins with relaxation of the external sphincter followed by relaxation and opening of the bladder neck and contraction of the detrusor. The normal detrusor contraction lasts long enough to empty the bladder. In the central nervous system there are highly integrated interrelations between the cerebral motor cortex, basal ganglia, cerebellum, pontine nuclei, and sacral cord nuclei that control voiding. Peripheral detrusor innervation is parasympathetic, mostly from S3 and some from S4. The trigone and bladder neck receive sympathetic output from T11 to L2. The external sphincter receives most of its input from S2 via the pudendal nerve. Disruption of any one of these pathways can result in a neurogenic bladder (see Table 4). Attempts to categorize the various neurologic bladder disorders have resulted in multiple systems of classification. The system devised by Lapides is one of the most useful for urologists because it describes bladder dysfunction as characterized by urodynamic evaluation.

Classification. The uninhibited neurogenic bladder is one that has uncontrolled detrusor contractions with filling. This overactive detrusor is often accompanied by decreased capacity but normal sensation and appropriate sphincter coordination. Patients complain of frequency, urgency, and urge incontinence. Neurologic lesions associated with this type of bladder interfere with the cerebral inhibition of bladder reflexes and include cerebral vascular accidents, tumors, cerebral palsy, dementia, and multiple sclerosis.

The reflex uninhibited bladder occurs as the result of suprasacral spinal cord lesions from trauma, transverse myelitis, cord tumors, or multiple sclerosis with cord involvement. In these patients, phasic uninhibited detrusor contractions occur and may be triggered by intrinsic or extrinsic stimulation. The sphincter is often dyssynergic and detrusor contractions can be unsustained, resulting in inefficient emptying. These patients have no sensation of bladder filling but may have autonomic reflex reactions to bladder distention such as sweating, headache, or lower extremity spasticity. Bladder compliance may be normal or decreased.

The autonomous neurogenic bladder shows no efficient voluntary or involuntary detrusor contractions on CMG. Voiding may be aided by increasing intra-abdominal pressure, but usually residual urine volume is large. Sensation is decreased or absent and compliance is variable. This type of neurogenic bladder results from damage to the sacral cord, conus medullaris, cauda equina, or sacral plexus from trauma, myelomeningocele, or pelvic surgery.

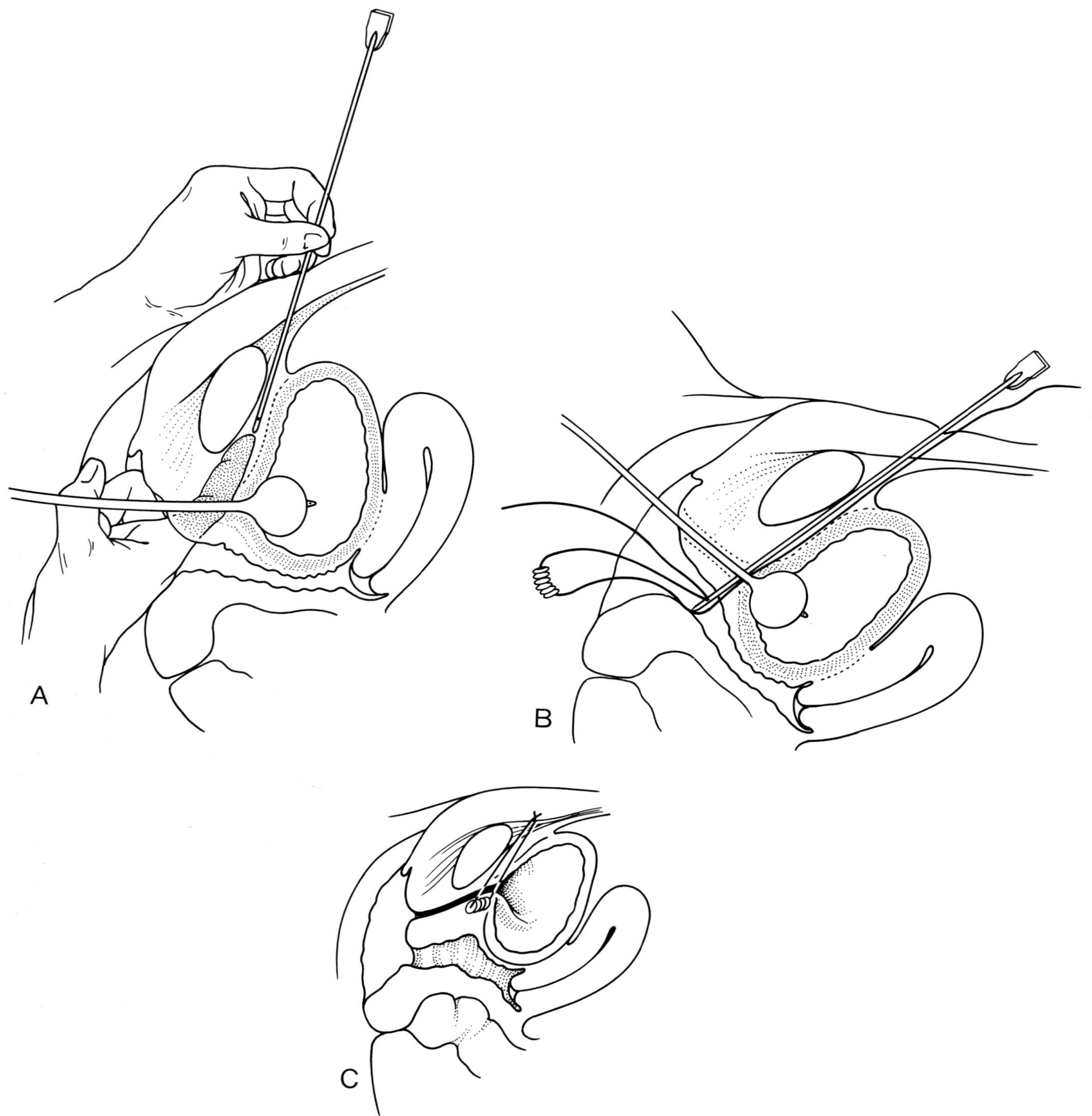

Figure 9.28. Stamey cystourethropexy. **A**, Lateral view showing passage of ligature carrier from the suprapubic incision, behind the pubic symphysis, and down to the vaginal incision (surgeon's finger is in the vaginal incision). **B**, Lateral view of ligature carrier with ready-to-pass second end of a suspension suture (note Dacron bolster). **C**, Lateral view of completed Stamey procedure with corrected position of bladder neck.

Table 9.4.
Effects of Neurologic Lesions on Bladder Function

Neurologic Lesion	Urodynamic Findings
Lesions above the brain stem	Involuntary bladder contractions
Complete lesions of the spinal cord above S2	Involuntary bladder contractions with smooth sphincter synergia and striated sphincter dyssynergia
Brain tumors	Detrusor hyperreflexia and urinary incontinence
Parkinson's disease	Detrusor hyperreflexia, urgency, frequency, urge incontinence
Shy-Drager syndrome	Detrusor hyperreflexia
Lesions above T6	Autonomic dysreflexia
Multiple sclerosis	Detrusor hyperreflexia, urgency, frequency
Diabetes mellitus	Impaired bladder sensation, decreased bladder contractility, impaired uroflow, residual urine
Tabes dorsalis	Loss of bladder sensation and decreased bladder contractility
Herpes zoster	Urgency, frequency, urinary retention
Disc disease	Detrusor areflexia
Radical pelvic surgery	Urinary retention
Myelodysplasia	Urinary retention, bladder dysfunction

The sensory neurogenic bladder is one with diminished or absent sensation, no detrusor hyperreflexia, and a large capacity. It results from interruption to sensory pathways from the bladder either in the sacral reflex arc or in the long afferent spinal tracts. It is associated with tabes dorsalis, diabetes, syringomyelia, and pernicious anemia.

A motor paralytic bladder occurs only rarely. Patients with this condition have no detrusor function but have normal sensation and either normal or increased capacity. This type of neurogenic bladder can be caused by poliomyelitis, trauma, meningomyelocele, or other congenital abnormalities.

Evaluation. Urodynamic evaluation of the neurogenic bladder takes several forms. Detrusor function is determined by cystometrogram to evaluate the strength and timing of detrusor contraction and bladder compliance. The CMG will also reveal uninhibited or hyperreflexic detrusor contractions. Sphincter function is evaluated with urethral pressure studies and electromyography. Efficiency of voiding is assessed by postvoid residual measurements. Fluoroscopic voiding studies show the anatomic position of the bladder and urethra, assess bladder neck function and coordination, and detect the presence of vesicoureteral reflux. Sensory function is appraised by questioning the patient about the sensation of filling and urgency during a CMG. In addition to urodynamics, renal ultrasound or IVP should be performed to check for hydronephrosis and renal scarring. Serum creatinine and urea nitrogen and, when necessary, nuclear renal scans should be performed to evaluate renal function.

Treatment. The therapeutic goals in the management of neurogenic bladder dysfunction are (*a*) to preserve renal function by preventing renal damage and (*b*) to normalize urinary tract function as much as possible, especially in respect to continence, bladder emptying, and infection prevention. Anticholinergics can be useful in suppressing uninhibited detrusor contractions and improving compliance. Sphincter resistance can be improved with α-adrenergic compounds like ephedrine. On the other hand, α-adrenergic blocking agents like phenoxybenzamine or antispasmodics such as baclofen, diazepam, or dantrolene will relax a spastic sphincter and improve emptying. Infections can be prevented by chronic low-dose prophylactic antibiotics.

Clean intermittent catheterization has proven to be an efficient, relatively easy, and safe method of ensuring bladder emptying with a wide range of applications. Because it has a significantly lower rate of infection, it is preferred over chronic urethral or suprapubic catheter drainage. In male patients with hyperfunction of the sphincter refractory to medical and other nonsurgical forms of management, transurethral sphincterotomy can be of benefit. Many patients require a combination of medicines and manipulations. Some patients have bladders that empty poorly and have high intravesical pressures. If these elevated pressures are long-term, ureteral drainage is impaired and vesicoureteral reflux can occur. Poor upper tract drainage, reflux, and infection can lead to renal damage and even renal failure. Other patients have difficulty with repeated episodes of cystitis and severe incontinence, debilitating and potentially life-threatening problems. They may require bladder augmentation with detubularized bowel or urinary diversions in order to preserve renal function and simplify urologic management. Regardless of the regimen used, patient compliance and close follow-up are essential. At minimum these patients need an annual evaluation of renal function and upper tract anatomy. Early evaluation and therapy is also necessary for suspected urinary tract infections or deterioration in bladder function. Urodynamic evaluation should be repeated as necessary to detect deleterious changes in bladder function that require a change in management.

Malignant Diseases

Bladder carcinoma, the fifth most frequent malignancy in the American population, is two-and-a-half times more common in males. It is about five times more prevalent among cigarette smokers and is associated with truck drivers and with rubber and oil refinery workers. Transitional cell carcinoma represents approximately 85–90% of tumors. Adenocarcinomas also occur, often in association with patent urachus and tumors at the bladder dome.

Evaluation. Gross painless hematuria is a common presenting sign. However, approximately 20% of patients may present with only microscopic hematuria. Diagnosis is made by intravenous pyelography (which shows a defect in the bladder), urinary cytology, and—especially—cystoscopy. Newer studies such as cell ploidy (the state of a cell nucleus with respect to the number of genomes it contains) have been found to yield a high correlation between positive urinary cytology and bladder carcinoma.

Bladder cancer can be staged according to whether it is superficial or muscle invading.

Stage O = Superficial, limited to mucosa
Stage A = Extends to lamina propria
Stage B = Invades muscle
Stage C = Extends into the perivesical fat
Stage D = Metastatic either to pelvic lymph nodes or viscera

Treatment. Management of bladder carcinoma depends on whether the tumor is superficial, involving only the mucosa and lamina propria, or whether it is deeper, involving the muscularis. For superficial bladder carcinoma, transurethral resection of the tumor is often the only treatment required. However, if the superficial bladder carcinoma is recurrent, intravesical chemotherapy with agents such as Thiotepa, BCG, and mitomycin-C becomes necessary. Use of these agents often reduces the recurrence rate by half. Patients with transitional cell carcinoma of the bladder have an increased incidence of tumors occurring at other sites in the bladder, ureter, or renal pelvis. Surveillance is mandatory since the recurrence rate in the bladder may be as high as 50% at 5 years. Surveillance protocols include cystoscopy and urinary cytologies every 3–4 months, with appropriate treatment where indicated. Approximately 10–20% of these patients will develop muscle invasion in the bladder.

If the bladder tumor penetrates the muscularis, treatment must be more aggressive. Treatment options include radiotherapy and surgical removal of the bladder. Cure rates for surgery exceed those for radiation by twofold. The 5-year survival rate of patients who have undergone surgical extirpation is approximately 60%.

Radical cystectomy is currently the treatment of choice for muscle invasive transitional cell carcinoma of the bladder. The entire bladder and pelvic lymph nodes are removed. In addition, the prostate is removed in males and pelvic exenteration may be done in females, depending on the depth of penetration of the tumor. Cystectomy is always carried out with some form of urinary diversion. Either an incontinent ileal loop diversion is performed or, in younger patients, a continent urinary reservoir is created using loops of bowel or colon.

Several types of urinary diversions are possible, the standard being the cutaneous ureteral ileal conduit. The ureters are reimplanted into a small section of the ileum that is brought out to the skin as a cutaneous stoma. Because it acts as a conduit, not a reservoir, patients must wear a ureterostomy bag.

Other types of urinary diversion that have become accepted include continent urinary reservoirs that use large sections of either the small bowel (the Kock pouch) or of the large bowel (the Indiana pouch, the Florida pouch, or the Ohio State pouch). The pouch is made of a large section of the right colon, cecum, or midportion of the transverse colon, which is detubularized to prevent spontaneous massive contractions and incontinence. The borders are reimplanted into the colon so that they will not reflux, and a resistance tube is made and anastomosed to the skin. This tube allows easy catheterization and offers passive resistance to the flow of urine. These patients often can then be managed with a small 4 × 4 dressing on the skin, eliminating the need for a stomal appliance. The success rate concerning reimplantation and reflux prevention approaches 95%. The expected and achieved continence rate approaches 90%. Patients with continent urinary reservoirs, however, have a higher incidence of reoperation (10–30%) than those with the standard ileal conduit. Approximately 58% of patients choose the standard ileal conduit, probably for two reasons. First, most patients requiring cystectomy are in their 60s or 70s and may not tolerate the extra hour-and-a-half in surgery necessary to construct the continent urinary reservoir. Second, these patients are willing to accept the urostomy bag and have no desire for a continent urinary reservoir. Support groups throughout the country help patients cope with their urostomies. Most patients engage well in normal activities.

The last type of urinary diversion that should be mentioned is for male patients, in whom the bladder is removed and the new reservoir connected directly to the urethra. While these patients are usually managed by clean intermittent catheterization, some void spontaneously. Unfortunately, many of these patients are incontinent at night and require an external catheter to avoid soilage.

The Penis

Anatomy

The penis is composed of two corpora cavernosa and the corpus spongiosum, which are bound by fibrous tissue and covered by skin (Fig. 9.29). Each corpus cavernosum has a thick fibrous capsule, the tunica albuginea, which forms around the cavernous sinuses. Distal to the symphysis pubis, the corpora cavernosa run side-by-side divided by a septum. More proximally, the corpora cavernosa separate and fuse to the ischial rami. The corpus spongiosum is positioned ventrally with its distal portion expanding to form the glans penis. The urethra is enclosed by the corpus spongiosum, traverses the glans penis, and opens as the external ure-

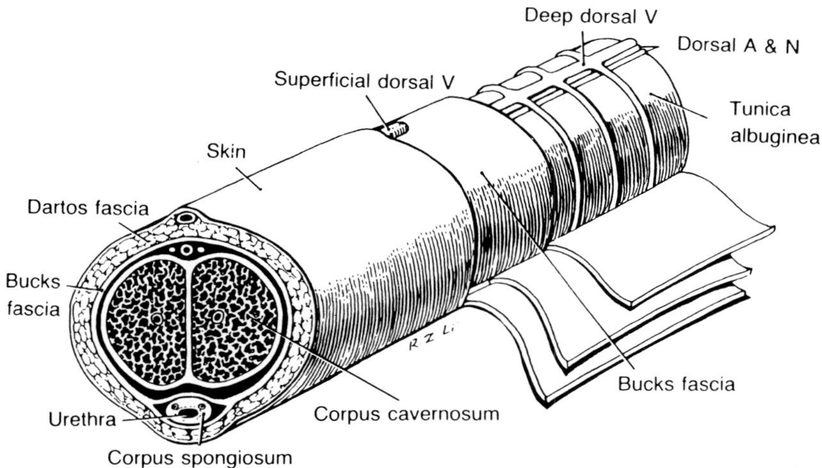

Figure 9.29. Anatomy of the penis.

thral meatus. The corpora cavernosa and corpus spongiosum are enveloped by Buck's fascia and covered with skin that is virtually hairless and devoid of fat. The penile skin extends over the glans to form the prepuce or foreskin.

The major blood supply of the penis is the internal pudendal artery, a branch of the internal iliac artery. Venous drainage from the penis is into the iliac veins by way of the deep and superficial dorsal veins. The lymphatics of the glans penis, corpus spongiosum, and distal corpus cavernosum drain into the external iliac, superficial, and deep inguinal lymph nodes. The proximal corpus cavernosum and posterior urethra drain into the internal iliac lymph nodes.

Traumatic Injuries

Penile injury may result from blunt or penetrating trauma, avulsion, strangulation, burns, and occasionally biting. Evaluation of cutaneous and underlying soft tissue damage, including assessment of urethral and testicular integrity, is mandatory. A careful physical examination is of prime importance. Retrograde urethrography is indicated in all cases of suspected urethral injury, and testicular ultrasound is helpful when testicular injury is suspected.

Blunt penile trauma can result in a contusion or a fracture. The injury is a contusion if there is minor soft tissue injury without associated urethral or testicular damage. Hematoma formation is usually small and limited by Buck's fascia or the dartos fascia of the scrotum. Management is supportive and consists of analgesics, bed rest, and scrotal support and elevation. Morbidity may be significantly reduced by drainage of large hematomas, even though most resolve with time. Fracture of the penis involves rupture of the tunica albuginea of the corpus cavernosum. Penile fracture usually occurs following trauma and during erection when the protective thickness of the tunica albuginea is reduced 4 to 8 times compared to the flaccid state. The patient typically reports experiencing a cracking sensation or noise followed by pain, detumescence, and rapid penile shaft swelling. Concomitant urethral injury occurs in about one-third of patients, requiring immediate exploration, evacuation of hematoma, closure of the tunica albuginea, and urethral catheterization or suprapubic cystotomy. In the absence of urethral injury, conservative management consisting of ice packs, elevation, and oral estrogens to inhibit erections will produce a satisfactory result in the majority of patients. Immediate surgical exploration with evacuation of the hematoma and repair of the tunica albuginea may reduce subsequent penile curvature.

Penetrating penile injuries may be due to gunshot or knife wounds. Low velocity gunshot wounds without involvement of the urethra may be cleaned and left open. High velocity gunshot wounds are associated with significant tissue destruction and usually require surgical management. Knife injuries resulting in superficial lacerations may be closed if the wound is clean. Repair of complete penile amputations using microsurgical techniques can be attempted up to 18 hours after injury if contamination is minimal and the penis has been properly preserved in cold saline. If repair of the amputated penis is not feasible, then partial penectomy is performed. Injuries that involve the urethra or testis require surgical exploration.

Avulsion injury to the penis may be caused by the patient's clothing becoming entrapped in rotating machinery or by suction devices used for sexual excitement. Usually, the skin and loose areolar tissue superficial to Buck's fascia are avulsed and deeper tissues are left intact. Small noncircumferential penile avulsions are closed primarily with a full-thickness preputial skin graft or a split-thickness skin graft. With circumferential penile avulsions, complete interruption of the lymphatic drainage results in chronic lymphedema of skin distal to the injury. Superior cosmetic results will be obtained if the skin distal to the injury is removed up to the coronal sulcus and replaced with a split-thickness skin graft (Fig. 9.30).

Constricting objects placed around the penis have resulted in penile strangulation. A variety of such objects

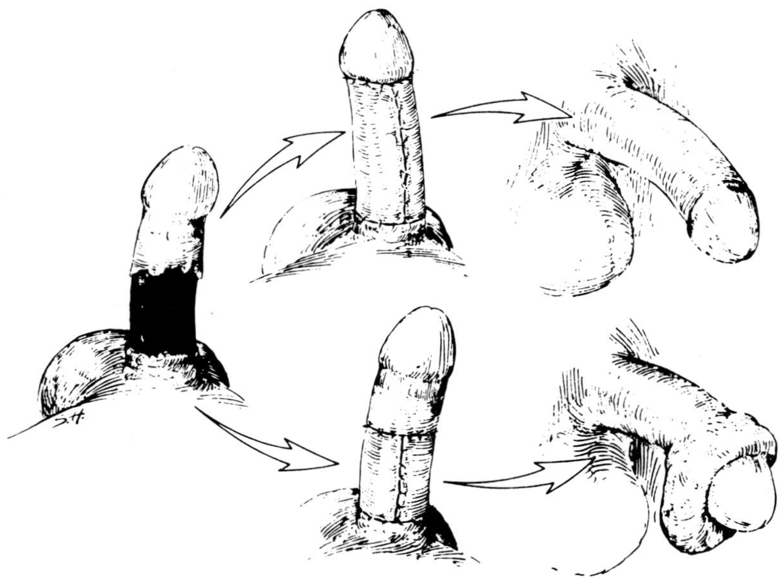

Figure 9.30. Correct (above) and incorrect (below) management of partial penile avulsion. If distal remnant of penile skin is left in place, chronic lymphedema of the remnant will occur.

Table 9.5.
Premalignant Penile Lesions

Penile Lesion	Gross Characteristics	Microscopic Characteristics	Treatment
Leukoplakia	White plaque	Acanthosis, hyperkeratosis, and parakeratosis	Excision
Balanitis xerotic obliterans	White, atrophic red lesion of glans and/or prepuce	Abundant, amorphous collagen and lymphocyte infiltrate of reticular dermis	Excision, topical steroids
Bowen's disease	Solitary, red plaque on penile shaft	Carcinoma in situ	Laser fulguration, excision, topical 5-FU[a]
Erythroplasia of Queyrat	Raised, red velvety lesion of glans or coronal sulcus	Carcinoma in situ	Laser fulguration, excision, topical 5-FU
Giant condyloma acuminatum	Large, exophytic lesion	Similar to condyloma acuminatum with invasion into underlying tissue	Excision

[a]5-Fluorouracil

has been reported, including hair, string, rubber bands, metal washers, and bottles. Following removal of the constricting band, the cutaneous and underlying soft tissue is evaluated. When the skin is nonviable, it is debrided and replaced by a split-thickness skin graft. If the deeper soft tissues are necrotic, initial management should include suprapubic cystostomy and application of topical antimicrobials. Debridement or partial penectomy is delayed until nonviable tissue is clearly defined.

Penile burns may be caused by thermal, chemical, or electric injury, and are managed similarly to burns in other areas of the body. Because penile preservation is the prime objective, extensive debridement should be approached cautiously. Topical antimicrobials are applied to thermal burns in an open or dressed fashion. A urethral catheter or suprapubic cystostomy is usually necessary to monitor urinary output. Chemical burns are typically superficial; after copious irrigation with saline, they are managed as thermal burns. Although electrical burns cause minimal skin damage, extensive deep soft tissue injury may occur. Conservative management is recommended until the full extent of tissue injury has been demarcated.

Neoplasms

Premalignant Lesions. Five penile lesions have been identified as premalignant: leukoplakia, balanitis xerotica obliterans, Bowen's disease, erythroplasia of Queyrat, and giant condyloma acuminatum (Table 9.5). Leukoplakia appears grossly as a white plaque and is characterized microscopically by acanthosis, hyperkeratosis, and parakeratosis. The treatment is local excision. Balanitis xerotica obliterans (lichen sclerosus et atrophicus) presents as white, atrophic, edematous lesions involving the glans penis and/or prepuce. Histo-

Table 9.6.
Squamous Cell Carcinoma of the Penis: Jackson Classification

Stage I	Tumor limited to the glans penis and/or prepuce
Stage II	Tumor with invasion of the corpora, but not involving nodes and without distant metastasis
Stage III	Tumor as in stage II but with proven regional node involvement
Stage IV	Tumor with distant metastasis

Table 9.7.
TNM Classification of Penile Carcinoma

T—Primary Tumor		
Tis	Preinvasive carcinoma (carcinoma in situ)	
T0	No evidence of primary tumor	
T1	Tumor 2 cm or less in its largest dimension, strictly superficial or exophytic	
T2	Tumor larger than 2 cm but not more than 5 cm in its largest dimension with minimal infiltration	
T3	Tumor more than 5 cm in its largest dimension, or tumor of any size with deep infiltration, including into the urethra	
T4	Tumor infiltrating neighboring structures	
N—Regional Lymph Nodes		
	The clinician may record whether palpable nodes are considered to contain growth	
N0	No palpable nodes	
N1	Movable unilateral nodes	
	N1a	Nodes not considered to contain growth
	N1b	Nodes considered to contain growth
N2	Movable bilateral nodes	
	N2a	Nodes not considered to contain growth
	N2b	Nodes considered to contain growth
N3	Fixed Nodes	
M—Distant Metastases		
M0	No evidence of distant metastases	
M1	Distant metastases present	

logically, the dermis is composed of abundant amorphous collagen and a lymphocytic infiltrate in the underlying reticular dermis. Treatment consists of local excision and topical steroids. Bowen's disease typically appears as a solitary, erythematous plaque on the penile shaft. Approximately 25% of patients with Bowen's disease will have a concomitant visceral malignancy. Erythroplasia of Queyrat consists of raised, red, velvety, well-marginated areas of the glans penis or coronal sulcus. Both Bowen's disease and erythroplasia of Queyrat histologically appear as carcinoma in situ and may be treated by neodymium-YAG (yttrium-argon-garnet) laser fulguration, local excision, or topical application of 5-fluorouracil. Giant condyloma acuminatum (Buschke-Löwenstein tumor, verrucous carcinoma) is a large exophytic lesion often grossly indistinguishable from squamous cell carcinoma. Histologically, these lesions are similar to condyloma acuminatum except that the tumor extends into the underlying tissue. Local excision is required, often necessitating partial or total penectomy.

Squamous Cell Carcinoma. Although rare in the United States, penile cancer is common in men living in hot, humid regions. Poor personal hygiene and retained phimotic foreskin have been implicated in the etiology of penile carcinoma. Penile cancer is extremely rare in men circumcised at birth, with fewer than 10 cases reported. Squamous cell carcinoma of the penis occurs most commonly in the sixth decade. The symptoms are related to ulceration, necrosis, suppuration, and hemorrhage of the penile lesion. The clinical evaluation of patients with penile cancer includes physical examination with palpation of the inguinal region, liver function tests, chest radiograph, CT of the abdomen and pelvis, and bone scan. The most widely used staging system is that proposed by Jackson (Table 9.6). The TNM staging system is also used (Table 9.7).

Small penile cancers limited to the prepuce can be treated by circumcision alone. Partial penectomy with at least a 2-cm margin of normal tissue is used to treat smaller (2–5 cm) distal penile tumors (Fig. 9.31). The remaining penis should be long enough to permit voiding in the standing position. The 5-year cure rate for patients treated with partial penectomy is 70–80%. Larger distal penile lesions or proximal tumors require total penectomy and perineal urethrostomy. If the scrotum, pubis, or abdominal wall is involved, radical en bloc excision may be necessary.

Most patients will have inguinal lymphadenopathy at presentation. However, inguinal lymph node enlargement before excision of the primary tumor is usually the result of infection and not the result of metastatic disease. Thus, clinical assessment of the inguinal region should be delayed 4–6 weeks, during which time the patient is treated with antibiotics. If inguinal lymphadenopathy persists or subsequently develops, there is a high likelihood of metastatic lymph nodal disease and ilioinguinal lymphadenectomy should be performed. However, if inguinal lymphadenopathy resolves, most surgical oncologists would not perform prophylactic lymph node dissection because it does not enhance survival and is associated with considerable morbidity, particularly lower extremity lymphedema.

An alternative approach to the management of regional lymph nodes was proposed by Cabanas. He suggested that the sentinel lymph nodes located at the junction of the saphenous and femoral veins represent the first site of inguinal lymph node metastases. Further treatment may be based on bilateral sentinel lymph node biopsy. Negative biopsy is associated with a 5-year survival rate of approximately 90%, and thus ilioinguinal lymph node dissection is not necessary. However, a positive biopsy is an indication for ilioinguinal lymphadenectomy. A 5-year survival rate for patients with unilateral and bilateral inguinal lymph node involvement is 56% and 9%, respectively. Involvement of the iliac nodes is uniformly fatal.

Radiation of the primary tumor and regional lymph nodes is an alternative to surgery in patients with small (<2 cm), low-stage tumor. The advantage of radiotherapy over surgery is preservation of the penis. However, control rates are slightly lower than those of surgical excision. Similarly, radiotherapy can cure patients with

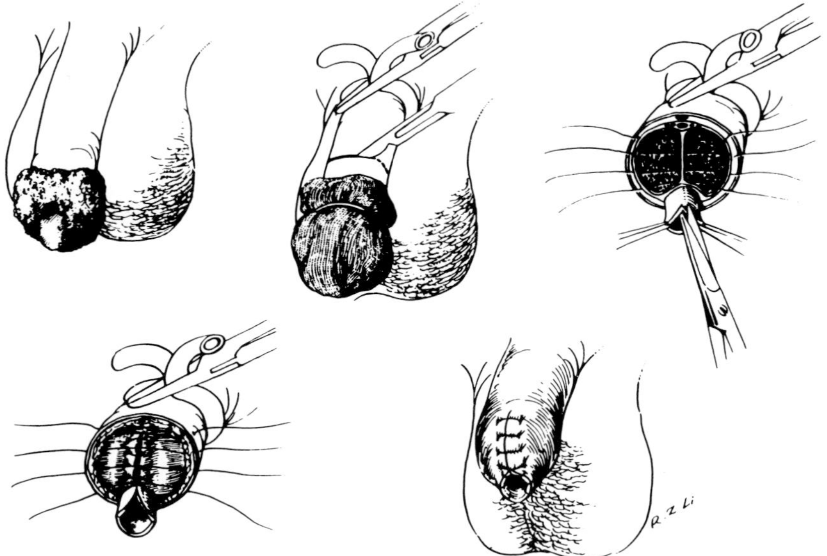

Figure 9.31. Technique of partial penectomy.

inguinal nodal metastases, but at a lower rate than with ilioinguinal lymphadenectomy.

Acquired Disorders

Priapism. Priapism is the pathological prolongation of penile erection. Unlike normal tumescence, only the corpora cavernosa are turgid, while the corpus spongiosum (including the glans penis) remains flaccid. Priapism results from obstruction of penile venous outflow, which produces sludging and thrombosis of cavernosal blood. Left untreated the corpora cavernosa become fibrotic and the patient becomes impotent. In the majority of patients the etiology of priapism is idiopathic. However, sickle cell anemia, trauma, leukemia, metastatic disease, and intracorporal injection of vasoactive substances for the treatment of impotency have been implicated in the pathogenesis of this disease.

The treatment of patients with sickle cell anemia and neoplasms should be directed at the underlying cause. Sickle cell patients should be treated with hydration, alkalinization, analgesics, and transfusions with packed red blood cells. Patients with malignancies should be treated with radiation therapy and/or chemotherapy. Surgery is reserved for nonresponders. Patients with priapism caused by intracorporal injection of vasoactive substances such as papaverine may respond to intracorporal injection of phenylephrine.

Surgical treatment consists of cavernosal irrigation to remove sludged blood followed by the formation of a fistula between the corpus cavernosum and corpus spongiosum,thus creating a shunt. Most often this can be accomplished using a Travenol biopsy needle (Winter procedure) as illustrated in Figure 9.32. Alternatively, surgical excision of windows of tissue (Quackles and Al-Ghorab procedures), or a corpus cavernosum - saphenous vein shunt may be performed (Grayhack procedure). Despite prompt treatment, about 50% of patients will have permanent erectile impotence.

Phimosis. Phimosis is the fibrotic contracture of the foreskin prohibiting retraction of the prepuce over the glans penis. The etiology is poor hygiene or infection beneath redundant foreskin resulting in chronic irritation. When phimosis causes urinary retention, calculus formation, and/or balanoposthitis (acute inflammation of the foreskin), acute treatment is required. Minor infection usually responds to sitz baths and topical antibiotics. Urinary retention and calculus require a dorsal slit or circumcision.

Paraphimosis. When mild prepucial contracture is present, the retracted foreskin forms a constricting band that over a prolonged period of time results in paraphimosis (Fig. 9.33), a painful constriction of the glans penis by phimotic foreskin that has been retracted behind the corona. Initially, venous occlusion results in edema, which subsequently leads to arterial occlusion and eventually glandular gangrene. Manual compression of the glans usually decreases the edema allowing the foreskin to be reduced. If manual compression fails, the constricting prepucial band of tissue requires incision. Circumcision should follow resolution of edema and inflammation.

Peyronie's Disease. Peyronie's disease is an inflammatory process involving the tunica albuginea of the corpora cavernosa resulting in fibrous plaques that may calcify or even ossify. Peyronie's plaques may be multiple and are typically located on the dorsal penile surface. The disease usually causes painful erections and variable degrees of penile curvature that may be sexually incapacitating. No one treatment of Peyronie's disease is uniformly successful. Conservative approaches include vitamin E, potassium p-aminobenzoate (Potaba), or intralesional injections of antiinflammatory steroids. If conservative management fails, the fibrous

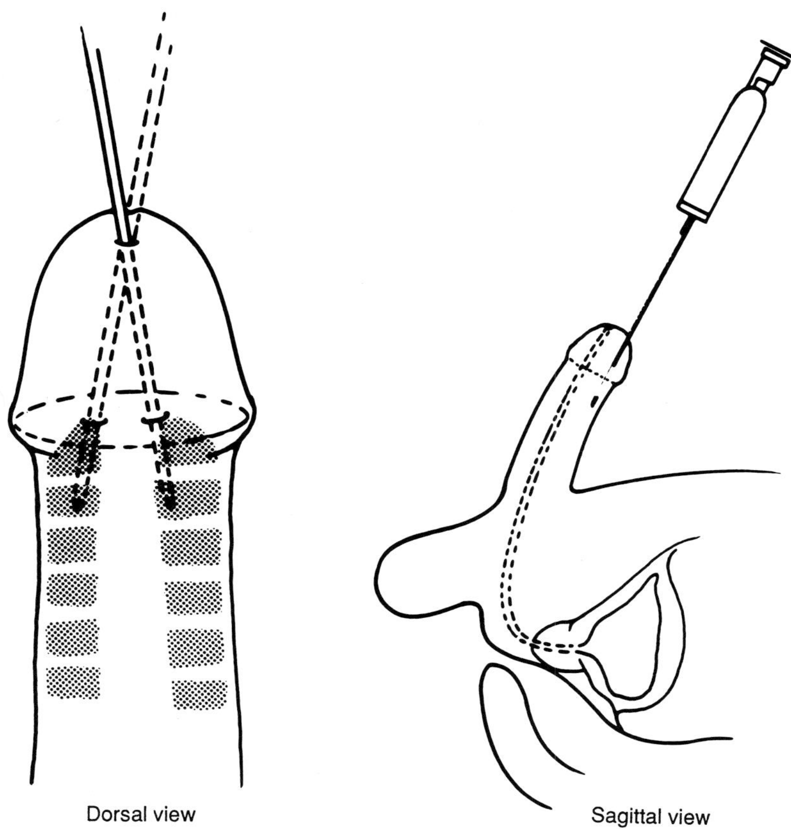

Figure 9.32. Winter shunt for the treatment of priapism. A Travenol biopsy needle is used to create fistulae between the glans penis (corpus spongiosum) and the corpora cavernosa. **A**, Dorsal view; **B**, sagittal view.

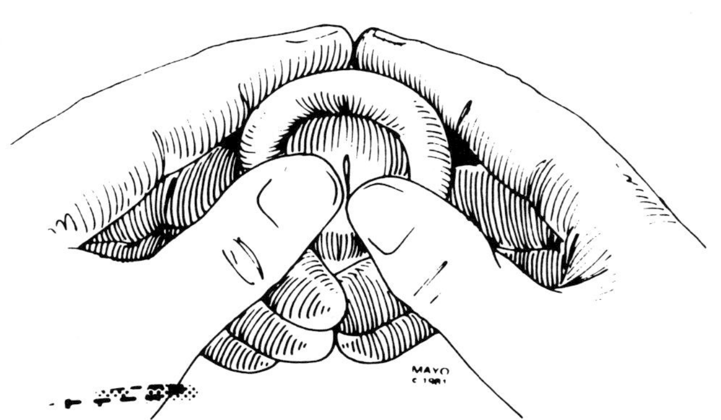

Figure 9.33. Manual reduction of paraphimosis.

plaque may be excised and replaced by a free dermal or synthetic graft. A semirigid penile prosthesis is sometimes placed to correct impotency and assure penile straightening.

Congenital Penile Disorders

Isolated penile congenital anomalies are rare. Agenesis of the penis results when the genital tubercle fails to develop. The urethra opens in the perineum near the anus. Sex reassignment should be performed, which includes castration, vaginoplasty, and estrogen therapy at puberty. Bifid penis results from failure of the genital tubercle to fuse. Micropenis is a normally developed penis that is unusually small. It is defined as a penis that is less than 2 standard deviations from the normal length (less than 2 cm stretched length at birth). If the patient has a female karyotype, an intersex evaluation should be initiated. A patient with a male karyotype should have serum luteinizing hormone, follicle-stimulating hormone, and testosterone determinations. Patients with low testosterone levels may respond to hormonal manipulation; otherwise, gender reassignment should be considered.

Sexually Transmitted Infectious Diseases

Syphilis. Syphilis is caused by the spirochete *Treponema pallidum*. The natural history of syphilitic infections is divided into three stages. Following an average incubation period of 3 weeks, the primary stage is heralded by the appearance of a painless ulcer (chancre) that has a smooth base and indurated border and appears chiefly on the glans penis and prepuce. Secondary syphilis begins as the chancre starts to heal, usually 6–8 weeks after exposure. Bilateral symmetrical macular, papular, or papulosquamous eruptions are the hallmarks of secondary syphilis. Additionally, mucous membrane lesions, lymphadenopathy, fever, alopecia, or local organ involvement may occur. Both primary

Table 9.8.
Treatment of Sexually Transmitted Diseases

Type or Stage	Drug of Choice	Dosage	Alternatives
Gonorrhea urethritis or cervicitis[a]	Ceftriaxone	250 mg i.m. once	Amoxicillin 3 g p.o. once, plus probenecid 1 g once Penicillin G procaine 4.8 million U 1.m.[b] once, plus probenecid 1 g p.o. once Spectinomycin 2 g i.m. once
Syphilis			
Early (primary, secondary, or latent less than 1 year)	Penicillin G benzathine	2.4 × 10^6 U i.m. once	Tetracycline 500 mg p.o. q.i.d. for 14 days Erythromycin 500 mg p.o. q.i.d. for 14 days
Late (more than 1 year's duration; cardiovascular)	Penicillin G benzathine	2.4 × 10^6 U i.m. weekly for 3 weeks	Tetracycline 500 mg p.o. q.i.d. for 30 days Erythromycin 500 mg p.o. q.i.d. for 30 days
Neurosyphilis	Penicillin G	2.4 × 10^6 U i.v. q.4h. for 10 days	Tetracycline 500 mg p.o. q.i.d. for 30 days
	Penicillin G procaine	2.4 × 10^6 U i.m. daily plus probenecid 500 mg p.o. q.i.d. both for 10 days	Erythromycin 500 mg p.o. q.i.d. for 30 days
	Either treatment above followed by penicillin G benzathine	2.4 × 10^6 U i.m. weekly for 3 weeks	
Chancroid	Ceftriaxone Erythromycin	250 mg i.m. once 500 mg p.o. q.i.d. for 7 days	Trimethoprim-sulfamethoxazole DS[c] tablets p.o. b.i.d. for 7 days
Lymphogranuloma venereum	Doxycycline Tetracycline Erythromycin	100 mg p.o. b.i.d. for 21 days 500 mg p.o. q.i.d. for 21 days 500 mg p.o. b.i.d. for 21 days	
Granuloma inguinale	Doxycycline	100 mg p.o. b.i.d. for 21 days	Gentamicin 1 mg/kg i.v. b.i.d. for 21 days
	Tetracycline	500 mg p.o. q.i.d. for 21 days	Chloramphenicol 500 mg p.o. t.i.d. for 21 days
	Ampicillin Trimethoprim-sulfamethoxazole	500 mg p.o. q.i.d. for 12 weeks DS[c] tablets b.i.d. for 21 days	
Genital herpes	Acyclovir	200 mg p.o. q.4h. for 10 days 5% ointment q.3h. for 7 days 5 mg/kg i.v. q8h.	
Chlamydia trachomatis urethritis or cervicitis	Doxycycline	100 mg p.o. b.i.d. for 2 days	Sulfisoxazole 500 mg p.o. q.i.d. for 10 days
	Tetracycline Erythromycin	500 mg p.o. q.i.d. for 7 days 500 mg p.o. q.i.d. for 7 days	
Trichomoniasis	Metronidazole	2 gm p.o. once or 250 mg p.o. t.i.d. for 7 days	
In pregnancy	Clotrimazole	100 mg intravaginally at bedtime for 7 days	

[a]Many authorities recommend a 7-day course of tetracycline or doxycycline for treatment of possible coexisting *Chlamydia trachomatis* infection.
[b]Divided into two injections at one visit.
[c]Each tablet contains 80 mg of trimethoprim and 400 mg of sulfamethoxazole.

and secondary syphilitic lesions heal spontaneously. The patient then either enters a latent period, which may last indefinitely, or proceeds to tertiary syphilis in which the cardiovascular and central nervous systems frequently are involved.

A positive dark field examination confirms the diagnosis of syphilis. However, its application is limited because it requires the exudate of a primary or secondary syphilitic lesion. Serologic tests such as the VDRL (Venereal Disease Research Laboratory) or the RPR (rapid plasma reagin) may become reactive 4 weeks after a patient has contracted the infection. Immunofluorescent treponemal antibody absorption (FTA-ABS) or microhemagglutination (MHA-TP) tests should be performed if a reactive serological test cannot be substantiated by dark field examination. When neurosyphilis is suspected, a lumbar puncture should be done to obtain spinal fluid for examination of VDRL reactivity, cell count, and total protein measurement. Treatment for primary, secondary, and latent (duration of less than 1 year) syphilis is given in Table 9.8.

Chancroid. Chancroid is caused by *Hemophilus ducreyi*. Following an incubation of 1–5 days, multiple vesicular or papular lesions develop on the genitalia, perineum, and thigh. These lesions rapidly become pustular and rupture, resulting in the soft chancre, which is a nonindurated ulcer with an overhanging edge, necrotic base, and foul-smelling exudate. A week or two following the appearance of the primary lesion, matted inguinal adenopathy (bubo) occurs. In about half of cases the bubo of chancroid suppurates. The diagnosis is made on Gram's stain of the lesion or bubo aspirate, which show Gram-negative rods in parallel arrangement. The treatment of chancroid is given in Table 9.8.

Lymphogranuloma Venereum. Several immunotypes of *Chlamydia trachomatis* are responsible for the development of lymphogranuloma venereum. The primary lesion is a small, painless herpetiform vesicle or ulcer, which rapidly resolves, is often overlooked, and appears 3 days–3 weeks after exposure. Regional adenopathy becomes evident 2–6 weeks after exposure. With progressive lymphadenopathy, the inelastic inguinal ligament will cause a depression creating the almost pathognomonic "sign of the groove." Untreated, most involved lymph nodes will suppurate. Involvement of the perirectal lymphatics may result in pararectal abscesses, rectovaginal fistula, and rectal strictures. Elephantiasis of the genitalia caused by lymphatic obstruction is not uncommon.

The diagnosis is made by isolating the organism from the bubo aspirate. Complement fixation and microimmunofluorescent serological tests may also be used. Treatment regimens are given in Table 9.8.

Granuloma Inguinale. Granuloma inguinale (donovanosis) is caused by *Calymmatobacterium granulomatis* (formerly *Donovania granulomatis*). Eight to 12 weeks after inoculation papules form on the genitalia. The papules progress to nontender ulcers with raised edges and a beefy-red exuberant granulation base. Secondary infection leads to cicatricial healing and keloid-like scarring. Lymphatic obstruction may result in elephantiasis. The diagnosis is made on biopsy of the granulation tissue demonstrating bipolar Gram-negative bacilli within histiocytes (Donovan bodies). Treatment is given in Table 9.8.

Genital Herpes. Genital herpes is caused by herpes simplex virus (HSV). Most cases results from HSV type I, but HSV type II infection may also be causative. Vesicular lesions may be identified 3–6 days after inoculation and rupture 1–4 days later forming painful ulcers. Viral shedding occurs until a dry crust forms. Extragenital sites of herpetic involvement are common. Systemic manifestation of HSV infection includes myalgias, malaise, and headache. The diagnosis is made from examination of the vesicular fluid or by viral culture. Multinucleated giant cells containing intranuclear inclusion bodies are seen from scrapings of lesions examined by *Papanicolaou* smear or immunofluorescence. A negative serologic test may exclude HSV infection, but a positive test is useful only in demonstrating prior infection. Treatment is listed in Table 9.8.

Condyloma Acuminatum. Condyloma acuminatum (venereal wart) is caused by the human papilloma virus. The external genitalia and perineum are the most common sites of infection. About 5% of patients with warts on external genitalia also have intraurethral involvement. The incubation period ranges from several weeks to months. Usually, the diagnosis is obvious from gross appearance. Although podophyllin is still widely used, its cure rate is low. Liquid nitrogen, surgical excision, electrocautery, and laser fulguration are more successful. Treatment with interferon is not recommended because of its relatively low efficacy, high incidence of toxicity, and high cost. Intraurethral warts are best treated by laser fulguration and/or 5% 5-fluorouracil cream applied after voiding up to 6 times daily for 7 days.

Circumcision and Dorsal Slit

Circumcision is the most common operation performed on males in the United States (Fig. 9.34). Indications include parental decision, phimosis, cosmetic effect, and malignancy. Contraindications to circumcision include myelodysplasia and hypospadias. In the newborn, a Gomco clamp or plastibell is usually used. If circumcision is not performed shortly after birth, it should be delayed until age 1, because a general anesthetic is required. Adults obtain excellent anesthesia from a local penile block; circumcision may be performed as an outpatient procedure.

After appropriate preparation and draping, a straight hemostat is placed on the middle of the dorsal surface of the prepuce. The hemostat is removed and a dorsal slit is performed by cutting the crushed foreskin proximally to within 1 cm of the coronal sulcus. The prepuce should now easily retract to expose the glans penis. If only a dorsal slit is to be performed, the cut edges are hemostatically approximated by absorbable interrupted sutures. If a circumcision is to be done, the cut edges of the dorsal slit are not sutured. A similar incision is made in the ventral surface of the prepuce to the frenulum. Occasionally, bleeding from a frenular artery will require ligature. With the foreskin divided in two, redundant prepuce is excised. Hemostasis is secured with electrocautery and/or absorbable sutures. The mucosal and cutaneous surfaces of the foreskin are then approximated using interrupted absorbable sutures. The incision is protected by antibiotic ointment and a loose dressing. The dressing is removed the following morning and warm sitz baths may be started. Intercourse should be avoided until the suture line is well healed.

The Urethra

Anatomy

The male urethra, approximately 20 cm in length, is divided by the urogenital diaphragm into posterior and anterior portions (Fig. 9.35). The posterior portion includes the prostatic urethra, which continues through the urogenital diaphragm as the membranous urethra. The anterior portion consists of a proximal bulbous ure-

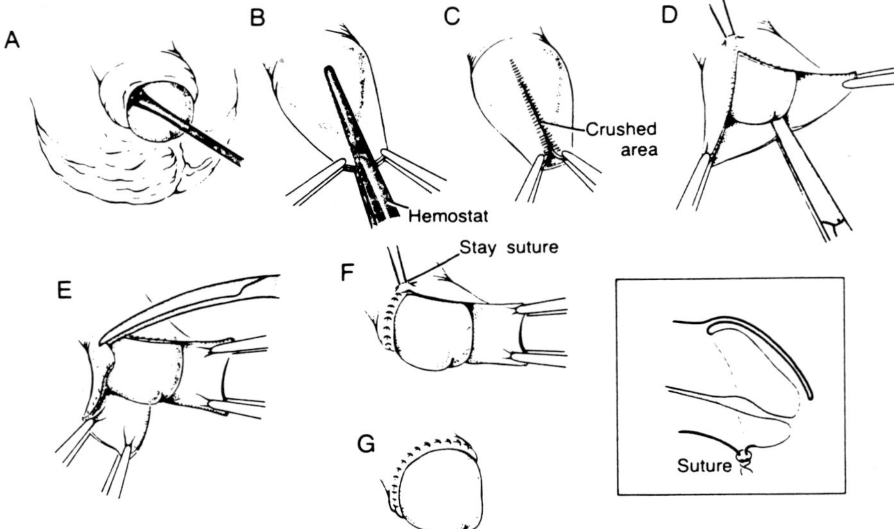

Figure 9.34. Freehand circumcision.

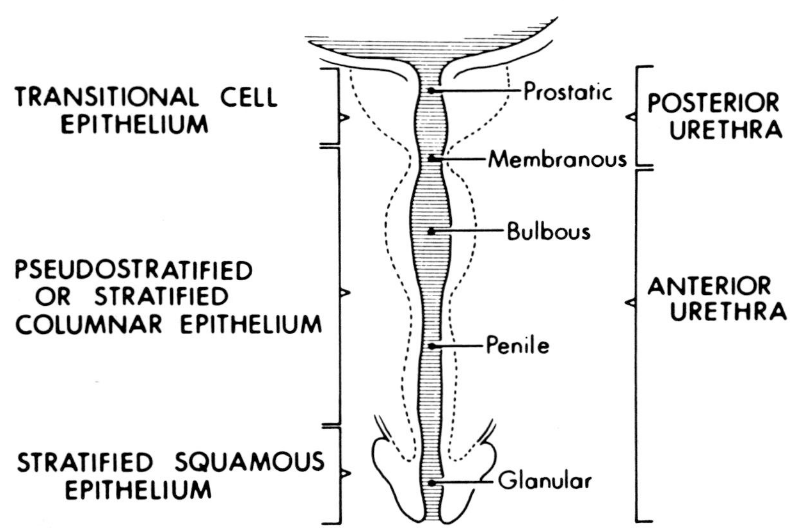

Figure 9.35. Anatomy and cell types lining the male urethra.

thra, and a distal penile urethra that terminates as the external urethral meatus. The prostatic urethra is lined by transitional epithelium; the membranous, bulbous, and penile sections of the urethra are lined by pseudostratified or stratified columnar epithelium; the external urethral meatus is lined by squamous epithelium. Paired bulbourethral (Cowper's) glands, located in the urogenital diaphragm, produce a clear viscous fluid (sometimes called the preejaculatory fluid) and secrete into the bulbous urethra. Multiple glands of Littre, which also produce a preejaculatory fluid, line the penile urethra. Their exact function is unknown, but it is believed these secretions favorably alter the urethra for sperm transport during ejaculation. The lymphatic drainage of the posterior urethra is directly into the obturator and iliac nodes, while that of the anterior urethra is through the deep inguinal nodes into the iliac nodes.

The female urethra, about 4 cm long (Fig. 9.36), lies immediately anterior to the vagina; its external urethral meatus opens 2 cm posterior to the clitoris. Transitional epithelium lines the proximal third of the female urethra and stratified squamous epithelium lines the distal two-thirds. The periurethral glands of Skene are homologues of the male urethral glands and empty into the distal urethra. The proximal female urethra drains into the iliac lymph nodes and the distal portion into the inguinal lymph nodes.

Urethral Trauma

Urethral injuries occur more frequently in males than in females because the male urethra is fixed to the pubis by the puboprostatic ligaments and the suspensory ligament of the penis. Tearing occurs at these fixed areas. The urogenital diaphragm is the anatomic landmark

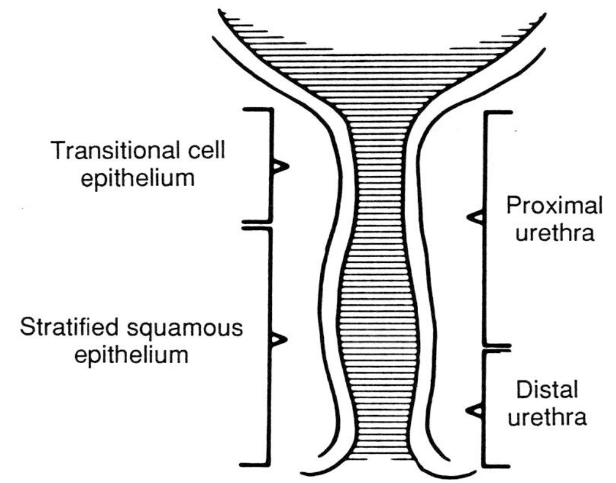

Figure 9.36. Anatomy and cell types lining the female urethra.

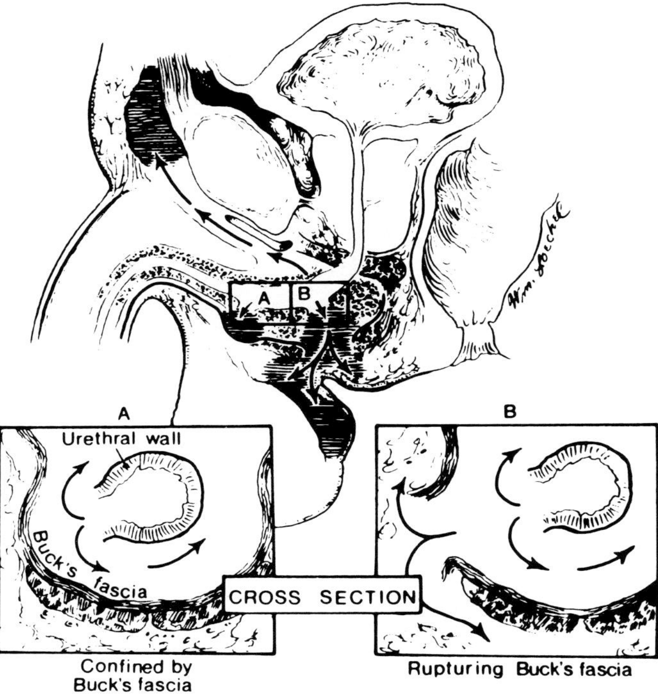

Figure 9.37. Straddle injury to the bulbous urethra demonstrating pathways of blood and urine extravasation.

that divides anterior (bulbar and pendulous) from posterior (prostatic and membranous) urethral injuries. Both anterior and posterior urethral injuries may be secondary to blunt, penetrating, and iatrogenic trauma.

Anterior urethral injuries usually result from blunt trauma, such as straddle injuries, in which the bulbous urethra is crushed against the pubic rami. Although 90% of posterior urethral injuries have simultaneous pelvic fractures, only 10% of pelvic fractures have associated posterior urethral injury. Urethral injury should be suspected in patients with blood at the urethral meatus, inability to void, or penile/perineal edema and ecchymosis. If Buck's fascia remains intact, extravasation of blood and urine are confined to the penile shaft (Fig. 9.37). However, disruption of Buck's fascia allows extravasated contents into a space limited by Colles' fascia. Posteriorly, Colles' fascia attaches to the triangular ligament and laterally, to the deep fascia of the thigh; anteriorly it is continuous with Scarpa's fascia. Thus, extravasations limited by Colles' fascia form a scrotal and perineal "butterfly" hematoma that can extend up the abdominal wall under Scarpa's fascia. If digital rectal examination reveals a superiorly displaced prostate gland, a pelvic hematoma with urethral injury must be considered and evaluated.

Diagnosis. When urethral injury is suspected, radiographic evaluation should *precede* urethral catheterization. Otherwise, attempts to pass a urethral catheter may convert a simple urethral laceration or incomplete rupture into a complete transection. Because most patients with urethral injury have concomitant trauma to other organ systems, they require a complete evaluation of the entire urinary system. Intravenous pyelography (IVP) should precede retrograde urethrography or cystography, since extravasation of contrast from intraperitoneal bladder rupture may obscure IVP findings. Often a urethral catheter is passed before consultation and radiographic evaluation have been obtained. In such an instance, retrograde urethrography should be performed through a second, smaller catheter which is inserted alongside the original catheter. On retrograde urethrography, a partial urethral rupture is suggested when there is both urethral extravasation and passage of contrast into the bladder. Extravasation without passage of contrast into the bladder indicates complete urethral rupture (Fig. 9.38).

Treatment. Small, incomplete anterior urethral ruptures with extravasation limited by Buck's fascia are treated by draining with a urethral catheter for 2–3 weeks or by performing a suprapubic cystostomy. When extravasation is large or Buck's fascia has been violated, however, surgical drainage is usually indicated. Complete anterior urethral ruptures require primary surgical repair. In the unstable patient, suprapubic cystostomy and subsequent surgical repair may be the most prudent approach.

Partial posterior urethral ruptures are treated by suprapubic cystostomy, urethral catheterization, and retroperitoneal drainage. The urethral catheter is left for 2–4 weeks. Complete posterior urethral rupture is managed by either immediate or delayed surgical repairs. With immediate repair the bladder is opened, hematoma and bony fragments removed, concomitant bladder ruptures repaired, and a suprapubic cystostomy performed. A catheter is passed retrograde from the meatus to the bladder in order to realign the disrupted urethral segments. The actual posterior urethral rupture is not sutured since mobilization and dissection of the prostatic and membranous urethra results in an increased incidence of stricture, incontinence, and impotence. Delayed repair involves suprapubic cystostomy without urethral realignment, followed by definitive surgery 3–6 months later. Although delayed repair inevitably results in urethral stricture, incontinence and impotency rates (5% and 8%, respectively) are signifi-

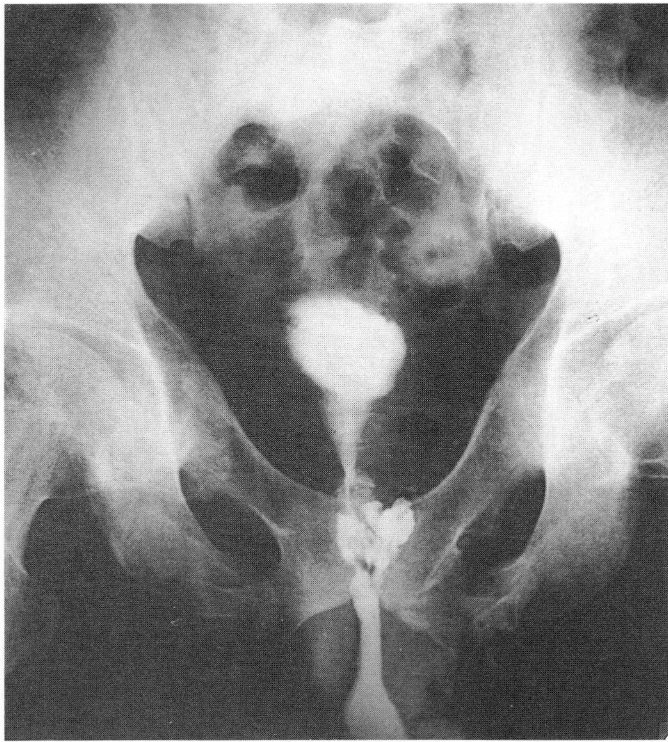

Figure 9.38. Retrograde urethrogram showing retroperitoneal extravasation of contrast due to a traumatic posterior urethral rupture.

cantly lower than those in patients treated by immediate repair (50% and 33%, respectively).

Neoplasms

Male Urethral Carcinoma. Urethral carcinoma is less common in males than in females: approximately 600 cases have been reported in males compared with 1400 cases in females. Although the disease may occur at any age, it usually occurs after 60 years of age. While the etiology remains undetermined, about 50% of cases have been associated with urethral stricture, probably because stricture and its concordant inflammation may induce squamous metaplasia and subsequent malignant transformation. A patient should be evaluated for urethral carcinoma when a urethral mass is palpable, obstruction does not respond to conventional stricture management, a urethral abscess and/or fistula occurs, hematuria is present, or inguinal adenopathy becomes evident.

Female Urethral Carcinoma. Although the etiology of female urethral carcinoma remains obscure, there is an association with urethral malakoplakia and urethral caruncles. Most patients are white and over 50 years of age. The usual presenting symptom is a papillary or fungating urethral mass. Local tumor extension into the vagina and bladder neck is common. Lymphatic spread of distal urethral lesions is by way of the inguinal nodes, while that of proximal urethral tumors is by way of the iliac nodes. When present, inguinal lymphadenopathy usually indicates metastatic disease.

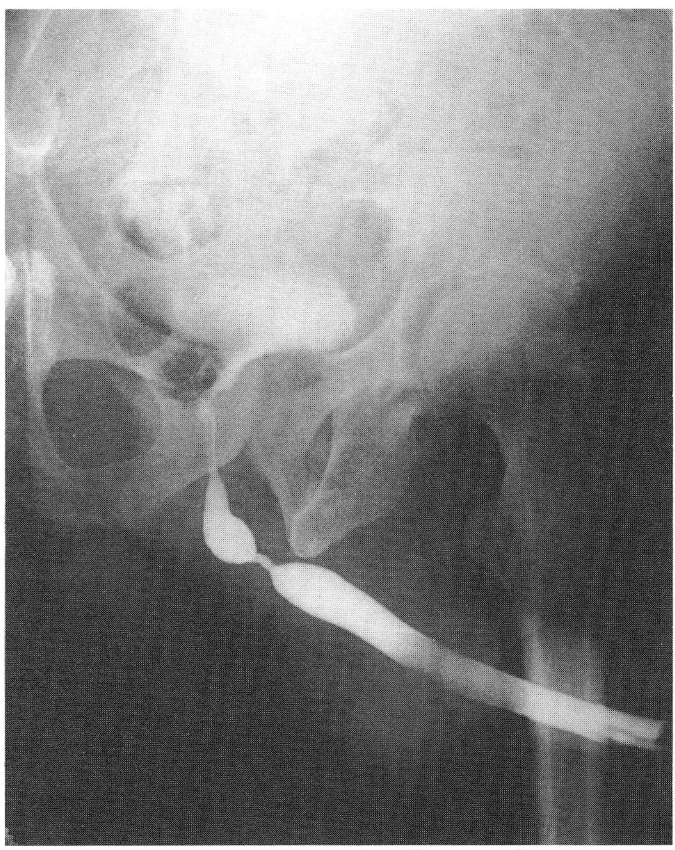

Figure 9.39. Retrograde urethrogram showing bulbar urethral stricture.

Urethral Strictures

Urethral strictures may be congenital or acquired. Congenital strictures typically occur in the fossa navicularis or membranous urethra; acquired urethral strictures, usually the result of trauma or infection, most frequently occur in the bulbomembranous urethra. Obstructive voiding symptoms such as those encountered with prostatism are common presenting complaints. Occasionally, urinary tract infection or inability to pass a urethral catheter may be the initial symptom. A history of prior urethral trauma, urethral instrumentation, or gonorrhea may be elicited. On physical examination an indurated area may be palpable in the urethra.

A urine flow study is a noninvasive method of initiating the diagnostic evaluation. A mean flow rate of >10 mL urine/sec or a peak flow rate of >15 mL urine/sec is indicative of obstruction. A retrograde urethrogram may reveal a narrowed urethral segment (Fig. 9.39). Occasionally, a voiding cystourethrogram performed through a suprapubic cystostomy tube may demonstrate the strictured urethral segment. Although urethroscopy permits direct visualization of the stricture, estimating the extent of strictured urethra may be difficult.

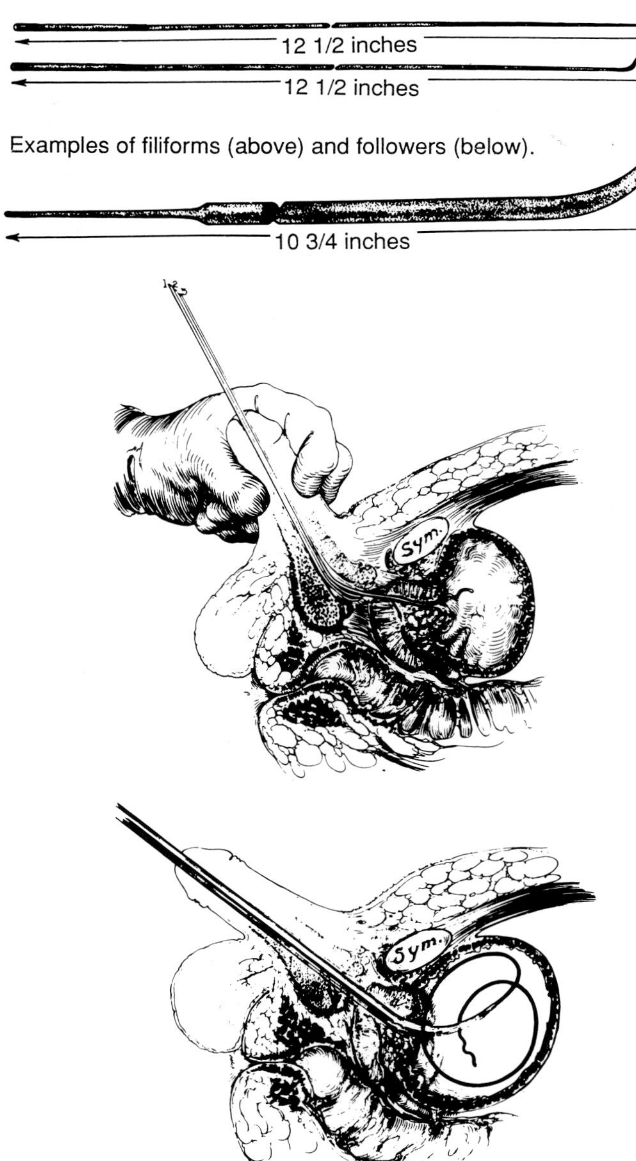

Figure 9.40. Technique of passing filiforms and followers to dilate a urethral stricture. **A**, After urethral lubrication, a filiform is passed through the urethral stricture into the bladder. **B**, A follower is screwed into the end of the filiform and advanced into the bladder. This process is repeated using successively larger diameter followers.

Treatment of urethral stricture disease must be tailored to the type of stricture and the patient's condition. Urethral dilatation is usually performed by distending the urethra with a water-soluble lubricant. A flexible plastic filiform (4–6 French) catheter is passed through the strictured area and into the bladder (Fig. 9.40). A larger follower is screwed into the distal end of the filiform and passed through the stricture. The filiform serves to guide the follower and harmlessly coils in the bladder. This process is repeated using successively larger followers until the stricture is dilated to about 24 French (8 mm in diameter). A urethral catheter is then passed into the bladder and left indwelling for several days. Most strictures will recur after dilatation. Short strictures may be cut using a knife blade passed through a cystoscopic instrument. This procedure is called *direct vision internal urethrotomy*. About 75% of properly selected patients have initial and long-term improvement in voiding symptoms.

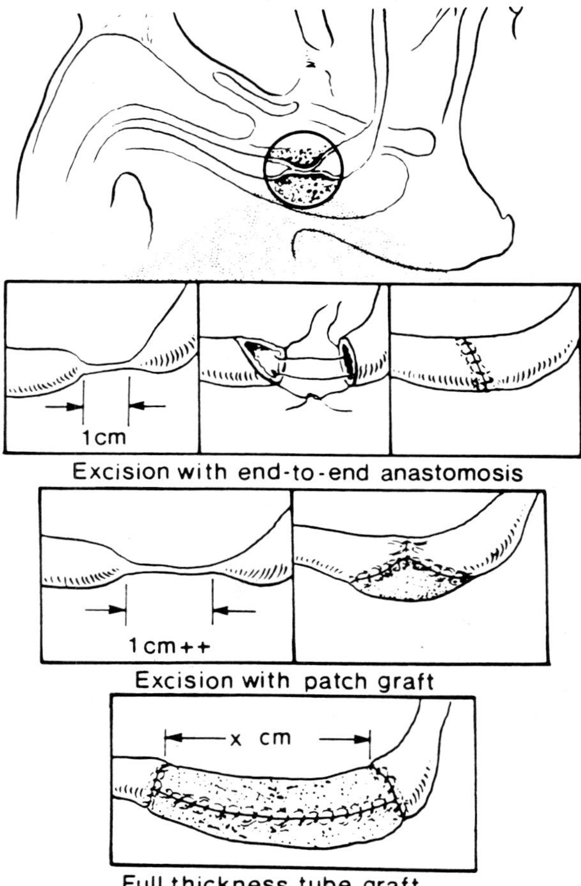

Figure 9.41. Common techniques of urethroplasty.

If the stricture recurs after dilatation or direct vision internal urethrotomy, or if the stricture is complex, open surgical reconstruction may be necessary (Fig. 9.41). Short strictures may be treated by simple excision of the involved urethral segment and primary end-to-end anastomosis. A variety of surgical procedures exists for more complex urethral strictures. Repair of the urethra (urethroplasty) may be performed in one operation (single staged) or may require multiple surgeries (multistaged). Tenets of urethroplasty involve excision of the strictured urethral segment and construction of a new segment using either a patch graft or a tube graft. Foreskin, which is devoid of hair and subcutaneous fat, is an ideal graft.

Congenital Disorders

Posterior Urethral Valves. The most common type of posterior urethral valve anomaly (Type I) consists of paired folds of mucous membranes that extend from the distal portion of the prostatic verumontanum and

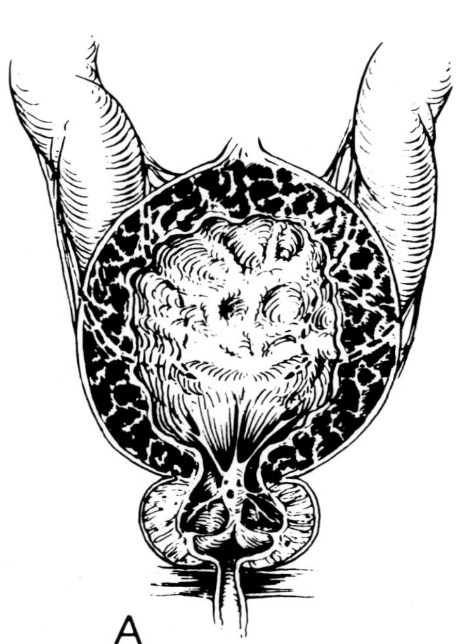

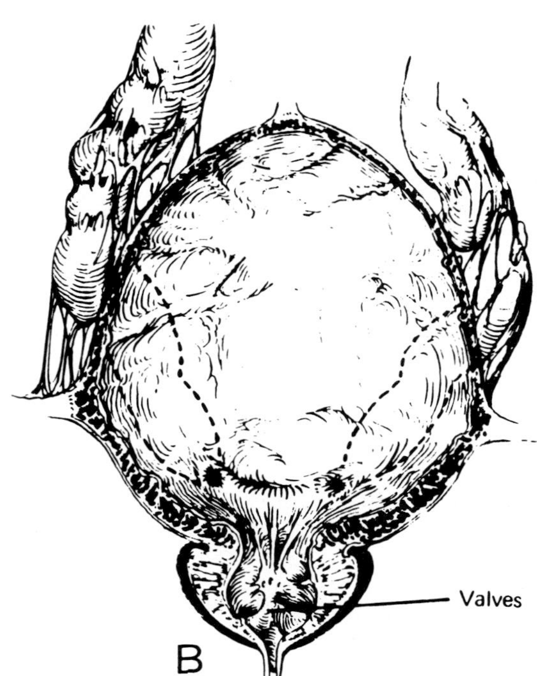

Figure 9.42. Posterior urethral valves. **A**, Dilation of the prostatic urethra, hypertrophy of vesical wall, and trigone in stage of compensation; bilateral hydroureters due to trigonal hypertrophy. **B**, Attenuation of bladder musculature in stage of decompensation; advanced ureteral dilation and tortuosity, usually secondary to vesicoureteral reflux.

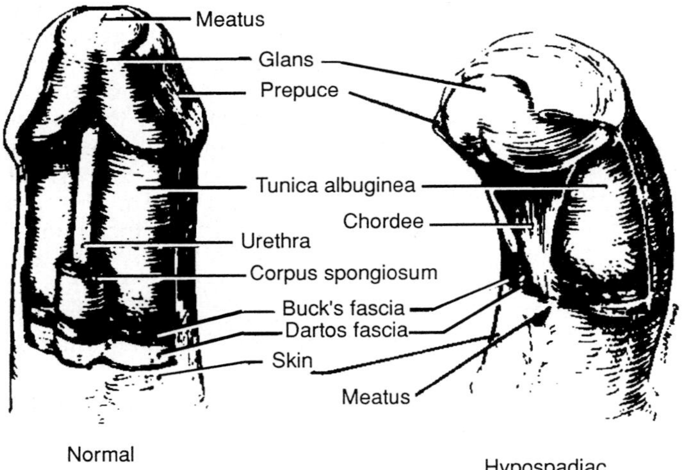

Figure 9.43. Comparison of normal and hypospadiac penis. Asterisk (*) indicates chordee.

meet anteriorly in the membranous urethra (Fig. 9.42). Posterior urethral valves cause a variable degree of urethral obstruction with resultant bladder distention, vesicoureteral reflux, hydroureteronephrosis, and renal insufficiency. The diagnosis is suggested in newborns with poor urinary streams or inability to void, and suprapubic or flank masses. Ultrasonography demonstrates bladder distention and hydronephrosis. A voiding cystoureterogram may show the valves, but a more consistent finding is a dilated posterior urethra, with secondary findings of bladder and upper urinary tract obstruction.

Initial treatment consists of placing either an 8 French infant feeding tube as a urethral catheter or a percutaneous suprapubic tube. Fluid, electrolyte, and acid-base status must be optimized. After the patient is stable, endoscopic valve ablation may be performed; alternatively, the bladder dome may be opened onto the lower abdomen (cutaneous vesicostomy) and endoscopic valve ablation performed another time.

Hypospadias. Hypospadias is one of the most common congenital anomalies, occurring in 1:300 live male births. In hypospadias the urethral meatus is located on the ventral penile surface proximal to its normal position at the tip cf the glans penis (Fig. 9.43). Classification is based on the location of the meatus, which may be perineal, penoscrotal, penile, coronal, or glandular. Usually the prepuce is incompletely developed and is present only on the dorsal aspect. Additionally, remnants of the corpus spongiosum distal to the urethral meatus form fibrous bands called chordee, producing ventral penile curvature. When the chordee are released during hypospadias repair, the meatus often retracts more proximally, resulting in a greater distance between the hypospadiac and the normal meatal positions. In boys with perineal hypospadias, the scrotum is bifid (resembling labia majora), the testes are often undescended, and the penis is small (resembling a hypertrophied clitoris); gender assignment may be difficult.

The goals of hypospadias repair are twofold. First is the correction of penile curvature, which is usually accomplished by releasing the chordee. Second is the creation of a new urethra to bridge the gap between the hypospadic meatus and the tip of the penis. Numerous techniques of hypospadias repair exist; the principles are similar to those of urethroplasty discussed in the urethral stricture section of this chapter. To minimize the psychological effects of genital surgery, it is best that hypospadias repair be performed before the child is 2–2 1/2 years of age.

Infectious Diseases

Gonococcal Urethritis. Gonorrhea is caused by the pathogen *Neisseria gonorrhoeae*, an anaerobic Gram-negative diplococcus, which is transmitted during sexual intercourse. Following an incubation period of 2–14 days, most men present with a yellowish urethral discharge caused by anterior urethritis. Other symptoms may include dysuria, urethral itching, and urinary frequency. About one-fourth of infected males remain asymptomatic and serve as a reservoir. If rectal or oral intercourse is suggested by the history, rectal and pharyngeal cultures are recommended. Complications of gonorrheal infection include epididymitis, prostatitis, urethral structure, and—less frequently—ophthalmia, endocarditis, hepatitis, and meningitis.

A Gram's stain of urethral exudate, which demonstrates typical Gram-negative intracellular diplococci, is sufficient to make the diagnosis of gonorrhea. Otherwise, a culture specimen using Thayer-Martin medium must be obtained. A concomitant serologic test for syphilis is also obtained. If a presumptive diagnosis of gonococcal urethritis is made, patients and their sexual contacts are treated without waiting for the culture reports. Current treatment recommendations reflect the emergence of tetracycline- and penicillin-resistant *N. gonorrhoeae*. Ceftriaxone 250 mg given once intramuscularly is considered the treatment of choice. Alternative therapy includes a single 3 g dose of amoxicillin or 4.8 million units of aqueous procaine penicillin G i.m. divided in two injections, both preceded by 1 g of probenecid. All therapies are followed by a 7-day course of doxycycline or another tetracycline to prevent postgonococcal urethritis caused by coexistent *Chlamydia trachomatis*.

All men should undergo a repeat culture 7–10 days after treatment has been completed. Positive repeat cultures are tested for penicillinase-producing *N. gonorrhoeae*. Patients with penicillin-resistant gonococcal infections are treated with one dose of spectinomycin, 2 g intramuscularly.

Nongonococcal Urethritis. Nongonococcal urethritis is characterized by dysuria, urinary frequency, periurethral itching, and a clear or white mucoid discharge. *Chlamydia trachomatis* and *Ureaplasma urealyticum* are the most common causative agents; both pathogens have an incubation period of 1–3 weeks. Less common causative agents are mycoplasma and *Trichomonas vaginalis*. Because patients with gonococcal urethritis treated with penicillin often develop a postgonococcal urethritis caused by a penicillin-insensitive chlamydia, all patients treated for gonorrhea should receive a 7-day course of doxycycline or another tetracycline to treat chlamydia as well.

The diagnosis of nongonococcal urethritis is made by cultures of the urethral swab, not the exudate. Because cultures are technically difficult to perform, most clinicians base therapy on Gram's stain findings. The presence of polymorphonuclear lymphocytes in the absence of intracellular Gram-negative diplococci is sufficient indication to treat the patient for presumptive nongonococcal urethritis. Regardless of the causative pathogen, patients and their sexual partners should be treated. Both *C. trachomatis* and *U. urealyticum* are sensitive to doxycycline, 100 mg given orally twice daily, or oral erythromycin, 500 mg, for 7 days. Alternatively, sulfisoxazole, 500 mg given orally for 10 days, may be used. Occasionally, wet-mount examination will disclose *Trichomonas*. Treatment is metronidazole, either a single 2-g oral dose or the more effective 250-mg oral dose given three times daily for 7 days. If symptoms persist despite adequate treatment, cystoscopy is performed to exclude an intraurethral lesion.

The Testes, Male Infertility, and Impotency

The Testes

Embryology and Anatomy. The testes develop embryologically from a long band of mesoderm on the posterior abdominal wall, the genital ridge. This band parallels the mesonephric kidney, and together they make up the mesonephric ridge. At the 4th week of gestation, gonocytes migrate from the endoderm of the yolk sac into the developing genital ridge; if a Y chromosome is present a testicle is formed. Twelve to 15 of the mesonephric tubules abutting the testicle join the rete testes and form the ductuli efferentes. These join the caudal extremity of the mesonephric duct to form the vas deferens and epididymis. A remnant of the mesonephros is attached to the head of the epididymis as the appendix epididymis, while a remnant of the paramesonephros (mullerian duct) becomes the appendix testes. This structure may become infarcted in later life to mimic testicular cord torsion.

Due to differential growth, the testicle lies just inside the internal inguinal ring by the 7th month. The gubernaculum ("rudder") is a thick, inelastic structure connecting the lower pole of the testicle to the genital eminence and, in an unknown fashion, leads the testicle through the inguinal canal into the scrotum during the 8th month. During its descent, the testicle becomes invested with a number of coverings (Fig. 9.44). The peritoneum surrounds the anterior four-fifths of the testicle and becomes the tunica vaginalis. The superior portion remains as the tubular processus vaginalis, which shortly collapses and obliterates. The internal oblique fascia becomes the cremasteric ("suspender") fibers, which act as a thermoregulator, elevating the testicle during periods of cold.

The main arterial supply to the testicle, the internal spermatic artery, arises from the aorta below the renal artery and pierces the tunica medial to the epididymis. Additional arterial inflow arises from the deferential ar-

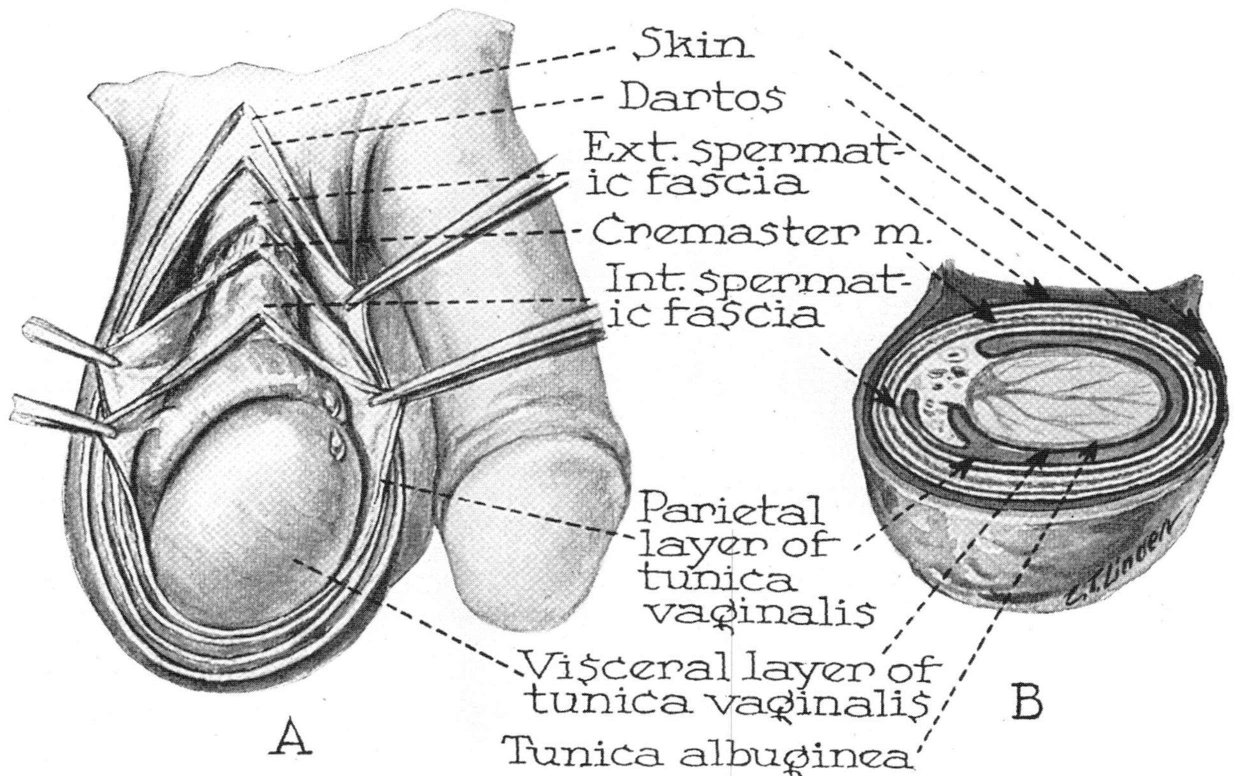

Figure 9.44. Coverings of the testicle.

tery, a branch of the inferior vesical artery, and from the external spermatic (cremasteric) artery, a branch of the inferior epigastric artery. The venous drainage parallels the arterial supply with a deferential vein draining into the hypogastric vein, an external spermatic vein draining into the epigastric vein, and an internal spermatic vein draining into the vena cava on the right and the renal vein on the left. Due to the juxtaposition of the mesonephric and genital ridges, the lymphatic drainage of the testicles is to the preaortic and precaval region, not, as commonly thought, to the inguinal or pelvic nodes. This knowledge is essential in considering the spread of testicular malignancy.

The vas deferens and epididymis form from the caudal extension of the mesonephric (wolffian) duct. The epididymis pierces the tunica albuginea of the posterolateral upper pole of the testicle. It is approximately 2 inches in length and composed of the globus major (head), the corpus (body), and globus minor (tail). The 12–15 ductuli efferentes coalesce into a single convoluted tubule within the epididymis that is estimated to be 28 feet in total length. The globus minor becomes the vas deferens, composed of middle circular and outer and inner longitudinal muscles. The initial portion of the vas is extremely convoluted and lacks the sheath that invests the remainder of the vas and carries the nerves, lymphatics, and vasculature. The vas travels through the inguinal canal and internal ring, at which point it leaves the accompanying spermatic vessels to cross the ureter and external iliac artery. It then travels behind the bladder, medial to the seminal vesicle, and sacculates as the ampulla before it pierces the prostate as the ejaculatory ducts.

Congenital Abnormalities. Cryptorchidism. One of the more common abnormalities seen in newborn boys is a nonpalpable testicle (cryptorchidism). The incidence of this abnormality decreases with age, from 3.4% seen in term infants to 0.7% seen at 9 months of age. If an empty scrotum is found, anorchia, nondescent, or retractile testis is possible. The student is encouraged to refer to EGS2, Chapter 15 for the various types of hernias that may present in this region in association with cryptorchidism.

Anorchia occurs in 3–5% of all cases explored for nonpalpable testes. Most are caused by prenatal torsion or vascular accidents, rarely by agenesis. At exploration, a vas deferens is found adjacent to the spermatic vessel, with a bud of scar representing the infarcted testicle (blind ending vas). Unilateral anorchia is of minimal concern; the contralateral testicle is usually larger and spermatogenesis and hormonal function do not appear to be affected. Bilateral anorchia leads to sterility and the need for hormonal replacement at puberty.

Retractile testes are caused by overactivity of the cremasteric musculature. They are easily pulled into the scrotum, but retract promptly into the groin. Most descend properly at puberty. This phenomenon underlines the need to examine the infant in a warm environment with gentle manipulation of the inguinal region.

Undescended testicles usually lie along the usual course of descent, from the retroperitoneum to the external inguinal ring. Rarely, the testicular descent is aberrant and the testicle may be found in the perineum in front of the anus. Most commonly, if the undescended testicle is not palpable within the inguinal canal, it is found just inside the internal inguinal ring. If neither testicle is palpable, but present, a stimulatory test with human chorionic gonadotropin (HCG) will cause a rise in serum testosterone. If no surge is noted, the diagnosis of intersex should be entertained. If a surge is noted with bilateral and sometimes unilateral cryptorchidism, treatment with exogenous HCG may lead to descent. CT or ultrasound may be used to locate nonpalpable testicles. A nonpalpable testicle must be explored because the undescended testicle has a 48-times greater incidence of testis malignancy. The contralateral descended testicle also has an increased risk of malignant degeneration. Unfortunately, surgical orchidopexy (movement of the testicle into its normal position) does not decrease these risks, but does allow earlier diagnosis of future malignancies. Men with a history of testicular maldescent also have an increased risk for subfertility. A number of epididymal abnormalities are also seen with testicular nondescent, including an elongated epididymis, detachment from the testicle, and partial disruption.

Patent Processus Vaginalis. The processus vaginalis, the tube of peritoneum extending from the abdominal cavity to the tunica vaginalis, usually closes and involutes before birth. When it does not, the child presents with an inguinal hernia. A patent processus vaginalis is found in 4.4% of full-term and up to 13% of premature infants. If the processus is completely open, herniation of abdominal viscera may occur with possible strangulation, dictating emergency surgical correction. If the processus partially closes, a hydrocele forms, which increases in size if the infant is upright or cries. If a hydrocele is not apparent, gentle examination may reveal a fuller cord on one side. A hydrocele is present if rubbing the cord between the thumb and forefinger gives the sensation of silk rubbing on silk (silk glove sign) when the peritoneal sac is palpated. Spontaneous obliteration of the processus vaginalis may occur after birth. Only if the hydrocele persists after age 2 is repair necessary. Repair consists of simple high ligation of the patent processus vaginalis at the internal inguinal ring.

Testicular Cord Torsion. Neonates who present with an acutely hard, enlarged scrotal mass that does not transilluminate may have incarcerated inguinal hernia, torsion of a testicular appendage, trauma-induced scrotal hematoma, or testicular torsion. In the newborn, torsion is extravaginal; that is, the epididymis, testicle, and tunica vaginalis all twist within the internal spermatic fascia with resultant organ infarction. Examination of the scrotum in the early phase of torsion will sometimes demonstrate a testicle lying in the transverse plane rather than in the normal longitudinal position. Occasionally, the epididymis may be palpable in the abnormal anterior position rather than in the normal posterior medial position. Loss of cremasteric reflex can be seen in 95% of patients with testicular torsion. An incarcerated hernia can sometimes be diagnosed with ultrasound or with stethoscope. Auscultation of bowel sounds in the scrotum indicates trapped bowel contents.

Intravaginal torsion occurs more commonly in the adolescent period. In this entity the tunica vaginalis surrounds the testicle instead of being fixed posterolaterally. The testicle is then free to twist inside the tunica, similar to the clapper within a bell. The patient presents with an acutely swollen, tender testicle that may preclude examination. The testicle may be retracted high in the scrotum, or the epididymis may be in an abnormal position. A thorough history may elicit previous episodes of transient testicular pain. Torsion may follow vigorous activity, but rarely is caused by it. Differential diagnosis includes trauma, epididymoorchitis, torsion of a testicular appendage, scrotal insect bites, viral orchitis (chickenpox, mumps, *Coxsackievirus*, infectious mononucleosis), or testicular cord torsion. Torsion of a testicular appendage may present with a "blue dot sign" in which the infarcted appendage is seen through the scrotal skin as a blue infarcted area. Epididymoorchitis is extremely rare in the adolescent age group and in the absence of pyuria should not be considered.

If the diagnosis is in doubt, a technetium radionuclide scan showing a central radiolucent pattern indicates a testicular cord torsion. If testicular cord torsion is a possible diagnosis, the patient should be explored surgically. Temporizing maneuvers of icing the scrotum, blocking the cord with an anesthetic, or attempting manual detorsion may be used while awaiting operating room availability. Because prolonged torsion (greater than 6 hours) may lead to irreversible testicular damage with resultant subfertility, correction should proceed quickly. If a bell clapper deformity is noted at surgery, it is assumed to be present bilaterally and a simultaneous contralateral testicular fixation can prevent subsequent contralateral torsion.

Testicular Trauma. Although the testicles hang freely within the scrotum and are relatively resistant to trauma, a direct blow to the organ may lead to injury. A contusion of the testicle is the most commonly seen injury and presents with pain and a scrotal mass. If the mass does not transilluminate, however, blood is probably within the tunical space. A real-time ultrasound examination should be performed to assure the integrity of the tunica albuginea and epididymis. If a fracture has occurred, scrotal exploration should be performed with removal of defunctionalized seminiferous elements and closure of the tunical tear. If the testicle cannot be salvaged, orchiectomy should be performed to remove all defunctionalized tissue. A contused testicle responds to bed rest, ice, and analgesia.

Scrotal Infections. The scrotal skin is subject to the same types of localized infections seen elsewhere on the body. An environment particularly conducive to bacterial and fungal infections is created by the moisture produced by abundant sweat glands that is then trapped by hair follicles and scrotal rugations. Local abscesses can present quickly but respond well to surgical drainage. The presence of tubercular or syphylitic abscesses may lead to chronic scrotal fistulae. Periurethral and perirectal infections may extend into the scrotum and become resistant to local care unless the underlying disease is treated aggressively.

Fournier's gangrene, a rare disorder occurring in otherwise normal individuals, is marked by acute gangrenous changes within the scrotum. Without aggressive surgical management, the disorder can lead to the patient's death. It is considered idiopathic but thought to be caused by an underlying infection of microaerophilic coccus or anaerobic bacillus. The scrotum becomes erythematous, tense, and moist. The gangrene spreads rapidly and the patient evidences early constitutional symptoms. Wide debridement and drainage of the affected area as well as administration of broad-spectrum antibiotics are essential.

Because the testicle has a rich vascular and lymphatic supply, it rarely is the sole site of infection but can become infected secondary to an adjacent epididymitis. Infection is transmitted through the lumen of the vas deferens and usually originates as a urethritis, prostatitis, or following instrumentation or catheterization. When the testicle is involved the patient is acutely ill with a high fever, leukocytosis, nausea, and often vomiting. The scrotum is swollen, red, and tender. A hydrocele may be present, and in later stages the scrotum may be fixed and indurated. Urine and urethral cultures should be taken to determine whether the patient needs treatment for a Gram-negative infection. Gonoccocal smears and cultures should also be obtained. The patient should respond within 48 hours; otherwise, an abscess should be suspected and a real-time ultrasound of the testicle obtained. If the testicle is spared and only the epididymis involved, the epididymis is swollen, tender, and indurated. *Chlamydia* is the most likely organism in patients under 35 years of age; otherwise, *E. coli* is the most common organism. Treatment consists of elevating the scrotum, bed rest, localized heat, and antibiotics. Extensive epididymitis may lead to pressure on the nearby spermatic artery with aseptic infarction of the ipsilateral testicle. Before antibiotics, the epididymis was surgically opened (epididymotomy) to relieve local pressure.

Traumatic epididymitis is characterized by epididymal pain, induration, and swelling. The condition seems to be related to trauma in that it is commonly seen in young military men following a forced march or vigorous activity. It may be secondary to urine refluxing into the epididymis with resultant pressure or chemical irritation. Traumatic epididymitis does not respond to antibiotic treatment but usually responds to nonsteroidal antiinflammatory agents, bed rest, and elevation. As with infectious epididymitis, it may become chronic because of sperm invasion of the paraepididymal tissue and foreign body reaction. If chronic, the only viable treatment may be surgical excision.

Orchitis occurs in 18% of mumps infection cases. This viral complication occurs 4–6 days after parotid gland involvement and presents with symptoms similar to those of other forms of orchitis:a reactive hydrocele, pain, swelling, and constitutional reactions. Testicular involvement is unilateral in 79% of cases, with organ loss or atrophy in 50% of cases. Treatment is supportive, although gamma globulin, steroids, adrenocorticotropic hormone (ACTH), and high-dose estrogens have been used. None of these treatments has been shown to alter the devastating effects of mumps orchitis.

Neoplasms

Evaluation. Testicular cancer is the most common solid malignancy in men between the ages of 18 and 35. Finding a scrotal mass is a frightening experience for a young man, and fear of malignancy may lead to denial. Physicians need to teach all young men the need for and technique of testicular self-examination.

The patient presenting with a scrotal mass should be questioned as to how long the mass has been present and whether it is increasing in size, painful, or has been preceded by infection, trauma, or surgery. After the scrotum is examined manually, a bright light is placed behind the mass in an attempt to transilluminate it. Transillumination implies fluid with probable hydrocele or spermatocele as the etiology. If the testes are seen to "float" in the middle of the cystic mass, the mass is a hydrocele, caused by decreased absorption of fluids by the parietal layer of the tunical vaginalis, leading to a fluid collection between the two leaves of the tunica. If, however, the mass sits above or below the testes, it is probably a spermatocele caused by local extravasation of sperm from the epididymis, usually the head. Both entities are benign, but the distinction is important if surgical correction is entertained. If the mass is adjacent to the spermatic cord and is tubular with a "bag of worms" sensation, it is probably a varicocele: a dilated segment of internal spermatic vein. Varicoceles are seen in approximately 19% of all men and need correction only if there is ipsilateral pain, testicular atrophy, or subfertility. The etiology of this abnormality is unknown, but because of its predilection for left-sided occurrence, a valve abnormality (or "nutcracker" phenomenon by the inferior mesenteric vein) has become a popular explanation. If the mass does not transilluminate but appears to be localized to the head or tail of the epididymis, it most likely is a sperm granuloma, an epididymal cyst, a benign epididymal adenomatoid tumor, or—rarely—a mesothelioma of the epididymis, which has malignant potential.

A mass that involves the testicle has a high probability of malignancy and should be treated as such. Real-time ultrasonography of the mass can be performed to help differentiate the various causes of scrotal masses, but surgical exploration is usually necessary for both diagnosis and treatment. Because of the lymphatic drainage of the testicle, a scrotal incision is contraindicated. If a malignancy is present, lymphatic drainage patterns are altered and future treatment compromised. Therefore, a groin incision should be made in the region of

Table 9.9.
Staging of Germ Cell Tumors

Stage I	Metastatic workup is negative; preoperative markers, if positive, normalize. Tumor is isolated to the testicle.
Stage IIA	Microscopic retroperitoneal disease.
Stage IIB	Minimal retroperitoneal disease on radiographic studies (<5 mL).
Stage IIC	Bulky retroperitoneal disease (>5 mL).
Stage III	Disease beyond retroperitoneal lymph drainage, or positive markers after retroperitoneal lymph node dissection.

the mid-inguinal canal. The spermatic cord is atraumatically occluded and the testicle brought into the surgical field and exposed. If a tumor is present, the cord structures are ligated with a silk suture and the testicle is removed. Before removal, frozen sections are obtained if the lesion appears to involve only the tunica albuginea or to be a hematoma from previous trauma.

Treatment. Testicular malignancies can be divided into germ cell tumors (which arise from the germinal elements) and nongerminal tumors (which arise from the mesodermal elements of the testicle). Only germ cell tumors, the most common, are discussed below.

Germ cell tumors of the testicle are divided into seminomas and nonseminomas. Seminomas do not undergo further neoplastic transformation, while nonseminomas differentiate along extraembryonic lines (choriocarcinoma or yolk-sac tumors) or intraembryonic lines (teratoma). Prior to radical orchiectomy, certain tumor markers are obtained. Classically, these are α-fetoprotein (AFP) and β-human chorionic gonadotropin (BHCG), although recent evidence indicates that lactate dehydrogenase (LDH), carcinoembryonic antigen (CEA), and human chorionic somatomammotropic hormone (HCS) may also serve as markers. These markers, like CEA in colon cancer, aid not in diagnosis but in evaluating response to therapy or onset of recurrences. Following radical orchiectomy (removal through an inguinal incision), tumor staging is performed with retroperitoneal computerized tomographic scanning (supplanting lymphangiography), chest radiographs (with or without a CT scan or tomograms), and IVP. Clinical and pathologic staging is complicated, but generally follows the outline in Table 9.9.

Seminomas usually cause diffuse enlargement of the testis. The cut tissue is glistening white. Microscopically there is a monotonous overgrowth of large, round cells with clear cytoplasm. Lymphocytic infiltration is found in 20% of cases. Since AFP is produced by endodermal cells lining the yolk sac, it will not be elevated in a pure seminoma. BHCG, however, is produced by the syncytiotrophoblastic cell and may be found in 30–40% of seminomas. After the histologic diagnosis is made, staging is completed (according to Table 9.9). Treatment of seminoma is as follows.

Stage I. Currently, the mainstay treatment of seminoma isolated to the testis remains radiation therapy to the paraaortic and ipsilateral iliac nodal areas. If the scrotum was violated during orchiectomy, the ipsilateral hemiscrotum is irradiated. Approximately 95% of these patients will be cured of their disease.

Stages IIa and IIb. The mainstay of treatment is radiation therapy to the paraaortic and ipsilateral iliac nodes with increased radiation given to the affected nodal tissue. The disease-free survival rate at 5 years is 95%.

Stages IIc and III. In the past, patients with advanced retroperitoneal nodal disease or extranodal metastases were treated with radiation therapy. Unfortunately, relapses were difficult to treat because bone marrow suppression limited chemotherapy. These patients, now treated with chemotherapeutic regimens based on platinum or etoposide, have an 85% complete response and cure rate for greater than 5 years.

Nonseminomatous germ cell tumors are divided according to their extra- or intraembryonic differentiation into embryonal, endodermal sinus, choriocarcinoma, or teratoma. Initial treatment and staging is similar to that for seminomas. Prognosis of these tumors varies, but because they are treated similarly they will be discussed as a group.

Stage I. Unlike seminomas, these tumors are radioresistant and require toxic chemotherapeutic regimens. Surveillance protocols for stage I nonseminomatous tumors with normal postorchiectomy markers have been established. Of patients with these tumors, 20% will relapse (80% within 1 year), but over 90% can be saved with chemotherapy. Surveillance may avoid repeat surgery, expense, and the toxicity of chemotherapy, as well as the reduced fertility associated with both surgery and chemotherapy. Should the patient not be a candidate (follow-up is demanding) nor desire surveillance, a modified or selective retroperitoneal node dissection is performed. Unlike complete bilateral node dissections, which in the past led to near 100% loss of ejaculation capabilities, modified dissections may preserve, in greater than 85% of cases, the sympathetic chains that allow normal ejaculation.

Stages IIa and IIb. The exact tumor burden that limits surgical extirpation before chemotherapeutic intervention is not known. However, patients with less than 5 mL of nodal disease may be served best by surgery. These patients undergo retroperitoneal lymph node dissection and, if markers return to normal and all disease is thought to be removed, are followed monthly with markers, chest x-rays, and CT scans. Recurrences are treated with 3–4 courses of a chemotherapy regimen using platinum or etoposide.

Stages IIc and III. Advanced nodal or extranodal disease is treated with cytoreductive chemotherapy. Four courses of platinum or etoposide regimen over a 12-week period are instituted. Of patients so treated, 30% will have residual disease while 60% will have a teratomatous differentiation or fibrosis. Retroperitoneal surgical dissection is necessary to determine those who require further chemotherapy.

Male Infertility

Of all newly married couples, 15% experience difficulty conceiving a child. Statistics show that 60% of fertile couples will conceive within 3 months of unpro-

Table 9.10.
Standards for Adequate Semen Analysis[a]

Ejaculate volume	1.5–5.0 mL
Sperm density	>20 million/mL
Motility	>60%
Grade of motility	>2 (scale 1–4)
Morphology	>60% normal

[a]As determined by the World Health Organization.

tected intercourse, and 90% within 1 year. Therefore, each partner merits evaluation if no pregnancy occurs within 1 year of unprotected intercourse. This section will limit itself to male infertility. A male factor is causative in 40% of cases, and partially responsible in an additional 20%.

Evaluation. A complete history should include: (*a*) childhood illnesses (such as mumps) and previous groin, scrotal, or bladder surgical procedures; (*b*) problems with delayed or premature puberty; (*c*) previous viral illnesses, since spermatogenesis takes approximately 90 days; (*d*) medications that may cause fertility abnormalities (cimetidine, Macrodantin, Azulfidine); (*e*) toxin exposure and marijuana or cigarette smoking; (*f*) knowledge of fertility timing (the couple may be having intercourse too frequently, not frequently enough, or timing it incorrectly); (*g*) use of lubricants (some are spermicidal).

The physical examination includes examining (*a*) the genitalia; (*b*) body habitus for Klinefelter's syndrome; (*c*) visual fields and olfactory sense to ascertain possible pituitary or hypothalamic lesions; (*d*) the breasts for gynecomastia; (*e*) the abdomen for a male escutcheon and any scars; (*f*) the penis for lesions and the urethral meatus for position and size; (*g*) the vas deferens and epididymis, which are palpated for any abnormalities; (*h*) the testicles, which also are palpated and sized with an orchidometer, noting consistency and any abnormalities. A varicocele is elicited by asking the patient to stand during the history taking. If no varix is felt, a deep Valsalva maneuver or a Doppler ultrasound examination may be necessary.

Semen Analysis. The mainstay off male evaluation is the semen analysis. Since the findings of this analysis may vary, three fresh ejaculates, obtained after 24 hours of sexual abstinence, are examined within 1 hour of collection. The complete ejaculate is collected in a wide-mouthed glass jar (plastic may be spermicidal) and is kept at body temperature until analyzed. If masturbation is not possible, nonspermicidal condoms (Mylex) may be used. Semen analysis results should be discussed in terms of "adequacy" as determined by the World Health Organization (see Table 9.10), rather than in terms of "average" or "normal."

While sperm density is important, morphology and motility may be even more important factors in predicting fertility or infertility. If the sperm move in a haphazard fashion rather than in a straight direction, or if a significant percentage of the sperm is malformed or immature, fertility can be impaired. In patients with azoospermia or oligospermia, a fructose test is performed. Fructose is normally produced by the seminal vesicles; its absence in the ejaculate indicates obstruction either in the ejaculatory duct or in the seminal vesicles. Fresh semen is coagulum that liquefies within 30 minutes of ejaculation. If liquefaction does not occur, impaired sperm motility may result. Sperm agglutination may indicate antisperm antibodies, a condition that requires further evaluation.

Treatment. Most patients have combined deficits in their semen analysis, usually decreased density and motility. If a varicocele is present, ligation or transcutaneous embolization leads to improvement in semen quality in 64% of men, with a resultant impregnation rate of 35%. Many theories have been proposed for this unproven but apparent effect of varicocele, the most accepted being temperature elevation and blood flow alteration leading to decreased intratesticular hormone production.

Many empiric drug therapies have been tried in the subfertile male, but none has been shown effective in double-blind, cross-over studies.

Male Impotency

It is estimated that at least 10 million men in the United States, during more than half of their sexual encounters, suffer from an inability to obtain or maintain erections satisfactory for vaginal intercourse. In the past, most of these men were thought to have an underlying psychological abnormality. However, recent advances in knowledge of the mechanisms of erections have led to findings of physical abnormalities in over 90% of these men.

Erections occur by two different mechanisms, reflex and psychogenic. Reflex erections occur from genital stimulation and are transmitted by way of the pelvic and cavernosal nerves (parasympathetic). Psychogenic erections are caused by a compilation of cortical and midbrain stimuli affecting the thoracolumbar sympathetic penile pelvic nerves. These two mechanisms act in concert for normal erections. It has been proposed that sympathetic tonic stimulation maintains constriction of smooth muscle endothelial-like cells within the corpora cavernosal bodies. With stimulation, there may be a decrease in sympathetic tone as well as parasympathetic-induced dilation of these sinusoidal endothelial cells. This effect causes dilation of lacunar spaces, with a subsequent increase in blood flow to the corporal bodies that results in increased intracavernosal pressure. The pressure increase causes compression of the subtunical veins with resultant decrease in venous outflow, allowing intracavernosal pressure to approach systemic pressure. Rhythmic contractions of ischiocavernosal and bulbocavernosal muscles cause further inflow, with ultimate pressures reaching 2–3 times systolic pressure.

Erectile impotence is classified according to four main categories: vasculogenic, endocrinologic, psychogenic, and neurogenic. Evaluation of the impotent male consists of studies to elicit abnormalities in one or more of these categories.

Vasculogenic. Vasculogenic disorders probably are the most common cause of erectile dysfunction. Arterial insufficiency is worsened by hypertension, hyperlipidemia, diabetes mellitus, and cigarette smoking. Pelvic trauma and irradiation are less common causes of this abnormality. Many patients have normal arterial inflow but are unable to either dilate the intracavernosal trabecular smooth muscles or constrict the venous outflow, resulting in a "venous leak" with either early loss of erections or poor erectile capacity. Plethysmography, radionuclide washout, or pressure cuff measurements have been used to evaluate arterial inflow.

Endocrinologic. Endocrinologic syndromes causing erectile dysfunction include: hypogonadotrophic hypogonadism, hypergonadotrophic hypogonadism, and hyperprolactinemia. In the majority of cases the testicles are small and soft. Signs of feminization may be present, and the patient usually complains of decreased libido. The first study is a serum testosterone level, keeping in mind the circadian nature of testosterone release. A low testosterone level should be checked against a second early morning level or a "pooled" specimen obtained over a 45-minute period. If hypogonadism is found, gonadotrophins and prolactin levels are drawn. Hyperprolactinemia may be caused by a pituitary lesion, which is suspected if there are alterations in visual fields, an abnormal film of the sella turcica, or an abnormal CT scan. Treatment of hypogonadism involves injection of a depo-testosterone such as enanthate or cyprionate given every 2–3 weeks. Oral androgens should not be used because of their variable uptake and possible hepatotoxicity.

Psychogenic. Psychogenic abnormalities in erection capability are difficult to evaluate. When REM sleep was found to be associated with erections in normal men, many felt that nocturnal penile tumescence testing would accurately diagnose men with psychogenic etiology. Although this testing is helpful, it is expensive, time-consuming, and may not be accurate. Psychogenic etiologies rarely respond to psychotherapy. The treatment of men so afflicted should nevertheless not be dismissed, and psychotherapy should be offered.

Neurogenic. Neurogenic impotence may be caused by disorders that affect the efferent peripheral fibers to the penis, suprasacral lesions, or nerve transmission. The most common neuropathic lesions are caused by spinal cord injury, multiple sclerosis, alcoholism, and diabetes. Patients may present with voiding disabilities in addition to erectile dysfunction. Complete peripheral nerve evaluation is important. Previous pelvic surgery that has interfered with peripheral autonomic nerves may also cause a neurogenic impotence.

SUGGESTED READINGS

Abrams P, Feneley R, Torrens M. Urodynamics. Clinical practice in urology. Berlin: Springer Verlag, 1983.

Carson CC, Dunnick NR, eds. Endourology. New York: Churchill Livingstone, 1985.

Dekernion JB, Paulson DF. Genitourinary cancer management. Philadelphia: Lee & Febiger, 1987.

McAninch JW, ed. Trauma management: Vol II, Urogenital trauma. New York: Thieme-Stratton, 1985.

Smith DR. General urology. 9th ed. Los Altos, California: Lange Medical Publications, 1978.

Strauss MB, Welt LG, eds. Diseases of the kidney. 2nd ed. Boston: Little, Brown, 1963.

Prostate

Smith JA Jr. Management of localized prostate cancer. Cancer 1992;70:302–306.

Cooner WH, Mosley BR, Rutherford CLJ, Beard JH, Pond HS, Terry WJ, Igel TC, Kidd DD. Prostate cancer detection in a clinical urological practice by ultrasonography, digital rectal examination, and prostate specific antigen. J Urol 1990;143:1152–1154.

Catalona WJ, Smith DJ, Ratliff TL. Measurement of prostate specific antigen as a screening test for prostate cancer. N Engl J Med 1991;324:1156–1161.

Foote JE, Crawford ED. Total androgen suppression: are there any advantages? Sem Urol 1988;6:291–302.

Pfau A. Prostatitis: a continuing enigma. Urol Clin N Amer 1986;13:695–715.

Oesterling JE. Prostate specific antigen: a critical assessment of the most useful tumor marker for adenocarcinoma of the prostate. J Urol 1991;145:907–923.

Stoner E, Bracken RB, Stein E, et al. The clinical effects of 5-alpha reductase inhibitor, finasteride, in BPH. J Urol 1992;147:1292–2302.

Kidney

Nora PF, ed. Operative surgery. 3rd ed. Philadelphia: WB Saunders, 1990:ch 45.

Walsh PC et al, eds. Campbell's urology. 5th ed. Philadelphia: WB Saunders, 1986:chs 7, 26, 29, 38, 62.

Bladder

Galloway NTM. Classification and diagnosis of neurogenic bladder dysfunction. Prob in Urol 1989;3:1–22.

Hayes EE, Sandler CM, Corriere JN Jr. Management of the ruptured bladder secondary to blunt abdominal trauma. J Urol 1983;129:946.

Herschorn S. The management of neurogenic bladder dysfunction, emphasis on pharmacologic manipulation and intermittent catheterization. Prob in Urol 1989;3:23–29.

Kelalis PP. Surgical correction of vesicoureteral reflux. In: Kelalis PP, King LR, Belman AB, eds. Clinical pediatric urology. Philadelphia: WB Saunders, 1985.

Levitt SB, Weiss RA. Vesicoureteral reflux: natural history, classification and reflux nephropathy. In: Kelalis PP, King LR, Belman AB, eds. Clinical pediatric urology. Philadelphia: WB Saunders, 1985.

Peters PC, Bright TC III. Management of trauma to the urinary tract. In: Longmire WP Jr, ed. Advances in surgery. Vol 10. Chicago: Year Book Medical Publishers, 1976.

Raz S. Modified bladder neck suspension for female stress incontinence. Urology 1981;18:82.

Scott FB, Light JK, Fishman I, West J. Implantation of an artificial sphincter for urinary incontinence. Contemp Surg 1981;18:11.

Shortliffe LMD, Stamey TA. Infections of the urinary tract: introduction and general principles. In: Walsh PC et al, eds. Campbell's urology. 5th ed. Philadelphia: WB Saunders, 1986.

Stamey TA. Endoscopic suspension of the vesical neck for urinary incontinence in females: report on 203 consecutive cases. Ann Surg 1980;192:465.

Penis

Penile Trauma

Jordan GH, Gilbert DA. Male genital trauma. AUA Update Series. American Urologic Association, 1985;Lesson 20(4):2–7.

Jordan GH, Gilbert DA. Management of amputation injuries of the male genitalia. Urol Clin North Am 1989;16:359–367.

McAninch JW. Management of genital skin loss. Urol Clin North Am 1989;16:387–397.

Orvis BR, McAninch JW. Penile rupture. Urol Clin North Am 1989;16:369–375.

Penile Cancer

Cabanas RM. An approach to the treatment of penile carcinoma. Cancer 1977;39:456–466.

Crawford ED, Dawkins CA. Cancer of the penis. In: Skinner DG, Lieskovsky G, eds. Diagnosis and management of genitourinary cancer. Philadelphia: WB Saunders, 1988.

Fair WR, Perez CA, et al. Cancer of the urethra and penis. In: DeVita VT, Hellman S, eds. Cancer principles and practice of oncology. Philadelphia: JB Lippincott, 1989.

Srinivas V, Morse MJ, Herr HW, et al. Penile cancer: relation of extent of nodal metastasis to survival. J Urol 1987;137:880–882.

Acquired Disorders

Devine CJ Jr. Surgery for Peyronie's disease. In: Novick AC, Streem SB, eds. Operative urology. Baltimore: Williams & Wilkins, 1989.

Hanno PM. Priapism. AUA Update Series. City?:American Urologic Association, 1984;Lesson 20(3):2–7.

Kramer SA. Circumcision. In: Glenn JF, ed. Urologic surgery. Philadelphia/Toronto: JB Lippincott, 1989.

Testes

Johnson DE, Zagars GK. Testicular seminoma. In: Resnick MI, Kursch E, eds. Current therapy in genito-urinary surgery. Toronto/Philadelphia: BC Decker, 1987.

Kaufman DG, Nagler HM. Specific non-surgical therapy in male infertility. Urol Clin North Am 1987;14:489–498.

Krane RG, Goldstein I, et al. Impotence. N Engl J Med 1989;321:1648–1653.

Levine SB, Althof SE, et al. Side effects of self-administration of intracavernosal papaverine and phentolamine for treatment of impotence. J Urol 1989;141:54–57.

Swerdloff RS. Physiology of male reproduction. In: Walsh, PC, et al, eds. Campbell's urology. 5th ed. Philadelphia: WB Saunders, 1986.

Urethra
Urethral Trauma

Klosterman PW, McAninch JW. Urethral injuries. AUA Update Series. American Urologic Association, 1989;Lesson 32 (8):250–255.

Morehouse DD, MacKinnon KJ. Management of prostatomembranous urethral disruption: 13 years' experience. J Urol 1980;123:80–82.

Pierce JM, Jr. Disruption of the anterior urethra. Urol Clin North Am 1989;16:329–334.

Turner-Warwick R. Prevention of complications resulting from pelvic fracture urethral injuries—and from their surgical management. Urol Clin North Am 1989;16:335–358.

Urethral Cancer

Ahlering TE, Lieskovsky G. Surgical treatment of urethral cancer in the male patient. In: Skinner DG, Lieskovsky G, eds. Diagnosis and management of genitourinary cancer. Philadelphia: WB Saunders, 1988.

Grabstald H. Tumors of the urethra in men and women. Cancer 1973;32:1236–1255.

Levine RL. Urethral cancer. Cancer 1980;45:1965–1972

Schellhammer PF. Urethral carcinoma. Semin Urol 1983;1:82–89.

Skinner EC, Skinner DG. Management of carcinoma of the female urethra. In: Skinner DG, Lieskovsky G, eds. Diagnosis and management of genitourinary cancer. Philadelphia: WB Saunders, 1988.

Urethral Strictures

Turner-Warwick RT. Urethral stricture surgery. In: Glenn JF, ed. Urologic surgery. Philadelphia: JB Lippincott, 1983.

Webster GD, Sihelnik S. The management of strictures of the membranous urethra. J Urol 1985;134:469–473.

Congenital Anomalies

Glassberg KI. Current issues regarding posterior urethral valves. Urol Clin North Am 1985;12:175–185.

Kroovand RL. Hypospadias and chordee. In: Resnick MI, Kursh E, eds. Current therapy in genitourinary surgery. Toronto/Philadelphia: BC Decker, 1987.

Woodhouse CRJ, Kellett MJ. Anatomy of the penis and its deformities in exstrophy and epispadias. J Urol 1984;132:1122–1124.

Infectious Diseases

Abramowicz M, Aaron H, et al. Treatment of sexually transmitted diseases. In: Kallet A, Aaron H, eds. The Medical Letter on drugs and therapeutics. New York: The Medical Letter, 1987.

Churchill RD, Hewitt SM, et al. 1989 Sexually transmitted diseases treatment guidelines. Morbid Mortal Weekly Rep, Sept 1, 1989;38 Suppl:8.

Skills

1. Given a patient with acute urinary retention, demonstrate physical examination findings (such as an enlarged prostate and palpable bladder).
2. Demonstrate an understanding of the use of Foley catheters in patients with urinary obstruction and the ability to place such a catheter using sterile technique.
3. Demonstrate an understanding of the use of ultrasound and prostatic biopsy in diagnosing prostate cancer.
4. On rectal exam, be able to distinguish among a normal prostate, one with benign prostatic hypertrophy, and one with a nodule or mass.
5. Demonstrate the ability to interpret an intravenous pyelogram, a urine flow rate, and a urinalysis.
6. Indicate a renal mass on CT scan.
7. Perform a workup for a patient with a renal mass lesion; indicate when to operate and when to observe a particular mass.
8. Demonstrate cystoscopy and enumerate the basic tests and examinations that can be done with the cystoscope.
9. Demonstrate the ability to evaluate a patient with suspected bacterial urinary tract infection:
   a. List the indications for further evaluation the the tests involved in such an evaluation
   b. List an adequate differential diagnosis for a patient with the symptoms of a urinary tract infection
10. For vesicoureteral reflux:
    a. Describe its pathophysiology
    b. Outline the evaluation of a patient with reflux
    c. Outline the difference between the patients who require surgical repair and those who can be treated nonsurgically
    d. Describe some of the different modes of ureteral reimplantation and the indications for each
11. Demonstrate the ability to transilluminate a testicular mass and be able to distinguish between a cystic and a noncystic lesion on that basis.

12. In a patient seen without a testicle in the scrotum, be able to evaluate the inguinal canal for the presence of a palpable undescended testicle or retractile testicle.
13. Demonstrate the proper transscrotal or inguinal examination for evaluation of a hernia and be able to distinguish between a direct and indirect hernia.
14. Demonstrate the ability to outline a workup of the male for a couple with primary infertility.
15. Demonstrate the ability to interpret properly a semen analysis.
16. Demonstrate the ability to evaluate the genitalia for a male with possible male factor infertility.
17. Demonstrate the ability to outline a workup for a man with erectile dysfunction.

CATHETER INSERTION: MALE

1. Before inserting a urethral catheter into a male, make certain the patient does not have a history or urethral stricture, trauma to the urethra, or prior prostatic surgery. If the patient admits to any of the preceding conditions, it is best to proceed slowly or call for a urological consultation.
2. The patient should be in a supine position with thighs slightly abducted.
3. If a catheter insertion kit is available, open it under sterile conditions and place the sterile drape over the patient's genitalia.
4. Pour the enclosed Betadine packet into the sterile receptacle. Do not pour the Betadine over the cotton swabs that usually accompany these kits.
5. Open the lubricant packet in the kit and squeeze sterile lubricant onto the sterile field.
6. If the patient is uncircumcised, retract the foreskin with your left hand. Then prep the glans with a sweeping motion away from the urethral meatus. The entire penis and puba penile area should be prepped. Inject sterile topical analgesic lubricant into the urethra, if available.
7. Hold the catheter with the right hand while stretching the penis upwards.
8. Liberally lubricate the catheter.
9. Insert the catheter into the urethral meatus and pass catheter into the urethra. The catheter should be grasped close to the glans to minimize bending.
10. Expect some resistance at the external sphincter area. Asking the patient to void if you encounter difficulty will relax the sphincter and facilitate passage of the catheter.
11. Pass the catheter up to the level of the valve.
12. Wait a few seconds for urine to drain. If no urine drains, gently irrigate the catheter with sterile saline. Once urine returns, inflate the balloon slowly. For a male inflate at least 10 mL of sterile water or saline, do not inflate air.
13. Gently tug on the catheter until resistance is met assuring that the balloon is tucked up against the bladder neck.
14. If there is any question of correct catheter position, instill 50 mL of sterile saline under gravity without irrigating. If there is no obstruction to the lumen of the catheter there will be free flow of the saline into the bladder. Then allow the catheter to drain. If there is no obstruction the same amount of fluid should drain readily from the bladder.
15. In young males you may encounter more resistance at the sphincter. Slow gentle pressure will usually overcome the resting pressure of the sphincter.
16. In general, passing a larger catheter (18 F to 20 F) is easier and less traumatic than passing a smaller catheter (14 F to 16 F).

CATHETER INSERTION: FEMALES

1. Position the patient in the supine position with thighs and knees slightly flexed.
2. Prepare the catheter tray as above for male catheterization.
3. With you left hand prep the external labia.
4. Spread the labia majora and gently prep the vaginal and urethral introitus.
5. If sterile analgesic lubrication is available, inject into the urethral meatus.
6. Pass catheter into urethra.
7. Inflate balloon and gently retract it against bladder neck.
8. Urine should flow freely. In some elderly females there is prolapse of the urethral meatus into the vagina. Occasionally a blind insertion will be required. For very obese women catheter insertion requires an assistant to expose the urethral meatus and retract redundant tissue.

RECTAL EXAMINATION

1. A digital rectal examination is best preformed with the patient bending over or in the knee-chest position.
2. Lubricate the finger well and apply gentle pressure to the anal sphincter.
3. Slowly insert finger into the rectum. The prostate gland will be palpable below your finger.
4. Begin examination on the right side of the prostate gland and with a sweeping motion of your finger examine the prostate from right to left. Seminal vesicles are not normally palpable so no effort should be made to try to examine these organs.
5. A normal prostate gland in a young male is approximately the size of walnut. In a male above 40 the prostate gland may be the size of a ping pong ball. It is not unusual to find enlarged glands two to three times the size of glands in younger males in older patients.
6. The consistency of the prostate gland should be evaluated. Normal prostate gland consistency is that of a

soft rubber eraser. Normal prostate consistency has also been compared to the tissue of the thenar eminence. A median furrow may be palpable in some patients. Any firm or indurated area should be noted. Any obvious prostatic nodules should be noted.

7. Bogginess is a very subjective finding.
8. Any tenderness elicited during prostatic examination should be further evaluated to rule out prostatitis.
9. Occasionally small calcifications are palpable below the surface of the prostate. These are clinically insignificant.

TESTICLE EXAMINATION

1. Patient should be standing for the examination. If possible the room should be warmed to prevent testicle retraction into the upper scrotum. This is the cremasteric reflex.
2. The scrotum should be observed for any difference in size or position of the testicles. The adult male scrotum demonstrates transverse rugae with normal coloration. Loss of rugae on either side with an enlarged hemi scrotum may indicate a mass or tense hydrocele.
3. Either testicle may be examined first. The left testicle should be examined with the right hand and the right testicle examined with the left hand.
4. Either hemi-scrotum is palpated to identify the vas deferens just above the testicle. The vas can be followed distally to the posterior aspect of either testicle. The epididymitis is a soft tube-like structure located along the posterior aspect of the testicle. The testicle itself should be smooth, soft, and non-tender. Any firm mass or firm area should be considered suspicious. A large tense scrotal mass may be transilluminated with a flash light. A hydrocele can be diagnosed with transillumination.
5. A firm testicular mass should be considered tumor until proven otherwise. A mass in the epididymitis either in the head or tail or body of the epididymitis is usually soft, non-tender, and round. Spermatoceles or epididymal cysts are the most common benign epididymal masses. Occasionally they can be identified using transillumination.
6. A tender indurated firm epididymitis usually indicates epididymitis.
7. A proliferation of small or large veins in the epididymal area or above the testicle indicates varicocele.
8. An indirect hernia may be present in the scrotum. This may be diagnosed by palpation or exudation of bowel sounds in the scrotum. An incarcerated scrotal hernia usually presents with scrotal tenderness, erythema, and abdominal tenderness.

Study Questions

PROSTATE

1. Identify the anatomical zones of the prostate and their significance.
2. Differentiate bacterial from nonbacterial prostatitis and the clinical signs and symptoms of each.
3. Describe the indications for treatment in patients with benign prostatic hypertrophy.
4. List the therapeutic options for treatment of BPH.
5. What are the methods for early detection of prostate cancer?
6. Describe the relationship of prostate specific antigen levels to benign prostate hypertrophy and carcinoma of the prostate.
7. Outline the staging systems for the primary tumor in patients with prostate cancer.
8. What are the surgical procedures for definitive treatment of prostate cancer?
9. Define the role of hormonal therapy in men with metastatic prostate cancer and the therapeutic options.

KIDNEYS

1. Describe the evaluation and treatment of patients with renal trauma.
2. Describe causes of and treatment for a nonfunctioning kidney.
3. Discuss the techniques for reimplantation of the ureter and the treatment of ureteral injuries secondary to surgical misadventure.
4. Discuss treatment of upper tract urinary stones, renal pelvis stones, and ureteral stones.
5. List indications for endourologic procedures of the renal pelvis and ureters.
6. Discuss the causes of ureteral stones.
7. Outline the basic workup for a patient with an obstructed ureter; differentiate between a stone and other causes of obstruction.
8. Discuss the mechanisms involved in renal maintenance of acid-base balance.

BLADDER

1. Describe the evaluation and treatment of the following patients:
   a. A 42-year-old female with 5 culture-proven urinary tract infections in the last 6 months
   b. A 35-year-old male with an episode of bacterial cystitis
   c. A 57-year-old female with dysuria, frequency, and nocturia but multiple negative urine cultures
2. A 19-year-old male involved in a motor vehicle accident complains of severe lower abdominal discomfort. He is not able to void nor does he feel the urge to

void. Outline evaluation and possible treatment options.

3. A 65-year-old male, status postcardiac transplantation, complains of lower abdominal pain, burning dysuria, purulent urine, and occasionally passing air when he voids. Outline evaluation and possible treatments.

4. Discuss the possible etiologies, evaluation, and treatment of a 45-year-old female with incontinence associated with rising from a sitting position, coughing, sneezing, and lifting heavy objects.

5. Outline the evaluation, treatment, and long-term follow-up of a 19-year-old male, complete T10 paraplegic.

6. Describe the evaluation, treatment, and follow-up of the following patients:
   a. 2-year-old female with unilateral grade II vesicoureteral reflux
   b. 24-year-old female with grade II vesicoureteral reflux and recurrent urinary tract infections
   c. 4-year-old male with grade IV vesicoureteral reflux

7. Describe the anatomy and pathophysiology of the following conditions:
   a. Exstrophy of the bladder
   b. Persistent urachal remnants
   c. Congenital and acquired bladder diverticula
   d. Recurrent urinary tract infection in females
   e. Chronic interstitial cystitis
   f. Bladder rupture as a result of blunt trauma
   g. Stress urinary incontinence
   h. Vesicoureteral reflux

8. Describe the sequence of events in normal micturition.

9. List and describe the tests that can be involved in a urodynamic evaluation. Mention their normal results.

10. List the medications used in the treatment of neurogenic bladder dysfunction. Describe their effects.

PENIS

1. Draw the cross-sectional anatomy of the penis.

2. Describe the management of:
   a. Blunt penile trauma
   b. Fractured penis
   c. Gunshot wounds and knife wounds to the penis
   d. Penile avulsion injury
   e. Penile strangulation
   f. Penile burns

3. List five premalignant penile lesions, their characteristics, and their treatment.

4. A 64-year-old male has a 1-cm exophytic lesion of the penile glans. An incisional biopsy has confirmed squamous cell carcinoma. Discuss further therapeutic options for the primary tumor.

5. A 59-year-old male has had a partial penectomy for squamous cell carcinoma. The patient initially had inguinal lymphadenopathy that was treated with antimicrobials for 6 weeks. Discuss further management of the inguinal lymph node region if:
   a. Inguinal lymphadenopathy persists despite antimicrobial therapy
   b. Inguinal lymphadenopathy resolves after antimicrobial therapy

6. A 23-year-old male presents with a prolonged, painful erection.
   a. Outline pertinent points in history taking
   b. Outline specific features to be looked for on physical examination
   c. What is the proper therapeutic management?

7. An obtunded 74-year-old man presents to the emergency room with a distended bladder. Attempts at placing a urethral catheter are unsuccessful because of a very tight phimosis. What is the proper management of this patient?

8. A patient presents with a penile ulcer:
   a. Outline the pertinent points in history taking
   b. Formulate a differential diagnosis
   c. Describe which diagnostic tests should be ordered
   d. Describe proper therapeutic management

URETHRA

1. Draw a sketch demonstrating the clinical anatomy of the male and female urethra.

2. Explain how a pelvic fracture could result in extravasation of urine into the upper chest wall and axilla.

3. Describe the pros and cons of immediate repair versus delayed repair and suprapubic cystostomy in men with complete posterior urethral rupture secondary to trauma.

4. Describe the lymphatic drainage of the male and female urethra.

5. A 62-year-old male has a biopsy positive for urethral cancer:
   a. Where is the most likely site of the biopsy?
   b. What is the most likely histologic cell type?

6. In men, what is the surgical treatment of:
   a. Small anterior urethral tumors?
   b. Larger anterior urethral tumors?
   c. Posterior urethral tumors?

7. A 50-year-old female has a biopsy positive for urethral cancer:
   a. Where is the most likely site of the biopsy?
   b. What is the most likely histologic cell types?

8. In women, what is the surgical treatment of:
   a. Tumors involving the distal one-third of the urethra?
   b. Tumors involving the proximal one-third of the urethra?

9. Describe the evaluation of a patient suspected of having a urethral stricture.

10. Compare gonococcal and nongonococcal urethritis in terms of:
    a. Pathogens
    b. Symptoms

c. Diagnostic evaluation
d. Treatment

THE TESTES, MALE INFERTILITY, AND IMPOTENCY

1. A 13-year-old male presents with left testicular pain:
   a. Outline pertinent points in history taking
   b. Describe appropriate physical examination points
   c. List the appropriate laboratory studies
   d. Discuss appropriate therapy
2. A 22-year-old white male presents to your office with the finding of a right scrotal mass on self-examination:
   a. Describe the appropriate physical examination
   b. Discuss the differential diagnosis of a transilluminated testicular mass
   c. If the mass is not transluminal discuss the proper workup and diagnosis
   d. Discuss the staging and therapy for testicular carcinoma
3. Discuss the rationale for and against "expectant" therapy for stage I nonseminomatous germ cell tumors.
4. A 26-year-old white male presents with a history of 2 years of unprotected intercourse without an ensuing pregnancy:
   a. Describe the appropriate history and physical examination
   b. Discuss a typical "adequate" semen analysis
   c. List the indications for testicular biopsy
   d. Describe the use of antisperm antibody testing
   e. Describe the Huhner test
   f. Discuss varicocele ligation with its indications and benefits
   g. Discuss the surgical options associated with male infertility
5. A 55-year-old white male states that he has not been able to obtain erections for the last 2 years:
   a. Describe an appropriate history and physical examination
   b. Outline a diagnostic plan
   c. Discuss the possible therapeutic options for this patient

Glossary

abduction—movement of the eye away from the primary position.

accommodation—process of ciliary muscle contraction that leads to an increase in the power of the lens of the eye.

acoustic neuroma—inner ear neoplasm causing hearing loss; hallmark symptom is unilateral sensorineural hearing loss with poor word discrimination.

adduction—movement of the eye toward the nose.

afterload—impedance or resistance against which the heart must eject blood.

Allen test—a test performed on physical examination to determine the patency of the radial and ulnar arteries as they contribute to the circulation of the hand.

allograft—a graft between members of the same species.

amaurosis fugax—a temporary blindness that may result from a transient ischemia due to carotid artery insufficiency or to centrifugal force.

amblyopia—poor or decreased vision in an eye that is anatomically normal.

analgesia—relief of pain.

anginal equivalent—symptoms of cardiac ischemia in the absence of or in addition to typical cardiac chest pain—it may be heart failure, nausea, syncope, or arrhythmia.

angle-closure glaucoma—glaucoma caused by an anatomic proximity of the iris to the cornea; may be acute.

anisometropia—unequal refractive error between the two eyes.

annular pancreas—a ring of pancreas encircling the duodenum, produced when the ventral pancreatic bud fails to rotate around and become incorporated into the dorsal bud. The duodenum may become partially or completely obstructed.

anosmia—loss of the sense of smell.

anotia—congenital absence of the ear.

anterior chamber angle—area of the eye where the iris meets the cornea; contains trabecular meshwork where aqueous leaves the eye.

anxiolysis—relief of anxiety.

aphakia—absence of the lens of the eye.

astigmatism—a refractive error in which the defect is not the same in all meridians.

avascular necrosis—pathologic death of one or more cells, or of a portion of tissue or organ due to deficient blood supply axial length—measurement from the cornea to the back of the eye.

axial pattern flap—a flap that is vascularized by a specific artery and vein enabling the flap's length to significantly exceed the flap's width.

background diabetic retinopathy—early retinal changes associated with diabetes; may include microaneurysm, hemorrhage, exudate.

bandage contact lens—extended-wear lens that can remain in the eye.

Battle' sign—ecchymosis overlying the mastoid process, associated with a basilar skull fracture.

Bier block—intravenous regional anesthesia, achieved by exsanguinating a limb and filling the venous system of that limb with a dilute solution of local anesthetic.

bifascicular block—electrical obstruction to conduction along two of the three major cardiac conduction pathways—usually right bundle branch block and left anterior hemiblock.

biliary atresia—sclerotic obliteration of the extrahepatic biliary ducts, occurring at about the time of birth. Usually the entire ductal system, but occasionally only a portion, is affected. The intrahepatic ducts are involved to some extent as well. The condition causes cholestasis and jaundice, and may progress to cirrhosis.

bioprosthetic valves—artificial heart valves synthesized from living animal or human tissue.

Bjerrum scotoma—glaucoma defect wedge-shaped or similarly shaped.

bladder neck—inferior part of the bladder, where the base and inferolateral surfaces converge. In the male, the neck of the bladder rests on the prostate gland.

blepharitis—inflammation of the eyelids.

blepharoplasty—aesthetic contouring of the eyelids.

blepharospasm—involuntary contraction of the orbicularis muscle.

blind spot (scotoma)—nonseeing area within the visual field.

blow-out fracture—an isolated fracture of the orbital floor.

Bowman's membrane—layer of the cornea just under the epithelium.

boxer's fracture—a fracture of the distal fifth metacarpal.

branchial cleft cyst—a fluid-filled subcutaneous structure arising from failure of complete resorption of the branchial clefts and arches. Most commonly located along the anterior border of the sternomastoid muscle as a remnant of the second branchial cleft.

branchial cleft cysts—persistent, painless (unless infected) masses just anterior to the middle third of the sternocleidomastoid muscle. These masses or tracts are subject to recurrent infection.

Bruch's membrane—innermost layer of the choroid just under the retinal pigment epithelium.

canthus—area formed by the junction of the upper and lower eyelids.

carcinomatous meningitis—seeding of carcinoma by spread within the cerebrospinal fluid.

cardiac bypass—provision for circulation and respiration by the heart-lung machine: a pump (heart) and oxygenator (lung).

cardiac reserve—the work that the heart is able to perform beyond that required under ordinary circumstances.

cardioplegic—solution that electrochemically paralyzes the heart muscle resulting in cardiac arrest in diastole; used in heart surgery to provide a quiet operative field.

cataract—any cloudiness in the crystalline lens of the eye.

cathode stimulation principle—cardiac pacing utilizing electrical stimulation of the negative pole of a bipolar electrical system—which is more efficient than anodal (positive) stimulation.

cat scratch fever—regional granulomatous lymphadenitis, often follows the scratch or bite of a cat. The adenopathy may resolve spontaneously.

cauda equina syndrome—dull pain in upper sacral region with anesthesia or analgesia in buttocks, genitalia, or thigh; accompanied by disturbed bowel and bladder function.

centrocecal scotoma—central visual loss that includes the fixation area.

cerebellopontine angle—the recess lying lateral to the junction of cerebellum and pons.

cerebral perfusion pressure—the blood pressure in excess of that sufficient to permit perfusion of the brain.

cervicofacial rhytidectomy—a face lift.

chemical peel—a method of treating small wrinkles of the face by the application of a caustic solution (e.g., phenol).

chemosis—edema of the conjunctiva.

Chlamydia trachomatis—a species of bacteria that produces glycogen (detectable by iodine stain) and is susceptible to sulfadiazine. Various strains cause trachoma, inclusion and neonatal conjunctivitis, lymphogranuloma venereum, mouse pneumonitis, nonspecific urethritis, epididymitis, cervicitis, salpingitis, proctitis, and pneumonia.

choanae—posterior nasal apertures; these open into the nasopharynx.

choanal atresia—congenital failure to open of one or both choanae.

choledochal cyst—dilatation of the extrahepatic ductal system with distal obstruction. May be congenital or acquired, and may produce obstructive jaundice.

cholesteatoma—tumor-like mass of keratinizing squamous epithelium and cholesterol in the middle ear, usually resulting from chronic otitis media.

circumcision—the operation of removing part or all of the prepuce, or foreskin.

cochlea—cone-shaped cavity in the petrous portion of the temporal bone, forming one of the divisions of the labyrinth or internal ear.

coin lesion—a round mass within lung parenchyma—actually it is three-dimensional with volume as well as length and breadth.

Colles' fracture—fracture of the lower end of the radius with displacement of the distal fragment dorsally; sometimes called a reversed Colles' fracture or Smith's fracture when volar displacement of the distal fragment occurs at the same location.

comminuted—broken into several pieces; denoting especially a fractured bone.

compartment syndrome—condition in which increased pressure in a confined anatomical space adversely affects the circulation and threatens the function and viability of the tissues therein. Four leg compartments are: anterior, deep posterior, lateral, and superficial posterior.

conductive hearing loss—problem in the middle or external ear; usually treated medically or surgically.

congenital—existing at birth, referring to certain traits, malformation, diseases, etc.; may be either hereditary or due to some influence occurring during gestation.

congenital bicuspidization—a heart valve with two instead of three leaflets—a deformity from birth rather than being acquired.

congenital diaphragmatic hernia—the protrusion of abdominal contents into the chest through a developmental defect in the diaphragm. Bochdalek's hernia is the most common, in which the defect is in the posterolateral diaphragm, most often on the left side.

corneal guttata—excrescences on Descemet's membrane.

cricothyrotomy—cricothyroidotomy; incision through the skin and cricothyroid membrane for relief of respiratory obstruction.

croup—laryngotracheobronchitis in infants and young children; caused by parainfluenza viruses 1 and 2; characterized by difficult and noisy respiration and a hoarse cough.

cryptorchidism—failure of the testicle to descend fully into the scrotum, an event that normally takes place between the seventh and ninth months of gestation.

cycloplegia—paralysis of the ciliary body.

cystic hygroma (lymphangioma)—a congenital malformation of the lymphatic vessels characterized by multiloculated cystic masses lined with endothelium and filled with lymph. Most commonly found within the posterior triangle of the neck and the axilla.

cystic hygromas—soft, painless, often very large multiloculated masses that are usually evident at birth or are seen in the first or second year of life.

cystoid macular edema—swelling of the macular region usually following surgery.

Dacron—artificial cloth material used to fabricate blood vessel prosthetic grafts.

decerebrate posturing—extensor posturing (nonpurposeful and stereotyped) of all four limbs whether spontaneous or in response to stimulation.

decorticate posturing—flexor posturing (nonpurposeful and stereotyped) of the upper limbs, usually accompanied by extensor posturing of the lower limbs.

decortication—operative removal of a restrictive or infected peel or rind trapping the lung.

dental occlusion—the manner in which the maxillary and mandibular teeth come in contact with one another.

depolarizing neuromuscular blocking agent—a drug that interrupts neuromuscular transmission by depolarizing the postsynaptic junction, resulting in transient muscle contraction, and then occupying the receptor to prevent further depolarization. Example: succinylcholine.

dermabrasion—mechanical sanding of irregular areas of skin contour.

Descemet's membrane—layer of cornea formed by the endothelium.

diaphysis—shaft of a long bone, as distinguished from the epiphyses, or extremities, and apophyses, or outgrowths.

diplopia—double vision.

dislocation—complete displacement of apposing joint surfaces.

dopaminergic—responding to the neurotransmitter dopamine.

drawer sign—in a knee examination, the forward or backward sliding of the tibia indicating laxity or tear of the anterior (forward slide) or posterior (backward slide) cruciate ligaments of the knee.

dribbling—to drool, slaver, dribble. To fall in drops, as the urine from a distended bladder.

Dupuytren's disease—progressive palmar fascitis and contraction.

dysraphic—fused in a defective fashion as a result of a congenital, usually midline, malformation.

echocardiography—use of ultrasound to image the heart; reflected sound waves projected to give form and shape to cardiac structures.

enchondroma—benign tumor originating in cartilage; commonly, metaphysis of tubular bones of hands and feet.

endourology—within the urinary tract in both male and female and within the genital organs in the male.

enophthalmos—the posterior displacement of the globe in the orbit.

entropion—inward rotation of the eyelid.

epidural hematoma—blood clot lying outside the dura (extradural) but inside the skull cavity or spinal canal.

epiglottis—inflammation of the supraglottis; may cause respiratory obstruction, especially in children; frequently due to *Haemophilus influenzae*.

epikeratophakia—refractive corneal procedure in which a graft is placed on the patient's cornea: "living contact lens."

epiphysis—part of a long bone developed from a center of ossisfication distinct from that of the shaft and separated at first from the latter by a layer of cartilage.

epistaxis—nasal bleeding.

erectile impotence—inability to have an erection of the penis.

escharotomy—an incision within an eschar to release the constriction of the eschar.

esophageal atresia—a congenital interruption in the continuity of the upper and lower portions of the esophagus. It usually occurs in association with a fistula of the lower esophageal segment to the trachea.

esophoria—tendency of the eye to drift inward.

esotropia—misalignment of the eyes in which one of the eyes deviates toward the other eye.

exophoria—tendency of the eye to drift outward.

expressive (nonfluent) aphasia—inability to say some or all words due to a problem with cerebral function rather than articulation—characterized by sparse speech.

exsanguinating—emptying blood.

external fixation—a method of fracture fixation that utilizes pins through the bone attached to an external frame.

extracorporeal membrane oxygenation (ECMO)—a form of prolonged cardiopulmonary bypass through which gas exchange occurs in an external circuit containing the patient's flowing blood. ECMO can provide complete or partial respiratory and cardiac support.

exudate—fluid with a higher protein concentration than serum.

Ewing's sarcoma—malignant tumor originating in bone marrow; commonly, diaphysis of femur, ilium, tibia, humerus, fibula, ribs.

familial polyposis—an autosomal dominant disorder, characterized by numerous adenomatous polyps in the colon. It usually presents in the second decade of life with abdominal pain and rectal bleeding; malignant transformation is inevitable in adulthood.

felon—a suppurative infection of the distal finger pulp.

Fogarty catheter—a balloon-tipped plastic tube utilized to entrap and thereby remove clots and debris from within blood vessels.

fortified antibiotics—antibiotics that are more concentrated than standard commercial products.

fractional excretion of sodium (FENa)—used to measure renal function. It is a percentage derived by dividing the amount of sodium entered by the amount of sodium filtered. FENa greater than 1% is seen in renal damage, such as acute tubular necrosis.

fracture—a break or loss of structural continuity in a bone.

free flap—flap of skin, muscle, or bone that is transferred to a distant anatomic location using a microvascular anastomosis of the blood vessels.

gamekeeper's thumb—ulnar collateral ligament of the thumb metacarpophalangeal joint; vulnerable to thumb abduction stress.

ganglion cyst—a common benign tumor of the hand originating from the joint spaces.

gastrografin—a water soluble, radiopaque contrast agent with a very high osmolarity.

gastroschisis—a congenital defect in the abdominal wall to the side of the umbilical cord, through which abdominal viscera protrude. The exposed abdominal contents have no covering sac.

genu valgum—knock knee; tibia valga; deformity marked by abduction of the leg in relation to the thigh.

genu varum—bowleg; bandy leg; tibia vara; outward bowing of the legs.

germ cell tumor—a neoplasm composed of cells of primordial spermatic or ovum cell origin.

Gore-Tex—a non-wettable artificial fabric used for vascular prostheses.

greenstick fracture—bending of a bone with incomplete fracture involving the convex side of the curve only.

heart—the four-chambered muscular organ responsible for pumping blood within the human circulation.

hemangioma—a histologically benign vascular tumor characterized initially by cellular proliferation, followed in many cases by involution. Commonly located in the head and neck but may be found anywhere and usually appearing within the first few weeks after birth.

hematospermia—also hemospermia. The presence of blood in the seminal fluid.

hemianopia—loss of vision in one half-field.

hemianopsia—defect in one half of the visual field.

hepatoblastoma—the most common malignant tumor of the liver in childhood, composed of tissue resembling fetal or mature liver cells or bile ducts.

histamine-releasing effects—physiologic release of histamine from body stores.

Hirschsprung's disease—a congenital disorder producing functional partial or complete intestinal obstruction due to the absence of ganglion cells are from the distal intestinal tract. The transition zone is most often at the rectosigmoid colon but can occur anywhere, with the entire colon or even the small intestine being aganglionic.

homonymous hemianopia—loss of vision in the same half-field of each eye.

hydrocele—a collection of serous fluid in a widened portion of a partly or completely patent processus vaginalis. Clinically presents as fluid around, or less often above, the testicle.

hypercarbia—elevated tension of carbon dioxide in arterial blood, usually considered greater than 45 mm Hg.

hyperopia—farsightedness; an eye that is "too short" or underpowered. Corrected by adding power by "plus" lenses.

hypertrophic pyloric stenosis—progressive enlargement of the musculature of the pylorus in infancy, leading to gastric outlet obstruction.

hypertrophic scar—a raised, reddened scar that does not extend beyond the boundaries of the original scar.

hypesthesia—decreased appreciation of touch.

hypopharynx—division of the pharynx that lies below the upper edge of the epiglottis and opens into the larynx and esophagus.

hypopyon—collection of pus (white cells) in the anterior chamber.

hypotony—low intraocular pressure.

hypoxemia—lower than normal (for age) tension of oxygen in arterial blood.

impotence—weakness, lack of power. Inability of the male to achieve and/or maintain penile erection and thus engage in copulation; a manifestation, usually, of a neurological or psychomotor dysfunction.

inotropes—medications that enhance the contractile state of the myocardium: they increase the strength of cardiac contractility and increase cardiac output.

internal fixation—a method of fracture fixation in which the hardware is completely contained within the body.

intussusception—a telescoping of one portion of the intestine into another.

iridocyclitis—inflammation of the anterior segment of the eye.

keloids—exuberant scar tissue that mushrooms out and extends beyond the boundaries of the normal scar.

keratitis—inflammation of the cornea.

keratoacanthoma—a rapidly growing, benign skin tumor.

keratoconjunctivitis sicca—dry eye syndrome.

keratometer—a device used for measuring corneal curvature.

keratomileusis—lamellar keratoplasty where patient's own cornea is lathed.

keratoplasty—corneal transplantation.

Kanavel's sign—four signs used to diagnose tenosynovitis: fusiform form of swelling of the finger, finger held in a slighted flexed position, pain over the tendon sheath, and pain on passive extension of the finger.

KUB—kidney, ureter, and bladder.

Ladd's bands—the peritoneal attachments of an incompletely rotated cecum, which crosses the duodenum; may obstruct the duodenum by extrinsic compression.

laryngomalacia—softness/flaccidity of the epiglottis and aryepiglottis folds as seen in congenital laryngeal stridor.

laryngopharynx—part of the pharynx that is posterior to the larynx.

laryngospasm—a pathological state of adduction of the vocal cords or contraction of the intrinsic muscles of the upper airway that precludes entry of air into the trachea.

lateral humeral epicondylitis (tennis elbow)—overuse injury of wrist extensor muscle origin.

LeFort classification—a method of characterizing fractures of the maxilla according to the level at which they occur.

Legg-Calvé-Perthes disease—epiphysial aseptic necrosis of the upper end of the femur.

lipemia retinalis—creamy coloring of the blood vessels secondary to high lipid level.

liposuction—a technique of removing fat utilizing small cannulas connected to a suction apparatus.

Luschka's joints—small synovial joints between adjacent lateral lips of the bodies of the lower cervical vertebrae.

Macintosh laryngoscope blade—a gently curved laryngoscope blade designed to expose the vocal cords for endotracheal intubation under direct vision when the tip is placed in the vallecula, between the epiglottis and the base of the tongue.

mallet (baseball) finger—avulsion, partial or complete, of the long finger extensor from the base of the distal phalanx.

malleus—one of three middle ear bones, called auditory ossicles; others are incus and stapes.

malocclusion—abnormal occlusion usually resulting from a fracture of developmental abnormality.

malrotation—failure during embryonic development of normal rotation of the intestinal tract. Normally the vertical midgut rotates 270° in a counterclockwise rotation, placing the cecum in the right lower quadrant and the duodenojejunal junction in the left upper quadrant. In malrotation, the cecum may be located high in the right abdomen, or completely in the left abdomen, with the duodenojejunal junction to the right of the midline. There is a resulting predisposition to obstruction by midgut volvulus or extrinsic compression from congenital Ladd's bands.

mastopexy—an aesthetic operation aimed at lifting the breast by removing excess skin, also known as a dermal mastopexy.

Meckel's diverticulum—a blind sac located at the distal ileum, found in 2% of the population. It represents a remnant of the vitelline duct, and can cause inflammation, bleeding, or obstruction.

meconium—the first bowel movement of a new born infant, usually occurring within 24 hours of birth. The material is greenish in color and consists of epithelial cells, mucous, intestinal and pancreatic enzymes and bile.

meconium ileus—congenital obstruction in the distal ileum due to impaction of sticky, inspissated meconium. It occurs in 10% of patients with cystic fibrosis, due to the abnormal enzymes secreted by the exocrine pancreatic and intestinal glands.

Ménière's disease—(endolymphatic hydrops)—auditory or labyrinthine vertigo; affliction categorized clinically by vertigo, nausea, vomiting, tinnitus, and progressive deafness.

metaphysis—growth zone between the epiphysis and diaphysis during development of a bone.

microtia—congenitally small or partially absent ears.

midgut volvulus—a twisting of the small intestine around the two closely fixed points from which it is suspended in cases of malrotation. Most common in the first month after birth, midgut volvulus can obstruct the duodenum and produce ischemic infarction of the entire small intestine, if not corrected early.

Miller laryngoscope blade—a straight narrow laryngoscope blade with a curved tip designed to expose the vocal cords for endotracheal intubation under direct vision when the tip is used to elevate the epiglottis.

myocardial compliance—passive or diastolic stiffness of the ventricle of the heart, usually the left ventricle.

myocutaneous flap—a reconstructive flap that consists of muscle and the overlying skin.

myopia—nearsightedness; an eye that is essentially too strong. Rays of light are focused in the vitreous.

myositis ossificans—deposit of bone in muscle with fibrosis, causing pain and swelling in muscles.

myringotomy—tympanotomy; tympanostomy; paracentesis of the tympanic membrane.

myxomatous degeneration—alteration in heart valve tissue that diminishes its strength and character resulting in stretching of tissues or tearing of chordae tendinea leading to valvular regurgitation.

nasopharynx—part of the pharynx that is posterior to the nose and superior to the soft palate.

necrotizing enterocolitis—a type of hemorrhagic necrosis of the intestinal mucosa, which can progress to infarction of the entire bowel wall. It occurs exclusively in the neonatal period, most often in premature infants.

neuroblastoma—a malignant neoplasm derived from embryonal neural crest tissue. It can arise anywhere in the sympathetic nervous system, and is the most common extracranial solid tumor of childhood.

neuroectoderm hyphema neuroectodermal tumors—tumors of the central or peripheral nervous system.

neuroendocrine—the means by which the brain controls glandular function.

nevus—a benign usually pigmented skin lesion (e.g., "mole").

nociceptive impulses—neural transmission that results in the physiological or conscious perception of pain.

nondepolarizing neuromuscular blocking agent—a drug that interrupts neuromuscular transmission by altering prejunctional transmitter release and/or occupying the postsynaptic receptor to prevent depolarization, without first depolarizing the muscle. Example: *d*-tubocurarine.

omphalocele—a congenital defect in the center of the abdominal wall, through which the abdominal viscera protrude. The herniated abdominal contents are covered with a membranous sac.

orchidopexy—surgical treatment of an undescended testicle by freeing it and implanting it into the scrotum.

oropharynx—part of the pharynx that is posterior to the mouth; it contains the palatine tonsils.

osteochondroma—solitary osteocartilaginous exostosis; a benign cartilaginous neoplasm that consists of a pedicle of normal bone covered with a rim of proliferating cartilage.

osteoid osteoma—benign bone tumor usually occurring in femur and tibia.

osteomalacia—adult rickets; disease characterized by gradual softening and bending of the bones with varying severity of pain; softening is due to inadequate bone mineralization, sometimes due to lack of vitamin D.

osteoporosis—reduction in quantity of bone or atrophy of skeletal tissue; occurs in postmenopausal women and elderly men.

otitis media—inflammation of the middle ear.

otosclerosis—new formation of spongy bone around the stapes and fenestra vestibuli (ovalis), resulting in progressively increasing deafness, without signs of disease in the eustachian tube or tympanic membrane.

Paget's disease—osteitis deformans; a generalized skeletal disease, frequently familial, of older persons; bone resorption and formation are both increased, leading to thickening and softening of bones.

papillitis—optic disc swelling caused by inflammation.

paraneoplastic syndrome—endocrine and systemic malfunction in association with certain lung cancers.

paronychia—an infection of the perionychium or lateral nail fold.

patient-controlled analgesia—a system of acute pain control where the patient triggers infusion of a dilute narcotic solution from a programmed intravenous pump according to that individual's need.

percutaneous transluminal coronary angioplasty (PTCA)—balloon dilation of atherosclerotic narrowing of a coronary artery—luminal widening occurs by compressing atheroma or "evoking" mural plaque.

Peutz-Jeghers syndrome—generalized multiple polyposis of the intestinal tract, consistently involving the jejunum, associated with the melanin spots of the lips and buccal mucosa; autosomal dominant inheritance.

Phalen's sign—tingling in some or all radial three and one-half fingers on holding the wrist flexed.

photocoagulation—laser-induced scarring.

photophobia—light sensitivity.

pinna—the projecting part of the ear lying outside the head (auricula).

plantar fasciitis (heel spur)—inflammation of the sole of the foot.

plasma cholinesterase—a circulating enzyme that breaks down certain ester bonds, most notably those in succinylcholine and ester-based local anesthetics. This is distinct from acetylcholinesterase, which is present in cholinergic synapses and in the neuromuscular junction and breaks down acetylcholine to terminate transmission.

plasma imbibition—an initial phase of skin graft healing where the skin graft absorbs plasma from the recipient bed.

pleural cap—radiographic opacity over the apex of the lung caused by extrapleural dissection of a hematoma—a hallmark of traumatic aortic transection.

pneumotachograph—a monitor that measures respiratory rate or the velocity of air flow by sensing changes in turbulence.

polyhydramnios—an excess in the amount of amniotic fluid. May occur in association with congenital obstructions of the upper alimentary tract.

porphyria—one of several autosomally inherited metabolic diseases resulting from lack of enzymes involved in hemoglobin formation, most of which result in neurologic damage.

posterior fossa—the skull cavity below the tentorium.

preload—the load (or volume) to which a muscle is subjected before shortening (cardiac contraction).

premature infant—born less than 37 weeks of gestation; birth weight is not considered a criteria.

presbycusis—progressive loss of ability to perceive or discriminate sounds as a part of the aging process.

presbyopia—lack of accommodative ability that comes with loss of elasticity of the crystalline lens.

prostatism—a clinical syndrome, occurring mostly in older men, usually caused by enlargement of the prostate gland and manifested by irritative (nocturia, frequency, decreased voided volume, sensory urgency, and urgency incontinence) and obstructive (hesitancy, decreased stream, terminal dribbling, double voiding, and urinary retention) symptoms.

prostatodynia—pain in the prostate gland.

prosthetic endocarditis—infection on an artificial heart valve.

pseudophakia—an eye with an artificial lens.

pseudophakic bullous keratopathy—permanent corneal clouding after intraocular lens implant surgery.

ptosis—a dropping, often referring to a dropping of the upper eyelid.

pulmonary artery catheter—a plastic tube, carried by an inflatable balloon through the veins, right atrium and right ventricle into the pulmonary artery with the ability to measure intravascular pressure, certain gas tensions, and temperature gradients for cardiac output determinations.

pulmonary reserve—the difference between normal ventilation and the maximum breathing capacity.

pulse oximeter—a device that provides continuous measurement of the percentage of oxygen saturation of hemoglobin by assessing the differential light absorption of oxygenated and reduced hemoglobin, using a light shined through the distal part of an extremity. This noninvasive instrument has replaced the need to sample arterial blood for its oxygen content in many situations.

radionuclide angiography—heart and blood vessel imaging by counting radioactive output from intravascular isotope injections with computer synthesis of reproductions of cardiovascular structures.

random pattern skin flap—a skin flap that does not contain a specific artery and vein, thus, limiting the length of the flap to not much greater than that of the width of the flap.

receptor blockade—interruption of synaptic neurotransmission because of inactivation of a specific receptor by a pharmacologic agent.

renal pedicle—constricted portion or stalk by which a nonsessile tumor is attached to normal tissue. Anatomically fixed in the retroperitoneum, the renal pedicle is susceptible to injury in blunt trauma.

retrobulbar—behind the globe within the orbit.

rhabdomyosarcoma—a diverse group of tumors derived from primitive mesenchymal cells that may appear anywhere in the body. It represents the most common soft tissue sarcoma in children.

rhegmatogenous—hole in the retina.

rheumatic valvulitis—inflammation of heart valves by an immune phenomenon initiated by streptococcal infection.

rhinitis—nasal catarrh; inflammation of the nasal mucous membrane.

rhinoplasty—an operation that reshapes and recontours the nose.

rhinorrhea—drainage from the nose.

rhytidectomy—an operation designed for the removal of wrinkles.

Rinne's test—comparison of hearing when a vibrating tuning fork's handle tip is held in contact with the mastoid process (bone conduction) with the normally louder perception when the tuning fork's prongs are held close to the external auditory meatus (air conduction).

Salter-Harris classification—classification of epiphysial fractures into five groups (I to V), according to different prognoses regarding the effects of the injury on subsequent growth and subsequent deformity of the epiphysis.

Schlemm's canal—channel that collects aqueous from the trabecular meshwork.

scleral buckle—surgical procedure for retinal detachment.

scoliosis—lateral curvature of the spine. Scoliosis may be flexible (correctable) or fixed (structural).

semicircular canals—the three bony tubes (anterior, posterior, and lateral) in the labyrinth of the ear within which the membranous semicircular ducts are located. They lie in planes at right angles to each other.

sensorineural hearing loss—problem in the inner ear; usually treated with a hearing aid.

sick sinus syndrome—abnormally fast or slow initiation of sinoatrial cardiac conduction causing either bradyarrhythmia, tachyarrhythmia or both.

sleep apnea—interrupted respiration during sleep or sedation caused by upper airway obstruction or a decrease in the central drive mechanisms.

spinal headache—a postural headache (occurring only when the patient is in the upright position) that follows lumbar puncture and loss of CSF pressure.

spinal stenosis—encroachment of spinal canal or foraminal contents by degenerative hypertrophic spondyloarthritic changes.

spinal stenosis—narrowing of the spinal canal with or without stenosis of its foramina.

spondylolysis—osteoarthritis; degeneration of the articulating part of a vertebrae.

stapedius—muscle of the middle ear.

Stensen's duct—arises anteriorly, approximately 1 cm below the zygoma. It is the duct of the parotid gland, which is the largest salivary gland.

stereotaxic—three-dimensional localization, usually provided by means of a frame (to provide coordinates) and an imaging device such as MRI or CT.

strabismus—malalignment of the eyes.

strain fracture—tearing off, by a sudden force, a piece of bone attached to a tendon, ligament or capsule; the force may be exogenous or endogenous.

stress fracture—fatigue fracture occurring usually from sudden, strong, violent, endogenous force.

struvite calculi—stones in which the crystalloid component consists of magnesium ammonium phosphate. These are treatable with ESWL (extracorporeal shock wave lithotripsy); however, most of these stones are large staghorns requiring percutaneous nephrostomy.

subdural hematoma—blood clot lying outside the brain and arachnoid but inside the dura within the skull cavity or spinal canal.

subglottic stenosis—respiratory obstruction.

subluxation—partial displacement of apposing joint surfaces.

supratentorial—pertaining to the skull cavity above the tentorium.

syndactyly—a congenital webbing of the fingers.

talipes equinovarus (clubfoot)—t. equinus and t. varus combined; the foot is plantar flexed, inverted, and adducted.

tamponade—squeezing of the heart within a confined space, thereby impeding diastolic filling of the heart, diminishing cardiac output.

tenosynovitis—an infection of the tendon sheath, usually of the hand.

teratoma—a benign or malignant neoplasm composed of multiple tissues of kinds foreign to the parts in which it arises. This latter definition replaces the time-honored requirement that a teratoma must contain all three germinal layers. Frequently occurs in the gonads or near the midline of the body.

thermal dilution—use of small temperature gradients and mathematical algorithms to calculate cardiac output.

Thompson test—determines whether the gastrocnemius-soleus complex is intact. Examiner squeezes the calf muscle belly and the foot responds with plantar flexion. Lack of plantar flexion indicates torn Achilles tendon.

thyroglossal duct cyst—a fluid-filled sac in the midline of the neck due to failure of the thyroglossal duct to obliterate after the thyroid gland descends embryologically from the base of the tongue.

thyroglossal duct cysts—soft, painless, persistent midline neck masses seen in first or second decade of life.

Tinel's sign—tingling in part or all of the sensory distribution of a peripheral nerve elicited by tapping over a portion of the nerve; e.g., the median nerve at the wrist in cases of compression at that site.

tinnitus—noises (ringing, whistling, booming, etc.) in the ears; the third most common inner ear disorder.

tissue expansion—a method of stretching tissue for reconstructive purposes utilizing an inflatable device buried beneath the tissue to be expanded.

tonometry—measurement of the pressure within the eye, usually expressed in terms of millimeters of mercury.

TRAM flap—transverse rectus abdominis myocutaneous flap: a method of breast reconstruction that utilizes the lower abdominal tissue to create the breast mound.

transudate—fluid with essentially the same protein content as serum.

trifascicular block—impedance of cardiac electrical conduction is one of the three major tracts.

TRUS (transrectal ultrasonography)—imaging test for prostate cancer. TRUS is usually performed in patients with an abnormal PSA or a palpable abnormality of the prostate.

turbinate—bone shaped like a top; superior, middle, and inferior nasal conchae (turbinates) are found on the lateral wall of the nasal cavity.

tympanic membrane—thin, semitransparent, oval membrane (8–9 mm in diameter) at the medial end of the external acoustic meatus, separating it from the middle ear.

umbilical hernia—a protrusion of bowel or omentum through the abdominal wall under the skin of the umbilicus.

umbo—most depressed point of the tympanic membrane.

ureterovesical—junction of ureter with bladder.

uveitis—inflammation of any portion of the uvea, the iris, ciliary body, and/or choroid.

uvula—conical projection from the posterior edge of the middle of the soft palate.

velopharyngeal region—the soft palate and the posterior nasopharyngeal wall.

venous oxygen saturation—percentage of filling of the available sites on the hemoglobin molecule by oxygen, in the venous circulation.

ventricular hypertrophy—enlargement of cardiac muscle fibers.

Vogt's ring—benign, crescent shaped white opacity at the limbus on the cornea.

Weber's test—the application of the tip of the handle of a vibrating tuning fork to the midline (e.g., forehead) to ascertain which ear has the best hearing with bone conduction. If sound conduction through the ossicles is defective, hearing will be greater on that side. If there is an injury to the auditory nerve or its sensory apparatus, the sound will be heard better in the opposite ear.

wheal and flare—the typical cutaneous manifestation of local histamine release, consisting of a central whitish raised fluid-filled wheal surrounded by an area of redness with intense itching.

Wilms' tumor—an embryonal neoplasm of the kidney, often associated with other anomalies such as hypospadias, hemihypertrophy, and aniridia.

Wisconsin-Hipple laryngoscope blade—a straight blade, shorter and wider than the Miller, designed to lift the epiglottis to expose the vocal cords for endotracheal intubation. Also called Wisconsin, Wis-Forreger, and Wis-Hipple.

YAG laser—neodymium-yttrium-aluminum-garnet yields an amplified light beam, parallel in nature, the wavelength of which finds use in coagulating and vaporizing various tissues within the body; utilized to remove inflammatory tissue as well as malignant tissue.

zonules of Zinn—fibers that suspend the lens and attach it to the ciliary body.

z-plasty—an operation used to reorient a scar by lengthening the scar at the expense of width. The incisions resemble a Z.

Figure and Table Credits

Figures

Figure 2.26. From Rickham PP, Soper RT, Stauffer UG. Synopsis of pediatric surgery. Stuttgart: Year Book Medical Publishers, 1975.
Figure 2.27. From Mulliken JB, Young AE. Vascular birthmarks. Philadelphia: WB Saunders, 1988.
Figure 2.31. From Coren CV. Burn injuries in children. Pediatr Ann 1987;16(4):328–339. original perhaps in Surg Gyn Obstet 1944;78: 463.
Figure 3.1. Modified from Grant JCB. Grant's atlas of anatomy. Baltimore: Williams & Wilkins, 19.
Figure 3.14. From Sheilds MB. A study guide for glaucoma. Baltimore: Williams & Wilkins, 1982:137.
Figure 3.15. From Sheilds MB. A study guide for glaucoma. Baltimore: Williams & Wilkins, 1982:464. Portions reprinted with permission from Opthal Surg 1980;11:498.
Figure 3.16. From Sheilds MB. A study guide for glaucoma. Baltimore: Williams & Wilkins, 1982:137.
Figure 3.17. From Sheilds MB. A study guide for glaucoma. Baltimore: Williams & Wilkins, 1982:478.
Figure 3.18. From Sheilds MB. A study guide for glaucoma. Baltimore: Williams & Wilkins, 1982:489.
Figure 3.31. Modified from Jones LT, Wobig JL. Surgery of the eyelids and lacrimal system. Birmingham: Aesculapius Publishing, 1976.
Figure 3.32. From Doxanas MT, Anderson RL. Clinica! orbital anatomy. Baltimore: Williams & Wilkins, 1984:58.
Figure 3.33. From Doxanas MT, Anderson RL. Clinical orbital anatomy. Baltimore: Williams & Wilkins, 1984:26.
Figure 3.34. From Doxanas MT, Anderson RL. Clinical orbital anatomy. Baltimore: Williams & Wilkins, 1984.
Figure 3.35. From Doxanas MT, Anderson RL. Clinical orbital anatomy. Baltimore: Williams & Wilkins, 1984:51.
Figure 6.3. From Braunwald E. A textbook of cardiovascular medicine. Philadelphia: WB Saunders, 1980:378.
Figure 6.8. Reproduced with permission from Starek P. Heart valve replacement and reconstruction. Chicago: Mosby Yearbook, 1987. Data from: Rowe JC, Bland EF, Sprague HB, White PD. The course of mitral stenosis without surgery: ten- and twenty-year perspectives. Ann Intern Med 1960;52: 741 (black square); Oleson KH. The natural history of 271 patients with mitral stenosis under medical treatment. Brit Med J 1962;24: 349 (black circle); Munoz S, Gallardo J, Diaz-Gorrin JR, et al. Influence of surgery on the natural history of rheumatic mitral and aortic disease. Am J Cardiol 1975;35:234 (black triangle); Rapaport E. Natural history of aortic and mitral valve disease. Am J Cardiol 1975;35:221 (white circle).
Figure 6.10. From Soto B et al. Classification of ventricular septal defects. Br Heart J 1980;43:332.
Figure 6.11. Reproduced with permission from Sabiston DC, Spencer FC, eds. Surgery of the chest. Philadelphia: WB Saunders, 1990.
Figure 6.16. Modified from Seymour G. Medical assessment of the elderly supine patient. Rockville, Maryland: Aspen Publishers, 1986:123.
Figure 6.19. From Oldham HN Jr, Sabiston DC Jr. The mediastinum. In: Sabiston DC Jr, ed. Textbook of surgery. 13th ed. Philadelphia: WB Saunders, 1986.
Figure 7.1. B and **C** modified from Rockwood C, Green D. Fractures in adults. 3rd ed. Philadelphia: JB Lippincott, 1982:1193.
Figure 7.9. Modified from American Orthopaedic Association. Manual of orthopaedic surgery. 6th ed. Park Ridge, Illinois: Amer Acad Ortho Surg, 1985. Letter "L" added by Berg.
Figure 7.10. From Rang MC, Children's fractures. 2nd ed. Philadelphia: JB Lippincott, 1983.
Figure 7.17. American Academy of Orthopaedic Surgeons. Athletic training and sports medicine. 2nd ed. Park Ridge, Illinois: Amer Acad Ortho Surg, 1991:277.
Figure 7.18. B, from Rockwood C, Green D. Fractures in adults. 3rd ed. Philadelphia: JB Lippincott, 1982:1092.
Figure 7.21. From Rockwood C, Green D. Fractures in adults. 2nd ed. Philadelphia: JB Lippincott, 1982.
Figure 7.24. A, from American Academy of Orthopaedic Surgeons. Athletic training and sports medicine. 2nd ed. Park Ridge, Illinois: Amer Acad Ortho Surg, 1991:235. **B**, modified from Rowe CR. The shoulder. New York: Churchill Livingstone, 1988:142.
Figure 7.25. Modified from Wilson FC, ed. The musculoskeletal system: basic processes and disorders. 2nd ed. Philadelphia: JB Lippincott, 1983.
Figure 7.26. From American Academy of Orthopaedic Surgeons. Athletic training and sports medicine. 2nd ed. Park Ridge, Illinois: Amer Acad Ortho Surg, 1991.
Figure 7.29. From American Academy of Orthopaedic Surgeons. Athletic training and sports medicine. 2nd ed. Park Ridge, Illinois: Amer Acad Ortho Surg, 1991:365.
Figure 7.30. From American Academy of Orthopaedic Surgeons. Athletic training and sports medicine. 2nd ed. Park Ridge, Illinois, 1991:151.
Figure 7.31. From American Academy of Orthopaedic Surgeons. Athletic training and sports medicine. 2nd ed. Park Ridge, Illinois, Amer Acad Ortho Surg, 1991:151.
Figure 7.33. From Rodeo SA. Turf toe: an analysis of metatarsal-phalangeal joint sprains in professional football. Am J Sports Med 1990;18(3):284.
Figure 7.36. From Wilson FC, ed. The musculoskeletal system: basic processes and disorders. 2nd ed. Philadelphia: JB Lippincott, 1983.
Figure 7.37. Modified from Crenshaw. Campbell's operative orthopaedics. 7th ed. St. Louis, Missouri: CV Mosby, 1986:2725.
Figure 7.38–39. From Staheli L. Rotational problems of the lower extremities. Orthop Clin North Am 1987;18(4):506.
Figure 7.40. Modified from Kling T. Angular deformities of the lower limb in children. Orthop Clin North Am 1987;18(4):514.
Figure 7.41. From American Orthopaedic Association. Manual of orthopaedic surgery. 6th ed. Park Ridge, Illinois: Amer Acad Ortho Surg, 1985:106.
Figure 7.43. Modified from Salter RB. Textbook of disorders and injuries of the musculoskeletal system. 2nd ed. Baltimore: Williams & Wilkins, 1983.
Figure 7.44. Modified from Salter RB. Textbook of disorders and injuries of the musculoskeletal system. 2nd ed. Baltimore: Williams & Wilkins, 1983.

Figure 7.48. Modified from American Academy of Orthopaedic Surgeons, Athletic training and sports medicine. 2nd ed. Park Ridge, Illinois: Amer Acad Ortho Surg, 1991: 515.

Figure 7.49. From Wilson FC, ed. The musculoskeletal system: basic processes and disorders. 2nd ed. Philadelphia: JB Lippincott, 1983.

Figure 7.50. Modified from McNab I, McCullough J. Backache. 2nd ed. Baltimore: Williams & Wilkins, 1990.

Figure 7.58. Modified from Phillips WA. The child with a limp. Orthop Clin North Am 1987;18(4):490.

Tables

Table 1.16. Modified from Standards for intraoperative monitoring. In: American Society of Anesthesiologists: directory of members. Park Ridge, Illinois: American Society of Anesthesiologists, 1992.

Table 2.2. From Greene MG, ed. The Harriet Lane handbook. St. Louis, Missouri: Mosby Year Book, 1991.

Table 3.1. From Brady SE, Rapauno CJ, Arentsen SE, et al. Clinical indications for and procedures associated with penetrating keratoplasty, 1983–1988. Am J Ophth 1989;108: 118.

Table 6.6. From Mountain CF. A new international staging system for lung cancer. Chest 1986;89(suppl):2255–2335.

Table 6.7. Modified from Ginsberg RJ, Hill LD, Eagan RT, et al. Modern 30-day operative mortality for surgical resections in lung cancer. J Thorac Cardiovasc Surg 1983;86: 654–657.

Table 9.2. American Joint Committee for Cancer Staging and End-results Reporting of the American College of Surgeons. Manual for staging of cancer. 2nd ed. Philadelphia: JP Lippincott, 1983:177.

Table 9.3. Modified from Dairiki L, Stamey T. Infections of the urinary tract. In: Walsh PC et al, eds. Campbell's urology. 5th ed. Philadelphia: WB Saunders, 1986.

Index

Page numbers followed by "f" indicate figures; those followed by "t" indicate tables.